Practical Guide to the Assessment of Clinical Competence

THIRD
Edition

Practical Guide to the **Assessment** of Clinical Competence

Edited by

Eric S. Holmboe, MD

Professor Adjunct, Medicine
Yale University
New Haven, Connecticut
Adjunct Professor of Medical Education
Feinberg School of Medicine, Northwestern University
Chicago, Illinois
United States

Steven J. Durning, MD, PhD

Professor and Vice Chair, Department of Medicine
Director, Center for Health Professions Education (CHPE)
Uniformed Services University
Bethesda, Maryland
United States

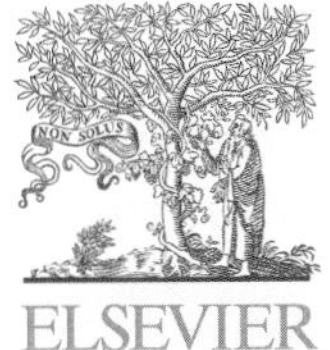

ELSEVIER

Elsevier
1600 John F. Kennedy Blvd.
Ste 1800
Philadelphia, PA 19103-2899

PRACTICAL GUIDE TO THE ASSESSMENT OF CLINICAL COMPETENCE, THIRD EDITION ISBN: 978-0-443-11226-3

Notice

Practitioners and researchers must always rely on their own experience and knowledge in evaluating and using any information, methods, compounds or experiments described herein. Because of rapid advances in the medical sciences, in particular, independent verification of diagnoses and drug dosages should be made. To the fullest extent of the law, no responsibility is assumed by Elsevier, authors, editors or contributors for any injury and/or damage to persons or property as a matter of products liability, negligence or otherwise, or from any use or operation of any methods, products, instructions, or ideas contained in the material herein.

Previous editions copyrighted 2018 and 2008

Publisher: Elyse W. O'Grady
Senior Content Development Specialist: Vaishali Singh
Publishing Services Manager: Shereen Jameel
Project Manager: Gayathri S
Design Direction: Patrick C. Ferguson

Printed in India

Last digit is the print number: 9 8 7 6 5 4 3 2 1

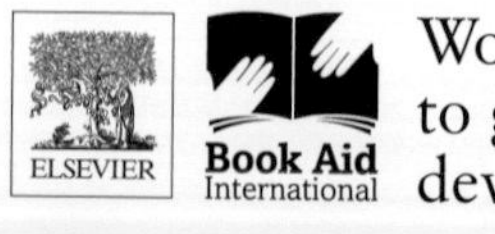

Preface

Assessment of health professionals across the continuum of medical education and practice is essential for advancing high-quality and safe healthcare and improving health for patients and the public. Assessment of clinical competence is a core element of educational professionalism and underlies effective professional self-regulation; it is essential for fulfilling our professional obligation as educators to assure the public that the graduates of health professions education training programs are truly prepared to enter the next stage of education and/or practice. Despite substantial attention to the quality and safety of healthcare over the past 25 years, major deficiencies and concerns persist in healthcare fields. The transformation of medical education, and the education of all healthcare professionals, is appropriately seen as part of the solution. Effective assessment is a vital component of this difficult transformation that is only further challenged by a once-in-a-century pandemic.

First and foremost, medicine is a service profession. As medical educators, it is vital that we develop and use high-quality assessment methods embedded within effective assessment systems to meet our primary obligation to the public and patients we serve. Furthermore, effective assessment provides the necessary data for robust feedback, coaching, and guidance to support professional growth and development. Learners are entitled to no less; without assessment, feedback, and coaching, the attainment of mastery, the ultimate goal of outcomes-based education, is nearly impossible.

It has been more than 5 years since the second edition of this book, and much has changed during this relatively brief period. We have seen an encouraging acceleration of the development of assessment tools, methods, and research despite the COVID-19 pandemic. Competency-based medical educational (CBME) models are being implemented more widely but variability in the uptake of CBME continues across the globe. However, most health professions educational systems have recognized the value of an outcomes-based approach using CBME models. The philosophical underpinnings of CBME continue to inform curricular and programmatic assessment changes, accreditation and certification approaches, and the credentialing of healthcare professionals. CBME has highlighted the importance of rebalancing more traditional methods of assessment with other methods of assessment, especially in the workplace. Fully implemented, CBME frameworks embrace holistic and constructivist approaches to assessment; successful assessment programs will need to incorporate a diverse range of educational and assessment theories and methods.

We are pleased to be able to share changes and advances in assessment that have occurred since 2018. Many readers let us know that one of the main benefits of both editions of this book was the practical suggestions in each chapter that could be implemented in training programs. We have attempted to stay true to that philosophy by adding new chapters and more supplemental material. All other chapters have undergone extensive revision to be up to date and practical.

Both of us have spent much of our professional lives thinking, learning, and teaching about assessment. Like many of you, much of our initial learning was through trial and error, occurring as a result of being assigned positions of responsibility in determining the competence of students and residents in internal medicine. We have also had the privilege to work within national organizations involved in the assessment of physicians across the continuum. Assessment is not routinely seen by physicians and other health professionals as a welcome activity, especially when it comes from an external entity. Yet without assessment, feedback and coaching are almost impossible and continuous professional growth is difficult. We hope that by sharing part of our own journey and the journey of our colleagues who contributed chapters and their expertise, we can help the reader address important assessment challenges they are facing in their own context and also contribute to larger conversations around assessment as a mechanism to improve healthcare and health for all.

The primary purpose of this book is to provide a *practical* guide to developing assessment programs using a systems lens. No single assessment method is sufficient to determine something as complex as clinical competence. Educators will need to develop programs of assessment (i.e., programmatic assessment) by choosing the optimal combination of methods, based on the best evidence available, for their local context. This book has been organized around the various assessment methods and instruments and how individuals with responsibilities for assessment can apply these methods and instruments in their own setting. We have provided an overview of key educational theories applicable to help the reader understand how best to use the assessment method and its purpose. Each chapter provides information on the strengths and weaknesses of the assessment method, along with information about specific tools. Many chapters provide examples of assessment instruments along with suggestions on faculty development and effective implementation of the assessment method. Each chapter also contains an annotated bibliography of helpful articles for additional reading.

Chapter 1 provides an overview of basic assessment principles with a focus on the rise and impact of competency-based education and the core components of CBME to achieve desired educational and clinical care outcomes. Chapter 2 provides a useful primer on key theories and aspects of psychometrics, a discipline that remains essential to effective assessment. Chapter 3 is a new chapter on programs of assessment, or programmatic assessment, using a systems approach. Chapter 4 explores the evolving approaches to the use of rating scales, especially developmental and entrustment scales, a common component of assessment forms and surveys, highlighting the importance of appropriate frameworks and anchors. Direct observation in the workplace, especially of clinical skills, is the focus of Chapter 5 with multiple practical suggestions on how to better prepare faculty in this essential assessment skill, and this chapter also provides access to multiple videos that can be used for practice and faculty development. Chapter 6 explores the assessment of clinical skills with standardized patients, another form of direct observation in controlled settings.

Chapter 7 provides an extensive overview on the effective use of the traditional written, standardized tests of medical knowledge and clinical reasoning, still an essential part of an assessment program. However, the need for high-quality assessment of clinical reasoning in the workplace has grown in importance with the recognition of the persistent and pernicious problem of diagnostic and management errors in clinical practice. This is the focus of Chapter 8. Chapter 9 covers the assessment of procedural competence in the workplace, another area experiencing new approaches and of major interest for medical educators in an era of concerns about appropriate supervision and patient safety.

Chapter 10 addresses the importance of assessing evidence-based practice, an essential competency in a time of rapidly expanding medical knowledge and growing use of clinical decision support at the point of care, an area that is also being buffeted by advances in clinical support tools and augmented intelligence. Chapter 11 focuses on the multiple ways to assess performance in clinical practice using different types of quality and safety measures. The growing use of these measures, now mostly extracted from electronic medical records, is an established part of medical practice across the globe. Chapter 12 provides updated guidance on the effective use of multisource feedback, an approach essential to patient-centered care and interprofessional practice.

Chapter 13 is a complement to Chapter 5, covering the expansive field of simulation outside standardized patients. Simulation, depending on the discipline, should increasingly become a standard component of an assessment program and is being increasingly used in mastery-based educational approaches. Chapter 14 is an expanded chapter on practical approaches to feedback with the inclusion of new tools and resources.

The final three chapters help the reader "put it all together." Portfolios, covered in Chapter 15, offer a comprehensive approach to supporting an assessment program. This chapter provides practical advice on how to design and implement portfolios. Chapter 16 is a new chapter on the use of group process, commonly called clinical competency committees, that is rapidly becoming an essential component of programmatic assessment. Chapter 17 provides a systematic approach to working with the struggling learner (i.e., the learner in difficulty). These learners require an assessment program and systematic approach using multiple assessment methods. The final chapter, Chapter 18, covers the important role of programmatic evaluation as part of an effective educational program. Up-to-date concepts and approaches to program evaluation are provided.

In sum, effective assessment requires a multifaceted approach using a combination of assessment methods. This is the rationale behind the organization and design of this book. Effective assessment also depends upon collaboration among a *team* of faculty and other educators; thus any change to an assessment system must include not only buy-in from others, but also the investment to train educators to use assessment methods and tools effectively. A CBME system must also include the learners as "active agents" in their own learning and assessment, meaning assessment activities need to be, at a minimum, a coproduced process. Leaners, along with patients and families, are the ultimate stakeholders in health professions education. Interprofessional faculty, program leaders, and learners need to work together to cocreate and coproduce assessment to maximize educational, and ultimately, clinical outcomes.

It is essential to remember that the true assessment instrument is the individual using it, not the instrument itself. Assessment tools are only as good as the individual using them. If done well, assessment can have a profoundly positive effect on patients, learners, and faculty. That has not changed since the first edition of this book in 2008 and likely never will. Nothing can be more satisfying than knowing each and every one of your graduates is truly ready to move to the next career level. The public expects no less, and we should expect no less from ourselves. In that spirit, we welcome comments from you, the reader, on how we can improve upon this book.

Eric S. Holmboe
Steven J. Durning

Contributors

Loai Albarqouni, MD, MSc, PhD
Assistant Professor
Institute for Evidence-Based Healthcare
Faculty of Health Sciences & Medicine
Gold Coast, Australia

James G. Boyle, MBChB, MD, MSc, FRCP
Associate Professor
Glasgow Royal Infirmary
School of Medicine, Dentistry & Nursing
University of Glasgow
United Kingdom

Brian E. Clauser, EdD
Distinguished Research Scientist
Office of Research Strategy
National Board of Medical Examiners
Philadelphia, Pennsylvania
United States

Susannah Cornes, MD
Professor
Department of Neurology
University of California San Francisco
San Francisco, California
United States

Brigid M. Dolan, MD, MEd
Associate Professor
Assistant Dean of Assessment
Department of Medicine and Medical Education
Feinberg School of Medicine
Northwestern University
Chicago, Illinois
United States

Steven J. Durning, MD, PhD
Professor and Vice Chair, Department of Medicine
Director, Center for Health Professions Education (CHPE)
Uniformed Services University
Bethesda, Maryland
United States

Andem Ekpenyong, MD, MHPE
Associate Professor
Department of Internal Medicine
Rush University Medical Center
Chicago, Illinois
United States

Stanley J. Hamstra, PhD
Professor and Vice-Chair of Clinical Teaching, Department of Surgery, University of Toronto, Toronto, Canada;
Senior Scientist, Holland Bone and Joint Program, Sunnybrook Research Institute, Toronto, Canada;
Research Consultant, Milestones Research and Evaluation, Accreditation Council for Graduate Medical Education, Chicago, Illinois, United States;
Adjunct Professor, Department of Medical Education, Northwestern University Feinberg School of Medicine, Chicago, Illinois, United States

Karen E. Hauer, MD, PhD
Associate Dean for Competency Assessment and Professional Standards
University of California, San Francisco School of Medicine
San Francisco, California
United States

Eric S. Holmboe, MD
Professor Adjunct, Medicine
Yale University
New Haven, Connecticut
Adjunct Professor of Medical Education
Feinberg School of Medicine, Northwestern University
Chicago, Illinois
United States

Dragan Ilic, PhD
Professor
Deputy Head of School (Education)
Director, Teaching & Learning
Head, Medical Education Research & Quality (MERQ) unit
Monash University, Australia

William Iobst, MD, FACP
Senior Scholar at ACGME
Emeritus Professor of Medicine at Geisinger Commonwealth School of Medicine
Scranton, Pennsylvania
United States

Benjamin Kinnear, MD, MEd
Associate Professor
Department of Pediatrics
University of Cincinnati College of Medicine
Cincinnati, Ohio
United States

Jennifer R. Kogan, MD
Professor of Medicine
Associate Dean, Student Success and Professional Development
Perelman School of Medicine at the University of Pennsylvania
Philadelphia, Pennsylvania
United States

Jocelyn M. Lockyer, PhD
Professor Emerita and Adjunct Professor
Community Health Sciences
Cumming School of Medicine
University of Calgary
Calgary, Alberta
Canada

Melissa J. Margolis, PhD
Senior Measurement Scientist
Center for Advanced Assessment
National Board of Medical Examiners
Philadelphia, Pennsylvania
United States

Celia Laird O'Brien, PhD
Assistant Dean of Program Evaluation and Accreditation
Assistant Professor
Department of Medical Education
Feinberg School of Medicine
Northwestern University
Chicago, Illinois
United States

Patricia S. O'Sullivan, MS, EdD
Director of Research and Development in Medical Education
Center for Faculty Educators;
Professor of Medicine and Surgery
University of California
University of California San Francisco
San Francisco, California
United States

Louis N. Pangaro, MD, MACP
Professor of Medicine
Professor of Health Professions Education
Uniformed Services University School of Medicine
Bethesda, MD

Joan M. Sargeant, PhD
Professor
Continuing Professional Development and Medical Education
Faculty of Medicine
Dalhousie University
Halifax, Nova Scotia
Canada

Ross J. Scalese, MD
Professor of Medicine and Medical Education
Director of Educational Technology Development
Michael S. Gordon Center for Simulation and Innovation in Medical Education
University of Miami Miller School of Medicine
Miami, Florida
United States

Daniel J. Schumacher, MD, PhD, MEd
Professor with Tenure
Department of Pediatrics
Cincinnati Children's Hospital Medical Center
Cincinnati, Ohio
United States

Michael Soh, PhD
Assistant Professor
Center for Health Professions Education
Uniformed Services University of the Health Sciences
Bethesda, Maryland
United States

David B. Swanson, PhD
Professor, Department of Medical Education
University of Melbourne Medical School
Melbourne, Victoria
Australia

Olle ten Cate, PhD
Professor
Center for Research and Development of Education
University Medical Center Utrecht
Utrecht, Netherlands

Toshiko Uchida, MD
Associate Professor
Department of Medicine and Medical Education
Feinberg School of Medicine
Northwestern University
Chicago, Illinois
United States

Karen M. Warburton, MD
Associate Professor of Medicine
Department of Medicine
University of Virginia School of Medicine
Charlottesville, Virginia
United States

Thilan Wijesekera, MD, MHS
Assistant Professor
Department of Internal Medicine
Yale School of Medicine
New Haven, Connecticut
United States

Acknowledgments

We wish to acknowledge the talent and dedication of all the authors whose effort and expertise resulted in this book. We also wish to thank the countless trainees and faculty who we have worked with over the years and who continue to inspire and challenge us. We hope this book, in a small way, can help improve the educational experience of all health professions educators and learners and, ultimately, patients.

Eric S. Holmboe and Steven J. Durning

Dedication

In memory of my incredibly supportive parents, Dr. Kenneth C. and Mrs. Bette M. Holmboe.

All my love and appreciation to my wife and best friend of 41 years, Eileen Holmboe, and my two amazing children who bring so much joy, Ken and Lauren. Finally, to all my family who keep me grounded and remind me what is most important.

Eric S. Holmboe

To my wife of over 30 years, Kristen, and my three wonderful sons, Andrew, Daniel and Malik, for their love and support. To my parents and my in-laws for their wisdom and encouragement.

Steven J. Durning

Contents

Video Contents

1

Assessment in the Era of Outcomes-Based Education

ERIC S. HOLMBOE, MD, OLLE TEN CATE, PHD, AND STEVEN J. DURNING, MD, PHD

CHAPTER OUTLINE

The Rise of Outcomes-Based Medical Education

Despite major biomedical and technical advances, medical care across the globe continues to suffer from pernicious quality and safety gaps that result in substantial harm and ineffective care for too many patients each year. The COVID-19 pandemic only exacerbated this situation, further exposing serious problems in healthcare equity and the care of vulnerable populations. It is estimated that over 20 million people had died from COVID-19 worldwide by the end of 2022.[1–3] The Institute of Medicine (now called the National Academy of Medicine, NAM) published a seminal report on the serious quality and safety issues in healthcare and codified the six aims of quality: care that is effective, efficient, safe, patient centered, timely, and equitable.[4–6] More recently, the Quadruple Aim of quality in patient experience (defined by the six aims), health of a population, cost stewardship, and wellness of the healthcare workforce has become the overarching driving framework for the US and other healthcare systems.[6,7] Some are calling for healthcare equity to be its own aim.[8]

Data from multiple sources, such as the Organisation for Economic Co-operation and Development (OECD), the World Health Organization (WHO), and the Commonwealth Fund, demonstrate persistent problems in morbidity and mortality that are amenable to better and safer healthcare delivery.[9–11] While a number of factors contribute to this state of affairs, many medical educators and policymakers accept the premise that the medical education enterprise bears some responsibility through insufficient preparation of trainees for 21st-century practice.[12] In conjunction with these concerns about healthcare quality and safety has been the growing focus on the *outcomes* of education. Specifically, educators are now most concerned with the abilities of a graduate rather than whether a trainee simply completes a prescribed educational program.[13,14] These and other factors have led to the global spread of outcomes-based medical education using competencies as a foundational outcomes framework for educational programs, or competency-based medical education (CBME).[15–18]

In 1978, McGaghie and colleagues described a rationale for an approach to health professions education founded on the acquisition of defined competencies using mastery-based learning principles. "The intended output of a competency-based programme," they wrote, "is a health professional who can practise medicine at a defined level of proficiency, in accord with local conditions, to meet local needs."[15] Educational leaders and policymakers worldwide produced multiple reports lamenting that medical education systems were not producing physicians with the abilities needed to meet the complexities of modern practice, leading to the realization that reforms in undergraduate, graduate, and continuing medical education were urgently needed. In the United States, reviews call attention to the inadequate preparation of our graduates to practice effectively in our evolving healthcare system, especially around transitions from undergraduate medical education (UME; i.e., medical school) to graduate or postgraduate medical education (GME or PGME) training, to clinical practice.[19–21]

These findings and other factors ultimately led to the development of competency frameworks in several countries as part of initiatives to implement CBME to achieve better educational and clinical care outcomes. The first iteration of the CanMEDS Roles by the Royal College of Physicians and Surgeons of Canada (RCPSC) was produced in 1996.[22,23] Recognizing similar needs and issues, the Accreditation Council of Graduate Medical Education (ACGME), the American Board of Medical Specialties (ABMS), the National Academy of Medicine (NAM), the General Medical Council of the United Kingdom, the Royal Australasian College of Surgeons, the Dutch College of Medical Specialties, and other national professional entities produced competency frameworks.[23–27] Two key features of these competency frameworks stand out. One is a redefinition of the doctor to include many more important and relevant abilities and constructs beyond medical knowledge and technical skill that had been dominating training in the previous decades. The other feature is the intention to better monitor doctors in training and to ensure that they meet predefined competency standards upon graduation to unsupervised practice.[23–28]

Several major reports and initiatives have sought to move CBME toward broader implementation. The International CBME Collaborators (ICBME), a group of medical educators and leaders convened by the RCPSC, produced in 2010 an initial series of articles on the history, definitions and concepts, and challenges to implementation of CBME, including needed changes to assessment, across the continuum of medical training.[29–31] That same year, Frenk and a group of international leaders published an influential position paper in *The Lancet* on the need to accelerate transformation in medical education, grounded in the principles of CBME.[12] The Carnegie Foundation, on the 100th anniversary of the Flexner report (1910), released recommendations for medical education that embraced many of the key principles and goals of CBME.[16] Finally, the ICBME released a second series of articles on evolving concepts and recommendations for CBME based on a growing body of experience with CBME implementation. All of these reports have highlighted the critical and continued need for better *assessment*.[32–39]

The primary purpose of this third edition is to provide practical guidance to educators and program leaders on the frontlines for building and implementing better procedures, programs, and systems of assessment, using the best evidence and information available. Assessment is essential for effective learning and for achieving desired educational and clinical outcomes. As the adage goes, assessment drives learning and learning should drive the right form of assessment, all connected to the ultimate outcome of achieving the Quadruple Aim (Fig. 1.1).

CBME represents the latest phase of what should be a continuous commitment to improve educational programs and, by extension, the quality and safety of care that patients and populations receive. This introductory chapter will present an overview of the drivers of change in the assessments used during clinical education, frameworks for such assessments, criteria for choosing assessment methods, elements of an effective faculty development effort, and the need to shift to developmental assessment approaches using competencies, Milestones, and Entrustable Professional Activities (EPAs). Before moving on to fundamental issues of assessment in a CBME world, we will first review some key definitions and elements of CBME.

Competency-Based Medical Education

A focus on the educational process has now shifted to an emphasis on what a physician is able to actually do at the end of training and at important junctures during the training process. Competencies have become a primary mechanism for defining the educational outcomes of individuals. Outcomes-based education starts with "the end in mind"; in other words, a specification of the competencies (i.e., abilities) that are expected of a physician and are needed for the healthcare tasks to be done. These educational outcomes should determine the requirements for the content, context, and structure of the curriculum; the selection and deployment of teaching and learning methods; the site of training; and the abilities needed of the teachers. Assessment plays a central role in determining whether students, residents, and fellows (or any learner in PGME) have achieved the competencies that have been specified and whether the educational program has been effective in producing the desired outcomes. CBME highlights the importance of integrating curriculum with assessment; competencies are not independent

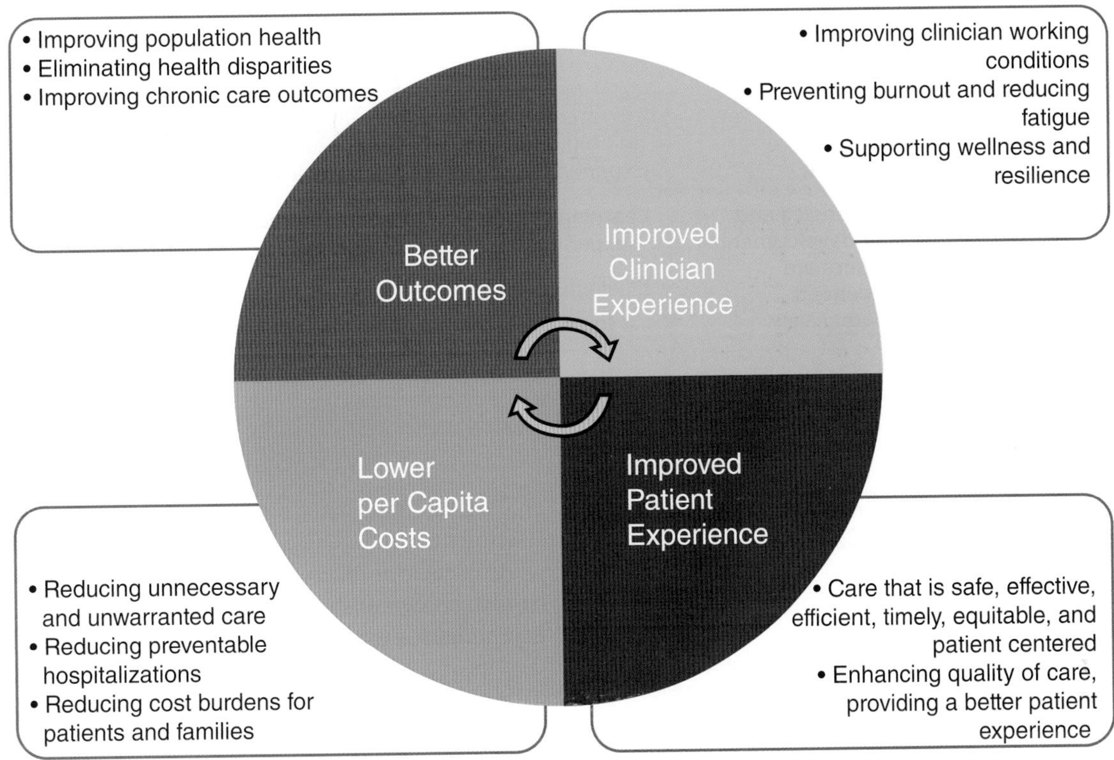

• **Fig. 1.1** The Quadruple Aim.

abilities, but rather, all competencies should be integrated as part of an overall educational system and program of assessment. This change in thinking and the need to assess the diverse and interdependent competencies of the physician has been an important factor in the development of new methods of assessment, especially the work-based assessments covered in detail throughout this book.

CBME is an outcomes-focused approach to and philosophy of designing the explicit developmental progression of health professionals to meet the needs of those they serve. Among its fundamental characteristics (see Table 1.1) is a shift in emphasis away from time-based programs based solely on exposure to experiences such as clinical rotations in favor of an emphasis on needs-based graduate *outcomes*, authenticity, and learner centeredness.[18,32] As defined by Frank and colleagues, CBME is "an outcomes-based approach to the design, implementation, assessment, and evaluation of medical education programs, using an organizing framework of competencies."[18] While outcomes are now the primary driver, that does not mean educational structures and processes are not important. The famous Donabedian equation for quality, Structure × Process = Outcomes, highlights that the desired outcomes depend on effective structures and processes.[40] However, we are also learning that the relationship between structure and process is quite complex and nonlinear in its actual execution.[41] Chapter 18 provides helpful guidance on how to embrace complexity as part of program design and evaluation. Assessment is a critical part of the complex interaction between structure and process in an educational program.

TABLE 1.1 Fundamental Characteristics of Competency-Based Medical Education

1. Graduate outcomes in the form of achievement of predefined desired competencies are the goal of CBME initiatives. These are aligned with the roles graduates will play in the next stage of their careers.
2. These predefined competencies are derived from the needs of patients, learners, and institutions and organized into a coherent guiding framework.
3. Time is a resource for learning, not the basis of progression of competence (i.e., time spent on a ward is not the marker of achievement).
4. Teaching and learning experiences are sequenced to facilitate an explicitly defined progression of ability in stages.
5. Workplace curricula are individualized, with learning tailored to the learner's individual progression in some manner.
6. Numerous observations and focused feedback contribute to effective learner development of expertise.
7. Assessment is planned, systematic, systemic, and integrative.

In 2019, Elaine Van Melle and colleagues, using a rigorous stepwise process, identified and elaborated five core components of CBME (Table 1.2, Fig. 1.2):[42]

1. Competencies required for practice are clearly articulated.
2. Competencies and their developmental markers are arranged and sequenced progressively.
3. Learning experiences are tailored to facilitate the progressive development of competencies.

TABLE 1.2 Core Components Framework

Outcome Competencies	Sequenced Progression	Tailored Learning Experiences	Competency-Focused Instruction	Programmatic Assessment (Using Systems Thinking)
Competencies required for practice are clearly articulated.	**Competencies and their developmental markers are sequenced progressively.**	**Learning experiences** **Facilitate . . .**	**Teaching practices promote . . .**	**Assessment practices support and document . . .**
		. . . the developmental acquisition of competencies.		

From Van Melle E, Frank JR, Holmboe ES, et al. A core components framework for evaluating implementation of competency-based medical education programs. *Acad Med.* 2019 Jul;94(7):1002-1009. doi:10.1097/ACM.0000000000002743.

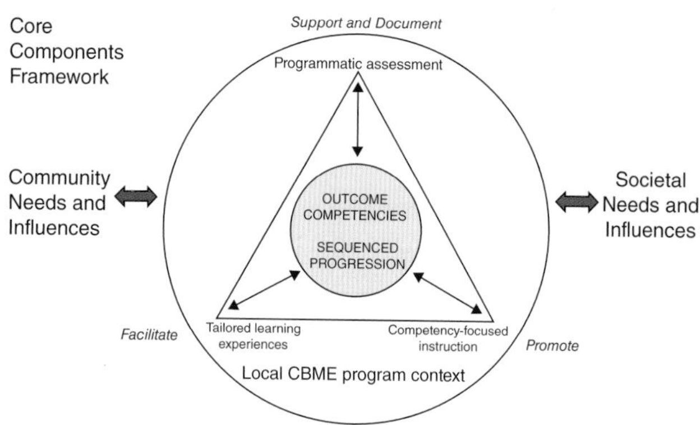

• Fig. 1.2 Core components framework for competency-based medical education.

4. Teaching practices promote the progressive development of competencies.
5. Assessment practices support and document the progressive development of competencies (i.e., programmatic assessment).

This core components framework (CCF) is increasingly considered a useful characterization of CBME. Two aspects of the CCF merit highlighting. First is the strong focus on development; a recognition that educating health professionals is an intensely developmental process. The CCF is grounded in a mindset of growth and motivation and is fully cognizant of the individualized trajectories each learner will experience. Growth mindset—that is, a learner's intrinsic will to develop—should be the foundation for a significant redesign of instructional methods, learning experiences, and assessment practices.[42–46] Training programs should focus on promoting and providing space for learner growth and development in the desired competencies through frequent formative (lower-stakes) assessment that is rich in both feedback and individualized coaching. Educators and programs must therefore design assessment tools that support the developmental trajectories of learners and integrate them into a program of assessment, thus supporting the learner's professional development. Second, programmatic assessment uses a systems lens as an essential component, and Chapter 3 provides specific guidance on creating, implementing, and maintaining programmatic assessment.

Assessment is an essential activity (i.e., process) that can be used to demonstrate outcomes of interest. This is not a new insight—assessment has always been critically important in any educational endeavor. However, the problems with assessment in medical education, and generally all of health professions education, have been long-standing and persistent and include lack of direct observation of learner performance and meaningful feedback; overreliance on testing for assessment of medical knowledge; lack of attention to other essential competencies that address our graduates' abilities to function effectively in our healthcare systems, such as interprofessional teamwork and quality improvement; and ineffective use of assessment methods and tools by faculty, to name just a few. In the remainder of the chapter, we will explore fundamental issues in assessment, followed by how all programs can more effectively operationalize competencies through Competency milestones and EPAs and how these developmental assessment constructs can support a program of assessment. Throughout the chapter we will refer the reader to other chapters in the book to help the reader create and revise their own program of assessment.

A Brief History of Assessment in Medical Education

Through the early 1950s, physicians were assessed in limited ways.[47] Medical knowledge was evaluated with essays and other open-ended question formats that were graded by an instructor. Clinical skill and judgment were tested using an oral examination that often required the student to go to the bedside, gather patient information, and present it along with a diagnostic list and treatment plan to one or more examiners who asked questions. Because these were the only generally accepted methods available, they were applied to most assessment problems even if they were not completely suitable to the task and were often unreliable. That may have been acceptable at a time when supervisors had much more control over the healthcare process, the therapeutic and diagnostic armamentarium was much more limited, and supervisors had natural checks for everything learners reported. Healthcare is now far too complex to warrant this type of "on-the-fly," ad hoc approach. For example, length of stay in hospitals has dropped dramatically, the number and type of diagnostic and therapeutic tools has exploded, and faculty have multiple competing responsibilities.

From that point to the present, there have been extensive changes in the way assessment is conducted. Methods have proliferated, as have the requirements for their appropriate use. Much progress has been made in the assessment of medical knowledge with a variety of written and computer-based techniques now offering reliable and valid results regarding the capability of learners (see Chapter 7). In the past few decades, considerable gains have been made in defining and enhancing the psychometric qualities of standardized performance assessments that control for context, such as objective structured clinical examinations (OSCEs), particularly around their use for higher-stakes purposes (see Chapter 6). However, while assessments in the context of caring for actual patients in clinical units (e.g., wards, operating theaters, ambulatory clinics) have vastly improved, especially in the areas of patient care skills such as medical interviewing, informed decision-making, and clinical reasoning, much work remains, especially in competencies such as interprofessional teamwork, care coordination, and abilities in quality improvement and patient safety.[38,48]

Equally important, the methods that have been developed to support clinical education often rely on faculty who are inexperienced in their use, do not share common standards or mental models of the competencies of importance, and have not been trained to apply them in a consistent fashion. In addition, faculty now experience substantial time pressures, including caring for more patients, higher degrees of comorbidity among hospitalized patients, and increasing personal administrative responsibilities. Perhaps more concerning are persistent findings that one of the principal drivers of faculty assessment relates to their own clinical skills (i.e., self as frame of reference or standard), with several studies highlighting important deficiencies in practicing physician clinical skills such as medical interviewing, physical examination, and communication[49,50] (see Chapter 5). Finally, many faculty are also being asked to assess and judge competencies, such as care coordination, quality improvement, use of clinical performance measures, reflective practice, patient safety, and use of information technology—areas in which they themselves were never formally trained. Compounding this state of affairs has been insufficient or ineffective faculty development approaches and models to address these new clinical and educational methods, although thankfully this situation is improving[51–54] (see Chapter 11).

Drivers of Change in Assessment

The increased public focus on the medical education enterprise is important; medical education should always be in *service* of individual patients, families, and the public. Using a service logic can help educators develop assessment programs that meet public, patient, and learner needs.[55] Fig. 1.3 provides an example of a logic model based on implementing competency milestones (discussed later in the chapter). Many programs globally are implementing curricular changes that embrace competencies and outcomes, supported by improvements in technology, psychometrics, and evolving work-based assessment approaches that increasingly incorporate more qualitative techniques and systematic judgment.

Accountability and Quality Assurance

The movement to CBME has been accompanied by significant efforts to enhance the accountability of physicians.[3] Motivated by the need to improve quality and safety—and in part by high-profile cases of derailed physicians in the 1990s such as Michael Swango (USA) and Harold Shipman (UK), and more recently neurosurgeon Christopher Duntsch (USA)—the public has continued to pressure medicine to increase its level of oversight and eliminate the "bad apples."[56,57] Medical educators are also more keenly aware that too many trainees graduate with substantial deficiencies in foundational knowledge as well as clinical skills and other core competencies (e.g., professionalism, interpersonal skills, and communication) important to succeed in our healthcare system[58–60] (see Chapter 5). Effective quality assurance of promotion decisions depends on robust assessment programs and is critically important to ensure that graduates of medical education programs are truly ready for the next stage of training and, ultimately, unsupervised practice. Promoting trainees who lack competence erodes, if not destroys, the trust between the medical profession and the public. When the focus shifts from promotion based on time-in-training to promotion based on competence, adequate assessment become even more key.[61]

Quality Improvement Movement

At the same time, a variety of efforts have focused on continuously improving the quality of healthcare. The urgency to improve healthcare and achieve the Quadruple Aim has only accelerated because of the COVID-19 pandemic.[62–64] These efforts have relied on methods devised by workers in the field of quality improvement science and engineering and, in some cases, have been used successfully in industry for over 60 years to drive continuous improvement in healthcare and are now increasingly being used in medical education programs. Central to quality improvement is assessment—it is very hard to improve without *meaningful* measurement and data. Assessment offers a means of identifying those whose overall performance is well below expectations and identifying areas for improvement for all learners in the medical education system, helping to drive the continuous quality improvement process. These developments have helped fuel the creation of multiple new methods of assessment and increase the use of other methods already available. For example, the

TABLE 1.3 The Competencies and Subcompetencies of Physicians as Described by Four Organizations

Competency Domain	Subcompetencies
CanMEDS (Canada)	
Medical expert	1. Practice medicine within their defined scope of practice and expertise. 2. Perform a patient-centered clinical assessment and establish a management plan. 3. Plan and perform procedures and therapies for the purpose of assessment and/or management. 4. Establish plans for ongoing care and, when appropriate, timely consultation. 5. Actively contribute, as an individual and as a member of a team providing care, to the continuous improvement of healthcare quality and patient safety.
Communicator	1. Establish professional therapeutic relationships with patients and their families. 2. Elicit and synthesize accurate and relevant information, incorporating the perspectives of patients and their families. 3. Share healthcare information and plans with patients and their families. 4. Engage patients and their families in developing plans that reflect the patient's healthcare needs and goals. 5. Document and share written and electronic information about the medical encounter to optimize clinical decision-making, patient safety, confidentiality, and privacy.
Collaborator	1. Work effectively with physicians and other colleagues in the healthcare professions. 2. Work with physicians and other colleagues in the healthcare professions to promote understanding, manage differences, and resolve conflicts. 3. Hand over the care of a patient to another healthcare professional to facilitate continuity of safe patient care.
Leader	1. Contribute to the improvement of healthcare delivery in teams, organizations, and systems. 2. Engage in the stewardship of healthcare resources. 3. Demonstrate leadership in professional practice. 4. Manage career planning, finances, and health human resources in a practice.
Health advocate	1. Respond to an individual patient's health needs by advocating with the patient within and beyond the clinical environment. 2. Respond to the needs of the communities or populations they serve by advocating with them for system-level change in a socially accountable manner.
Scholar	1. Engage in the continuous enhancement of their professional activities through ongoing learning. 2. Teach students, residents, the public, and other healthcare professionals. 3. Integrate best available evidence into practice. 4. Contribute to the creation and dissemination of knowledge and practices applicable to health.
Professional	1. Demonstrate a commitment to patients by applying best practices and adhering to high ethical standards. 2. Demonstrate a commitment to society by recognizing and responding to societal expectations in healthcare. 3. Demonstrate a commitment to the profession by adhering to standards and participating in physician-led regulation. 4. Demonstrate a commitment to physician health and well-being to foster optimal patient care.
General Medical Council (United Kingdom)	
Competency Domain	**Subcompetencies**
Professionalism in action	Domain 1 describes six principles and expectation of all physicians.
Domain 1: Knowledge, skills, and performance	1. Develop and maintain your professional performance. 2. Apply knowledge and experience to practice. 3. Record your work clearly, accurately, and legibly.
Domain 2: Safety and quality	1. Contribute to and comply with systems to protect patients. 2. Respond to risks to safety. 3. Risks posed by your health.
Domain 3: Communication, partnership, and teamwork	1. Communicate effectively. 2. Work collaboratively with colleagues. 3. Teaching, training, supporting, and assessing. 4. Continuity and coordination of care. 5. Establish and maintain partnerships with patients.

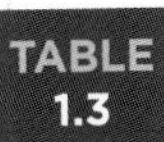

TABLE 1.3 The Competencies and Subcompetencies of Physicians as Described by Four Organizations—cont'd

General Medical Council (United Kingdom)	
Competency Domain	**Subcompetencies**
Domain 4: Maintaining trust	1. Show respect for patients. 2. Treat patients and colleagues fairly and without discrimination. 3. Act with honesty and integrity a. Communicating information b. Openness and legal or disciplinary proceedings c. Honesty in financial dealings
ACGME/ABMS General Competencies (United States)	
Competency Domain	**Subcompetencies**
Patient Care	Residents must be able to perform all medical, diagnostic, and surgical procedures considered essential for the area of practice.Subcompetencies vary by specialty and often target specific conditions (e.g., chronic illness) or settings (e.g., ambulatory clinic), and includes: 1. Medical interviewing 2. Physical examination 3. Procedural care
Medical Knowledge	Residents and fellows must demonstrate knowledge of established and evolving biomedical, clinical, epidemiological, and social-behavioral sciences, as well as the application of this knowledge to patient care. Subcompetencies vary by specialty, may target specific conditions (e.g., chronic illness) or specific domains of knowledge (e.g., pathophysiology, etc.), and include: 1. Clinical reasoning in the clinical care space
Systems-based Practice	1. Patient safety and quality improvement 2. System navigation for patient-centered care 3. Physician role in healthcare system
Practice-based Learning and Improvement	1. Evidence-based and informed practice 2. Reflective practice and commitment to personal growth
Professionalism	1. Professional behavior and ethical principles 2. Accountability/conscientiousness 3. Self-awareness and help-seeking
Interpersonal Communication Skills	1. Patient and family-centered communication 2. Interprofessional and team communication 3. Communication with healthcare systems
Institute of Medicine (now National Academy of Medicine; United States)	
1. Employ evidence-based practice. 2. Work in interdisciplinary teams. 3. Provide patient-centered care. 4. Apply quality improvement. 5. Utilize informatics.	

ABMS, American Board of Medical Specialists; *ACGME*, Accreditation Council for Graduate Medical Education; *CanMEDS*, Canadian Medical Education Directions for Specialists.

competency milestones, first implemented in the United States in 2014, describe competencies in narrative, developmental terms and use the principles of continuous quality improvement as part of their foundation to improve GME. The Milestones initiative can be viewed through the lens of "action- or practice-based research" to learn and develop evidence over time.[65,66] There is no single "holy grail" of assessment. All assessments have strengths and weaknesses, and programs need to build in ongoing evaluation of their assessment activities (see Chapter 18).

Technology

Over the past 60 years, the availability of increasingly sophisticated technology has changed the testing of medical knowledge and judgment in fundamental ways.[67,68] The introduction of the computer heralded an era of large-scale testing by encouraging the use of multiple-choice questions (MCQs), the answers to which could be scanned by machine, turned into scores, and then reported in an efficient and objective fashion.

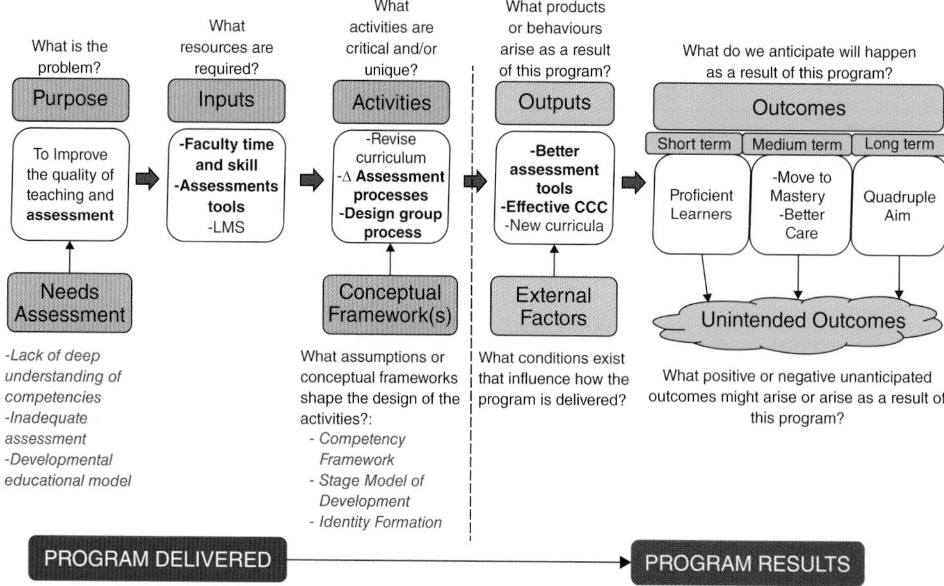

• **Fig. 1.3** Logic model for assessment. Courtesy Elaine Van Melle.

More recently, the intelligence of the computer has improved assessment in important ways:

1. It has enabled the application of significant psychometric advances to the assessment of medical knowledge. Specifically, the computer's intelligence has improved efficiency by allowing the selection of questions that are targeted to the ability of particular examinees. Sequential testing and adaptive testing permit gains in efficiency and precision.
2. It has improved the assessment of higher cognitive abilities, including clinical reasoning, by permitting the use of interactive item formats that more closely simulate the types of judgments physicians need to make in practice (see Chapters 7 and 8).
3. It has enabled new approaches to assessment that leverage the science of retrieval practice to enhance long-term retention, such as progress testing and confidence-based learning platforms.[69]

While the impact of technology on assessment of clinical skills has been slower to develop, advances in simulation and computer technology have led to the development of approaches and tools that re-create aspects of the clinical encounter with considerable fidelity. These methods have a growing impact on assessment, especially in the area of procedural skills, where mastery models are beginning to gain traction and have been shown to translate to the bedside.[70–74]

Finally, technology, especially through smartphone and tablet applications, is beginning to change the way assessment data is obtained and processed. For example, tools designed for assessment through direct observation are increasingly being converted into smartphone applications[75] (see Chapters 5 and 9). Natural language processing (NLP) is enabling more feasible collection of narrative assessments, and NLP software shows substantial promise in analyzing narrative assessments for levels of developmental bias. Learning management systems, increasingly used by programs, are also beginning to incorporate mobile apps into their platforms.[75] These portable applications hold substantial promise to reduce data collection burden while guiding the assessment activity of the faculty to attend to critical competencies.

Psychometrics

While the technology has improved, there have been significant advances in psychometrics, the basic science of assessment. Classical test theory, prominent from the mid-20th century, has gradually given way to measurement models based on strong assumptions about test items and examinees. The family of item response theory models now makes it possible to produce equivalent scores even when examinees take tests made up of different questions.[76] They also support the computer-based administration of examinations that are tailored to the ability level of individual test-takers; this allows tests to be shortened by as much as 40%.[77] The ability to shorten tests has cost and validity implications; less test material exposure decreases the likelihood that future examinees are familiar with examination content.[78] Generalizability theory makes it possible to help identify how much error is associated with different facets of measurement (e.g., raters, patients).[79] Based on this information, assessments can be prospectively designed to make the best use of resources, such as faculty time, while maintaining the reliability of the results.

In addition to these major developments, there have been several other advances. For example, a variety of systematic methods are available for setting standards on tests and for identifying when test questions are biased against particular groups of examinees.[80,81] Test development methods have gotten better, as has the means for judging whether particular items are working properly. Overall, these advances have improved both the quality and efficiency of assessment.

Qualitative Assessment and Group Process

Although advances in psychometrics have clearly helped improve assessment in medical education and will remain a core science for assessment for the foreseeable future, many have noted significant limitations of the traditional psychometric approach in today's complex clinical and educational environment.[82] Often referred to as qualitative assessment or narrative assessment, use of the written word has grown in importance. For example, many of the new smartphone apps contain NLP capabilities that allow for the capture of narrative assessment and feedback through dictation. Milestones, discussed in more detail later in the chapter, are more robust narrative descriptors of stages of development, bringing both quantitative and qualitative aspects of measurement closer together.[74] Recent work has also found that applying rigorous qualitative methodology to assess narrative assessments can produce high levels of reliability. Ginsburg and colleagues noted: "Using written comments to discriminate between residents can be extremely reliable even after only several reports are collected. This suggests a way to identify residents early on who may require attention. These findings contribute evidence to support the validity argument for using qualitative data for assessment." They also noted that reliability coefficients above 0.8 are possible with narrative assessment.[83]

Group process, commonly conducted by entities called clinical competency committees (CCCs), has also become an important and established part of assessment process and programs (see Chapter 16). Effective group process can lead to better judgments around competence, especially needed for summative decisions.[84–88] Finally, qualitative research techniques have been shown to have value in judging aggregate assessment information, such as that contained within a portfolio (see Chapter 15). Again, a rigorous approach to application of qualitative research techniques and principles helps enhance the reliability and validity of judgments.[89–91]

Framework for Assessment

As methods of assessment have proliferated, so has the need to use them efficiently and effectively as an integrated combination in a system of assessment. Developing, implementing, and sustaining effective systems for the assessment of clinical competence in medical school, residency, fellowship, and all graduate and postgraduate health professions educational programs requires consideration of what competencies need to be assessed, how best to assess them, and the developmental level of the trainee being assessed. Consequently, a three-dimensional framework for structuring an assessment system can help medical educators make better judgments about learner development. Along the first dimension are the competencies (i.e., abilities) that need to be assessed, the second is the type of assessment required, and the third is the trainees' stage of development.

Dimension 1: Competencies

As shown in Table 1.3, there are several schemes for describing the knowledge, skills, and attributes of the physician.[24–27] The Canadian Medical Education Directives for Specialists (CanMEDS) model, developed and periodically updated by the RCPSC, describes the competencies in terms of the roles of a physician and was last updated in 2015 with plans to again review and revise in 2025. Good Medical Practice, which was created by the General Medical Council in the United Kingdom, describes the elements of good practice and was revised in 2019 to highlight the problem of discrimination. In the United States, two influential groups developed a set of core competencies. The ACGME and the ABMS adopted six general competencies in 2001 and have recently revised and updated these competencies as subcompetencies within the Milestones framework. These competencies comprise the educational outcomes framework for residency and fellowship training as well as maintenance of certification programs throughout a physician's career in the United States. The NAM (formerly the Institute of Medicine) recommended five core skills, or competencies, that create a framework for evaluating performance and stimulating the reform of education. CanMEDS, the ACGME/ABMS General Competencies, and Good Medical Practice also highlight how the competency frameworks evolve with time and changing science as all three frameworks are now structured with subcompetencies that reflect the multitude of abilities needed and complexities of being a physician. They are intended to improve professional education and practice with a goal of enhancing the safety and quality of healthcare. Although there are some differences among the schemes, there is also significant overlap in these descriptions of a physician (Table 1.3).

These competencies are intended as the first step in identifying the key educational outcomes of individual healthcare professionals that should inform learning objectives, assessment, and curriculum of graduate training programs, adapted to the content, education, and practice of the particular specialty/subspecialty. As we will see in the section, Dimension 3: Assessment of Progression, Milestones and EPAs are constructs and concepts, specified and adapted by specialties that can facilitate the implementation of competency-based training. The data produced by the assessment of competencies serve as a basis for judging the quality of the trainees and their training, as well as supporting the continuous improvement of both.

Dimension 2: Levels and Types of Assessment

The multifaceted nature of the competencies makes it apparent that no single method could provide a sufficient basis for making judgments about learners in health professions education. In an organized approach to this problem, George Miller proposed a classification scheme in 1990 that stratifies assessment methods based on what they require of the trainee and has stood the test of time. Often referred to as Miller's pyramid (Fig. 1.4), it is composed of four levels: knows, knows how, shows how, and does.[92]

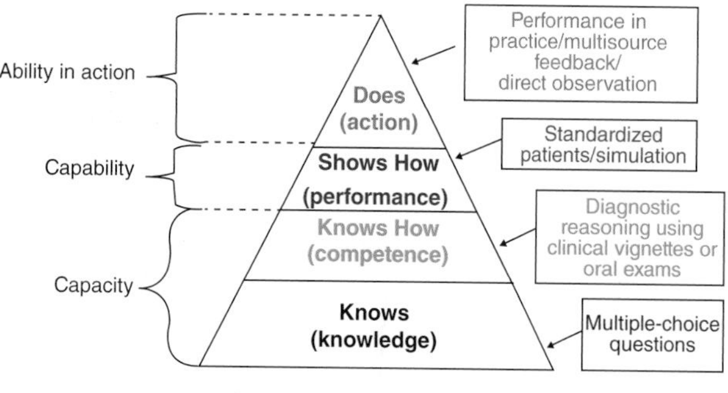

• **Fig. 1.4** Miller's pyramid.

Miller's Pyramid

Knows. This is the lowest level of the pyramid and it contains methods that assess what a trainee "knows" in an area of competence. Forming the base of the pyramid, knowledge represents the foundation upon which clinical competence is built. Most MCQ examinations focus on biologic and clinical domains. However, an MCQ-based examination composed of questions focused on ethics and principles of patient confidentiality would provide an assessment of what a trainee "knows" about key tenets of professionalism.

Knows how. To function as a physician, a good knowledge base is necessary but insufficient. It is important to know how to apply this knowledge in the acquisition of data, the analysis and interpretation of findings, and the development of management plans. Oral examinations, still in use by some certification boards, are one example of a high-stakes "knows how" assessment. In the United States, the surgical certification boards use oral examinations to assess how recent residency and fellowship graduates would approach a clinical condition (e.g., trauma). As another example, a training program used for professionalism might pose a moral dilemma, asks trainees to reason through it, and evaluate the sophistication of their moral thinking.

Shows how. Although trainees may know and know how, they may not be able to integrate these skills into a successful performance with patients. Consequently, certain assessment methods require the trainee to show how they perform with patients. For example, standardized patients may be used to assess clinical skills such as informed decision-making and breaking bad news. As another example, a standardized patient presenting with an ethical challenge would offer the trainee an opportunity to "show how" they would respond to a professionalism challenge. Miller referenced this level as "performance," akin to an actor on a stage performing under controlled conditions.

Does. No matter how good traditional assessment methods become, there remains the concern that what happens in a controlled testing environment does not generalize directly or predict what happens in practice. This is evident in studies of high-stakes MCQ examinations that find, at best, only a modest correlation of test scores and quality of care provided to actual patients.[93] The highest level of Miller's pyramid therefore focuses on methods that provide an assessment of routine performance, or what Miller called *action*. For example, the development and use of multisource feedback tools, patient experience surveys, and critical incident systems, such as the one currently used in some residencies and medical schools, offers an assessment of what learners actually do in terms of interpersonal skills and professionalism.

Miller's pyramid is a useful framework for considering differences and similarities among assessment methods. However, the fact that it is a pyramid might imply to some that methods addressing the higher levels are better, or conversely, that the larger area occupied by the base of the pyramid implies that knowledge assessment is most important. Instead, superior methods are those best aligned with the purpose of the assessment. For example, if an assessment of foundational medical knowledge is needed, a method associated with that level (e.g., MCQs) is likely better than a method associated with another level (e.g., standardized patients).

Two groups have advocated for changes to Miller's pyramid. Cruess and colleagues argued to add "Is" to the top of the pyramid to recognize the importance of professional identity formation, but it is not yet clear where this fits into an assessment program.[94] More recently, ten Cate and colleagues extended the pyramid, placing "Entrusted with future care" at the top as the ultimate assessment decision.

The Cambridge Model

As physicians near the end of training and enter practice, external forces and context come to play a very large role in performance. The Cambridge Model, a variation on Miller's pyramid, proposes that performance in practice (the highest level of the pyramid) is influenced by two large forces beyond competence.[95] Systems-related factors, such as government programs, clinical microsystems (i.e., the clinical units where learners care for patients), institutional care delivery practices, patient expectations, and guidelines, among other factors, strongly influence what physicians do. Similarly, factors related to the individual physician such as state of mind, physical and mental health, and relationships with peers and family have a significant effect. Consequently, assessment becomes more difficult because it is harder to disentangle the effects of the context (e.g., context specificity; see Chapter 8) of care from the competence of the individual physician. Here, a focus on healthcare processes and outcomes as a measure of what a physician "does" can provide a robust assessment of a physician's ability to integrate multiple competencies within a complex social context.

However, processes and outcomes are still impacted by system factors that can affect patient preferences and thus impact the measurement of processes of care such as the availability of specific services that may also impact outcomes. Fig. 1.5 highlights the complex, interdependent interactions and relationships involved in caring for patients. Assessment programs must consider the impact of these relationships when designing and implementing assessment programs because of the significant intersection and dependence of educational outcomes and quality of care provided to patients.[54,96,97]

Dimension 3: Assessment of Progression

Acquiring competence is not an overnight process. Trainees progress through a series of stages that begin in undergraduate medical education and continue throughout their careers. Educators must be able to recognize when a trainee has attained sufficient knowledge, skills, and attitudes to enter the next stage and this requires appropriate standards and benchmarks for the transition. Hurbert Dreyfus and Stuart Dreyfus created a developmental model of learning applicable to the health professions that proposes five stages of educational development (Table 1.4).[24,97]

The characteristics of learners and the steps they must go through to acquire competence will change over the five stages of development, and each step, or stage, does not occur in a linear fashion (Fig. 1.6). Necessarily, the methods of assessment applied at each developmental level will likely also evolve. For example, at the level of the novice, an MCQ-based knowledge test might be most appropriate, but a standardized patient–based examination might be better suited to learners who are in the competence or proficiency stage depending on the competency of interest. It is important to realize that learners are typically at different stages for different competencies, depending on the content and context of the task and competency being assessed. This observation

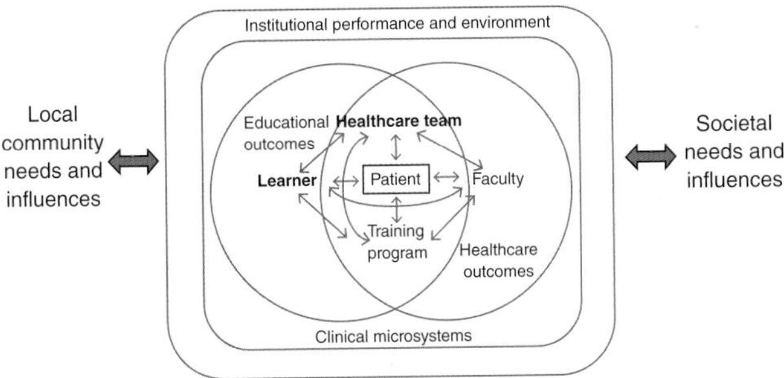

• **Fig. 1.5** Changing perspective: patients at the intersection of educational and healthcare outcomes.

TABLE 1.4 The Stages of Learning as Proposed by Dreyfus

Stage of Learning	Method of Learning (Teaching Style)	Learning Steps	Learner Characteristics
1. Novice	Instruction (instructor) Breaks skill into context-free, discrete tasks, concepts, rules	Recognizes the context-free features Knows rules for determining actions based on these features	Learning occurs in a detached analytic frame of mind
2. Advanced beginner	Practice (coach) Experiences coping with real situations Points out new aspects of material Teaches rules and reasoning techniques for action	Recognizes relevant aspects based on experience that makes sense of the material Learns maxims about actions based on new material	Learning occurs in a detached, analytic frame of mind
3. Competence	Apprenticeship (facilitator) Develops a plan or chooses perspective that separates "important" from "ignored" elements Demonstrates that rules and reasoning techniques for choosing are difficult to come by Role models also emotionally involved in making decisions	Volume of aspects is overwhelming Performance is exhausting Sense of what's important is lacking Stands alone in making correct and incorrect choices Coping becomes frightening, discouraging, elating	Learner is emotionally involved in the task and its outcome Too many subtle differences for rules; student must decide in each case Makes a mistake, then feels remorse Succeeds, then feels elated Emotional learning builds competence
4. Proficiency	Apprenticeship (supervisor) Gains more specific experience with outcomes of one's decisions Applies rules and maxims to decide what to do	Rules and principles are replaced by situational discrimination Emotional responses to success or failure build intuitive responses that replace reasoned ones	Learner immediately sees the goal and salient features Learner reasons how to get to the goal by applying rules and principles
5. Expertise	Independence (mentor) Experiences multiple, small random variations Observes other experts or experiences nonrandom simulations Working through the cases must emotionally matter	Gains experience with increasingly subtle variations in situations Automatically distinguishes situations requiring one response from those requiring another	Immediately sees the goal and what must be done to achieve it Builds on previous learning experiences

From Dreyfus HL. On the Internet. *Thinking in Action Series*. Routledge; 2001.

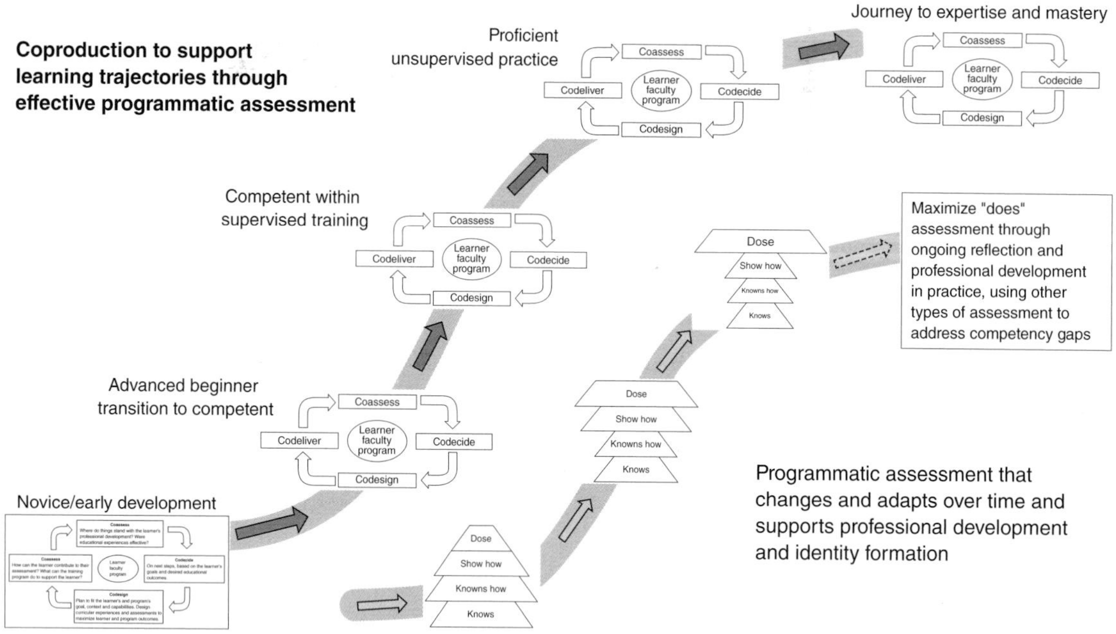

• **Fig. 1.6** Coproduction to support learning trajectories through effective programmatic assessment.

has been clearly seen in the US Milestones data and other studies of learning curves.[98] For example, a resident may be seen as "proficient" in working up a patient with chest pain, but at the "advanced beginner" level in counseling a patient regarding end-of-life care. Likewise, many students achieve competence with regard to medical knowledge, or perhaps communication skills, before they acquire the same level in more challenging systems-based practice domains such as care coordination or cost-conscious care delivery.

Pusic and colleagues have noted that learning curves, or trajectories, are in fact sigmoidal, and that learners during UME and GME training will spend almost the entirety of their time on the steep part of the curve.[98] Ultimately, work-based assessment will need to be the predominate component in a program of assessment, especially for postgraduate programs and ongoing professional development in practice. Educators need to recognize this developmental sequence when designing an assessment system and it will be critical to ensure that the chosen method is suitable to the task. Finally, programs and educational leaders should adopt a coproduction mindset that is aligned with the core components framework described earlier. Coproduction sees learner as partners in the educational program and sees assessment as something faculty do *with* learners instead of *to* them. This involves a series of coproduced learning cycles to support learners' professional development.

Criteria for Choosing an Assessment Method

Decisions about which method of assessment to use in a particular circumstance have traditionally rested on validity and reliability. *Validity* is the degree to which the inferences based on the results of an assessment are correct. Valid inferences regarding a particular test score or assessment result depend upon the *reliability* of these outcomes, and reliability is a component in more "modern" concepts of validity such as those by Kane and Messick, discussed in Chapter 2.

For purposes of assessment in medical education, Van Der Vleuten added educational impact, cost-effectiveness, and acceptability as other key factors in their utility index to guide the choice or revision of assessments. The utility index is represented by the equation Validity × Reliability × Educational Impact × Cost-Effectiveness × Acceptability = Utility.[99] Utility is a useful concept as programs choose and implement assessment methods. It is also important to note that Utility is a multiplicative construct; if any of the terms, or variables, are zero, utility is, by definition, zero.

In terms of *educational impact*, Van Der Vleuten argues that trainees will work hard in preparation for an assessment.[90] Consequently, the method should direct them to study in the most relevant way. For example, if an educational objective is for trainees to know the differential diagnoses for a particular chief complaint, then assessment using extended matching questions will likely induce better learning than assessment based on standardized patients.

Cost-effectiveness is the extent to which an assessment method is affordable and efficient. Although high-fidelity simulations might be a good way to assess procedural competence, the use of a method such as direct observation of procedural skills (DOPS), which is based on faculty observation, is likely to be more cost-effective in most graduate training settings.[100] *Acceptability* is the degree to which the trainees and faculty believe that the method produces valid results. This factor will influence motivation of faculty to use the method and enhance trainees' distrust of the results. It is important that educational leaders not underestimate trainees' knowledge and understanding of assessment and their ability to participate in decisions regarding assessment practices.

An international group of assessment experts updated the utility index and created a list of criteria for good assessment.[101] Validity and acceptability were retained as separate categories, and for validity the importance of *coherence* (a body of evidence that hangs together to support the results for a specific purpose) was highlighted. Reliability was essentially split into two new categories: (1) *reproducibility* (repeatability) and *consistency* (all items or components of the test intercorrelate in the same direction), and (2) *equivalence* (all students are treated equally). Educational impact was split into *educational effect* (the assessment motivates learners to prepare for it in a fashion that has educational benefit) and *catalytic effect* (the assessment provides results and feedback in a fashion that creates, enhances, and supports education; it drives future learning forward). Finally, the last new category was *feasibility*, namely that the assessment should be practical, realistic, and sensible.[101]

Educational Effect	**Catalytic Effect**
"The assessment motivates those who take it to prepare in a fashion that has educational benefit."	"The assessment provides results and feedback in a fashion that creates, enhances, and supports education; it drives future learning forward."

In addition to the factors highlighted in the two versions of criteria for good assessment, it is important to consider how a particular method fits into the overall system for assessment. The same method can (and arguably should) be used to assess more than one competency. For example, peer assessment can provide a measure of both professionalism and interpersonal skills. Likewise, two different methods can be used to capture information on the same competency, thereby increasing confidence in the results. For example, patient care can be assessed using both the single-encounter mini-CEX (clinical evaluation exercise) and summary ratings by attending physicians derived from a more longitudinal experience (e.g., clinical rotation).

Educational effect, catalytic effect, feasibility, and acceptability are not easily quantifiable, nor is the relationship among methods of assessment in a system. However, these factors plus reliability and validity should be weighed interactively when considering selection of a particular method.

Elements of Effective Faculty Development

Faculty members play a particularly critical role in assessment in the clinical setting because such assessment is often based on observation. And by faculty we mean any health professional, at a minimum, who participates in an assessment system. Recall that Miller placed "does," meaning the care of actual patients, at the top of the pyramid. Envision the pyramid as a spear and at the tip of that spear are patients. Using this metaphor helps faculty appreciate the central role of observation in both assuring trainee competence (at a minimum) and guaranteeing that patients receive high-quality, safe care in the context of training (see Chapter 5). Most important is the fact that the actual measurement instrument is the *faculty*, not the assessment tool. We cannot emphasize enough throughout this book that assessment in the workplace is essential and relies on informed, expert judgment (see Chapters 4, 5, and 9).

Assessment methods and tools are only as good as the individuals using them. Although there has been substantial progress in creating many new methods and tools, significantly less attention has been paid to the development of approaches to training faculty in how to use them most effectively. This omission continues to occur despite repeated studies over time demonstrating significant problems with the quality of faculty assessments[102–104] (see Chapter 5). There are three significant reasons why faculty training is urgently needed. First, to perform quality assessment, faculty members must possess sufficient knowledge, skill, and attitudes in the competency targeted by the assessment. For example, a decline of clinical skills teaching in the workplace was noted by George Engel in *1976*[105] and has resulted in many of today's educators failing to acquire a high level of clinical skills needed for effective care and teaching. This likely limits the degree to which they can validly assess clinical performance, and recent research adds evidence to the importance of the faculty's own underlying clinical skills.[49] Faculty development and subsequent teaching and assessment can restore this gap.

Second, competencies that are considered essential for every physician have evolved and will continue to evolve and change over time. Witness the birth of the competency domains of Practice-based Learning and Improvement and Systems-based Practice in the ACGME/ABMS competency framework, and the change of the role of manager in CanMEDS to that of leader in 2015.[106] The majority of faculty today never received during their training any formal instruction in many of the competencies and subcompetencies now needed for modern practice. Many faculty actually acquire new knowledge and skills alongside their trainees (i.e., through colearning).

Finally, assessment is a core tenet of professionalism for medical educators. Too often, faculty members view assessment as someone else's job, especially when a negative performance appraisal is involved (see Chapter 16). Faculty development reinforces the importance of assessment and provides medical educators the opportunity to develop common standards for performance. The medical profession has the obligation to uphold and protect its own standards, implying a commitment for physicians to evaluate themselves and their colleagues.[107]

To make effective use of the methods of assessment, educational institutions must commit the necessary resources for faculty development. However, too often faculty development translates into a project or a brief workshop. If faculty development is to be truly successful, medical educators need to embrace new strategies that embed faculty development in real-time teaching and clinical activities.

For example, Hemmer and colleagues embed faculty frame-of-reference training into formal evaluation sessions for students.[108] Faculty development, like quality improvement and maintenance of competence, must become a continuous process and appropriately rewarded. As noted earlier, the quality and safety of patient care depends on it (see Chapter 5).

Medical educators must also end their quest for the perfect assessment tool with the perfect rating form imbued with special powers to solve all measurement needs. Assessment is a sophisticated skill that requires hard work and a multifaceted approach. Lindy and Farr, in a landmark article in the performance appraisal field over 40 years ago, pleaded with researchers to redirect development efforts from a search for the perfect rating form to training the assessors.[109] Researchers in this field subsequently developed several rater training approaches that can lead to better assessments. Chapter 5 provides guidance on several practical faculty training methods.

Milestones and EPAs, described later in the chapter, require special consideration. Using Milestones and EPAs for curriculum development and assessment requires a shift in thinking among faculty and an infrastructure to support new assessment practices. Both individual faculty and committees must get acquainted and experienced with entrustment decision-making for EPAs and their conditions.[110] Training in the dimensions to be used in assessment and in the criteria for decisions is needed, and specific tools related to EPA-based assessment continue to be developed and implemented.[111,112] If anything, sufficient and adequate supervision and feedback is key to entrustment decisions, which requires longitudinal relationships with program leaders, advisors, and coaches.[113,114] This does not necessarily mean huge investments in time for advising, but an efficient use of any encounter that advisors and advisees have, for the benefit of learning. Group process will also likely enhance the effectiveness of Milestones and EPAs as part of an assessment system, and faculty will need training in effective group process (see Chapter 16).

Overview of Assessment Methods

Traditional Measures

(See Chapters 2 and 7.)

Traditional measures will continue to play an important role in the assessment of clinical proficiency. Specifically, written methods such as MCQs and standardized patients will be foundational components of assessment programs for the near future, especially in undergraduate medical education. All of these methods can be improved and work on each must continue.

Methods Based on Observation

(See Chapters 4–6, 8, and 9.)

Assessment methods based on the observation of routine encounters in the clinical setting offer a rich and feasible target for assessment. Continued refinement of the methods themselves is needed, as is faculty development, which is a key to their successful use. Furthermore, the opportunity for educational feedback and coaching as part of these methods is probably as important as their assessment potential.

Simulation

(See Chapters 6, 7, and 13.)

Improvements in technology have spurred the development of a series of simulators that re-create reality with high fidelity, but even lower-tech simulations can be very valuable. The use of simulation in assessment is growing, but much of the technology remains expensive and several developments are needed before their widespread adoption and use. Researchers will need to continue to focus on identifying appropriate scoring methods, optimizing the generalizability of scores, and ensuring their relevance to performance in practice.[115] Recent research of mastery-based simulation in specific skills such as central venous lines and other bedside procedures has clearly shown translation of skills acquired at a mastery-defined level in a simulation to the patient bedside. These methods offer the ability to test under a variety of conditions without concern for harm to patients and they improve care at the bedside. Evidence is growing that mastery-based approaches combined with simulation-based deliberate practice can translate into improve patient care and outcomes.[116–118] Educators will confront difficult decisions requiring them to balance the cost, variable fidelity of individual simulation methods, and potential risks to patients (and trainees) in making decisions regarding how best to assess procedural skills.[119]

Workplace-Based Assessment

(See Chapters 3–5, 8–12, 16, and 17.)

The assessment of physicians' performance at work (mostly the "does" level of Miller's pyramid) is the area of assessment undergoing the most change and development. While learners may try to "perform" when under direct observation ("show how"), most learners acclimate quickly, and even if what the faculty observe is "best behavior" there is still much utility in the assessment and ensuring that the patient receives safe, effective, patient-centered care. The day-to-day performance of physicians is being used increasingly in the settings of continuous quality improvement and physician accountability. Assessment in this context is a matter of identifying the basis for the judgments (e.g., outcomes, process of care), deciding how the data will be gathered, and avoiding threats to validity and reliability (e.g., patient mix, patient complexity, attribution, and numbers of patients).[120] The patient is also playing a much greater role in workplace-based assessment, predominantly through patient experience surveys.[121] In addition, patient-reported outcome measures (PROMs) are being increasingly used by health systems to judge functional outcomes for patients (see Chapter 11). While substantial research continues around quality and safety measures, patient experience surveys, and PROMs, much work remains to be done as noted earlier in this chapter. However, given this is ultimately what patients and the public care most about, educational programs need to embrace workplace-based assessments as part of an overall assessment program.

Emerging Directions in Assessment

Implementation of competency-based medical education models has been very challenging for many programs across the educational continuum.[37] One reason has been the difficulty in translating the language and concepts of competencies into educational practices and assessments. As a result, two new approaches, Competency milestones and Entrustable Professional Activities (EPAs), are being used in various health professions educational programs around the world. Both approaches continue to evolve as mechanisms to potentially facilitate more effective implementation of outcomes-based education using competency frameworks. While both of these newer approaches are grounded in robust educational theory, it is important for the reader to recognize that we are still in the early days of determining the utility, including validity, and impact of both Milestones and EPAs on educational and clinical outcomes. While early research is encouraging, much work remains to be done. However, given both competency milestones and EPAs are now part of multiple national systems of assessment across the globe, we provide some background in this chapter to help guide the reader in evaluating and exploring these concepts in their own assessment program.

Competency Milestones

The ACGME competency framework was inspired by the five "Dreyfus stages of development of skill," including Novice, Advanced Beginner, Competent, Proficient, and Expert, first described in 1986.[24] Competency milestones were adopted to promote shared mental models of the competencies, support the developmental assessment of learners in the workplace, and facilitate curricular change.[65,66] They are narrative, behavioral descriptions aligned with the five developmental steps to assist faculty in the assessment of medical trainees using a logical trajectory of professional development within competencies and subcompetencies. Developed as narrative benchmarks for effective assessment, ACGME Milestones were written for all US postgraduate medical disciplines and first published in the *Journal of Graduate Medical Education* in March 2013 and March 2014.[122] All specialties and subspecialties have now created "Milestones 2.0" based on qualitative and quantitative research on the experience with Milestones 1.0. Specialty Milestones are the framework programs used for semiannual review by clinical competency committees on resident progress. Fig. 1.7 shows, as an example, one of the 21 Milestone sets of the pediatric competencies.[123] Early research using US national data for a number of specialties has now demonstrated multiple elements of validity, including correlations with early career outcomes of graduates.[124–131] Milestones have also been reported to be helpful for earlier identification of residents in difficulty, better feedback to residents and fellows, and development of better assessment approaches and as a useful framework for faculty development.[130,65]

In the 2015 edition of CanMEDS, Milestones are also introduced and defined as "descriptions of the abilities expected of a trainee or physician at a defined stage of professional development" of each of the "enabling competencies" under the seven CanMEDS competency roles, to guide learners and educators in determining whether learners are "on track."[106]

Entrustable Professional Activities

The concept of EPAs was introduced in 2005.[92] Since an article about EPAs was published in *Academic Medicine* in 2007,[132,133] the concept has attracted substantial attention among postgraduate programs in the United States, Canada, and other countries. For example, EPAs are a core element of the RCPSC's Competence By Design initiative.[134,135] In the United States, the American Boards of Surgery and Pediatrics are implementing end-of-training EPAs as the mechanism program directors will use to attest to eligibility for certification. Finally, the Ministry of Health in Singapore is instituting EPAs for determination of readiness for practice. EPAs have also been used by several US and all Canadian medical schools as a basis for judging readiness for entry into residency.[136,137]

An *EPA* is a unit of professional practice that can be fully entrusted to a trainee as soon as they have demonstrated the necessary competence to execute this activity unsupervised. In contrast with competencies, EPAs are not a quality of a trainee, but a part of the work that must be done. Fig. 1.7 shows a typical competency domain (patient safety) with its Milestones, reflecting specific competencies such as *awareness* of patient safety issues and causes, *ability to communicate* with patients and families, and *ability* to initiate improvement projects. EPAs, in contrast, are concrete tasks that require that learners (and for that matter, professionals) possess such competencies, usually several, in an integrated and interdependent fashion, before they are allowed to perform the task on their own. In this example, a learner would be asked to be the one to disclose a medical error to a patient and their family (a task that could be an EPA) only if the learner's supervisors have become convinced that the learner is truly ready to do this unsupervised. This may be an *ad hoc entrustment decision* if it happens the first time, or a *summative entrustment decision* that qualifies the learner to act unsupervised from then on, requiring extensive and careful prior assessment and a decision of a competency committee. We will come back to this terminology. More specifically defined, EPAs are part of essential professional work in a given context. They (1) require that trainees possess adequate knowledge, skills, and attitudes in the pertinent competencies, and are generally acquired through training; (2) must lead to recognized output of professional labor; (3) should usually be confined to qualified personnel; (4) should be independently executable; (5) should be

Systems-Based Practice 1: Patient Safety and Quality Improvement				
Level 1	Level 2	Level 3	Level 4	Level 5
Demonstrates knowledge of common patient safety events	Identifies system factors that lead to patient safety events	Contributes to the analysis of patient safety events (simulated or actual)	Conducts analysis of patient safety events and offers error prevention strategies (simulated or actual)	Leads teams and processes to modify systems to prevent patient safety events
Demonstrates knowledge of how to report patient safety events	Reports patient safety events through institutional reporting systems (actual or simulated)	Participates in disclosure of patient safety events to patients and families (simulated or actual)	Discloses patient safety events to patients and families (simulated or actual)	Models the disclosure of patient safety events
Demonstrates knowledge of basic quality improvement methodologies and metrics	Describes local quality improvement initiatives (e.g., community vaccination rate, infection rate, smoking cessation)	Contributes to local quality improvement initiatives	Demonstrates the skills required to identify, develop, implement. and analyze a quality improvement project	Creates, implements, and assesses sustainable quality improvement initiatives at the institutional or community level

Comments:

Not Yet Complete Level 1

• **Fig. 1.7** Example of a Milestone for the US competency of Systems-based Practice.

executable within a time frame; (6) should be observable and measurable in their process and their outcome, leading to a conclusion ("done well" or "not done well"); and (7) should reflect one or more of the competencies to be acquired (see Appendix 1.1).[133]

Much of the work in healthcare can be captured by tasks or responsibilities that must be entrusted to individuals. EPAs require a practitioner to possess and integrate multiple competencies simultaneously from several domains, such as content expertise, skills in collaboration, communication, management, et cetera. Conversely, each competency domain is relevant to many different activities. Combining competencies (or competency domains) and EPAs in a matrix reveals which competencies a trainee must achieve before being trusted to perform an EPA.[133] The two-dimensional matrix in Fig. 1.8 provides specifications that are helpful for assessment and feedback, for individual development, and to ground entrustment decisions. This makes assessment based on EPAs a holistic or synthetic approach, rather than the analytic wish to evaluate competencies analyzed in great detail as stand-alone qualities of learners.[138] EPAs are not an alternative to competencies; they constitute a different dimension, with the purpose of grounding competencies in clinical practice.

EPAs have now been identified for most graduate medical education programs in multiple jurisdictions across the globe.[139–145] An example of an EPA is conducting an uncomplicated delivery. This activity, performed by family physicians and obstetrics-gynecology specialists, needs to be entrusted to a trainee at some point in their training, as the trainee eventually will need to conduct it without supervision. It requires specific knowledge, skills, and behaviors; proficiency is acquired through training; and it is directly observable and involves specific competencies. As this activity reflects the CanMEDS roles of medical expert, communicator, and collaborator, it exemplifies how EPAs integrate competencies. Other examples of EPAs are providing preoperative assessment, managing care of patients with acute common diseases across multiple care settings, providing palliative care, managing common infections in nonimmunosuppressed and immune-compromised populations, conducting a family education session about schizophrenia, conducting a risk assessment, serving as the primary admitting pediatrician for previously well children suffering from common acute problems, pharmacological management of an anxiety disorder, providing end-of-life care for older adults, and office-based counseling in developmental and behavioral paediatrics. A comprehensive set of EPAs should cover the core of a profession. Each EPA should be described well and include, next to an informative title, specification and limitations; an indication of risks when not performed well; a list of required competencies; elaboration of required experience, knowledge, and skills; suggestions for assessment; and an expiration date after the EPA has last been done[136,146] (see Appendix 1.1).

	EPA1	EPA2	EPA3	EPA4	EPA5	EPA6
Competency 1	•		•	•	•	
Competency 2		•	•	•		
Competency 3		•	•	•		•
Competency 4	•	•				
Competency 5	•	•	•		•	•
Competency 6			•			
Competency 7		•	•			•

• **Fig. 1.8** Overview of EPAs: competencies matrix.

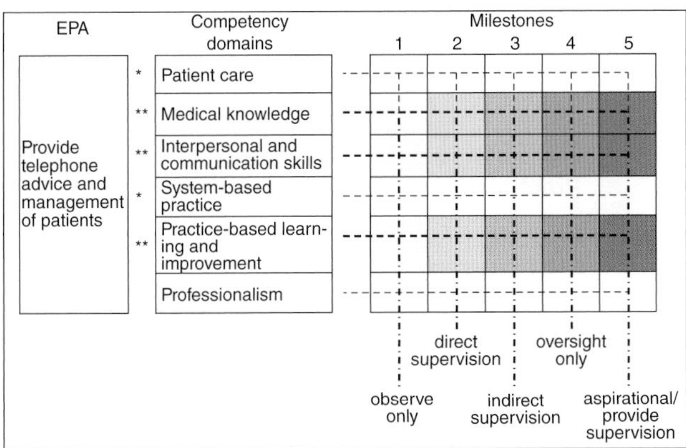

• **Fig. 1.9** Using Milestones to determine an appropriate level of supervision for an EPA.

Linked to the EPA construct is the purpose of *entrustment decision-making*. This process serves to acknowledge ability, to provide permission to act with limited supervision, and to enable duties in healthcare practice. True competency-based medical education grants certification as soon as competence is adequately demonstrated, irrespective of the time in training, and this requires a personalized and flexible approach to training programs. EPAs allow for making entrustment decisions for separate units of professional practice, resulting in more gradual, legitimate participation in professional communities of practice[147] rather than a full license to practice on the last day of training. Certification for EPAs is not a dichotomous process. As trust increases, the level of supervision can decrease. A model of five levels of supervision, entrustment, and permission has been proposed for postgraduate training and is shown in Fig. 1.9.[148]

Combining Competency Milestones and EPAs

While the implementation of competency milestones and EPAs, on top of using a competency framework, may feel to critics as another burden for programs and individual teachers, the competency milestones and EPAs are complementary. Eric Warm, program director of the University of Cincinnati Internal Medicine residency training, converted his assessments to entrustment scales and cross-walked the five Milestone developmental levels of competencies with the five supervision levels of EPAs (Table 1.5). Faced with the need to regularly report on Milestones for all residents, he asks clinicians to estimate trainees' readiness for direct supervision, indirect supervision, or unsupervised practice. This serves efficiency and conceptual elegance and allows faculty to use a more construct-aligned entrustment ratings scale (see Chapter 4). To take this approach one step further, the Dreyfus stage model of development, the broadly used RIME model (Reporter-Interpreter-Manager-Educator;[149] see Chapter 4), the competency milestones approach,[107] and levels of supervision can all be aligned as shown in Table 1.6. The model can be extended with more detailed representations of behavior

TABLE 1.5 Five levels of Supervision and Permission

1. Be present and observe, but not permitted to perform the EPA
2. Permitted to act under direct, proactive supervision, present in the room
3. Permitted to act under indirect, reactive supervision, readily available to enter the room
4. Permitted to act without qualified supervision in the vicinity; with distant supervision or clinical oversight; basically acting unsupervised
5. Permitted to supervise junior trainees regarding the EPA

and supervision,[150] but the core idea is that of alignment of frameworks. Moving from Milestone or supervision level 3 to 4 can be viewed as passing the threshold that allows for clinical oversight only or unsupervised practice at the end of training. It does not qualify a trainee to stop developing, as the journey to expertise and mastery must continue (Fig. 1.6), but would allow for a formal recognition of ability, permission, and duty to enact the EPA, sometimes called a STAR (statement of awarded responsibility) or a summative entrustment decision (discussed later in the chapter). As with many conceptual models, they are useful but have limitations. Nevertheless, Table 1.6 connects several developmental approaches together to help see the forest for the trees.

Given this alignment, an example may be given. Suppose a pediatric residency program has an EPA called "Provide telephone advice and management of patient" (taken from Jones et al.[150–152]). In the EPAs-Competencies Matrix, it has been determined that the most important domains of competence, from an assessment perspective, are Medical Knowledge, Interpersonal and Communication Skills, and Practice-based Learning and Improvement. Let us assume that for each of these domains Milestones have been described. A trainee must be assessed to determine whether indirect supervision—that is, not with a supervisor in the room or on the telephone or on a virtual visit—is justified. If the trainee meets the expected behavior at Milestone level 3 in all three domains, that decision seems justified. If the trainee does not yet show the behavior or skill expected at level 3 in either one of the competencies, additional close supervision will be necessary.

It is also important to note, however, that in reality all the general competencies are needed for effective provision of telemedicine visits, and this realization should be part of any curriculum for telemedicine. In the terminology of the RIME model, the learner would be evaluated as an adequate interpreter and beginning manager (see Chapter 4). Fig. 1.9 shows this relationship. Carraccio and colleagues performed a crosswalk of the competency milestones with the pediatric EPAs (see Appendix 1.2). Here you can see how the narrative descriptors of the competency milestones can be combined down to a competency milestone level to create a brief vignette, or story, of what the learner would actually be about to do at that level of development and entrustment.

TABLE 1.6 Alignment of Various Models of Development

Milestone Level	Dreyfus Model Stages	Learner Behavior	RIME Stages	Transition to Practitioner	Appropriate Level of Supervision and Permission
1	Novice	Doing what is told, rule driven	Reporter	Introduction to clinical practice	Observation, no enactment
2	Advanced beginner	Comprehension	Reporter/ interpreter	Guided clinical practice	Act under direct, proactive supervision
3	Competent	Application to common practice	Interpreter/ manager	Early independence	Act under indirect, reactive supervision
4	Proficient	Application to uncommon practice	Manager/educator	Full unsupervised practice	Clinical oversight
5	Expert	Experienced clinician	Educator	Aspirational growth after graduation	Provide supervision to others

RIME, Reporter-Interpreter-Manager-Educator.

The model can also be used in reverse order. Clinical educators may start with a holistic assessment that a trainee is ready for indirect supervision, based on their experience in various settings. Performing a quick check of the important competency domains may confirm this, and the conclusion may be drawn that the trainee meets Milestone level 3 of the relevant competencies. Both procedural and nonprocedural specialties have now reported success in organizing regular assessments of postgraduate trainees (e.g., residents, fellows, etc.) by scoring on an entrustment-supervision scale, assuming alignment with Milestones scales.[73,153,154]

EPAs – Competencies – Skills

While EPAs are units of work and competencies are descriptors of personal qualities and abilities, in common language educators tend to call "physical examination" a competency. Strictly speaking, the competency is not the physical examination itself; the *ability to perform a physical examination* is the skill and is a feature of the learner or professional. And it would be correct to say that physical examination skill, on a more detailed level, requires manual skills, visual skills, auditory skills, and even time management and communication skills. If a learner possesses these skills, or competencies, the learner may be granted the trust to do the physical examination without supervision. Simply put, health professionals require an integrated set of abilities (i.e., competencies) to effectively execute the clinical activity (i.e., EPA).[155]

EPAs Across the Continuum and Nested EPAs

Activities can be small or large. There is no easy answer to what is the "right" breadth of EPAs and consequently to the right number of EPAs. If the question is "What is the scope of responsibility that is covered when an EPA is entrusted to a trainee for indirect supervision?" then clearly big differences can arise depending on the stage of training of the trainee in question. The first EPA that may be entrusted to a junior medical student could be "Measuring blood pressure." If we consider this a unit of professional practice or activity that one can trust a trainee to complete without being checked by a supervisor, then it is a true EPA.

But clearly, at a later stage this responsibility is part of a full standard physical examination that is a more logical activity for entrustment for advanced medical students. The full standard physical examination, in turn, can be included in a broader EPA of a standard outpatient consultation that also includes the history. In technical terminology, smaller EPAs are nested within larger EPAs.

Among the Utrecht University undergraduate EPAs is the clinical consultation, and it is to be entrusted to any medical school graduate before graduation for indirect supervision. This is a relatively broad EPA, as it requires neurological, ENT, gynecological, psychiatric, and other history and physical examination skills. In the Utrecht curriculum, students are to be entrusted with a focused "neurological clinical consultation" at an earlier stage, and likewise for other specialities during a dedicated clerkship. Only in the final year do all these smaller EPAs become *nested* within a broader EPA, leading to full trust in the broad EPA of the clinical consultation and signed off separately in a subinternship for indirect supervision (Fig. 1.10).[156]

For EPA-based evaluation, it is therefore adequate to design EPAs for a particular course within the educational continuum (e.g., EPAs for undergraduate education, to be mastered before entering residency),[157] EPAs for the end of training in general surgery,[158] or EPAs for a fellowship.[159–161] This does not mean that the EPAs are only mastered at the end of that training period. Indeed, key to competency-based

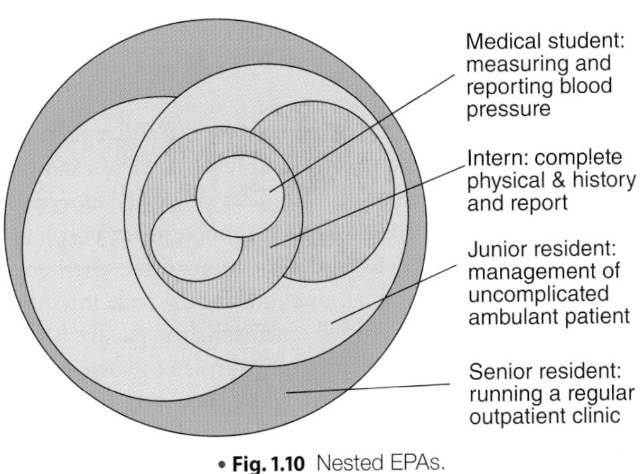

• **Fig. 1.10** Nested EPAs.

training is that EPAs may be mastered and awarded with a decrease in supervision and increase in autonomy as soon as the trainee demonstrates the required competence.

Entrustment Decision-Making as an Assessment Approach

Evaluating trainees with a focus on EPAs has the potential benefit that it aligns with the daily practice of clinician thinking. Much of it naturally focuses on whether clinical activities are carried out well, both their own activities in the care of patients and those care activities of others. Rewarding success in (1) diagnostic reasoning and therapeutic actions and (2) patient satisfaction is an important driver to monitor competence and quality of care.[162,163] From this, a series of recommendation can be derived. *Consider first focusing on EPA execution, then looking at competencies.*

When using EPAs, the primary focus of the learner assessment is whether a job is being done well enough (competently per Dreyfus) that direct supervision is no longer required. In many cases, there is little need to make detailed evaluations of all the competencies involved, but faculty using an EPA-based assessment must possess an up-to-date, evidence-based mental model of the clinical task. Failure to fully incorporate and understand *all* the key competencies needed places both patient and learner at risk: the patient may receive suboptimal care and the learner may receive suboptimal feedback and coaching as well as inappropriate supervision moving forward. For learners who do not perform optimally, systematically breaking down the deficiencies in specific competency domains can support a more effective analysis ("diagnosis" of the learning difficulties) and facilitate more effective remediation (see Chapter 17). In addition, understanding which competencies are most important for the EPA can support better feedback and coaching by providing specific language about what was done well and what areas for improvement might exist. Simply telling the learner they "did well" on the EPA is not helpful feedback (see Chapter 14). The EPAs-Competencies Matrix and Milestone descriptions may help identify weaknesses and coach learners to improve.

Distinguish Three Benchmarks or Frames of Reference for Assessment

Educators often struggle in assessing learners due to lack of clear standards, benchmarks, or appropriate frames of reference (see Chapters 3, 4, and 5). Often, educators struggle using criterion-referenced judgments (e.g., appropriate and effective care of the patient with multiple chronic conditions) versus normative-referenced judgments (e.g., is Robert as good as Jane at this stage of training?). Educators also often struggle in determining whether a learner should score higher because they made great progress after a previous observation, because they exerted extraordinary effort, or because they perform as well as the educator does (i.e., normative and self as frame of reference). This leads to three types of benchmarks being used for assessment and feedback provision: (1) comparison with evidence and standards of professional practice (expected performance based on best available evidence); (2) comparison with other trainees or self (how well do others do at similar stages of training or compared to the faculty's own standard of practice); and (3) comparison with past development (how much has the trainee progressed since the last assessment). Naturally, in competency-based training, evidence-based standards for adequate practice must form the benchmark for certification, which is a *criterion-referenced* measure. However, learners are usually evaluated with a mix of benchmarks because criterion referencing is not easy. In any case, assessors should at least be clear and transparent in expressing how the benchmarks are defined based on the context and purpose of assessment, and those being assessed should be aware of expectations for their performance.

Frame the Assessment as a Developmental Entrustment Decision

Trusting a learner to work unsupervised, if even occasionally, requires a broader view than simply measuring a skill in an examination. The question in the back of one's head is: Would I trust this trainee to execute this EPA tomorrow morning with a critical patient (or maybe a relative of mine) without a supervising professional present? This question about trust includes other features of the trainee besides their knowledge and skill, such as their discernment of their own limitations, willing to ask for help if needed, conscientiousness in carrying out clinical tasks, and truthfulness in communications to staff. Milestones 2.0 now includes a specific subcompetency of reflective practice.[66,123] While leniency bias is a known and common problem of workplace-based assessments (WBAs),[164–166] cautious entrustment decisions might lead to the opposite; that is, a stringency bias ("I will never fully trust a learner as long as they are in training"). But this clearly leads to graduates who are ill prepared for autonomous practice.[60] Recent studies in surgery also show that an increase in close supervision and a corresponding decrease in autonomy of trainees in the past decades has not particularly increased patient safety.[166–168]

On the contrary, entrustment with unsupervised practice for an EPA—that is, with only distant supervision as long as learners are in training—provides them with necessary autonomy experience before they leave training. Fig. 1.11 shows how, when the threshold of trust has passed and a summative decision of entrustment with unsupervised practice has been made, a learner can rise to higher levels of proficiency. "Competent" characterizes this threshold.

Entrustment Decisions Require the Acceptance of Risks

Core in the definition of trust is the "acceptance of risk and vulnerability, based on a positive expectation of the intentions and behavior of the other."[169–172] Ten Cate and colleagues further added that "trust involves the confident expectation that a person (i.e., the trainee) can be relied on to honor implied or established commitments to an individual and to protect the individual's (i.e., faculty *and* patient) interest. It renders the individual (faculty and patient) vulnerable to the extent (s)he cannot oversee or control the actions of the other, on whose expertise or integrity (s)he may depend." Trust in clinical trainees is an area of investigation that is sure to get more attention in the coming years, including the role of intuition, gut feelings, and heuristics in making entrustment decisions.[170,171] As noted earlier, the context needs to be considered when making entrustment decision. Risks may vary and range from breaching confidentiality and hurting and confusing the patient, to neglecting critical information, overestimating ability, inadequately testing diagnostics, and applying the wrong therapies and recommendations. These must all be avoided, but adverse events also depend on contextual variables and can never be fully excluded, and trainees must learn how to act when they arise.

Align Scales With Supervision Recommendation

Alignment of the constructs of clinical practice and assessment of learners is likely to lead to enhanced reliability. For example, Weller et al. used scales using the descriptors of "supervisor required in the theater suite – supervisor required in hospital – supervisor not required" for the evaluation of anesthesiology residents;[172] and George et al. used a (Zwisch) scale for surgical residents with "show and tell – active help – passive help – supervision only" signifying the required role of the supervisor during surgery.[173] Both authors report increased reliabilities when using these scales compared to a traditional one. The scale in Fig. 1.11 and Table 1.4 is a more general representation of this idea, but more detail may be added, depending on the stage of training or the setting or specialty (see Chapter 4).

Distinguish Ad Hoc Entrustment Decisions From Summative Entrustment Decisions

Entrustment decisions may be distinguished as *ad hoc entrustment decisions*, which happen every day in the moment, are usually taken by individual supervisors, and pertain to immediate permission for the trainee to act; or *summative entrustment decisions*, which are grounded in more systematic observation and lead to permission to act under a specified level of supervision, comparable to the driver's license that formalizes permission to drive unsupervised from that point onward, but may need to be reviewed at some later point in time. Ad hoc entrustment decisions per se do not have long-term consequences but may stimulate development and evaluation of trainee readiness for summative decisions. Conversely, a summative entrustment decision is a general statement that must be documented, awards a higher level of responsibility for future actions, and should be recognizable by third parties. Summative entrustment decisions should involve systematic processes and

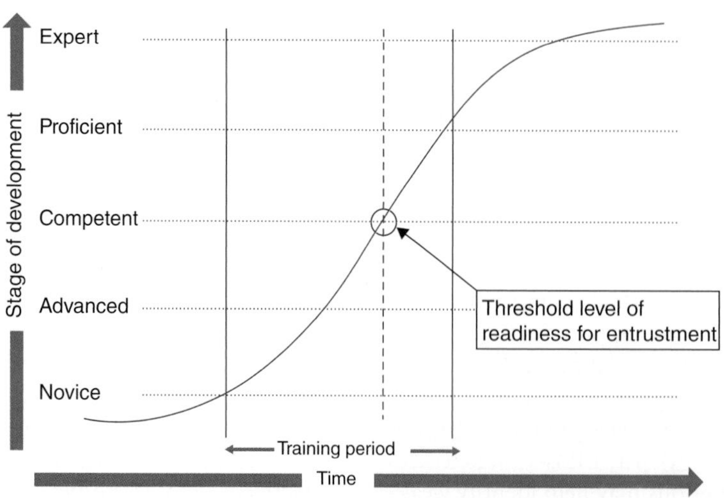

• **Fig. 1.11** Entrustment thresholds and stages of professional development.

practices (see Chapter 3). Both are important in EPA-based curricula. The ad hoc decision experiences of a supervisor may be documented in the trainee's portfolio (Was this a justified decision? If not, why not? Would the observer recommend a summative entrustment decision soon?).

Summative decisions may be informed by multiple ad hoc decisions supplemented with information gathered through other channels (multisource feedback, knowledge assessment, skills assessment). Summative entrustment decisions should be multisource decisions based on the summation of smaller elements of information. Summative entrustment decisions for level 4 over supervision may look like certifications, STARS, or digital badges that may be accessible for collaborators such as ward nurses or the outside world.[174] As these should signify current competence, a summative entrustment decision for level 4 of an EPA should potentially be retracted if the individual does not maintain the practice of the EPA, either within the training or after training. Renewed supervision should then be required as long as needed.

Finally, another form of an entrustment decision is the *scheduled or planned* entrustment. For example, many postgraduate medical education programs use night float systems where learners cover patient services overnight, often without direct faculty supervision (e.g., on-site supervision) being readily available. These night float rotations are usually baked into the learners' rotational schedule regardless of whether they are truly ready for this responsibility. This "level 4" entrustment decision is sometimes called "level 4a," meaning that a supervisor is on call and accessible through telephone if needed. As another example, changes in supervision are often based on the learner's year of postgraduate training regardless of whether the learner is truly ready. These types of entrustment decisions should ideally be based on robust assessment data and treated more as a summative type of assessment. In fact, entrustment decisions based on merely the time period in training contradicts the philosophy of competency-based education.

TABLE 1.7 Sources of Information to Support Summative Entrustment Decisions

Sources	Examples
1. Knowledge testing	Written or e-tests, case-based discussions, assessment of clinical reasoning in vivo, case-based discussions, chart-stimulated recall
2. Short practice observations	Mini-CEX, DOPS, handoffs, video, and other (119)
3. Long practice observations	Multisource feedback, review of shifts and rotations, daily shift cards
4. Simulation tests	OSCE, OSATS,[a] standardized patient tests
5. Work product evaluation	EHR entries, presentations, papers, reports, event analysis, review of quality and safety performance measures

[a]Can also be used as a direct observation tool.

CEX, Clinical evaluation exercise; *DOPS*, direct observation of procedural skills; *EHR*, electronic health record; *OSATS*, objective structured assessment of technical skill; *OSCE*, objective structured clinical examination.

Use Multiple Sources of Information to Support Entrustment Decisions

While ad hoc decisions to trust a trainee are usually taken by individuals and are very much situated in time and place, summative and planned entrustment decisions must be grounded in multiple identifiable sources of information (Table 1.7). The sources of information to inform entrustment decisions are not necessarily different for other WBAs. Chapter 3 provides guidance on programmatic assessment.

Entrustment Is an Approach to Assessment Requiring a Prospective Outlook

In most of education, the primary question is: Has the student met all the objectives and requirements that a school or program has set? In health professions education, an important additional question is: Is the learner ready to be licensed for practice? This essentially is an *entrustment* question. It is a question that forces one to stop and think of future situations, and not just look back at what a learner has done. Schools, programs, and clinical educators should, for instance, not graduate health professionals if they would not trust them to attend to their own family members.[175] Making entrustment decisions for smaller units of practice than a license means both weighing everything that is important for autonomous practice and a deliberate willingness to accept the risks that adverse events could happen. The breadth of healthcare with which graduates are entrusted may be more than supervisors have been able to observe, and could even be more than the graduate has encountered in training. This requires a shift in traditional thinking, from retrospective to prospective, and arguably even extending the "does" level of Miller's pyramid. Ready to be trusted with unfamiliar situations has led to suggest a fifth level of the pyramid[176] (see Fig. 1.12).

The evaluation of learners at this level includes features that many clinicians have acknowledged as important when trusting them with critical care tasks. Ten Cate and Chen reviewed several studies with this focus and concluded that, besides specific capability (knowledge and skill, experience, adaptive expertise), additional areas to assess include reliability (conscientious, predictable, accountable, responsible), integrity (truthful, good intentions, patient centered), humility (observing limits, willing to ask for help, receptive to feedback), and agency (self-confident; proactive toward work, team, safety, and development). To remember this with an acronym, they suggested thinking, prospectively, of A RICH entrustment decision (A = Agency; R = Reliability; I = Integrity; C = Capability; H = Humility).[177]

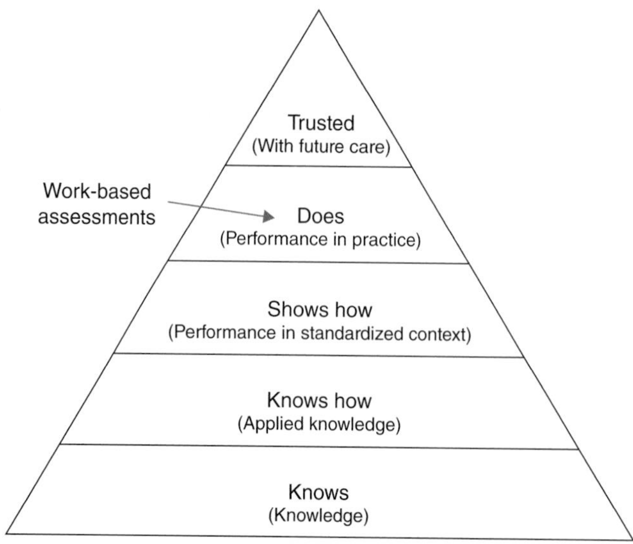

A new fifth level ("trusted") reflects the process for reaching the decision to award a learner an attestation of the completion of training, leading to a medical license or specialty registration or certification, that provides permission to act unsupervised and makes the grantors cognizant of the inherent risks.

• **Fig. 1.12** "Extended" Miller's pyramid with entrustment.

Systems of Assessment

(See Chapters 3 and 18.)

As the section on Competency milestones and EPAs clearly highlights, regardless of whether your program decides to utilize these developmental concepts, all medical education programs need a robust assessment *program* (i.e., programmatic assessment) using a multifaceted array of assessment methods embedded in an effective educational system. The movement toward outcomes-based education and assessment presents many challenges for medical educators. Educational leaders will need to integrate traditional and new assessment methods into their educational programs to ensure that individual trainees meet important educational and professional goals and to inform continued quality improvement of their programs. Assessment approaches must be clearly aligned with educational objectives and congruent with teaching and learning methods as highlighted by the core components framework. Assessment should be closely intertwined with instructional activities to optimize efficient use of resources and to consolidate learning. The assessment system will need to include multiple methods to capture each general competency and ideally to provide for the assessment of different aspects of each competency by different methods. Program and clerkship directors will need to prepare the assessors, through implementation of robust faculty development programs, and inform and engage trainees for the assessment system to succeed.

Beyond the performance of individual trainees, the assessment system will need to support the continuous collection and analysis of aggregate data to provide feedback regarding the quality of the educational program. This includes information from more traditional assessment methods, such as program-level subscores on MCQ examinations or aggregate case–level data from clinical skills examinations, as well as composite scores or ratings from newer methods such as multisource feedback, computer simulation–based exercises, and a robust combination of work-based assessments. It also involves collection and analysis of clinical information, such as adherence with evidence-based healthcare processes or patient health outcomes that can provide the impetus for curricular change or feedback on the quality of educational interventions. Establishing such a connection, at least at the institutional level, will facilitate conduct of needed research to elucidate the relationships between educational activities and healthcare practices and outcomes. Competency milestones and EPAs were created to facilitate this integration and connection.

In addition to compiling aggregate data within programs to inform quality improvement initiatives, assessment systems will need to enable information gathering regarding the performance of program graduates. As with concurrent measures, educational leaders will need to access and incorporate into their assessment systems information about the performance of the program's graduates to guide quality improvement efforts (see Chapter 18). Some information, such as licensure actions, in-training or board certification examination scores, or program director ratings, is available in some jurisdictions. For example, medical schools in the United States can access their graduates' first-year competency milestones data as one measure. Obtaining other sources of information, such as specific performance measures or clinical data, to provide additional feedback regarding educational program quality will require more effort. The formation of collaborative projects and networks linking professional and clinical outcomes across the spectrum of education and practice will facilitate understanding and incorporation of information critical to the continuous quality improvement of educational programs.

Conclusion

Public and professional pressure to increase accountability and quality improvement in clinical care has resulted in important changes in medical education and assessment. Delineation of essential physician competencies and widespread implementation of outcomes-based medical education, to varying degrees, has led to a critical review of the quality and methods used in the assessment of competence and performance. Advances in technology and psychometrics have supported continued refinement of traditional assessment modalities and the development of new approaches. Educational leaders now face challenges in developing and integrating assessment programs embedded within an effective system and overall educational program. The core components framework is a good place for programs to start examining their own "outcomeness"[42] (see Appendix 1.3 for worksheet). They must understand the psychometric and utility properties of various assessment tools, consider their relevance to trainee level as well as to instructional methods and educational objectives, and then balance these factors against program culture and resource availability in deciding what methods to use in their assessment system. Educators need to understand the evolving science of workplace-based assessment such as quality and safety measures, patient experience surveys, and PROMs. The use of qualitative assessments and judgment techniques, combined with group process, is also growing in importance for assessment programs. Finally, health professions educators must understand and use systems thinking (see Chapters 3 and 18). The chapters that follow are intended to help guide educational leaders in designing their assessment programs and systems to support evaluation of individual trainees and continuous quality improvement of their educational programs for the benefit of the trainee, program, and most importantly, patients and the public.

Acknowledgments

The authors wish to sincerely thank Dr. John Norcini for donating content from the first edition to this chapter. Finally, we wish to thank Dr. Rich Hawkins, one of the book's editors of the first and second editions. We are very appreciative of their graciousness and contributions to previous versions of this chapter and their contributions to medical education.

References

1. Hill L, Ndugga N, Artiga S. Key data on health and health care by race and ethnicity. Kaiser Family Foundation. Accessed March 19, 2023. at Key Data on Health and Health Care by Race and Ethnicity | KFF. https://www.who.int/data/stories/global-excess-deaths-associated-with-covid-19-january-2020-december-2021.
2. World Health Organization. Global excess deaths associated with COVID-19, January 2020 to December 2021. Accessed March 19, 2023. at Global excess deaths associated with COVID-19, January 2020 – December 2021 (Global excess deaths associated with COVID-19, January 2020 - December 2021 (who.int)). https://www.economist.com/graphic-detail/coronavirus-excess-deaths-estimates.
3. The Economist. The pandemic's true death toll. Accessed March 19, 2023. at The pandemic's true death toll | The Economist. (The pandemic's true death toll (economist.com)). https://www.ihi.org/resources/Pages/Publications/Free-from-Harm-Accelerating-Patient-Safety-Improvement.aspx.
4. Institute of Medicine. *To Err is Human: Building a Safer Health System*. National Academy of Health Sciences; 1999.
5. Institute of Medicine. *Crossing the Quality Chasm*. National Academy Press; 2001.
6. Berwick DM, Nolan TW, Whittington L. The triple aim: care, health cost. *Health Aff (Millwood)*. 2008 May-Jun;27(3):759–769. doi:10.1377/hlthaff.27.3.759.
7. Bodenheimer T, Sinsky C. From triple to quadruple aim: care of the patient requires care of the provider. *Ann Fam Med*. 2014 Nov-Dec;12(6):573–576. doi:10.1370/afm.1713.
8. Nundy S, Cooper LA, Mate KS. The quintuple aim for health care improvement: a new imperative to advance health equity. *JAMA*. 2022 Feb 8;327(6):521–522. doi:10.1001/jama.2021.25181.
9. National Patient Safety Foundation. Free from Harm: Accelerating Patient Safety Improvement Fifteen Years after To Err Is Human. May 28, 2016. Accessed September 30, 2023. Free from Harm: Accelerating Patient Safety Improvement Fifteen Years after To Err Is Human | IHI - Institute for Healthcare Improvement. https://www.commonwealthfund.org/sites/default/files/2020-12/International_Profiles_of_Health_Care_Systems_Dec2020.pdf.
10. Commonwealth Fund. 2020 International Profiles of Health Care Systems. Tikkanen R, Osborn R, Mossialos E, Djordjevic A, Wharton G, eds. Accessed March 19, 2023. at International Profiles of Health Care Systems: Australia, Canada, China, Denmark, England, France, Germany, India, Israel, Italy, Japan, the Netherlands, New Zealand, Norway, Singapore, Sweden, Switzerland, Taiwan, and the United States (commonwealthfund.org). https://www.gmc-uk.org/-/media/documents/good-medical-practice-english-20200128_pdf-51527435.pdf?la=en&hash=DA1263358CCA88F298785FE2BD7610EB4EE9A530.
11. World Health Organization. *World health statistics 2022: monitoring health for the SDGs, sustainable development goals*. Geneva: World Health Organization; 2022 License: CC BY-NC-SA 3.0 IGO. Accessed March 19, 2023, at World health statistics 2022: monitoring health for the SDGs, sustainable development goals (who.int).
12. Frenk J, Chen L, Bhutta ZA, et al. Health professionals for a new century: transforming education to strengthen health systems in an interdependent world. *Lancet*. 2010 Dec 4;376(9756):1923–1958. doi:10.1016/S0140-6736(10)61854-5.
13. Harden RM, Crosby JR, Davis M. An introduction to outcome-based education. *Med Teacher*. 1999;21(1):7–14. doi:10.1080/01421599978951.
14. Harden RM. Outcomes-based education: part 1–an introduction to outcomes-based education. *Med Teach*. 2009;21:7–14.
15. McGaghie WC, Miller GE, Sajid AW, Telder TV, Lipson L. *Competency-based curriculum development in medical education: an introduction*. World Health Organization Geneva; 1978.

16. Cooke M, Irby DM, O'Brien BC. *Educating Physicians. A call for Reform of Medical School and Residency*. Jossey-Bass; 2010.
17. Frank JR, Mungroo R, Ahmad Y, Wang M, De Rossi S, Horsley T. Toward a definition of competency-based education in medicine: a systematic review of published definitions. *Med Teach*. 2010;32(8):631–637. doi:10.3109/0142159X.2010.500898.
18. Frank JR, Snell LS, ten Cate O, et al. Competency-based medical education: theory to practice. *Med Teach*. 2010;32(8):638–645. doi:10.3109/0142159X.2010.501190.
19. Crosson FJ, Leu J, Roemer BM, Ross MN. Gaps in residency training should be addressed to better prepare doctors for a twenty-first-century delivery system. *Health Aff (Millwood)*. 2011 Nov 30;30(11):2412–2418. doi:10.1377/hlthaff.2011.0184.
20. Skochelak SE. A decade of reports calling for change in medical education: what do they say? *Acad Med*. 2010 Sep;85(9 Suppl):S26–S33. doi:10.1097/ACM.0b013e3181f1323f.
21. MedPAC. Graduate medical education financing: focusing on educational priorities. In *Report to the Congress: Aligning Incentives in Medicare*. Washington, DC: MedPAC; June 2010:103–128.
22. Frank JR, Jabbour M, Tugwell P, et al. Skills for the new millennium: report of the societal needs working group, CanMEDS 2000 Project. *Ann R Coll Phys Surg Can*. 1996;29:206–216.
23. Frank JR, ed. *The CanMEDS 2005 physician competency framework. Better standards. Better physicians. Better care*. Ottawa: The Royal College of Physicians and Surgeons of Canada; 2005.
24. Batalden P, Leach D, Swing S, Dreyfus H, Dreyfus S. General competencies and accreditation in graduate medical education. *Health Aff (Millwood)*. 2002 Sep-Oct;21(5):103–111. doi:10.1377/hlthaff.21.5.103.
25. General Medical Council. Good Medical Practice. 2019. Accessed March 19, 2023. Available at: Good medical practice-english (gmc-uk.org). https://www.surgeons.org/News/News/Updated-Surgical-Competence-and-Performance-Guide.
26. Institute of Medicine. *Health Professions Education: A Bridge to Quality*. National Academies Press; 2003.
27. Royal Australasian College of Surgeons. 2020. Accessed March 19, 2023. Surgical Competence and Performance. Available at: Updated Surgical Competence and Performance Guide | RACS (surgeons.org). https://www.pslhub.org/learn/investigations-risk-management-and-legal-issues/investigations-and-complaints/investigation-reports/other-reports-and-enquiries/the-shipman-inquiry-2002-2005-r867/.
28. Ten Cate O. Medical education in the Netherlands. *Med Teach*. 2007 Oct;29(8):752–757. doi:10.1080/01421590701724741.
29. Iobst WF, Sherbino J, ten Cate O, et al. Competency-based medical education in postgraduate medical education. *Med Teach*. 2010;32(8):651–656. doi:10.3109/0142159X.2010.500709.
30. Holmboe ES, Sherbino J, Long DM, Swing SR, Frank JR. The role of assessment in competency-based medical education. *Med Teach*. 2010;32(8):676–682. doi:10.3109/0142159X.2010.500704.
31. Campbell C, Silver I, Sherbino J, ten Cate O, Holmboe ES. Competency-based continuing professional development. *Med Teach*. 2010;32(8):657–662. doi:10.3109/0142159X.2010.500708.
32. Carraccio C, Englander R, Van Melle E, et al., on behalf of the ICBME Collaborators. Advancing competency-based medical education: a charter for clinician-educators. *Acad Med*. 2016 May;91(5):645–649. doi:10.1097/ACM.0000000000001048.
33. Caverzagie KJ, Nousiainen MT, Ferguson PC, et al. Overarching challenges to the implementation of competency-based medical education. *Med Teach*. 2017;39(6):588–593. doi:10.1080/0142159X.2017.1315075.
34. Englander R, Frank JR, Carraccio C, Sherbino J, Ross S, Snell L. Toward a shared language for competency-based medical education. *Med Teach*. 2017;39(6):582–587. doi:10.1080/0142159X.2017.1315066.
35. Frank JR, Snell L, Englander R, Holmboe ES. Implementing competency-based medical education: moving forward. *Med Teach*. 2017;39(6):568–573. doi:10.1080/0142159X.2017.1315069.
36. Harris P, Bhanji F, Topps M, et al. Evolving concepts of assessment in a competency-based world. *Med Teach*. 2017;39(6):603–608. doi:10.1080/0142159X.2017.1315071.
37. Holmboe ES, Sherbino J, Englander R, Snell L, Frank JR. A call to action: the controversy of and rationale for competency-based medical education. *Med Teach*. 2017;39(6):574–581. doi:10.1080/0142159X.2017.1315067.
38. Lockyer J, Carraccio C, Chan MK, et al. Core principles of assessment in competency-based medical education. *Med Teach*. 2017;39(6):609–616. doi:10.1080/0142159X.2017.1315082.
39. Nousiainen MT, Caverzagie KJ, Ferguson PC, Frank JR. Implementing competency-based medical education: what changes in curricular structure and processes are needed? *Med Teach*. 2017;39(6):594–598. doi:10.1080/0142159X.2017.1315077.
40. Donabedian A. *An Introduction to Quality Assurance in Health Care*. Oxford University Press; 2003.
41. Durning SJ, Lubarsky S, Torre D, Dory V, Holmboe E. Considering "nonlinearity" across the continuum in medical education assessment: supporting theory, practice, and future research directions. *J Contin Educ Health Prof*. 2015 Summer;35(3):232–243. doi:10.1002/chp.21298.
42. Van Melle E, Frank JR, Holmboe ES, et al. A core components framework for evaluating implementation of competency-based medical education programs. *Acad Med*. 2019;94(7):1002–1009. doi:10.1097/ACM.0000000000002743.
43. Richardson D, Kinnear B, Hauer KE, et al. Growth mindset in competency-based medical education. *Med Teach*. 2021;43(7):751–757. doi:10.1080/0142159X.2021.1928036.
44. Pusic MV, Boutis K, Hatala R, Cook DA. Learning curves in health professions education. *Acad Med*. 2015;90(8):1034–1042. doi:10.1097/ACM.0000000000000681.
45. Ericsson KA. Acquisition and maintenance of medical expertise: a perspective from the expert-performance approach with deliberate practice. *Acad Med*. 2015;90(11):1471–1486. doi:10.1097/ACM.0000000000000939.
46. McGaghie WC. When I say … mastery learning. *Med Educ*. 2015;49(6):558–559. doi:10.1111/medu.12679.
47. Norman GR. Research in medical education: three decades of progress. *BMJ*. 2002 Jun 29;324(7353):1560–1562. doi:10.1136/bmj.324.7353.1560.
48. Kogan JR, Holmboe ES. Realizing the promise and importance of performance-based assessment. *Teach Learn Med*. 2013;25(Suppl 1):S68–S74. doi:10.1080/10401334.2013.842912.
49. Kogan JR, Hess BJ, Conforti LN, Holmboe ES. What drives faculty ratings of residents' clinical skills? The impact of faculty's own clinical skills. *Acad Med*. 2010 Oct;85(10 Suppl):S25–S28. doi:10.1097/ACM.0b013e3181ed1aa3.
50. Kogan JR, Conforti LN, Iobst WF, Holmboe ES. Reconceptualizing variable rater assessments as both an educational and clinical care problem. *Acad Med*. 2014 May;89(5):721–727. doi:10.1097/ACM.0000000000000221.
51. Wong BM, Goldman J, Goguen JM, et al. Faculty-resident "co-learning": a longitudinal exploration of an inno-

vative model for faculty development in quality improvement. *Acad Med.* 2017 Aug;92(8):1151–1159. doi:10.1097/ACM.0000000000001505.
52. Hirpara DH, Wong BM, Safieddine N. Co-learning curriculum in quality improvement for surgical residents—five-year experience from the University of Toronto. *J Surg Educ.* 2022 Jan-Feb;79(1):46–50. doi:10.1016/j.jsurg.2021.08.001.
53. Wagner R, Weiss KB, Headrick LA, et al. Program Directors Patient Safety and Quality Educators Network: a learning collaborative to improve resident and fellow physician engagement. *J Grad Med Educ.* 2022 Aug;14(4):505–509. doi:10.4300/JGME-D-22-00490.1.
54. Wong BM, Holmboe ES. Transforming academic faculty to better align educational and clinical outcomes. *Acad Med.* 2016 Apr;91(4):473–479. doi:10.1097/ACM.0000000000001035.
55. Holmboe ES, Batalden P. Achieving the desired transformation: thoughts on next steps for outcomes-based medical education. *Acad Med.* 2015 Sep;90(9):1215–1223. doi:10.1097/ACM.0000000000000779.
56. Stewart JB. *Blind Eye: How the Medical Establishment Let a Doctor Get Away with Murder.* Simon and Shuster; 1999.
57. Name of Website. The Final Report of the Shipman Inquiry. 2005. Accessed September 30, 2023. The Shipman Inquiry (2002-2005) - Other reports and inquiries - Patient Safety Learning - the hub (pslhub.org). https://www.acgme.org/milestones/resources/.
58. Reilly BM. Physical examination in the care of medical inpatients: an observational study. *Lancet.* 2003 Oct 4;362(9390):1100–1105. doi:10.1016/S0140-6736(03)14464-9.
59. Jonker G, Ochtman A, Marty AP, Kalkman CJ, Ten Cate O, Hoff RG. Would you trust your loved ones to this trainee? Certification decisions in postgraduate anaesthesia training. *Br J Anaesth.* 2020;125(5):E408–E410. doi:10.1016/j.bja.2020.07.009.
60. Mattar SG, Alseidi AA, Jones DB, et al. General surgery residency inadequately prepares trainees for fellowship: results of a survey of fellowship program directors. *Ann Surg.* 2013 Sep;258(3):440–447. doi:10.1097/SLA.0b013e3182a191ca.
61. Gruppen LD, Ten Cate O, Lingard LA, Teunissen PW, Kogan JR. Enhanced requirements for assessment in a competency-based, time-variable medical education system. *Acad Med.* 2018;93(3 Competency-Based Time-Variable Education in the Health Professions):S17–S21. doi:10.1097/ACM.0000000000002066.
62. Nelson EC, Batalden PB, Godfrey MM. *Quality by Design: A Clinical Microsystems Approach.* Jossey-Bass; 2007.
63. Ogrinc GS, Headrick LA, Barton AJ, et al. *Fundamentals of Health Care Improvement: A Guide to Improving Your Patients' Care.* 4th ed. Joint Commission Resources and Institute for Healthcare Improvement; 2022.
64. Batalden M, Batalden P, Margolis P, et al. Coproduction of healthcare service. *BMJ Qual Saf.* 2016 Jul;25(7):509–517. doi:10.1136/bmjqs-2015-004315.
65. Holmboe ES, Yamazaki K, Edgar L, et al. Reflections on the first 2 years of milestone implementation. *J Grad Med Educ.* 2015 Sep;7(3):506–511. doi:10.4300/JGME-07-03-43.
66. Edgar L, McLean S, Hogan SO, Hamstra S, Holmboe ES. The Milestones Guidebook. Accessed March 19, 2023. Resources (acgme.org). https://www.abim.org/Media/ba2igl11/assessment-2020-final-report.pdf.
67. Bunderson CV, Inouye DK, Olsen JB. The four generations of computerized educational measurement. In: Linn RL, ed. *Educational Measurement.* American Council on Education; 1989.
68. Norcini JJ. Computers in physician licensure and certification: new methods of assessment. *J Educ Computing Res.* 1994;10:161–171.
69. Roediger HL 3rd, Butler AC. The critical role of retrieval practice in long-term retention. *Trends Cogn Sci.* 2011 Jan;15(1):20–27. doi:10.1016/j.tics.2010.09.003.
70. Griswold-Theodorson S, Ponnuru S, Dong C, Szyld D, Reed T, McGaghie WC. Beyond the simulation laboratory: a realist synthesis review of clinical outcomes of simulation-based mastery learning. *Acad Med.* 2015 Nov;90(11):1553–1560. doi:10.1097/ACM.0000000000000938.
71. George BC, Teitelbaum EN, Meyerson SL, et al. Reliability, validity, and feasibility of the Zwisch scale for the assessment of intraoperative performance. *J Surg Educ.* 2014 Nov-Dec;71(6):e90–e96. doi:10.1016/j.jsurg.2014.06.018.
72. Foundation for Excellence in Women's Healthcare. MyTIPReport. Accessed March 19, 2023. https://mytipreport.org/on
73. Bohnen JD, George BC, Williams RGProcedural Learning and Safety Collaborative (PLSC). The feasibility of real-time intraoperative performance assessment with SIMPL (System for Improving and Measuring Procedural Learning): early experience from a multi-institutional trial. *J Surg Educ.* 2016 Nov-Dec;73(6):e118–e130. doi:10.1016/j.jsurg.2016.08.010.
74. Spickard 3rd A, Ridinger H, Wrenn J, et al. Automatic scoring of medical students' clinical notes to monitor learning in the workplace. *Med Teach.* 2014 Jan;36(1):68–72. doi:10.3109/0142159X.2013.849801.
75. Marty AP, Linsenmeyer M, George B, Young JQ, Breckwoldt J, ten Cate O. Mobile technologies to support workplace-based assessment for entrustment decisions: guidelines for programs and educators. AMEE Guide 154. Medical Teacher 2023 Early Online.
76. Hambleton RK, Swaminathan H. *Item Response Theory: Principles and Applications.* Kluwer; 1985.
77. Green BF. Adaptive testing by computer. In: Ekstrom RB, ed. *Principles of Modern Psychological Measurement.* Jossey-Bass; 1983:5–12.
78. American Board of Internal Medicine. A Vision for Certification in Internal Medicine in 2020. September 2015. Accessed September 30, 2023. Assess2020_FinalReport_final.docx (abim.org). https://www.acgme.org/milestones/resources/.
79. Brennan RL. *Generalizability Theory.* Springer-Verlag; 2001.
80. Norcini JJ. Standard setting. In: Dent JA, Harden RM, eds. *A Practical Guide for Medical Teachers.* Elsevier Churchill Livingston; 2005:293–301.
81. Berk RA, ed. *Handbook of Methods for Detecting Test Bias.* Johns Hopkins Press; 1982.
82. Hodges BD, Lingard L. *A Question of Competence. Reconsidering Medical Education in the Twenty-First Century.* Cornell University Press; 2012.
83. Ginsburg S, van der Vleuten CPM, Eva KW. The hidden value of narrative comments for assessment: a quantitative reliability analysis of qualitative data. *Acad Med.* 2017 Nov;92(11):1617–1621. doi:10.1097/ACM.0000000000001669.
84. Hauer KE, Cate OT, Boscardin CK, et al. Ensuring resident competence: a narrative review of the literature on group decision making to inform the work of clinical competency committees. *J Grad Med Educ.* 2016 May;8(2):156–164. doi:10.4300/JGME-D-15-00144.1.
85. Andolsek K, Padmore J, Hauer KE, Ekpenyong A, Edgar L, Holmboe E. Clinical Competency Committees. A Guide

book for Programs. 2020. Accessed March 19, 2023. Resources (acgme.org). https://royalcollege.ca/rcsite/canmeds/canmeds-framework-e#:~:text=CanMEDS%3A%20Better%20standards%2C%20better%20physicians%2C%20better%20care%20CanMEDS,These%20abilities%20are%20grouped%20thematically%20under%20seven%20roles.
86. Gaglione MM, Moores L, Pangaro L, Hemmer PA. Does group discussion of student clerkship performance at an education committee affect an individual committee member's decisions? *Acad Med.* 2005 Oct;80(10 Suppl):S55–S58. doi:10.1097/00001888-200510001-00016.
87. Hauer KE, Edgar L, Hogan SO, Kinnear B, Warm E. The science of effective group process: lessons for clinical competency committees. *J Grad Med Educ.* 2021 Apr;13(2 Suppl):S59–S64. doi:10.4300/JGME-D-20-00827.1.
88. Kinnear B, Warm EJ, Hauer KE. Twelve tips to maximize the value of a clinical competency committee in postgraduate medical education. *Med Teach.* 2018;40(11):1110–1115. doi:10.1080/0142159X.2018.1474191.
89. Battistone MJ, Milne C, Sande MA, Pangaro LN, Hemmer PA, Shomaker TS. The feasibility and acceptability of implementing formal evaluation sessions and using descriptive vocabulary to assess student performance on a clinical clerkship. *Teach Learn Med.* 2002 Winter;14(1):5–10. doi:10.1207/S15328015TLM1401_3.
90. Van der Vleuten CPM, Schuwirth LWT. Assessing professional competence: from methods to programmes. *Med Educ.* 2005 Mar;39(3):309–317. doi:10.1111/j.1365-2929.2005.02094.x.
91. Van der Vleuten CP, Schuwirth LW, Driessen EW, et al. A model for programmatic assessment fit for purpose. *Med Teach.* 2012;34(3):205–214. doi:10.3109/0142159X.2012.652239.
92. Miller G. The assessment of clinical skills/competence/performance. *Acad Med.* 1990 Sep;65(suppl):S63–S67. doi:10.1097/00001888-199009000-00045.
93. Lipner RS, Hess BJ, Phillips RL Jr. Specialty board certification in the United States: issues and evidence. *J Contin Educ Health Prof.* 2013 Fall;33(Suppl 1):S20–S35. doi:10.1002/chp.21203.
94. Cruess RL, Cruess SR, Steinert Y. Amending Miller's pyramid to include professional identity formation. *Acad Med.* 2016 Feb;91(2):180–185. doi:10.1097/ACM.0000000000000913.
95. Rethans JJ, Norcini JJ, Barón-Maldonado M, et al. The relationship between competence and performance: implications for assessing practice performance. *Med Educ.* 2002;36:901–909.
96. Holmboe ES, Kogan JR. Will Any Road Get You There? Examining Warranted and Unwarranted Variation in Medical Education. *Acad Med.* 2022 Aug 1;97(8):1128–1136. doi:10.1097/ACM.0000000000004667.
97. Dreyfus HL. *On the Internet: Thinking in Action.* Routledge; 2001.
98. Pusic MV, Boutis K, Hatala R, Cook DA. Learning curves in health professions education. *Acad Med.* 2015 Aug;90(8):1034–1042. doi:10.1097/ACM.0000000000000681.
99. Van Der Vleuten CP. The assessment of professional competence: developments, research and practical implications. Adv Health Sci Educ Theory Pract. 1996 Jan;1(1):41–67. doi:10.1007/BF00596229.
100. Higgins R, Cavendish S. Modernising medical careers foundation programme curriculum competencies: will all rotations allow the necessary skills to be acquired? The consultants' predictions. *Postgrad Med J.* 2006 Oct;82(972):684–687. doi:10.1136/pgmj.2006.045419.
101. Norcini J, Anderson MB, Bollela V, et al. 2018 consensus framework for good assessment. *Med Teach.* 2018 Nov;40(11):1102–1109. doi:10.1080/0142159X.2018.1500016.
102. Herbers Jr JE, Noel GL, Cooper GS, Pangaro LN, Harvey J, Weaver MJ. How accurate are faculty evaluations of clinical competence? *J Gen Intern Med.* 1989 May-Jun;4:202–208. doi:10.1007/BF02599524.
103. Noel GL, Herbers Jr JE, Caplow MP, Cooper GS, Pangaro LN, Harvey J. How well do internal faculty members evaluate the clinical skills of residents? *Ann Intern Med.* 1992 Nov 1;117(9):757–765. doi:10.7326/0003-4819-117-9-757.
104. Kroboth FJ, Hanusa BH, Parker S, et al. The inter-rater reliability and internal consistency of a clinical evaluation exercise. *J Gen Intern Med.* 1992 Mar-Apr;7(2):174–179. doi:10.1007/BF02598008.
105. Engel GL. Editorial: are medical schools neglecting clinical skills? *JAMA.* 1976 Aug 16;236(7):861–863.
106. Royal College of Physicians and Surgeons of Canada. CanMEDS: Better standards, better physicians, better care. Accessed March 19, 2023. at CanMEDS Framework: The Royal College of Physicians and Surgeons of Canada. https://www.acgme.org/globalassets/pdfs/milestones/pediatricsmilestones.pdf.
107. Baron RJ, Coleman CH. Protecting the legitimacy of medical expertise. *N Engl J Med.* 2023 Feb 23;388(8):676–678. doi:10.1056/NEJMp2214120.
108. Hemmer PA, Dadekian GA, Terndrup C, et al. Regular formal evaluation sessions are effective as frame-of-reference training for faculty evaluators of clerkship medical students. *J Gen Intern Med.* 2015 Sep;30(9):1313–1318. doi:10.1007/s11606-015-3294-6.
109. Lindy FJ, Farr JL. Performance rating. *Psychological Bulletin.* 1980;87:72–107.
110. ten Cate O. Nuts and bolts of entrustable professional activities. *J Grad Med Educ.* 2013 Mar;5(1):157–158. doi:10.4300/JGME-D-12-00380.1.
111. ten Cate O, Hoff R. From case-based to entrustment-based discussions. *Clin Teach.* 2017 Dec;14(6):385–389. doi:10.1111/tct.12710.
112. Touchie C, Kinnear B, Schumacher D, et al. On the validity of summative entrustment decisions. *Med Teach.* 2021 Jul;43(7):780–787. doi:10.1080/0142159X.2021.1925642.
113. ten Cate O. Trust, competence, and the supervisor's role in postgraduate training. *BMJ.* 2006 Oct 7;333(7571):748–751. doi:10.1136/bmj.38938.407569.94.
114. ten Cate O, Hart D, Ankel F, et al. Entrustment decision-making in clinical training. *Acad Med.* 2016 Feb;91(2):191–198. doi:10.1097/ACM.0000000000001044.
115. Boulet JR, Swanson DB. Psychometric challenges of using simulations for high-stakes assessment. In: Dunn D, ed. *Simulators in Critical Care Education and Beyond.* Lippincott, Williams and Wilkins; 2004.
116. McGaghie WC, Barsuk JH, Cohen ER, Kristopaitis T, Wayne DB. Dissemination of an innovative mastery learning curriculum grounded in implementation science principles: a case study. *Acad Med.* 2015 Nov;90(11):1487–1494. doi: 10.1097/ACM.0000000000000907.
117. Barsuk JH, Cohen ER, Potts S, et al. Dissemination of a simulation-based mastery learning intervention reduces central line-associated bloodstream infections. *BMJ Qual Saf.* 2014 Sep;23(9):749–756. doi:10.1136/bmjqs-2013-002665.
118. McGaghie WC, Barsuk JH, Wayne DB, eds. *Comprehensive Healthcare Simulation: Mastery Learning in Health Professions Education.* Springer; 2020.

119. Ziv A, Wolpe RP, Small SD, Click S. Simulation-based medical education: an ethical imperative. *Acad Med.* 2003 Aug;78:783–788. doi:10.1097/00001888-200308000-00006.
120. Norcini JJ. Current perspectives in assessment: the assessment of performance at work. *Med Educ.* 2005 Sep;39(9):880–889. doi:10.1111/j.1365-2929.2005.02182.x.
121. Agency for Healthcare Quality and Research. CAHPS Toolkit. Accessed March 19, 2023. http://www.ahrq.gov/cahps/index.html.
122. Swing SR, Beeson MS, Carraccio C, et al. Educational milestone development in the first 7 specialties to enter the next accreditation system. *J Grad Med Educ.* 2013 Mar;5(1):98–106. doi:10.4300/JGME-05-01-33.
123. ACGME. Pediatrics Competency milestones. Accessed March 19, 2023. at pediatricsmilestones.pdf (acgme.org).
124. Bienstock JL, Shivraj P, Yamazaki K, et al. Correlations between Accreditation Council for Graduate Medical Education Obstetrics and Gynecology Milestones and American Board of Obstetrics and Gynecology qualifying examination scores: an initial validity study. *Am J Obstet Gynecol.* 2021 Mar;224(3):308.e1–308.e25. doi:10.1016/j.ajog.2020.10.029.
125. Hauer KE, Vandergrift J, Hess B, et al. Correlations between ratings on the Resident Annual Evaluation Summary and the Internal Medicine Milestones and association with ABIM Certification Examination scores among US internal medicine residents, 2013-2014. *JAMA.* 2016 Dec 6;316(21):2253–2262. doi:10.1001/jama.2016.17357.
126. Yaghmour NA, Poulin LJ, Bernabeo EC, et al. Stages of milestones implementation: a template analysis of 16 programs across 4 specialties. *J Grad Med Educ.* 2021 Apr;13(2 Suppl):14–44. doi:10.4300/JGME-D-20-00900.1 Erratum in: *J Grad Med Educ.* 2022 Dec;14(6):732. PMID: 33936531.
127. Holmboe ES, Yamazaki K, Nasca TJ, Hamstra SJ. Using longitudinal milestones data and learning analytics to facilitate the professional development of residents: early lessons from three specialties. *Acad Med.* 2020 Jan;95(1):97–103. doi:10.1097/ACM.0000000000002899.
128. Yamazaki K, Holmboe ES, Hamstra SJ. An empirical investigation into milestones factor structure using national data derived from clinical competency committees. *Acad Med.* 2022 Apr 1;97(4):569–576. doi:10.1097/ACM.0000000000004218.
129. Hamstra SJ, Cuddy MM, Jurich D. Exploring the association between USMLE scores and ACGME milestone ratings: a validity study using national data from emergency medicine. *Acad Med.* 2021 Sep 1;96(9):1324–1331. doi:10.1097/ACM.0000000000004207.
130. Hauer KE, Clauser J, Lipner RS, et al. The internal medicine reporting milestones: cross-sectional description of initial implementation in US residency programs. *Ann Intern Med.* 2016 Sep 6;165(5):356–362. doi:10.7326/M15-2411.
131. Beeson M, Holmboe E, Korte R, et al. Initial validity analysis of the emergency medicine milestones. *Acad Emerg Med.* 2015 Jul;22(7):838–844. doi:10.1111/acem.12697.
132. ten Cate O. Entrustability of professional activities and competency-based training. *Med Educ.* 2005 Dec;39(12):1176–1177. doi:10.1111/j.1365-2929.2005.02341.x.
133. ten Cate O, Scheele F. Competency-based postgraduate training: can we bridge the gap between theory and clinical practice? *Acad Med.* 2007 Jun;82(6):542–547. doi:10.1097/ACM.0b013e31805559c7.
134. Karpinski J, Frank JR. The role of EPAs in creating a national system of time-variable competency-based medical education. *Acad Med.* 2021 Jul 1;96(7S):S36–S41. doi:10.1097/ACM.0000000000004087.
135. Dagnone D, Stockley D, Flynn L, et al. Delivering on the promise of competency based medical education – an institutional approach. *Can Med Educ J.* 2019;10(1):e28–e38. doi:10.36834/cmej.43303.
136. Englander R, Flynn T, Call S, et al. Toward defining the foundation of the MD degree: core Entrustable Professional Activities for entering residency. *Acad Med.* 2016 Oct;91(10):1352–1358. doi:10.1097/ACM.0000000000001204.
137. Veale P, Busche K, Touchie C, Coderre S, McLaughlin K. Choosing our own pathway to competency-based undergraduate medical education. *Acad Med.* 2019;94(1):25–30. doi:10.1097/ACM.0000000000002410.
138. Pangaro L, ten Cate O. Frameworks for learner assessment in medicine: AMEE Guide No. 78. *Med Teach.* 2013 Jun;35(6):e1197–e1210. doi:10.3109/0142159X.2013.788789.
139. Scheele F, Caccia N, Van Luijk S, Van Loon K, De Rooyen C. *BOEG–Better Education for Obstetrics and Gynaecology. A national competency-based curriculum for obstetrics & gynaecology.* Utrecht, the Netherlands: Netherlands Association for Gynaecology and Obstetrics; 2013:1–61.
140. Gilhooly J, Schumacher DJ, West DC, Jones MD. The promise and challenge of Entrustable Professional Activities. *Pediatrics.* 2014 May 1;133(Supplement):S78–S79. doi:10.1542/peds.2013-3861H.
141. Caverzagie KJ, Cooney TG, Hemmer PA, Berkowitz L. The development of Entrustable Professional Activities for internal medicine residency training: a report from the Education Redesign Committee of the Alliance for Academic Internal Medicine. *Acad Med.* 2015 Apr;90(4):479–484. doi:10.1097/ACM.0000000000000564.
142. Shaughnessy AF, Sparks J, Cohen-osher M, Goodell KH, Sawin GL, Gravel J. Entrustable Professional Activities in family medicine. *J Grad Med Educ.* 2013 Mar;5(1):112–118. doi:10.4300/JGME-D-12-00034.1.
143. Schultz K, Griffiths J, Lacasse M. The application of Entrustable Professional Activities to inform competency decisions in a family medicine residency program. *Acad Med.* 2015 Jul;90(7):888–897. doi:10.1097/ACM.0000000000000671.
144. Boyce P, Spratt C, Davies M, McEvoy P. Using entrustable professional activities to guide curriculum development in psychiatry training. *BMC Med Educ.* 2011 Jan;11:96. doi:10.1186/1472-6920-11-96.
145. Fessler HE, Addrizzo-Harris D, Beck JM, et al. Entrustable professional activities and curricular milestones for fellowship training in pulmonary and critical care medicine: report of a multisociety working group. *Chest.* 2014 Sep 1;146(3):813–834. doi:10.1378/chest.14-0710.
146. ten Cate O, Taylor D. The recommended description of an entrustable professional activity, AMEE Guide 140. *Med Teach.* 2021 Oct;43(10):1106–1114. doi:10.1080/0142159X.2020.1838465.
147. Lave J, Wenger E. *Situated Learning. Legitimate Peripheral Participation.* Cambridge University Press; 1991.
148. ten Cate O, Snell L, Carraccio C. Medical competence: the interplay between individual ability and the health care environment. *Med Teach.* 2010 Jan;32(8):669–675. doi:10.3109/0142159X.2010.500897.
149. Pangaro L. A new vocabulary and other innovations for improving descriptive in-training evaluations. *Acad Med.* 1999

Nov;74(11):1203–1207. doi:10.1097/00001888-199911000-00012.
150. Hicks PJ, Schumacher DJ, Benson BJ, et al. The pediatrics milestones: conceptual framework, guiding principles, and approach to development. *J Grad Med Educ.* 2010 Sep;2(3):410–418. doi:10.4300/JGME-D-10-00126.1.
151. Chen HC, van den Broek WES, ten Cate O. The case for use of Entrustable Professional Activities in undergraduate medical education. *Acad Med.* 2015 Apr;90(4):431–436. doi:10.1097/ACM.0000000000000586.
152. Jones MD, Rosenberg A, Gilhooly JT, Carraccio CL. Perspective: competencies, outcomes, and controversy—linking professional activities to competencies to improve resident education and practice. *Acad Med.* 2011 Feb;86(2):161–165. doi:10.1097/ACM.0b013e31820442e9.
153. Warm EJ, Mathis BR, Held JD, et al. Entrustment and mapping of observable practice activities for resident assessment. *J Gen Intern Med.* 2014 Aug;29(8):1177–1182. doi:10.1007/s11606-014-2801-5.
154. Weiss PG, Schwartz A, Carraccio CL, et al. Achieving Entrustable Professional Activities during fellowship. *Pediatrics.* 2021 Nov;148(5):e2021050196. doi:10.1542/peds.2021-050196.
155. ten Cate O, Schumacher DJ. Entrustable professional activities versus competencies and skills: exploring why different concepts are often conflated. *Adv Health Sci Educ Theory Pract.* 2022 May;27(2):491–499. doi:10.1007/s10459-022-10098-7.
156. ten Cate O, Graafmans L, Posthumus I, Welink L, van Dijk M. The EPA-based Utrecht undergraduate clinical curriculum: development and implementation. *Med Teach.* 2018 May;40(5):506–513. doi:10.1080/0142159X.2018.1435856.
157. Englander R, Flynn T, Call S, et al. *Core Entrustable Professional Activities for Entering Residency—Curriculum Developers Guide [Internet].* Washington DC; 2014. www.aamc.org.
158. Lindeman B, Brasel K, Minter RM, Buyske J, Grambau M, Sarosi G. A phased approach: the general surgery experience adopting Entrustable Professional Activities in the United States. *Acad Med.* 2021;96(7):S9–S13. doi:10.1097/ACM.0000000000004107.
159. Leipzig RM, Sauvigné K, Granville LJ, et al. What is a geriatrician? American Geriatrics Society and Association of Directors of Geriatric Academic Programs end-of-training Entrustable Professional Activities for geriatric medicine. *J Am Geriatr Soc.* 2014 May;62(5):924–929. doi:10.1111/jgs.12825.
160. Rose S, Fix OK, Shah BJ, et al. Entrustable professional activities for gastroenterology fellowship training. *Gastrointest Endosc.* 2014 Jul;80(1):16–27. doi:10.1016/j.gie.2014.05.302.
161. Hennus MP, Nusmeier A, van Heesch GGM, et al. Development of entrustable professional activities for paediatric intensive care fellows: a national modified Delphi study. *PLoS ONE.* 2021;16(3):e0248565. doi:10.1371/journal.pone.0248565.
162. Crossley J, Johnson G, Booth J, Wade W. Good questions, good answers: construct alignment improves the performance of workplace-based assessment scales. *Med Educ.* 2011 Jun;45(6):560–569. doi:10.1111/j.1365-2923.2010.03913.x.
163. Kennedy TJT, Regehr G, Baker GR, Lingard L. Point-of-care assessment of medical trainee competence for independent clinical work. *Acad Med.* 2008 Oct;83(10 Suppl):S89–S92. doi:10.1097/ACM.0b013e318183c8b7.
164. Albanese M. Challenges in using rater judgements in medical education. *J Eval Clin Pract.* 2000 Aug;6(3):305–319. doi:10.1046/j.1365-2753.2000.00253.x.
165. Govaerts MJB, van der Vleuten CPM, Schuwirth LWT, Muijtjens AMM. Broadening perspectives on clinical performance assessment: rethinking the nature of in-training assessment. *Adv Health Sci Educ Theory Pract.* 2007 May;12(2):239–260. doi:10.1007/s10459-006-9043-1.
166. Oliver JB, McFarlane JL, Kunac A, Anjaria DJ. Declining resident surgical autonomy and improving surgical outcomes: correlation does not equal causality. *J Surg Educ.* 2023 Mar;80(3):434–441. doi:10.1016/j.jsurg.2022.10.009.
167. Tonelli C, Cohn T, Abdelsattar Z, Luchette F, Baker M. Association of resident independence with short-term clinical outcome in core general surgery procedures. *JAMA Surg.* 2023 Mar 1;158(3):302–309. doi:10.1001/jamasurg.2022.6971.
168. Kunac A, Oliver JB, Mcfarlane JL, Anjaria DJ. General surgical resident operative autonomy vs patient outcomes: are we compromising training without net benefit to hospitals or patients? *J Surg Educ.* 2021 Nov-Dec;78(6):e174–e182. doi:10.1016/j.jsurg.2021.09.017.
169. Earle TC. Trust in risk management: a model-based review of empirical research. *Risk Anal.* 2010 Apr;30(4):541–574. doi:10.1111/j.1539-6924.2010.01398.x.
170. Gigerenzer G. *GutFeelings. The Intelligence of the Unconscious.* Penguin Group; 2007.
171. Gigerenzer G, Gaissmaier W. Heuristic decision making. *Annu Rev Psychol.* 2011 Jan;62:451–482. doi:10.1146/annurev-psych-120709-145346.
172. Weller JM, Castanelli DJ, Chen Y, Jolly B. Making robust assessments of specialist trainees' workplace performance. *Br J Anaesth.* 2017 Feb;118(2):207–214. doi: 10.1093/bja/aew412.
173. DaRosa DA, Zwischenberger JB, Meyerson SL, et al. A theory-based model for teaching and assessing residents in the operating room. *J Surg Educ.* 2013 Jan-Feb;70(1):24–30. doi:10.1016/j.jsurg.2012.07.007.
174. Mehta NB, Hull AL, Young JB, Stoller JK. Just imagine: new paradigms for medical education. *Acad Med.* 2013 Oct;88(10):1418–1423. doi:10.1097/ACM.0b013e3182a36a07.
175. Jonker G, Ochtman A, Marty A, Kalkman CJ, ten Cate O, Hoff RG. Would you trust your loved ones to this resident? Certification decisions in postgraduate anesthesiology training. *Br J Anaesth.* 2020 Nov;125(5):E408–E410. doi:10.1016/j.bja.2020.07.009.
176. ten Cate O, Carraccio C, Damodaran A, et al. Entrustment decision making: extending Miller's pyramid. *Acad Med.* 2021 Feb 1;96(2):199–204. doi:10.1097/ACM.0000000000003800.
177. ten Cate O, Chen HC. The ingredients of a rich entrustment decision. *Med Teach.* 2020 Dec;42(12):1413–1420. doi:10.1080/0142159X.2020.1817348.

2

Issues of Validity and Reliability for Assessments in Medical Education

MELISSA J. MARGOLIS, PHD, BRIAN E. CLAUSER, EDD, AND DAVID B. SWANSON, PHD

CHAPTER OUTLINE

A proposition deserves some degree of trust only when it has survived serious attempts to falsify it.

—LEE CRONBACH

This chapter provides an overview of the concepts of validity and reliability as they apply to assessment in medical education. The discussion begins with a brief history of validity theory and a description of how the conceptualization of validity has changed over time. Michael Kane's approach to validity, in which the validation process is viewed as a structured argument in support of the intended interpretations and uses of test scores, will be the main focus of the chapter. Kane's approach is important because the view that the validation process is one of collecting evidence to construct a coherent argument in support of the intended interpretations leads to a notable conclusion: there is no such thing as a *valid test*! The score from any given test could be used to make a variety of decisions in different contexts and with different examinee populations; evidence to support the validity of one type of interpretation in one context with one population may or may not support the validity of a different interpretation in a different context with a different population. This point will be discussed in greater detail later; it is introduced here because it is central to understanding the argument that is made throughout the chapter.

The chapter continues by presenting the components of Kane's validity framework and, for each one, describing examples of the types of validity evidence that might be collected within three different medical education assessment contexts. The discussion of reliability will be presented within the context of generalizability theory, and the generalizability of scores will be considered in the context of the overall validity argument. The intent of this chapter is to provide the reader with a greater understanding of issues that are central to validity and reliability as these concepts pertain to assessment in medical education.

Historical Context

Practically speaking, the history of test theory as we know it began around the turn of the 20th century with Charles Spearman. Spearman's interest was in the study of intelligence rather than assessment, and to support his work he developed the field of correlational psychology. Most of the basic equations from classical test theory were developed by Spearman to aid his research on the presence of a common (g) factor shared by most—if not all—tests of mental proficiency.[1–4]

This groundwork laid the foundation for a science of testing that expanded explosively during World War I. The US Army had a monumental personnel problem: tens of thousands of recruits had to be placed in jobs. Testing provided a potentially effective and efficient means of determining appropriate job placements.[5] This effort established the practice of psychological testing in the United States; not surprisingly, the science of testing was used in an effort to boost educational and industrial efficiency after the war. In both military and industrial contexts, the question of interest was "How well do these tests predict performance on the job?" Evidence to justify the use of the test naturally conformed to the approach established by Spearman and took the form of a correlation between the test scores and an independent assessment of job performance.

The dramatic proliferation of placement testing did much to define the view of validity during the period from 1920 through 1950. Correlational evidence, referred to as *criterion validity*, was the standard during this period; in his 1951 chapter in the first edition of *Educational Measurement*, Edward Cureton defined validity "in terms of the correlation between the actual test scores and the 'true' criterion score."[6]

As a practical matter, criterion validity has obvious utility. In placement testing, it has clear relevance to the interpretation of the score and it provides an objective basis for comparing multiple assessments available for a given purpose. However, the strength of this approach is less apparent for applications beyond placement testing. One problem is that an obvious and practical criterion may not be available; no clear and objective external criterion is likely to exist for an achievement test. And if such a criterion is identified, the test developer would need to provide validity evidence to support its use.[7]

Questions about the appropriateness of criterion validity as a primary evaluation of assessments of academic achievement led to the development of procedures for assessing content validity. The purpose of such evidence is to establish that the content of the test reasonably represents the domain of interest. This type of evidence clearly is necessary, but it is not sufficient to establish the validity of interpretations for an achievement test. As Messick pointed out, evidence that the test content is relevant to the domain(s) of interest provides no direct support for inferences that are made based on the test scores.[8]

During the period after World War II, interest in personality testing and the development of testing instruments to standardize the process pushed researchers to continue considering the types of evidence required to support the use of these new instruments. Neither criterion nor content validity models provided a particularly good fit to these tests. It was in this context that Cronbach and Meehl introduced the idea of construct validity.[9] In the second edition of *Educational* Measurement,[10] Cronbach made the following comment when describing the underlying rationale for this new conceptualization of validity:

> *The rationale for construct validation (Cronbach and Meehl, 1955) developed out of personality testing. For a measure of, for example, ego strength, there is no uniquely pertinent criterion to predict, nor is there a domain of content to sample. Rather, there is a theory that sketches out the presumed nature of the trait. If the test score is a valid manifestation of ego strength, so conceived, its relations to other variables conform to the theoretical expectations.*

This approach to validation greatly expanded the types of evidence that could be considered when evaluating an assessment. For example, in the context of achievement testing, construct validation might argue for collecting evidence to demonstrate that learners with advanced training in the topic area outperform those with less training.

The 1950s brought two other important changes to the conceptualization of validity. First, Campbell and Fiske introduced the multitrait-multimethod matrix: a way to organize validity evidence about the relative strengths of the relationships between traits measured by a single method and measures of the same trait using different methods.[11] In the context of personality testing, examples of traits may have included extraversion and aggression; methods may have included individual examiner-administered assessments and group-administered paper-and-pencil assessments. Campbell and Fiske's matrix provided an empirical means of assessing the extent to which scores are impacted by otherwise irrelevant characteristics of the assessment method or format (signaled by relatively higher correlations between different traits measured by the same method compared with the same trait measured by different methods). This *method effect* relates to what was later to become known as construct-irrelevant variance, a concept that will be addressed in more detail later in this chapter. The second important change in the conceptualization of validity came when Loevinger focused attention on the proposed interpretation of test scores.[12] This represented an important shift in perspective from consideration of the relationship between the construct the test was designed to measure and the test score to consideration of the correspondence between what is measured by the test and the *proposed interpretations* of the test score.

By the time of publication of the third edition of *Educational Measurement*, Messick had developed a unified theory of validity.[8] Rather than being defined as "the correlation between the actual test scores and the 'true' criterion score,"[6] validity now was viewed as the ". . . degree to which empirical evidence and theoretical rationales support the adequacy and appropriateness of interpretations and actions based on test scores."[8] Messick's model built on the contributions of his predecessors; following Cronbach and Meehl,[9] Cronbach,[10] and Loevinger,[12] he emphasized the need to specify the intended meaning and use of the test score before validation. Consistent with Cronbach and Meehl and Campbell and Fiske,[11] Messick emphasized the importance of considering alternative hypotheses such as the impact of construct-irrelevant variance. Additionally, like his predecessors, Messick argued that the process of validation would involve an extended program of research.*

Messick's formulation is consistent with previous validity frameworks, although his conceptualization introduces a change in emphasis. In particular, he placed increased emphasis on evaluating the consequences of the testing program. He believed that both the actual and potential social consequences of a test must be evaluated. Considering as an example a test for medical licensure, at a minimum this requirement leads to examination of consequences such as the test's impact on what instructors choose to teach and what learners choose to learn. More broadly, consequential validity would require consideration of the test's impact on the availability of medical practitioners both for the community at large and, perhaps, specifically for underserved communities. Messick's view of consequential validity went beyond these considerations; he additionally required consideration of the impact that such an examination might have on the entrance of minority candidates into the profession. This broad definition of consequential validity emphasizes the importance of test developers and administrators accepting responsibility for their actions. The definition takes the validation process beyond the scientific evaluation of the assessment into the arena of social and political values.

By 1999, the role of consequences within the sphere of validity was sufficiently well established that it was included as one of the five sources of validity evidence referenced in the *Standards for Educational and Psychological Testing*.[13] They are presented here to provide continuity with previous secondary sources describing Messick's concept of validity theory. It is, however, important to remember that both Messick's unified theory of validity and the *Standards* emphasize that these are not different types of validity. Rather, they are different sources of evidence, each of which may be more or less important in providing support for a specific score interpretation.

The history of validity theory should make it clear that the definition of validity has expanded over time. The emphasis also has changed as the focus of testing has changed. Criterion validity (evidence based on relationships to other variables) has not been replaced; this type of evidence remains essential in evaluating admissions and employment tests. Similarly, content validity represents an important source of evidence in support of tests of achievement. The history of validity is a history of both an expansion in meaning and a shift in emphasis.

More recently, Kane has introduced an additional shift in perspective by representing validity as an argument in support of the proposed interpretations and uses of a test score.[7,14] As with previous phases in the evolution of validity theory, Kane's view does not deny the importance of the evidence and perspectives that have been discussed during the past half century; it provides a shift in perspective rather than a rejection of the basic arguments. That shift in perspective does have one important characteristic: it highlights the fact that the collection of evidence in support of the interpretations of test scores must form a structured and coherent argument that leads from the test administration to the interpretation. That structured argument is only as strong as its weakest component.

Kane's View of Validity

Implicit in the interpretation of a test score is a series of assertions and assumptions that support that interpretation. For example, the interpretation of a passing score on a medical licensing examination requires the assumption that the test was administered under standardized conditions and that the examinee did not have prior access to the test material. If the examinee cheated, no interpretation can be made about the score regardless of other characteristics of the test. Interpretation of the test score requires assumptions about the precision of the score; if the test score is not reproducible, there is no basis for making an interpretation. Interpretation of the score assumes that the test measures some relevant aspect of the overall set of knowledge, skills, and abilities required for the practice of medicine. It also assumes that the cut score (pass/fail standard) has been established in a way that supports the interpretation. If any one of these assumptions is unfounded, the strength of the others may be of little relevance.

Kane provides a structure for this validity argument that outlines four links in the inferential chain from the test administration to the final decision or interpretation.[7,14] He labels these four components *scoring*, *generalization*, *extrapolation*, and *decision*. Support for the *scoring* component of the overall argument includes evidence that the test was administered properly, examinee behavior was captured correctly, and scoring rules were appropriate and were applied accurately and consistently. The *generalization* component of the argument requires evidence that the observations were appropriately sampled from the universe of test items, clinical encounters, et cetera. Generalization also requires evidence that the sample of observations was large enough to produce scores with an acceptable level of precision. Broadly speaking, this stage in the argument asks the question: Is the test reliable? In this context, *generalization* refers to generalizing from the sample of behavior that was part of the test (the *observed* score) to the test-taker's *true score* or *universe* score. The *extrapolation* component of the argument requires evidence that the

*Throughout this chapter we argue that it is important to collect a range of evidence to evaluate the credibility of interpretations that are to be made based on test scores. We share the view of Cronbach, Messick, and Kane that this is likely to require a program of research. At the same time, it is clear that issues of practicality come into play. Although a test that contributes to a grade in a single class or clerkship may raise the same validity issues as a national licensing examination, the resources available to evaluate validity will be far greater in the latter context than in the former. In the case of the licensing examination, an extensive program of research certainly will be appropriate; in the case of a classroom test, the evaluation may be much more limited. That said, when educators introduce novel testing formats, they have a significant responsibility to provide empirical justification for the associated score interpretations and uses.

observations represented by the test score were relevant to the target competency or construct measured by the test. This requires a demonstration that the observations were relevant to the interpretation and that the scores were not unduly influenced by sources of variance that are irrelevant to the intended interpretation. Extrapolation also requires that the target competency that the test is intended to measure is reasonably well represented by the test score. The *decision* component of the argument requires evidence in support of any theoretical framework necessary for score interpretation or evidence in support of decision rules. For tests with a cut score, this evidence would include support for the procedure used to establish that cut score. Again, the score user can have confidence in an interpretation only if there is evidence for each component of the overall argument. The types of evidence required will vary with the purpose and characteristics of the assessment.

These last two sentences are critically important and warrant special comment because, since the last edition of this volume, there has been considerable interest within medical education in longitudinal assessment, formative assessment, and other forms of assessment for learning. There also have been numerous publications advocating the importance of including a broad range of assessment that allows for "triangulation."[15,16] These publications sometimes have drawn a distinction between tests designed to differentiate among individuals and those designed to identify strengths and weaknesses within an individual. They also have described these changes as leading to a "postpsychometric" era. To avoid confusion, we want to be clear that we believe richer sources of evidence are valuable regardless of the purpose of the assessment. At the same time, declaring that something represents a rich source of evidence does not make it so. Sources of feedback should be taken seriously when (and only when) there is evidence to support the validity of that feedback. This includes assessments that result in numeric scores *and* those that produce written or narrative feedback. Formative assessment of clinical competence is intended to support the development of expertise. That development requires practice; it also requires accurate and timely feedback. We will return to this issue throughout the chapter.

The next sections of the chapter will further explicate the four components of the validity argument as described by Kane. Within each section, content relevant to the particular component will be provided for three types of assessments that span a range of the types of assessments currently used in medical education: a multiple-choice examination, a performance assessment, and a workplace-based assessment (WBA). Multiple-choice examinations are ubiquitous in medical education from selection to medical school and through classroom assessment to credentialing. Performance assessments have a long history in medical education, with objective structured clinical examinations (OSCEs) and standardized-patient-based examinations being in common use within medical schools and having a history as part of licensure assessment.[17] WBAs are becoming an increasingly important part of assessment within medical education, particularly during residency training.[18–20] Table 2.1 provides examples of the kinds of questions that arise at each stage of the validity argument. The questions are provided as examples and are not intended to represent an exhaustive list. As you read what follows, we encourage you to think about the assessments that are presented, extrapolate to other assessments, and add your own questions to this list.

TABLE 2.1 Examples of Questions Supporting Each of the Four Components of Kane's Argument-Based Approach to Validity

Component	Questions
Scoring	1. Were the observations made or stimulus materials administered under standardized conditions? 2. Were the scores recorded accurately? 3. Were the scoring algorithms applied correctly? 4. Were appropriate security procedures implemented?
Generalization	1. What are the sources of measurement error that contribute to the observed scores on the assessment? 2. How similar would scores be across replications of the measurement procedure? 3. How similar would classification decisions be across replications of the measurement procedure? 4. To what extent are test forms constructed using a systematic process?
Extrapolation	1. To what extent do the scores correspond to real-world competencies of interest? 2. Are there factors that interfere with assessment of the competencies of interest? 3. Do scores predict real-world outcomes of interest? 4. Are there artificial aspects of the testing conditions that impact the scores?
Decision	1. Was the standard established through implementation of a defensible and properly implemented procedure? 2. Do examinees identified for remediation improve to meet the standard or benefit more from a remediation program than would those who were not identified?

Scoring

The *scoring* component of the validity argument must provide evidence that assessment data have been collected appropriately and scored accurately. This will include consideration of a variety of types of evidence, such as the extent to which the stated conditions of standardization have been implemented and the accuracy of the scoring process. As is true for each component of the validity argument, the specifics of the evidence that will be relevant to the scoring aspect of the argument will vary with the characteristics of the assessment. Again, it is important to remember that any argument for the validity of a score interpretation is only as strong as the weakest link in that argument!

Example 1: A Multiple-Choice Examination

Standardized tests have been developed to provide the strongest possible evidence for the *scoring* component of the validity argument. The multiple-choice format was developed in 1915 explicitly to support objective scoring.[21] Adherence to the conditions of standardization ensures that the data are collected in the same manner for all examinees. Factors such as the time allowed for the examination, the seating, the lighting, and the quality of the stimulus materials are controlled. To the extent that administration procedures require documentation of the violation of these conditions and annotation of score reports, the score user will have confidence in the conditions under which the test responses have been collected. Similarly, professionally administered and scored tests routinely will have quality control steps built into the scoring process. *Key validation*—statistical analyses of examinee responses designed to verify that the keyed answer is correct—provides evidence that the scoring rules have been applied accurately. This step includes activities such as (1) examining the proportion of examinees receiving credit for each item; and (2) comparing the probability of a correct response for examinees at different score levels.

A fundamental consideration for high-stakes[†] tests is security. In high-stakes settings, examinees may be motivated to cheat and may attempt to do so in any number of ways. When items are reused from one administration to another, it is possible for examinees testing earlier to steal (i.e., remember, copy, photograph) items and make them available to those testing on a later date. When computerized examinations are administered on a continuous basis, this threat to validity may be increased. Evidence about the size of the item pool and the frequency with which items are reused will support the user's confidence that prior exposure has not threatened the integrity of the score. For computer-based tests, encryption of test items at all times except when they are displayed on the screen may provide additional confidence in the security of the test material. Tests that are administered nationally or internationally are particularly likely to be targeted by individuals or groups interested in breaching security, but the same issues apply to tests developed and administered within a single medical school if items (or entire test forms) are used on multiple occasions.

Although these steps appear to fall under the heading of test development or test administration, they also are critical pieces of evidence to support the validity argument for standardized written examinations. Because they are a critical part of the validity argument, it is important that the steps in administration and scoring are verified and documented; it is not reasonable to assume that this is a given, even with professionally developed assessments.

Example 2: Performance Assessment

The reproducibility of the stimulus material and scoring procedures is, as previously noted, a strength of standardized tests comprising multiple-choice items. Relatively little effort is required to be satisfied that two examinees assigned to the same test form but sitting at different computers are seeing the same items and that those items are being scored in the same way. The same is not necessarily true for performance assessments such as standardized patient–based assessments or other formats that require humans to present and/or score the assessment. Adding the human element creates the possibility that two standardized patients trained to portray the same scenario may perform in a less-than-standardized manner; the same standardized patient may not portray the same scenario in the same way on two different occasions. The scoring phase of the validity argument will need to include evidence that standardized patients are trained to an acceptable standard, and it also will require evidence that standardized patients are monitored over time to ensure both inter- and intrapatient consistency. Similar issues arise with scoring for these tests; whether the scores are produced by a standardized patient or content expert, it will be necessary to assess the accuracy of the process. Again, this aspect of testing must be verified before testing begins and must continue to be monitored over time. It also is important to remember that collecting evidence of a high level of rater agreement during a small-scale pilot administration should not replace collecting the same evidence once the test is being administered operationally.

In addition to verifying that the overall error rate is low, both in standardized patient portrayal and in the scoring process, it will be important to provide evidence of a lack of significant relationship between examinee characteristics and standardized patients' portrayal or scoring. For example, the gender or ethnicity of a learner should have no impact on the way the scenario is portrayed and scored. If data suggest that learners *of otherwise equal competence* are likely to receive better scores if they are, for example, male rather than female, this would be a serious threat to valid score interpretation. This type of effect is more serious than random error in portrayal or scoring because

[†]High-stakes testing refers to situations in which the outcome of the test has important consequences for the examinee. In medical education, admissions tests and tests for licensing and certification have very high stakes. Tests that result in grades or pass/fail decisions also can be considered high stakes. A self-assessment would be considered low stakes.

random errors tend to average out across encounters; systematic effects do not.

Security issues also may be important with performance assessments. If the test is used to make important decisions, learners may attempt to improve their scores by gaining prior access to test information. In most circumstances, performance assessments (and standardized patient–based tests in paticular) are administered on multiple occasions. This creates the opportunity for learners who have completed the examination to share information with others who will test in the future; in most situations, prior knowledge about the specific tasks that will appear on a test should be expected to influence scores.[22] This threat to validity is analogous to the problem associated with the reuse of material on tests comprising multiple-choice items, but in the case of performance assessments it is much more difficult to produce large banks of test "items." When tests are administered during a relatively short period, sequestering examinees to prevent the sharing of information may provide evidence that this threat to validity has been controlled. With standardized patient–based tests, an additional threat to security exists in that standardized patients (or examiners, if they are used in test administration) themselves may share information with learners before or during the test administration.

Example 3: Workplace-Based Assessment

Assessment of a clinician or trainee through direct observation involves taking another step away from the completely standardized stimulus material of the multiple-choice examination and the partially standardized conditions that exist in performance assessment; it takes place in the largely *un*controlled conditions of the authentic clinical environment. To support the interpretations of scores produced in these settings, it will be necessary to produce evidence that different assessors working in different settings are, in fact, assessing the same construct in the same way. One way to provide such evidence would be to carefully define the characteristics of performance that will be rated. A combination of careful specification of what is being rated and thorough training of assessors may provide reasonable support for the assertion that individuals are being assessed on the same construct. The disadvantage of carefully defining the assessment content is that it may restrict what can be assessed to those aspects of the construct that can be defined easily; this will have an impact on the potential to extrapolate from the scores to the construct of interest. The alternative may be that each assessor defines the construct in their own way, but this approach clearly leaves the scoring aspect of the validity argument seriously weakened.

Even with careful attention to activities such as specifying the rating elements and assessor training, it will be important to collect evidence demonstrating that assessors are, in fact, assessing the same constructs. In a paper reporting on a WBA system implemented at 15 US residency programs, the authors describe several activities intended to strengthen the scoring component of the validity argument. In the early stages of instrument development, cognitive interviews were conducted with assessors in the roles that would be participating in the actual assessment. This allowed for collecting important information about how the items were being interpreted by different groups of assessors and led to targeted item revisions focused on decreasing the variability in individual interpretation and completion of items. In addition, as part of the instrument development process the researchers often would include a brief introduction to the item prior to the specific rating question. This was done in an attempt to provide a clear foundation for responding to the item and, by extension, to decrease the extent to which individual assessors responded to items based on their own interpretations of what question was being asked. The following provides an example of one of these items. There is an initial description of expectations for the person being assessed:

> *As a member or leader of a clinical team, a resident is counted on to keep interprofessional team members aware of: (1) patients' current status and potential for deterioration; and (2) any changes in status (e.g., physical exam, labs) that occur.*

And the scorable item follows:

> *Thinking about situations in which the resident would have been expected to inform the team about patient status, indicate the degree to which the resident kept you informed (rating scale: continuum between* did not keep me informed *and* kept me fully informed*).*

Providing specific examples to help assessors focus on the same construct when responding to assessment items is just one approach to addressing scoring-related considerations in WBA settings. Relevant considerations will differ based on the assessment context and the inferences that are to be made based on test scores. As such, a critical first step in the process is to ensure an understanding of the various factors that can impact the *scoring* component of the validity argument. This will help to ensure that the necessary validity evidence can be generated and collected.

As with other forms of assessment that do not lend themselves to machine scoring, careful training of assessors will be important with WBAs. That said, evidence to support the scoring component of the validity argument likely will include an evaluation of the accuracy of the scores rather than simply documentation of careful training.

Generalization

This stage of the argument focuses on the question of whether an examinee would receive the same score if the assessment were repeated. We would not waste our time standing on a scale if we discovered that the dial reported a wildly different weight when we stepped off and back on. Technically speaking, the generalization stage of the argument is focused on the relationship between the observed scores and the associated universe scores (or true scores). Both universe scores and true scores are conceptualizations. The universe score represents the score that an examinee would receive if it were possible for that examinee to respond to all items representing the universe of acceptable observations (i.e., if the examinee responded to all items in the domain). The true score is a closely related concept representing the mean score that the examinee would receive if they completed an unlimited number of randomly equivalent (parallel) forms of the test. (The observed score is the actual score that is recorded when an examinee completes a specific test form.) The details of these definitions and related theories are beyond the scope of this chapter; the interested reader is referred to Gulliksen[1] and Lord and Novick[23] for a detailed discussion of classical test theory and to Cronbach and associates[24] and Brennan[25] for discussions of generalizability theory.

Two kinds of evidence are required for this stage of the argument. First, it is necessary to show that the sample of items or observations made of the examinee are representative of the domain to which the score is to be generalized. Second, it is necessary to demonstrate that the sampling is sufficiently extensive to prevent the observed scores from being unduly influenced by sampling error. The extent to which the sample is representative will depend on the procedures used for test construction (a blueprint/sampling plan for data collection for WBAs); the adequacy of the sampling can be examined directly through a well-developed set of theory-based statistical procedures.

The samples will be representative to the extent that data collection follows specified rules. In some cases, random selection from a specified domain will be appropriate; in others, stratified sampling will be preferred. In some contexts, rules for the range of conditions under which observations may (or must) be made will replace the sampling of stimulus material.

The most developed aspect of test theory by far relates to evaluation of reliability; conceptually this methodology is designed to assess the relationship between observed scores and true scores or universe scores. The most common index of this relationship is the reliability coefficient; this coefficient represents the correlation between the observed test scores from two equivalent forms of the test. The square root of this value represents the correlation between observed scores and true scores on the test. In the classical test theory framework, the reliability coefficient also is directly related to the standard error of measurement, which represents the distribution of observed scores around a given true score.

Numerous approaches have been developed to estimate the relationship between observed scores and true scores; the usefulness of these procedures will depend on how one conceptualizes the meaning of "a replication of the measurement procedure."[26] Because the specific set of items and the specific time and date on which the test was administered rarely are central to how scores are to be interpreted, it is generally desirable to view "replication" as including measurements with different test forms on different occasions. This common condition makes correspondence between scores achieved on two forms of a test on different occasions a single standard for assessing replicability. The value of this standard rests on the assumption that the characteristic to be measured has not changed between administrations. This includes change in the narrow sense of learning as well as change in relevant conditions of observation such as motivation, fatigue, and familiarity with the test format.

When it is unlikely that *relevant* conditions of testing remain constant across occasions, it may be more appropriate to conceptualize a replication such that occasion is held constant. In the practical sense in which the test is administered twice on the same day, replication on the same occasion is open not only to the effects of fatigue but also to the effects of practice leading to increased familiarity with the format. In the literal sense of replication on the same occasion (in which two forms are administered simultaneously), these effects are absent but actual replication is not possible; only a conceptual or theoretical replication can exist.

For a test comprising multiple-choice items, the definition of replication should include consideration of occasion and the selection of items. For more complex testing formats, the definition of replication similarly will be more complex. Consider, for example, an essay examination in which the stimulus will be standardized but a replication may involve a different set of essay prompts to which an examinee will respond on a different occasion. Additionally, the responses may be scored by a different set of judges and the judges may evaluate the material on different occasions. The definition of a replication therefore will depend on which features are considered fixed and which are considered random. In this context, the definition of fixed and random variables is guided by the desired interpretation of scores. If score interpretation assumes that judgments were made by a specific group of experts and that all examinees were evaluated by the same experts, judges will be considered a fixed facet in the design.[‡] More commonly, it is appropriate to view judges as having been sampled from a larger group of similarly qualified and acceptable judges such that the judges should be viewed as a random facet. Similarly, if score interpretations assume a specific set of test items or other stimulus materials, this facet is fixed; alternatively, if the stimuli are viewed as sampled from a larger domain, items must be viewed as a random facet. Random facets will vary from one replication to the next; fixed facets will not. Again, it is uncommon for tasks to be fixed, but in certain situations, such as tests of specific procedural skills, this may be the case.

The appropriate methodology for examining the strength of the relationship between observed scores and true scores or estimating the standard error of measurement will depend on the complexity of the data collection design. When practicality allows, actually repeating the measurement procedure will provide a sound basis for assessing the relationship of interest. The correlation between scores produced across replications will provide an appropriate estimate of

[‡]In generalizability theory terminology, sources of variability—such as the sampling of items or judges—are referred to as *facets*. Facets are similar to factors used in analysis of variance.

the reliability of the test. Again, the square root of this value will represent the correlation between observed and true scores, and the well-known formula

$$\sigma_e = \sigma_x \sqrt{1 - r_{xx'}}$$

provides an estimate of the standard error of measurement in this situation. (In this formula, σ_x represents the standard deviation of the observed scores, σ_e represents the standard error, and $r_{xx'}$ represents the reliability of the test.)

In many circumstances, replication will not be practical; for example, candidates for licensure cannot be called upon to retest under the same high-stakes conditions after they have completed and passed an examination. Numerous procedures are available to evaluate the reliability (reproducibility, precision) of test scores based on a single examination administration. Nearly a century ago, Spearman and Brown introduced the first of these procedures based on the correlation between split halves (e.g., even- and odd-numbered items) of an examination.[4,27] Kuder-Richardson Formula 20 (KR-20)[28] and coefficient alpha[29] estimate a value equal to the average of all possible split halves. These procedures provide estimates of reliability based on the strength of relationship between items in a single test form. They work on the assumption that the strength of relationship (covariance) between item n and item m (n ≠ m) on a single test form will provide a good approximation of the strength of relationship between item "n" on test form 1 and item "m" on test form 2.

Coefficient alpha and the Kuder-Richardson formulas are useful tools for collecting evidence about the generalization of test scores. Unfortunately, they have become a kind of knee-jerk reaction to the question of score reliability. Too often, researchers appear to view estimating reliability as a requirement that allows them to report a coefficient that a journal editor will demand rather than as an opportunity to better understand the characteristics of their assessment. When applying these procedures, two important considerations arise. First and foremost, the evaluator must ask the question about what is meant by a replication in that specific context. The described estimation procedures are appropriate when generalization is viewed in terms of replication across items (or test forms) with all other conditions of measurement held constant. In the relatively simple context of tests based on multiple-choice items, this approach generally will underestimate the standard error of measurement that would be observed for replications across both test forms and testing occasions. For more complex testing formats, interpretation of the results from these procedures will be more difficult and often much more problematic.

A second important consideration in applying these procedures is related to the assumptions used in their derivation. The central assumption in interpreting coefficient alpha (or KR-20) is that, on average, the strength of relationship between any two items on a single test form is equal to that between any two items on different forms of the test. When this assumption is violated, the results may substantially misrepresent the actual reliability of the assessment. Typically, this violation will result in an overestimate of reliability. Consider, for example, the case in which a passage describing a clinical scenario is followed by several questions. It is common that the strength of relationship between questions associated with the same passage will be greater than the strength of relationship between items from different passages. Because scenarios typically will be different from one test form to the next, the average relationship between items across test forms will be best approximated by the relationship between items from different scenarios on a single test.

Another example of a situation in which these procedures may be misapplied occurs in assessments that require multiple raters to assess an examinee's performance on the same task. For example, consider the circumstance in which raters work in pairs to evaluate an examinee's interaction with a real patient. The assessment requires that each examinee interact with five patients, and each interaction is evaluated by a different pair of raters. If the raters score separately, the examinee will receive 10 scores. If all examinees have interacted with the same five patients and have been scored by the single set of raters assigned to that patient, the evaluator may be tempted to calculate coefficient alpha based on this set of 10 scores. Again, however, because the strength of relationship between scores from raters evaluating performance with the same patient typically will be greater than that between pairs evaluating performance with different patients, this approach will not appropriately approximate the strength of relationship between scores from different tests. In this instance, the error in estimation may be substantial (e.g., the estimated standard error may be 50% of the correct value) and may grossly overstate the reproducibility of the scores.

Lee Cronbach's coefficient alpha paper[29] may be the most cited paper in the history of educational measurement. As we mentioned, for many researchers it has become a kind of knee-jerk reaction to the measurement of reliability. Unfortunately, the interpretation of this coefficient also has been made mechanically, without consideration of the context. Too often a value of .80 has been viewed as a cut score to determine whether a test is reliable. Although there may be instances in which this is a reasonable target, the precision that is needed to make a specific inference based on a test score will depend on the inference itself.

Classical test theory divides observed scores into two components: true score and error. Because an examinee's true score is defined as uncorrelated with error, it follows that observed-score variance is composed of true-score variance and error variance. Generalizability theory expands this framework to divide (partition) the overall variance into multiple components. Consider as an example the simple testing situation in which examinees respond to essay prompts and the essays are scored by raters. To study the generalizability of the results, a researcher collected data for a group of examinees; all examinees responded to the same prompts, and all responses were scored by the same raters. In

TABLE 2.2 Sample Blueprint for a 200-Item Multiple-Choice Test in Internal Medicine

	Number of Questions per Clinical Task				
Disease Category/Organ System[a]	Making a Diagnosis	Making Therapeutic Decisions	Preventing Disease	Using Diagnostic Studies	Total
Cardiovascular disorders	10	9	5	6	30
Dermatologic disorders	4	2	2	2	10
Endocrine and metabolic disorders	7	6	3	4	20
Gynecologic disorders	3	3	2	2	10
Hematologic disorders	3	3	1	3	10
Immunologic disorders	3	3	2	2	10
Mental disorders	4	3	1	2	10
Musculoskeletal disorders	8	6	2	4	20
Neurologic disorders	6	4	2	3	15
Nutritional and digestive disorders	8	9	4	4	25
Renal, urinary, and male reproductive disorders	6	3	2	4	15
Respiratory disorders	8	9	4	4	25
Total	70	60	30	40	200

[a]Items related to infectious and neoplastic diseases are included in the affected organ system.

the framework of generalizability theory, essay prompts and raters become distinguishable sources of error variance. As in the classical test theory framework, it is possible to take data from a single administration, estimate the reliability (or generalizability) of the test, and project the expected reliability of the test with differing numbers of essay prompts. However, because generalizability theory provides a means of making explicit the error contributed by variability both in essay prompts and raters, this framework makes it possible to further project how the reliability of the test would change if the number of raters assessing performance on each prompt also is varied.

Example 1: A Multiple-Choice Examination

The focus of the *generalization* stage of the validity argument is on the extent to which scores will be comparable across replications of the assessment procedure. In the context of standardized multiple-choice–based assessments, the interpretation of scores typically will require that they are comparable across multiple test forms. For example, a licensing or certifying examination would lose credibility if the test forms to which examinees were assigned led to widely varying scores.

Viewed from a generalizability theory framework, this part of the argument will require several types of evidence. First, it will be necessary to demonstrate that the sampling procedure used for test construction supports the creation of comparable test forms. The simplest case of the construction of multiple forms would be based on random selection of items from an available pool of acceptable items. This is conceptually simple, but it is unusual for standardized tests. A more common approach would be to select items to meet the constraints of a table of specifications or test "blueprint." In this case, items may be randomly selected from each of a number of content categories (see Table 2.2 for a hypothetical 200-item multiple-choice test in internal medicine). When different item formats are included on the test, the table of specifications may indicate the number of items that should be included from each combination of format and category. A common variation on this theme is to write items for a new form of the test to meet the specifications of the previous form. When systematic differences exist in the test construction process across forms, estimation of the correlation between scores on multiple forms based on generalizability analysis of a single form will be inappropriate. When systematic test construction procedures are used, multiple-choice–based tests typically will have a reasonably simple data collection design, examinees typically will be the focus of the measurement procedure (referred to as the object of measurement in generalizability theory terminology), and the sampling of items will represent a potential source of measurement error. With this simple design, three sources of variance (referred to as variance components) can be estimated: a person variance component, which is conceptually equivalent to true-score variance in classical test theory; an item variance component, which represents the variability in item difficulty; and a person-by-item variance component, which represents residual variance not explained by the other two effects. The person-by-item variance component divided by the number of items will represent the error variance when comparisons are being made between examinees who have completed the same test form; when comparisons are being made between examinees who have completed different test forms, the definition of error variance is more complicated. If the test forms are constructed through a process that approximates random sampling from an undifferentiated item pool and there is no formal procedure to adjust the scores for difficulty differences, the appropriate error variance will be the sum of the item variance component and the person-by-item variance component both divided by the number of items. When statistical equating[§] procedures are used, the impact of the item variance component will be reduced; because equating is not likely to be error free, the error variance estimate based on the person-by-item variance component alone will represent a lower bound of the error variance when forms are equated.

When items are sampled from fixed content categories, the analysis becomes more complicated. In this situation, there are variance components for persons (p); content categories (c); items nested in content categories ($i{:}c$); persons by content categories ($p \times c$); and persons by items nested in content categories ($p \times i{:}c$). In this case, the c component will not contribute measurement error because this structure is fixed across test forms. Similarly, because the categories are fixed, the $p \times c$ variance component will contribute to universe variance. The $p \times i{:}c$ component will contribute to error, and when comparisons are made across forms the $i{:}c$ will contribute to measurement error. The impact of this latter component again will be mitigated to the extent that test forms are constructed or equated to be statistically equivalent. The stratification process typically will yield a smaller standard error and larger generalizability coefficient than analysis without stratification; this is one reason that coefficient alpha is referred to as a lower bound estimate of reliability. It should be noted, however, that in practice the difference in coefficients typically is modest.

The error variance estimates produced using generalizability theory provide a basis for estimating the standard error of measurement for the test; these are useful for providing confidence intervals around scores. Generalizability coefficients also may be produced as the ratio of the universe score variance divided by the sum of the universe score variance and the error variance. Although these indices are commonly reported, caution is required because they will be sensitive to the specific sample of examinees used in the estimation. Consider, for example, estimation of such an index for one of the Steps of the United States Medical Licensing Examination (USMLE); if the coefficient is estimated based on the relatively homogeneous group of US graduates taking the test for the first time, it may be several points lower than if it is estimated based on all examinees completing the test. In contrast, the standard error of measurement tends to be more stable across groups, making it a more interpretable and useful index of precision.[33]

Example 2: Performance Assessment

The logic of the argument described in the previous example holds in the context of performance assessments. To draw conclusions from analyses based on a single administration of the assessment, the rules employed in test construction must guarantee that there will not be systematic differences in test forms. The logistic realities of test delivery may make this more difficult when the "items" are people, but clearly generalization across test forms will be threatened if the tasks (e.g., standardized patients) on one form are systematically different than those on another. Important differences could include changes in the types of problems portrayed as well as changes in the level of experience and training of the patients.

The generalizability of standardized tests comprising multiple-choice items is relatively easy to evaluate, and even the simpler classical test theory models provide adequate tools for most situations. The complexity of performance assessments, however, makes evaluation of the generalizability of scores a more difficult matter. Consider a test in which examinees rotate through a set of stations and at each station they interact with a patient and complete a post-encounter note. The notes then are scored by a group of raters. When examinees complete the same set of stations and notes are rated by the same set of raters, variance components can be estimated for persons, stations, raters, persons by stations, persons by raters, stations by raters, and persons by stations by raters.** The evaluator will need to determine how much each component contributes to measurement error in the specific context. Interaction terms that include the person and station effect almost always will contribute to measurement error—regardless of the intended score interpretation—because the *generalization* argument is about the extent to which the score from this test form is comparable to the score from a similarly constructed test form. By contrast, generalization over raters may or may not be important. If the test is administered in a context in which the same group of raters rates all examinees, and if there is no intention to draw inferences about how the examinees may have performed with other raters (which is rarely true), then raters can be considered a fixed facet in the design. In this case, the rater and station-by-rater variance components will not contribute to measurement error and the person-by-rater component will contribute to universe score variance.

[§]A wide variety of procedures are in use for putting scores from different forms of the same test on a common scale. The simplest of these approaches is to administer the two test forms to the same group or to randomly equivalent groups of examinees and set the mean (or mean and standard deviation) for the two forms to be equal.[30] More sophisticated approaches include item response theory[31] and equipercentile equating.[32] Each approach is designed to minimize the differences in difficulty across test forms that are reflected in the item variance component.

**This is a relatively infrequent occurrence for large-scale OSCEs. Even if all examinees rotate through the same set of stations, multiple "circuits" with different standardized patients portraying case roles and different raters grading performance are commonly used, and this adversely affects precision.[21]

In most circumstances, however, users of test scores will want to draw inferences that extend beyond the group of raters scoring an examinee's performance, and these variance components are best viewed as contributing to measurement error (often substantially if the typical examinee is scored by a small number of raters).

At this point, it should be clear that when a facet in the design is considered fixed, the scores will have a smaller error variance and a higher level of generalizability. The evaluator may be tempted to try to increase the generalizability of scores by considering facets fixed. This strategy is without merit; it gives a promising answer to the wrong question.

Example 3: Workplace-Based Assessment

When examinees are observed in a practice setting, the *generalization* portion of the validity argument may be problematic. Although there may be explicit rules controlling the sampling of observations, the logistics of conducting a WBA could make it likely that the environmental factors and patient characteristics are more similar from one observation to another within versus between examinees. This may lead to an overly optimistic report on the generalizability of scores. In this setting, the scores will be influenced by the rater effect as well as an effect for the specific patient or task that provides the context for the observation. Depending on the design used to assign raters, it may be difficult to accurately estimate a rater effect. It also may be difficult or even impossible to fully differentiate between variance associated with the difficulty of the patient's presentation or other characteristics of the task and the residual variance.

It usually is the case that the generalizability of scores will decrease as the type of assessment changes from a highly structured format—such as a professionally developed multiple-choice test—to a performance assessment or workplace-based observational assessment. There are two reasons for this. First, it is possible to sample from the domain of interest more widely and efficiently with multiple-choice items because it takes relatively little time to respond to them and they are inexpensive to score. Second, both the sampling of content and the scoring can be more highly standardized with multiple-choice assessments so that the contribution of these factors to measurement error can be markedly reduced. At the same time, multiple-choice tests can assess only a limited range of skills, and it is important for the assessment format to have a good match to the skills to be assessed to avoid construct underrepresentation.

The potential to sample more widely reduces the impact of the examinee-by-item interaction as well as the effect of any higher-order interaction terms (including residual variance). There is a widely held view that the examinee-by-item interaction term in the typical person-by-item design represents "content specificity," or the tendency for physician knowledge to be highly problem specific. The pervasive nature of the effect is well documented: the examinee-by-item (or case) interaction term is routinely the largest single source of error variance. It is, however, less clear whether this term represents content specificity or other sources of uncontrolled variability in the design. There is relatively little research investigating how consistently examinees respond to the same items or cases on different occasions. To the extent that the effect of interest actually is content specificity, examinees completing the same multiple-choice items or completing the same performance task on multiple occasions would receive highly consistent scores. There is some evidence from outside the domain of assessment in medical education to suggest that scores may not be highly reproducible across occasions. Similarly, there is evidence that the generalizability of test scores can be improved by building test forms to consistently sample from fixed content categories; however, the absolute magnitude of this improvement generally is small.

As noted previously, a second reason for the lower generalizability of scores resulting from assessments using performance tasks or workplace observation is that the conditions of observation and scoring are more difficult to standardize. This argues for increasing the structure of the assessment, but this process requires careful thought. The decision to implement a less structured assessment instead of one that is more highly structured (e.g., a clinical rather than a multiple-choice examination) is based on the perceived need to more directly assess the construct of interest. The problem lies in the fact that changing the scoring procedure may increase the standardization of the assessment by altering what is being assessed; the focus of the assessment therefore may shift in the direction of competencies that are more easily quantified and away from its original intent. This is not to argue against making every effort to structure the assessment; the key is to structure the assessment with a careful eye on the intended interpretation of the scores. Inevitably, it will be necessary to strike a balance between the generalizability of scores and the extent to which one can extrapolate from those scores to the actual competencies of interest.

Additional Thoughts on Reliability

In the previous sections we have discussed generalization (reliability) issues for three testing contexts. There are, however, perspectives that have not been considered, some of which relate to the purpose of the test. For example, the same testing format (e.g., multiple-choice items, performance assessment) may be used in different ways, such as providing formative feedback to support learning or informing summative decisions about an individual. Similarly, a test may be used for low-stakes or high-stakes purposes. Generally, it is reasonable to argue that high-stakes decisions should be based on precise measurements; a summative decision that may lead to granting/denying an individual a license to practice requires a precise measurement to protect both the public and the test taker.

This does not imply that low-stakes summative assessments should be held to lower standards of precision. The required level of precision is dependent on the inference/use that is to be made of the test results. Medical professionals study and train to develop expertise. Decades of research on expertise have demonstrated that development of expertise is facilitated by accurate, timely, and specific feedback.[34] This would seem to argue for the importance of precision in formative feedback. Additionally, the need for reliability may be increased—rather than decreased—when decisions are made about relative strengths within rather than between individuals. One reason for this is that the correlations between competencies often are high. This, in part, explains why so much attention continues to be given to how and when we should report subscores,[35] but the problem has been recognized for nearly a century.[36] There is an extensive literature on the issues of measuring differences between correlated competencies and a similar literature on measuring change for individuals.[37] Both argue that the associated problems are complex and the need for precision may be substantially increased in these contexts.

In addition, if the primary purpose of an assessment system is formative—to identify an individual's areas of strength and weakness and to provide feedback that motivates trainees to remediate weaknesses, driving future learning forward[38]—the criteria for evaluating the utility of the assessment system logically should include its success in improving learning outcomes over time.[39] If assessment results are to be used for both formative and summative purposes—which often is true for assessments given during training, and more recently, for continuing certification[40]—then the reliability and validity considerations discussed in this chapter also must be addressed. The next section examines the *extrapolation* phase of the validity argument.

Extrapolation

The extrapolation phase of the validity argument focuses on examining a link between the scores collected as part of the assessment and performance in the real-world context of interest. Assessors rarely are interested in knowing about a learner's ability to answer multiple-choice questions or, for that matter, the learner's ability to interact with standardized patients. Instead, the interest is in competencies such as knowledge base, problem-solving skills, clinical judgment, and ability to communicate effectively. Assessment scores provide indirect evidence about how the learner is likely to perform in the context of interest; the *extrapolation* phase of the validity argument is concerned with that evidence.

This is the most difficult stage of the validity argument because the evidence is by nature inferential and the analytic framework is less well developed than that for the generalization argument. The *extrapolation* stage of the argument is every bit as vital as the *generalization* phase. A highly reliable score that measures the wrong characteristic is of little value. However, it is equally important to remember that the *appearance* that an examination measures the competency of interest is not a substitute for actual evidence supporing that assertion. Such "face validity" may support the political acceptability and, perhaps, the legal viability of an assessment,[41] but it does not contribute meaningfully to the validity argument.

As noted in the introduction to this chapter, the validity of inferences from test scores cannot be reduced to a correlation with a criterion measure because completely valid criteria are rarely (if ever) available. Nonetheless, information about the relationship between test scores and other relevant measures will contribute to the argument. Similarly, evidence about the content of the examination will be of interest. Beyond these two types of supportive evidence, the *extrapolation* argument must be guided by the quote from Cronbach that began this chapter: "A proposition deserves some degree of trust only when it has survived serious attempts to falsify it."[42] The evaluator will be called upon to assess both the extent to which scores are influenced by sources of variability that are not related to the competency of interest and the extent to which scores fail to reflect important aspects of the competency of interest; these two threats to validity are referred to as construct-irrelevant variance and construct underrepresentation.

The assessment format itself may be one potential source of construct-irrelevant variance. If a computerized test requires an examinee to manage a patient in a simulated patient-care environment (as does the computer-based case simulations component of USMLE Step 3), facility with the user interface may impact performance. Not only must examinees identify the next step in management; they must take that step in a potentially unfamiliar simulated world. Similarly, if the test format requires examinees to interact with a simulated electronic health record, scores may reflect the extent to which the health record is similar to the system they use in training or practice. The impact of such factors on test scores would be considered construct-irrelevant variance.

One way to evaluate the extent to which construct-irrelevant format effects are impacting scores is with the multitrait-multimethod matrix. For example, the ability to interview and examine a patient and to describe the critical features of the case could be evaluated based on typed responses and oral presentation by the examinee. These same response formats could be used to evaluate apparently distinct competencies. If scores across competencies within response format are more highly correlated than scores across formats within competencies, this would be a matter of concern.

One particularly problematic source of construct-irrelevant variance is systematic bias. Random errors—of the type we typically consider when assessing the generalizability of scores—tend to average out across items or judges. Systematic effects can be more problematic than random effects because they do not tend to sum to zero. This creates systematic error or bias. Aspects of the test format or administration can create this type of effect. For example, when time limits impact test scores, the effect is likely to vary across examinees. Examinees who need more time to respond to one item are more likely to need more time to respond to other items, and the effect accumulates as they move through the test. Of particular concern is that these effects might differentially impact distinct groups of examinees, such as non-native English speakers. Systematic effects also can impact scores when raters (e.g., standardized patients) allow characteristics such as examinee race, ethnicity, gender, or native language to impact scoring. Recently, considerable attention has been given to the potential for scoring systems driven by artificial intelligence (AI) to display bias because the data samples used to train the system do not represent the overall population variability.[43]

Example 1: A Multiple-Choice Examination

Tests of this sort typically assess a defined domain of interest. Extrapolation of test scores to performance in practice (or readiness for advancement in training) requires that the content of the test is matched appropriately to the demands of practice. Evidence for the content validity of the test will follow from the procedures used to define the domain and sample from it in assembling test forms. A job (or practice) analysis may be used to collect information about the requirements of practice, and additional studies may include collecting expert judgments about the relevance of items on actual test forms.[44]

Criterion-related evidence is conceptually central to the *extrapolation* stage of the validity argument. Certainly, it would be desirable to demonstrate that scores from a licensing examination were directly related to the learner's subsequent delivery of safe and effective treatment in practice. While some researchers have been successful in collecting this type of evidence, in general results of this sort have been limited. One reason for this is the lack of valid measures of the criterion of interest. For example, numerous studies have shown that learners with better performance on licensing examinations have a lower probability of being sanctioned by state medical boards.[45] These results generally are supportive of the use of these tests as part of licensure, but the tests are designed to measure medical knowledge or clinical judgment and the criterion measure is at best a very approximate measure of these competencies. Other researchers[46,47] have shown a relationship between test scores and patient outcomes or adherence to practice guidelines, but in general these criteria have been limited in scope and are somewhat removed from the actual competency the test is designed to measure.[48,49] In the case of licensing examinations, another limiting factor is the fact that examinees who fail are not able to practice, making it impossible to collect criterion measures. This is not to suggest that studies based on such criterion measures should not be pursued, but in the end, a more compelling argument may rest on less direct evidence demonstrating that the content of the examination reasonably represents the construct of interest and that scores are not unduly influenced by sources of construct-irrelevant variance.

Because logistic constraints necessitate administering high-stakes multiple-choice examinations within structured time limits, one potentially important source of construct-irrelevant variance with such tests is the impact of these time limits on outcomes (often referred to as speededness). It may be (and often is) the case that the ability to respond quickly is not a part of the construct of interest and is not consistent with the intended score interpretations.[††] The effects of speededness are another example of a potential source of construct-irrelevant variance.[50]

Example 2: Performance Assessment

The primary attraction of performance-based assessment formats is that they have the potential to more directly measure constructs of interest; weakening the *generalization* argument may be considered acceptable because the *extrapolation* argument is strengthened. However, even though simulation formats may be of high fidelity, there are likely to be aspects that are artificial. There has been relatively little research into the degree to which interactions with standardized patients differ from interactions with real patients, but it seems highly likely that differences exist. Even when standardized patients appear to be indistinguishable from actual patients, factors such as the choice of scoring approach may impact the extent to which the scores can be extrapolated to the performance of interest in practice. Checklists, for example, may fail to capture more subtle interviewing skills that facilitate information gathering. Similarly, knowledge that the interaction is being scored based on a checklist may alter an examinee's approach to interviewing in order to maximize score points.

The previous comments are intended to highlight the fact that the appearance of similarity between the assessment setting and the practice setting is not in and of itself validity evidence. Using an assessment task that closely approximates the practice setting has the potential to limit the effects of construct-irrelevant variance and construct underrepresentation, but this similarity does not ensure that the score appropriately represents the competency of interest.

Example 3: Workplace-Based Assessment

As with performance-based assessment formats such as those using standardized patients, direct observation is an attractive assessment approach because it has the potential to strengthen the *extrapolation* stage of the validity argument. Because observations are done in the practice setting, differences between the features of the assessment and those of practice may be minimized or eliminated. This characteristic may facilitate construction of an assessment that directly relates to real-world performance, but again it does not in and of itself make the argument for extrapolation. The act of observing may alter the environment. More importantly,

[††]In some areas of practice (e.g., emergency medicine, trauma surgery), speed of response may be critical in practice. In these areas it may seem attractive to include speed of response as part of the assessment. When this is done, it will be appropriate to collect evidence linking response speed on the test to response speed in practice.

the scoring algorithm will shape what is observed and how that observation is transformed into a score. Because it is the score and not the setting that is of interest, collecting observations in the practice setting does not ensure the elimination of construct-irrelevant variance or construct underrepresentation.

In the absence of highly structured scoring algorithms and/or careful training, assessments based on direct observation may be particularly susceptible to halo effects[51] and other sources of construct-irrelevant variance. Unfortunately, in an effort to more clearly define the behaviors to be assessed and avoid such effects, the focus of the assessment may shift from the construct of interest to a set of more easily defined behaviors. In an effort to avoid the effect of construct-irrelevant variance, the scores may suffer from construct underrepresentation. For example, the complex concept of physician–patient communication may be reduced to a set of descriptions, such as "asks open-ended questions" and "makes eye contact." This may leave out important aspects of the competency such as tone of voice or expressing compassion. When this happens, the knowledge, skills, behaviors, and attitudes that are included in the assessed competency will be a limited subset of those in the intended competency. Because of these issues, it is important to remember that even when the real-life behaviors of interest are directly observed, the resulting scores will be a function of the specifics of the instrument used to record the observation.

Decision/Interpretation

The *decision* stage of the validity argument provides support for the decision rules and theory-based interpretations that are applied to test scores. The most common decision rules will be simple pass/fail classifications based on a single cut score, but conjunctive or partially compensatory rules are not uncommon. Arguments supporting the reasonableness of these rules will be needed if the score interpretations associated with the resulting classification decisions are to be considered credible.

Similarly, score interpretations based on psychological theories about cognition, judgment, or decision-making will only be as credible as the theories themselves. For example, if a score is used to classify practitioners as experts or novices based on their patterns of data collection in reaching a diagnosis, the theory of expert judgment supporting scoring would be critical; if the theory were shown to be flawed, score interpretations would by extension be suspect.

Example 1: A Multiple-Choice Examination

When performance on multiple-choice tests is used to make a decision about eligibility for licensure or certification, the appropriateness of the cut score will be a critical part of any validity argument supporting the interpretation that failing candidates are likely to lack some competency that is necessary for safe and competent practice. That said, it must be remembered that standard setting decisions are policy judgments; they are not scientifically verifiable. Given this reality, Kane has argued that appropriate evidence to support the use of a cut score will demonstrate that the procedure used to establish the standard was appropriate.[52] Information about the choice of procedure, selection of judges, and implementation of the procedure will be central.

The credibility of the decision rule is central to score interpretation for high-stakes standardized tests, but this does not reduce the potential importance of theory-based assumptions. For example, the use of multiple-choice items may be based on the theoretical assumption that the knowledge and judgment required to respond to such items represent a necessary prerequisite for decision-making in practice. While high scores may not provide assurance of good performance in practice (because many other factors can have an influence), low scores on a well-designed test may indicate sufficiently serious knowledge deficits that are unlikely to allow for good performance in practice. These connections represent a theory about clinical decision-making: if the theory is shown to be flawed, the validity of the associated scores similarly will be undermined.

Example 2: Performance Assessment

Performance assessments (including standardized patient based examinations) sometimes are used to make classification decisions in medical schools or postgraduate education; and in these situations, failing examinees may be required to complete remedial training. When this is done, the assessment takes on the characteristics of a placement test because the test scores result in placing learners in either the standard education track or a remedial program. Evidence to support the decision rule(s) used in this setting might include results demonstrating that learners classified as requiring remediation will show differential improvement when exposed to the remediation program. Alternatively, evidence could be collected to demonstrate that learners so identified have a significantly greater chance of succeeding in future training if they complete the remediation program.

Scoring procedures for performance assessments also may be based, either implicitly or explicitly, on theoretical assumptions about how information is to be aggregated in drawing conclusions about competence. Decisions will need to be made about the relative value of thoroughness and efficiency. Similarly, decisions may need to be made about the importance of physical examination maneuvers. If the practitioner will confirm both negative and positive results with a diagnostic test, the theoretical basis for drawing conclusions about the learner's diagnostic ability based on their use of a nondiscriminating physical examination maneuver would be questionable at best. These comments are not intended to advocate for or against specific approaches to scoring such examinations; they are intended to highlight the fact that the structure of the scoring procedure ultimately rests on a theoretical view of the diagnostic process, and the strength of that model limits the extent to which scores can be interpreted with respect to the learner's diagnostic competency.

Example 3: Workplace-Based Assessment

As with the formats discussed previously, assessments based on direct observation will depend on theoretical assumptions. Assumptions about the nature of the construct being assessed will dictate the choice of process as opposed to product or outcome measures. Similarly, theories relating to expert-novice differences or cognitive theories about the nature of the medical diagnosis process—and, more broadly, medical decision-making—may influence the data that are collected, the way those data are aggregated, and the way the resulting scores are interpreted.

WBAs often are the basis for feedback to a learner. In this case, it may be that no explicit decision is made based on the scores. In other instances, however, promotional or other high-stakes decisions may be made based at least in part on the results of these assessments. In this circumstance, an implicit (if not explicit) cut score must exist. The argument for this use of the scores will require evidence to support the reasonableness of the cut score or, more broadly, the decision process. The fact that the implicit cut score may be built into the definition of the score scale rather than the result of a separate standard-setting process does not reduce the importance of this part of the validity argument. Such a circumstance might exist when the observer must rate a performance as "adequate" or "inadequate." The definition of the rating may make establishing a cut score unnecessary, but evidence that the definition of "adequate" corresponds to a skill level that is appropriate to support a specific decision still is needed.

Consequential Validity and Program Evaluation

In this chapter, the validity argument has been presented as the accumulation of scientific evidence to evaluate the credibility of intended score interpretations. We would, however, be remiss not to discuss the broader understanding of validity that has existed within the educational measurement community for the past 50 years.

Cronbach,[10] Messick,[8] and Kane[7] all emphasized the importance of what has come to be known as consequential validity. There has been debate over the years about whether the consequences associated with a testing program belong within the definition of validity. In the end, it may not matter whether evaluation of the consequences of a testing program are considered part of validity. What matters is the clear understanding that just as the test developer has a responsibility to evaluate the evidence that supports inferences made based on test scores, the test developer has a responsibility to evaluate the intended and unintended consequences of the testing program. Whether implemented within the classroom or on a national or international level, testing has consequences; programmatic review of the positive and negative consequences therefore is an important responsibility. The importance of evaluating the intended consequences should be obvious. If a licensing examination is implemented with the explicit purpose of protecting the health of the public from individuals who lack the knowledge, skills, and attitudes necessary to provide safe and competent care, it is reasonable to expect evidence indicating that the program is contributing to that outcome. Similarly, if a test is a part of a program of formative assessment intended to accelerate learning, good intentions are not sufficient. Evidence is needed to support the view that the assessment program leads to improved educational outcomes.

Reasonable program evaluation for a testing program must provide evidence about the extent to which the program is having the intended outcome; it also must examine the extent to which the program is producing unintended consequences. In the case of a licensing examination, one possible unintended consequence is the impact that the test content has on the curriculum of training programs (e.g., medical schools). Typically, a licensing examination will assess only a subset of the knowledge and skills needed for practice. If this leads to a narrowing of the curriculum, a program intended to ensure the competency of healthcare providers actually may have a negative impact on the training system. (It is worth noting that the same issue may arise with progress testing in medical schools.) Good intentions do not ensure uniformly good outcomes.

Test content, format, and scoring procedures all may have unintended consequences. Consider a test of clinical skills in which an individual's competence in taking a patient history is scored using a checklist that awards points for asking specific relevant questions of the patient. The checklist score might provide a useful surrogate for a more nuanced and complex approach to collecting evidence for competence in clinical reasoning. It also might motivate students to collect a patient history using a "shotgun" approach: asking a broad range of questions to maximize the score rather than focusing on a more appropriate history-taking approach that supports inferences about competency in diagnostic reasoning.

There is, of course, an important difference between consequential validity and the rest of the validity evidence we have discussed to this point: the evaluation of consequences requires value-based judgments. The intended consequences of the testing program will—at least in the eyes of those responsible for the program—have a positive valence. Unintended consequences could be happy surprises that increase the value of the program, or they could represent unanticipated costs. Both the valence and the associated magnitude may be a function of the policy driving the program and the values of those evaluating the program. Consider, as a hypothetical example, a test impacting acceptance to, advancement in, or graduation from medical school. This hypothetical test has ample evidence to support the inferences as described in the previous pages, and yet use of the test has led to a reduction in the number of minority candidates entering practice. The argument-based approach to validity described in this chapter would need to include evidence that the differential performance was the result of *actual* differences in the competencies the test was intended to measure and *not* construct-irrelevant variance in the test scores. The decision about when and how to use the scores would require value-based judgments, and these values may differ for different stakeholder groups.

Conclusion

In this chapter we have conceptualized validity as a systematic argument in support of score interpretations. Reliability has been viewed as a component of the overall validity argument. The details of the specific examples should be viewed as unimportant, and whether a specific piece of evidence is seen as part of the *extrapolation* stage or the *decision* stage of the argument is secondary. *The central issue is that the overall argument must be complete and coherent.* There is no such thing as a valid test; the validity argument must focus on intended interpretations of test scores. To construct such an argument, researchers and users of the test scores must systematically and self-critically collect a wide array of evidence that provides clear insight into the credibility of those interpretations.

Placement of this chapter at the beginning of the volume is intentional, as the included concepts are critical for any serious consideration of measurement. Reliability and validity are at once nuanced yet simple concepts. Reliability is an evaluation of the stability or precision of a measure. In this regard, an individual's weight, A1C level, and competence in clinical reasoning share one essential thing in common: we would not give credence to a measure of any of these characteristics if we believed that we would get widely disparate results if we stepped off and back on the scale, repeated the reading on the same blood sample, or implemented an equivalent form of our assessment of clinical reasoning. Similarly, validity might be reduced to the question, does the test measure what it was intended to measure? Clearly, if the answer is no, we should not use the measure. Unfortunately, the answer to that question is not always obvious—face validity can be deceiving. Simply speaking, the centrality of reliability, and validity more broadly, cannot be overstated.

It also is important to note that the importance of these concepts is not linked to the specifics of the measurement. These issues are critical in high-stakes and low-stakes testing, assessments that produce numeric scores and assessments that result in text-based feedback, tests intended to measure individual differences and tests intended to measure an individual's relative strengths, tests that break down complex constructs into components and tests that holistically evaluate performance, tests that are used for formative purposes, tests that are used for summative purposes, and tests that are used for both.

As we have described in this chapter, reliability and validity are the foundation of the psychometric requirement that the interpretations we make based on test results are supported by evidence. The place of evidence in the interpretation of test results—evidence-based measurement—is no different than the place of evidence in evidence-based medicine. In both cases, collecting the evidence is hard work, but it is essential work.

Annotated Bibliography

1. Kane MT. Validating the interpretations and uses of test scores. *J Educ Measure.* 2013 Mar 14;50:1–73. doi:10.1111/jedm.12000.
This publication provides a current, in-depth discussion of Michael Kane's approach to validity and validation, describing the validation process as a structured argument in support of the intended interpretations made based on test scores.
2. Clauser BE, Margolis MJ, Case SM. Testing for licensure and certification in the professions. In: Brennan RL, ed. *Educational Measurement.* 4th ed. American Council on Education/Praeger; 2006:701–731.
This chapter provides an overview of assessment methods commonly used in licensure and certification examinations in the professions. It includes an expanded discussion of the evolution of validity and validation over the past century, and discusses additional applications of Kane's framework to assessment methods commonly used in the professions.
3. Cook DA, Brydges R, Ginsburg S, Hatala R. A contemporary approach to validity arguments: a practical guide to Kane's framework. *Med Educ.* 2015 Jun;49(6):560–575. doi:10.1111/medu.12678.
This paper provides a very readable introduction to Kane's validity framework for both quantitative and qualitative assessment methods commonly used in medical education. As a part of the discussion, it highlights some of the parallels between validation work and evaluation of diagnostic studies in medicine.
4. Cook DA, Zendejas B, Hamstra SJ, Hatala R, Brydges R. What counts as validity evidence? Examples and prevalence in a systematic review of simulation-based assessment. *Adv Health Sci Educ Theory Pract.* 2014 May;19(2):233–250. doi:10.1007/s10459-013-9458-4.
5. Cook DA, Brydges R, Zendejas B, Hamstra SJ, Hatala R. Technology-enhanced simulation to assess health professionals: a systematic review of validity evidence, research methods, and reporting quality. *Acad Med.* 2013 Jun;88(6):872–883. doi:10.1097/ACM.0b013e31828ffdcf.
Using the frameworks proposed by Messick and Kane, these systematic reviews summarize sources of validity evidence from studies of technology-enhanced simulation-based assessments, identifying methodological and reporting shortcomings and recommending directions for improvement in future research.
6. Hatala R, Cook DA, Brydges R, Hawkins R. Constructing a validity argument for the Objective Structured Assessment of Technical Skills (OSATS): a systematic review of validity evidence. *Adv Health Sci Educ Theory Pract.* 2015 Dec;20(5):1149–1175. doi:10.1007/s10459-015-9593-1.
This systematic review uses Kane's framework to analyze the validity argument for the objective structured assessment of technical skills (OSATS). They found that, in general, validity evidence supports the use of OSATS for formative feedback, but more research is required to support use of OSATS for making higher-stakes decisions.
7. Hawkins RE, Margolis MJ, Durning SJ, Norcini JJ. Constructing a validity argument for the mini-clinical evaluation exercise: a review of the research. *Acad Med.* 2010 Sep;85(9):1453–1461. doi:10.1097/ACM.0b013e3181eac3e6.

This systematic review of research conducted from 1995 to 2009 uses Kane's validity framework to evaluate validity evidence related to the mini clinical evaluation exercise (mini-CEX). It concludes that scoring-related issues (e.g., leniency error and high interitem correlations) limit the utility of the mini-CEX for providing feedback to trainees, though evidence related to the generalization and extrapolation components is generally supportive of the validity of mini-CEX score interpretations.

References

1. Gulliksen H. *Theory of Mental Tests*. John Wiley & Sons; 1950. doi:10.1037/13240-000.
2. Spearman C. Proof of the measurement of association between two things. *Am J Psychol*. 1904;15:72–101. doi:10.2307/1412159.
3. Spearman C. "General intelligence" objectively determined and measured. *Am J Psychol*. 1904;15:201–292. doi:10.2307/1412107.
4. Spearman C. Correlation calculated with faulty data. *Br J Psychol*. 1910;3:271–295.
5. Yoakum CS, Yerkes RM. *Mental Tests in the American Army*. Sidgwick & Jackson; 1920. doi:10.1111/j.2044-8295.1910.tb00206.x.
6. Cureton EE. Validity. In: Lindquist EF, ed. *Educational Measurement*. American Council on Education; 1951:621–694.
7. Kane MT. Validating the interpretations and uses of test scores. *J Educ Measure*. 2013 Mar 14;50:1–73. doi:10.1111/jedm.12000.
8. Messick S. Validity. In: Linn RL, ed. *Educational Measurement*. 3rd ed. American Council on Education/Macmillan; 1989:13–103.
9. Cronbach LJ, Meehl PE. Construct validity in psychological tests. *Psych Bull*. 1955 Jul;52(4):281–302. doi:10.1037/h0040957.
10. Cronbach LJ. Test validation. In: Thorndike RL, ed. *Educational Measurement*. 2nd ed. American Council on Education; 1971:443–507.
11. Campbell DT, Fiske DW. Convergent and divergent validation by the multitrait-multimethod matrix. *Psych Bull*. 1959 Mar;56(2):81–105. doi:10.1037/h0046016.
12. Loevinger J. Objective tests as instruments of psychological theory. *Psych Rep*. 1957 Jun;3:635–694. doi:10.2466/pr0.1957.3.3.635.
13. American Educational Research Association, American Psychological Association, National Council on Measurement in Education. *Standards for Educational and Psychological Testing*. American Educational Research Association; 1999.
14. Kane M. An argument-based approach to validation. *Psych Bull*. 1992;112(3):527–535. doi:10.1037/0033-2909.112.3.527.
15. Hodges B. Assessment in the post-psychometric era: learning to love the subjective and collective. *Med Teach*. 2013 Jul;35(7):564–568. doi:10.3109/0142159X.2013.789134.
16. Schuwirth LWT, van der Vleuten CPM. A history of assessment in medical education. *Adv Health Sci Educ*. 2020 Dec;25(5):1045–1056. doi:10.1007/s10459-020-10003-0.
17. Swanson DB, van der Vleuten CP. Assessment of clinical skills with standardized patients: state of the art revisited. *Teach Learn Med*. 2013;25(Suppl 1):S17–S25. doi:10.1080/10401334.2013.842916.
18. Norcini J, Burch V. Workplace-based assessment as an educational tool: AMEE Guide No. 31. *Med Teach*. 2007 Nov;29(9-10):855–871. doi:10.1080/01421590701775453.
19. Hicks PJ, Margolis MJ, Carraccio C, et al. A novel workplace-based assessment for competency-based decisions and learner feedback. *Med Teach*. 2018 Nov;40(11):1143–1150. doi:10.1080/0142159X.2018.1461204.
20. Hicks PJ, Margolis MJ, Poynter SE, et al. The Pediatrics Milestones Assessment Pilot: development of workplace-based assessment content, instruments, and processes. *Acad Med*. 2016 May;91(5):701–709. doi:10.1097/ACM.0000000000001057.
21. Kelly FJ. *The Kansas Silent Reading Tests*. The Kansas Printing Plant; 1915. doi:10.1037/h0073542.
22. Swanson DB, Clauser BE, Case SM. Clinical skills assessment with standardized patients in high-stakes tests: a framework for thinking about score precision, equating, and security. *Adv Health Sci Educ Theory Pract*. 1999;4(1):67–106. doi:10.1023/A:1009862220473.
23. Lord FM, Novick MR. *Statistical Theories of Mental Test Scores*. Addison-Wesley; 1968. doi:10.1177/001316446802800439.
24. Cronbach LJ, Gleser GC, Nanda H, Rajaratnam N. *The Dependability of Behavioral Measurements: Theory of Generalizability for Scores and Profiles*. John Wiley & Sons; 1972. doi:10.1126/science.178.4067.1275.
25. Brennan RL. *Generalizability Theory*. Springer-Verlag; 2001. doi:10.1007/978-1-4757-3456-0.
26. Brennan RL. An essay on the history and future of reliability from the perspective of replications. *J Educ Meas*. 2001;38(4):295–317. doi:10.1111/j.1745-3984.2001.tb01129.x.
27. Brown W. Some experimental results in the correlation of mental abilities. *Br J Psych*. 1910;3:296–322. doi:10.1111/j.2044-8295.1910.tb00207.x.
28. Kuder GF, Richardson MW. The theory of estimation of test reliability. *Psychometrika*. 1937;2:151–160. doi:10.1007/BF02288391.
29. Cronbach LJ. Coefficient alpha and the internal structure of tests. *Psychometrika*. 1951;16:297–334. doi:10.1007/BF02310555.
30. Angoff WH. Scales, norms, and equivalent scores. In: Thorndike RL, ed. *Educational Measurement*. 2nd ed. American Council on Education; 1971:508–600.
31. Hambleton RK, Swaminathan H. *Item Response Theory: Principles and Applications*. Kluwer-Nijhoff Publishing; 1985. doi:10.1007/978-94-017-1988-9.
32. Kolen MJ, Brennan RL. *Test Equating, Scaling, and Linking. Methods and Practices*. 3rd ed. Springer; 2014. doi:10.1007/978-1-4939-0317-7.
33. Cronbach LJ. My current thoughts on coefficient alpha and successor procedures. *Educ Psychol Measure*. 2004;64(3):391–418. doi:10.1177/0013164404266386.
34. Ericsson A, Smith J. Prospects and limitations of the empirical study of expertise: an introduction. In: Ericsson A, Smith J, eds. *Toward a General Theory of Expertise: Prospects and Limits*. Cambridge University Press; 1991.
35. Zapata-Rivera D. *Score Reporting Research and Applications*. Routledge; 2018. doi:10.4324/9781351136501.
36. Kelley TL. *Interpretation of Educational Measurements*. World Book; 1927.
37. Lord FM. Elementary models for measuring change. In: Harris CW, ed. *Problems in Measuring Change*. Wisconsin Press; 1963.
38. Norcini J, Anderson B, Bollela V, et al. Criteria for good assessment: consensus statement and recommendations from the Ottawa 2010 Conference. *Med Teach*. 2011;33(3):206–214. doi:10.3109/0142159X.2011.551559.
39. Norcini J, Anderson MB, Bollela V, et al. Consensus framework for good assessment. *Med Teach*. 2018 Nov;40(11):1102–1109. doi:10.1080/0142159X.2018.1500016.
40. Price D, Swanson DB, Irons M, Hawkins RE. Longitudinal assessments in continuing specialty certification and lifelong learning. *Med Teach*. 2018 Sep;40(9):917–919. doi:10.1080/0142159X.2018.1471202.

41. Clauser BE, Margolis MJ, Case SM. Testing for licensure and certification in the professions. In: Brennan RL, ed. *Educational Measurement*. 4th ed. American Council on Education/Praeger; 2006:701–731.
42. Cronbach LJ. Validity on parole: how can we go straight? New directions for testing and measurement: measuring achievement over a decade. *Proceedings of the 1979 ETS Invitational Conference*. Jossey-Bass; 1980:99–108.
43. Norori N, Hu Q, Aellen FM, Faraci FD, Tzovara A. Addressing bias in big data and AI for health care: A call for open science. *Patterns (N Y)*. 2021 Oct 8;2(10):100347. doi:10.1016/j.patter.2021.100347.
44. Cuddy MM, Dillon GF, Clauser BE, et al. Assessing the validity of the USMLE Step 2 Clinical Knowledge Examination through an evaluation of its clinical relevance. *Acad Med*. 2004 Oct;79(10 Suppl):S43–S45. doi:10.1097/00001888-200410001-00013.
45. Cuddy MM, Young A, Gelman A, et al. Exploring the relationship among USMLE performance and disciplinary action in practice: a validity study of score inferences from a licensure examination. *Acad Med*. 2017 Dec;92(12):1780–1785. doi:10.1097/ACM.0000000000001747.
46. Norcini JJ, Lipner RS, Kimball HR. Certifying examination performance and patient outcomes following acute myocardial infarction. *Med Educ*. 2002 Sep;36(9):853–859. doi:10.1046/j.1365-2923.2002.01293.x.
47. Norcini JJ, Boulet JR, Opalek A, Dauphinee WD. The relationship between licensing examination performance and the outcomes of care by international medical school graduates. *Acad Med*. 2014 Aug;89(8):1157–1162. doi:10.1097/ACM.0000000000000310.
48. Tamblyn R, Abrahamowicz M, Dauphinee WD, et al. Association between licensure examination scores and practice in primary care. *JAMA*. 2002 Dec 18;288(23):3019–3026. doi:10.1001/jama.288.23.3019.
49. Swanson DB, Roberts TE. Trends in national licensing examinations in medicine. *Med Educ*. 2016 Jan;50(1):101–114. doi:10.1111/medu.12810.
50. Harik P, Feinberg RA, Clauser BE. How examinees use time: examples from a medical licensing examination. In: Margolis MJ, Feinberg RA, eds. Integrating Timing Considerations to Improve Standardized Testing Practices. Routledge; 2020: 73–89. doi:10.4324/9781351064781-6.
51. Margolis MJ, Clauser BE, Cuddy MM, et al. Use of the mini-CEX to rate examinee performance on a multiple-station clinical skills examination: a validity study. *Acad Med*. 2006 Oct;81(10 Suppl):S56–S60. doi:10.1097/01.ACM.0000236514.53194.f4.
52. Kane M. Validating the performance standards associated with passing scores. *Rev Educ Res*. 1994;64:425–461. doi:10.2307/1170678.

3

Programmatic Assessment Using Systems Thinking

ERIC S. HOLMBOE, MD

CHAPTER OUTLINE

Overview of Chapter

The introduction of competency-based medical education (CBME) has catalyzed advancements in assessment as highlighted throughout this textbook. Yet much work remains to be done to realize the full promise of CBME. Programmatic assessment provides the information needed for feedback, to support coaching, determine appropriate supervision levels, support the creation of individualized learning plans, inform progress decisions, and most importantly, help ensure that patients and families receive high-quality, safe care in the training environment and the future practice setting of graduates. Many training programs have not fully implemented programmatic assessment that includes assessment of all the key core competencies needed for effective clinical practice, such as a systems view of professionalism, interprofessional teamwork, quality improvement and patient safety, care coordination, systems thinking, and evidence-based practice (EBP), to name a few.

It is important to distinguish programmatic assessment from a simple, nonintegrated program of assessment. Programmatic assessment requires a systematic, longitudinal approach (i.e., systems thinking) in its design and execution. A key feature of programmatic assessment is the systematic approach to how data are synthesized and combined for purposes of judgment, feedback, and support of professional development. In many typical programs of assessment, data are often combined only when they have the same format to produce a score for a single competency domain or category of assessment (e.g., one objective structured clinical exam [OSCE] station with another OSCE station to produce a mean score or average outcome, or results from in-training multiple-choice exams).

Programmatic assessment seeks to synthesize, combine, and triangulate information so that it meaningfully contributes to a more holistic understanding of where the learner is in their journey and what they and the program can do with the learner to best support their longitudinal professional development. The term *programmatic* explicitly incorporates systems and developmental thinking. Finally, I want to briefly distinguish programmatic assessment from program evaluation (see Chapter 18). Program evaluation involves analyzing the performance of the educational system, training program, and all its interacting parts needed for changes in curriculum, assessment practices, and the learning environment; an educational system is made up of more than just its individual learners. Programmatic assessment of individual learners is thus one critical component of program evaluation. Many other sources of information will be important in formulating judgments about program quality and informing change and improvement strategies in the training program (see Chapter 18).

The chapters that follow will address specific assessment approaches needed to assess all the competencies (i.e., abilities) required for mastery in clinical practice. This chapter will guide the reader in how to improve assessment practices and assemble all the assessment components, or "parts," into an integrated and effective programmatic assessment approach to produce accurate entrustment decisions supported by strong validity evidence, and addresses the pernicious effects of bias. Although we have discussed important potential differences in terminology, "programs of assessment" will be interchangeable in this chapter with "programmatic assessment" with the understanding that both refer to a systematic, integrated, and longitudinal approach.

Overview of Programmatic Assessment

The growing recognition of serious deficiencies in healthcare in the late 20th century led to an examination of medical education's role in healthcare system performance. One result of this examination was to pressure the medical education enterprise to shift the focus and design of medical education programs to be outcomes based. However, uptake of an outcomes-based approach has varied around the world based on local needs and culture, and this is an important consideration for anyone implementing programmatic assessment.

Competency-based models are the primary approach to implementing outcomes-based medical education. Competencies, defined as "observable abilities of a health professional, integrating multiple components such as knowledge, skills, values and attitudes," are the predominant framework used to define learners' educational outcomes (see Chapter 1).[1] CBME depends on effective programmatic assessment to achieve the desired outcome goals of training. Using a systems lens, programmatic assessment can be defined as a group of integrated and related assessment *activities* (or methods) that are managed in a coordinated manner. These interdependent activities have a common goal or success "vision" under *integrated* management and are embedded in systems. Systems thinking acknowledges that the components and activities of an assessment program are *interdependent* and must work together to accomplish the shared aims of a training program.

Effective programmatic assessment, using a systems perspective, most importantly involves a *group of people who work together on a regular basis to perform assessment and provide feedback to a population of trainees over a period of time, and share:*[2]

- Educational goals and outcomes
- Linked individual learner assessments and program evaluation processes (see Chapter 18)
- Information about learner performance to support professional development
- A desire to produce a learner optimally prepared to enter the next phase of training and ultimately enable all graduates to deliver high-quality and safe care

The good news is that there have been meaningful advances in assessment practices and educators' assessment toolbox is more robust than ever. There have been substantial strides since the launch of multiple nationally based initiatives, such as the Graduate Medical Education (GME) Outcome project and the Undergraduate Medical Education (UME) Medical School Objectives Projects (MSOP) in the United States, the Canadian Medical Education Directives for Specialists (CanMEDS) initiative in Canada, and Good Medical Practice in the United Kingdom (and similar efforts in other countries) over the past 25 years (see Chapter 1). However, UME and GME training programs still face challenging barriers undermining the implementation of assessment programs that effectively integrate all assessments into a synthetic, holistic judgment about preparedness for the next stage of a professional's career.[3–6]

For example, too many UME and GME programs still rely heavily on processes designed and implemented based on a hypothesized equivalence between satisfactory completion of educational activity(ies) and competence. In this framing, faculty and programs mostly use assessments to determine whether satisfactory completion of the activity or program has occurred, and often rely on proxies, such as oral (case-based) patient presentations and multiple-choice in-training examination performance as evidence that a learner possesses sufficient knowledge, skills, and attitudes across core competencies. High-stakes testing, such as licensing and certification examinations, are another proxy assessment used to provide assurance that the learner has satisfactorily completed a stage of training. Abundant evidence now exists that overreliance on these assessment proxies produces variable educational outcomes and fails to adequately assess critical workplace-based abilities such as systems-based practice, professionalism, interprofessional teamwork, and practice-based learning and improvement competencies in the United States, and key competencies in other countries' frameworks (see Chapter 1 for the crosswalk among competency frameworks). Fundamentally, one major tension faced by health professions educational systems is between educational activities that may lead to better short-term performance on isolated, single assessments (as assessed within a traditional assessment program that relies heavily on examinations and other assessments *of* learning) and programmatic assessment designed to support professional developmental learning trajectories (with a predominant focus on assessment *for* learning).[7]

Training programs must embrace three core principles to realize the full potential of programmatic assessment to enable the achievement of desired medical education outcomes. This chapter will provide guidance on effective practices in creating programmatic assessment, along with tools the reader can use to judge their own programs of assessment. I will use a systems lens to help the reader build, review, and reflect on their programs of assessment.

Three Overarching Principles to Improve Programmatic Assessment

Programmatic Assessment Must Support Professional Development

Past and current assessment practices have and are overly focused on learners' demonstrations of knowledge or skills at limited, specific points in time. For example, the US medical education system especially places a heavy reliance on assessment proxies to determine clinical competence, such as single-point-in-time, high-stakes examinations or end-of-rotation summative assessments completed by faculty. This overreliance on point-in-time, summative assessments fails to support a developmental or growth mindset among learners, faculty, and training programs.[8,9]

It is well established that learners have different learning trajectories that vary by specific competencies within the individual.[10] The current design of most of our educational programs, from curriculum to assessment, disregards this reality and treats each individual learner as a monolithic product moving along a disjointed curricular and assessment assembly line. For example, most assessments fail to incorporate theories and empiric evidence for deliberate practice in attaining expertise, stage models of learner development, and mastery-based learning.[3,11,12] Using a developmental lens, assessment *for* learning is much more important than assessment *of* learning. Yet learners rarely have access to timely assessments, which prevents them from using assessment results to set goals and action plans. Learners must have full and ongoing access to their assessment information, ideally in the form of a learning portfolio, but also have ongoing support to meaningfully aggregate and synthesize their assessment information into learning plans and future activities (see Chapter 15). Programmatic assessment without some form of coaching/mentoring rarely works (see Chapter 14). Additionally, assessments in CBME must be developmentally designed where what the learner *cannot* do is as important to identify as what they *can* do.

A developmental approach that encourages a growth mindset should be the foundation for significantly redesigning instructional methods, learning experiences, and assessment practices.[8–12] Training programs should focus on promoting learner growth and development in the desired competencies through frequent assessment that is rich in feedback associated with individualized coaching.[13] In 2019, Elaine Van Melle and colleagues outlined five core components for CBME (see Chapter 1):

1. Competencies required for practice are clearly articulated.
2. Competencies and their developmental markers are arranged and sequenced progressively.
3. Learning experiences are tailored to facilitate the progressive development of competencies.
4. Teaching practices promote the progressive development of competencies.
5. Assessment practices support and document the progressive development of competencies.

Importantly, the core components framework is grounded in a growth mindset fully cognizant of the individualized trajectories each learner will experience.[13] Traditional assessment programs, and especially those that are still operating from the perspective of objectively measuring competence, start from a deficiency mindset model. In this model, outcomes of assessment are defined in terms of deficiency; for example, a student with a score of 75% on an examination or OSCE is more deficient than someone with a score of 85%. Everything that doesn't "load" onto a single scaled score is essentially ignored. Furthermore, while the score provides a judgment and ranking, the score alone is almost completely useless in providing the guidance needed to support future training activities and professional development.

In programmatic assessment, by combining multiple "bits" of information over time from various and multiple assessment sources, a personal narrative is produced that allows for a more diverse and holistic view of the developing learner. Programmatic assessment embraces a diversity model and therefore recognizes the individualized trajectories of each learner. Training programs should focus on frequent formative assessments that are rich in feedback and individualized coaching. Educators and programs must therefore design and use assessment tools that support the developmental trajectories of learners and integrate them into a program of assessment, or programmatic assessment, that supports the learner's professional development.[13] This is not meant to undermine the importance of a summative assessment around progression decisions such as whether a learner is ready to advance to the next level of training or ultimately graduate to unsupervised practice. In the end, if the training program treats the results (e.g., ratings, narrative comments, etc.) of each individual learner assessment event as formative ("here is where you are") and incorporates feedback and learning goals with subsequent results on the follow-up activities and assessments as the key inputs into summative judgments, you would still have an assessment *for* learning program.

Addressing Bias and Fairness in Programmatic Assessment

There is an urgent need to confront and address the persistent and pernicious effects of bias in medical education and assessment. Bias can occur at multiple levels. Structural bias involves institutional (e.g., medical schools, hospitals) patterns and practices that provide advantage to some groups and disadvantage to other groups based on personal and demographic characteristics and identity. At the individual level, explicit bias refers to *conscious* beliefs and attitudes one possesses about another person or groups. Implicit bias refers to an individual's "prejudicial attitudes towards and stereotypical beliefs about a particular social group or members therein."[14] These individual attitudes are often *subconscious*. A growing body of literature describes the factors contributing to, and the harmful effects of, implicit bias and educational inequity on learners who are underrepresented in medicine (URiM) or otherwise at risk for marginalization in assessment practices. It is also important to note that the makeup of URiM groups can vary by country.

Bias affects learners broadly—from the interpersonal dynamics of teaching dyads or teams to structural phenomena, such as standardized exams with grade cutoffs. Hagiwara et al. note that implicit bias has both affective and cognitive components and educators must recognize the distinction between prejudice and stereotyping when considering interventions to reduce implicit bias in assessment.[14] Prejudice relates to the negative attitudes individuals form toward other persons or groups often in advance or without any actual experience with the affected individuals. Stereotyping refers to rigid, fixed, and overgeneralized beliefs about a specific group of people. Prejudicial attitudes and stereotypical beliefs are often activated spontaneously and can produce changes in an individual's teaching and assessment behaviors. Likewise, structures and policies can recapitulate these ingrained behaviors to create a biased and inequitable learning environment.

Assessment occurs within the inextricably linked learning and working environments[15,16] where faculty responsibilities reside in the overlapping domains of patient care and education. Structural factors at the community and institutional levels can negatively affect the training of all learners in the combined learning-working environment. For example, inequities in community access to healthcare due to racism, xenophobia, and other biases produce suboptimal care for marginalized groups that may inculcate suboptimal clinical care behaviors in learners. Explicitly learning and understanding community-level factors affecting healthcare, a core tenet of systems-based practice in the United States, is crucial for learners. Institutions should routinely examine their own clinical care measures for evidence of bias and inequitable care and share that information with programs and learners to help drive improvement in both education and clinical practice.

When learners experience structural bias, it results in suboptimal learning environments, which compromise learners' well-being and ability to function at the top of their skills. Multiple studies have found that learners from groups historically URiM receive lower assessment ratings from faculty.[12,13] There are racial disparities in exam score grading and fewer admissions to honor's societies even when corrected for grades and other factors.[17–19] These effects are cumulative. Small differences in assessment translate to disparities in future opportunities, including training and employment, a phenomenon described as the amplification cascade.[20]

At the program level, conflicting priorities, time constraints, and burnout can lower the threshold for faculty to unconsciously apply their activated biases to their assessments of students. Bias affects learners and faculty through multiple phenomena that play themselves out intra- and interpersonally. Learners from URiM groups experience social isolation and heightened visibility that can lead to and reinforce stereotype threat and impostor syndrome.[21] Learners can also experience hostility and prejudice from patients and families, which may lead to sidelining or exclusion from patient care if teams are not equipped to handle difficult interpersonal dynamics with patients. Learners also experience different expectations in the preclerkship and clerkship settings.[22–25]

Fairness is another essential principle needed to reduce the harmful effects of bias. Valentine and colleagues have published several studies, including a systematic review, that have led to a conceptual model codifying what constitutes a fair program of assessment.[26–28] The model contains three interdependent domains: judgment decisions, individual assessor characteristics, and system factors (Fig. 3.1). Judgment decisions must be transparent, defensible, credible, and fit for purpose. Important individual characteristics include the need of narrative for the learner that supports defensibility, creditability, and transparency; evidence to support the assessment judgment, such as the link of a competency performance to better patient care; boundaries that specifically address what is *not* pertinent to an assessment decision such as race and ethnicity as discussed earlier; expertise in both clinical care and assessment; and finally, agility to manage and acknowledge ambiguity, uncertainty, and context in assessment events.

As noted at the outset of the chapter, systems thinking is essential for programmatic assessment. Systems fairness factors identified by Valentine and colleagues include procedural, such as due process in remediation decisions (see Chapter 17); documentation that is clear, robust and accessible to the learner; multiple opportunities for assessment; multiple assessors involved in providing assessment information; and ongoing and persistent pursuit of the validity evidence to support assessment judgments and assessment approaches used as part of programmatic assessment. To Valentine's model, I would add the need to use the core principles of translational (bench to bedside) science and quality improvement to mitigate individual and structural bias.[2,29]

Programmatic Assessment Must Use a Systems-Thinking Approach

Supporting professional development while reducing bias and enhancing fairness requires robust, thoughtfully designed programmatic assessment. Assessment programs are best viewed as a subsystem within a training program. A system can be simply defined as "two or more interdependent parts that work together to accomplish a shared aim."[30] Assessment programs possess a number of components or parts (called structures within a system), including people (learners, peers, faculty, interprofessional team members, and increasingly, groups of experts, commonly called clinical competency committees [CCCs], that judge learner progress), tools (e.g., exams, case presentations, faculty assessment forms, mini-clinical evaluation exercise [mini-CEX], etc.), and technology (e.g., learning management systems, smartphone apps). People are the most important components of a system. Fig. 3.2 provides an overview of

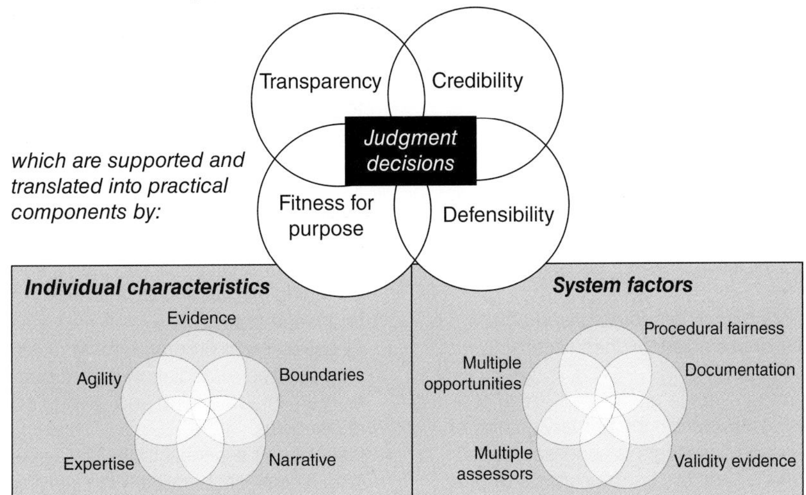

• **Fig. 3.1** Valentine framework for fairness in health professions education assessment. (From Valentine N, Durning S, Shanahan EM, Schuwirth L. Fairness in human judgement in assessment: a hermeneutic literature review and conceptual framework. *Adv Health Sci Educ Theory Pract*. 2021 May;26(2):713–738. doi:10.1007/s10459-020-10002-1.)

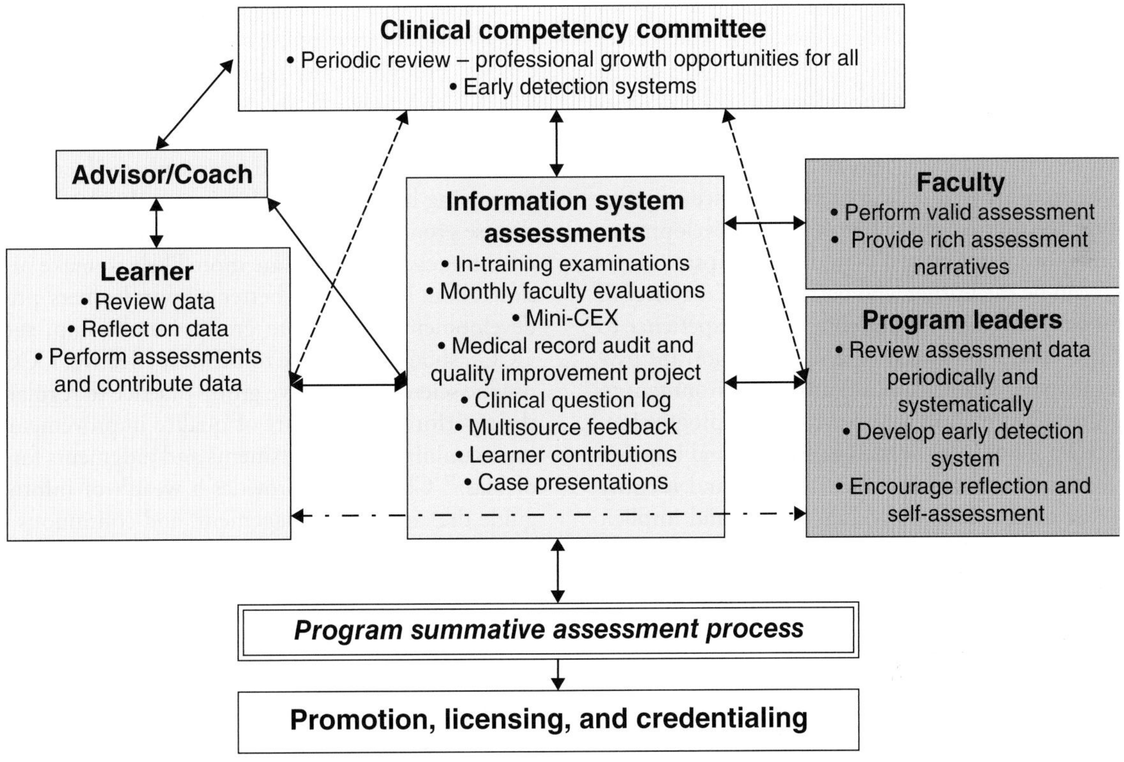

• **Fig. 3.2** Assessment structures: key components and actors.

some of the critical parts, or structures, of an assessment system and highlights the multiple connections, or interdependencies, among the components. The figure notes the centrality of the information "hub" that is typically housed within an electronic learning management system or portfolio. All the important agents in the system, such as the learner, faculty, clinical competency committees, and advisors, interact with the assessment information to support professional development.

Using systems thinking, an assessment program should function as a group of people, including the learners, who regularly work together to perform, review, and reflect on

• BOX 3.1 Core Principles of Effective Programmatic Assessment

- The training program has a centrally coordinated master assessment plan that aligns with and supports a curricular vision.
- Competence is specific, not generic. Assessment programs must sample across different clinical contexts *longitudinally* over training using multiple assessors.
- Use of quantitative (numeric) scales is not better than qualitative (words and narratives) data (see Chapters 5 and 6). Qualitative assessment can provide valuable information and insights. Since use of rating scales involves translating observations and/or questions into a numeric code, the numeric code is only useful if it is an accurate translation of developmental ability.
- Assessors must use credible clinical standards based on the best available clinical and systems science when assessing care provided to patients and families.
- Validity ultimately resides in the users (e.g., faculty, CCCs) of an assessment instrument as assessors are the primary source of variance. Training and preparing assessors is necessary to fully realize CBME's potential and reduce the harmful effects of bias.
- The assessment program must have a robust system for collecting information that is feasible and readily accessible to both learners and those performing the assessments.
- Learners should be provided opportunities to perform some of their own assessments and also be empowered to seek assessment from trusted faculty.
- Learners should have ready access to information-rich feedback to promote self-regulated learning. Learner access to assessment information supports transparency and the learner's agency—"nothing about me without me."[36]
- All assessments, especially lower-stakes assessments (i.e., formative assessments for learning), should always lead to meaningful feedback and coaching.
- All assessment programs should provide learners with advisors (see Fig. 3.2) who can serve as a sounding board and trusted partner in interpreting ("sense making") of assessment data and judgments.
- All assessment programs must possess systematic and personalized remediation for the purpose of supporting learners in addressing and closing competency gaps and deficiencies.
- Coaching is essential to facilitate effective use of assessment data for reflection and to plan learning.
- Expert groups, such as CCCs that use effective, bias-free decision-making practices, make decisions regarding learner progress and readiness for advancement.

CBME, Competency-based medical education; *CCCs*, clinical competency committees.

assessments, and provide feedback, coaching, and career guidance throughout training. The group must possess shared mental models of desired educational goals and outcomes and integrate individual assessments into holistic views of professional development.[31,32] This requires unbiased feedback and the feed-forward of learner performance to effectively support the learners' overall professional development. When training programs possess high degrees of psychological safety, it can be the learner who performs the majority of the feed-forward activity from one educational experience to the next. The institution and program must prioritize psychological safety within the clinical learning environment to effectively share information to support learner progression. Assessment data should also be used to evaluate and improve both the assessment program and curriculum and identify and address structural bias, individual explicit and implicit bias, and prejudice (see Chapter 18 on program evaluation). Van der Vleuten, Schuwirth, Hauer, and their colleagues have laid out the key principles that should guide the creation, development, and ongoing continuous improvement of programmatic assessment, summarized in Box 3.1.[33–35] In addition, involvement of the learner is essential, embracing a "nothing about me without me" mindset.[36]

Importance of Groups in Programmatic Assessment

When groups use effective practices, they make better judgments.[37] Having CCCs make judgments about learner development is an increasingly important design component of programmatic assessment.[37,38] Well-designed group processes enhance educational judgment by providing a mechanism for developing shared mental models of competencies through faculty training in assessment (see Chapter 16).[31] Conversely, poorly designed or implemented group processes can worsen educational judgments. Importantly, bias can be either mitigated or exacerbated by group process. A growing body of research suggests that high-performing, diverse groups (e.g., groups that implement evidence-based effective team practices) are more likely to make better decisions about learners and better support learners' professional development.[37] Therefore group membership, such as for CCCs, should be diverse to be most effective. CCCs should use the science of effective group practice to regularly review their performance as part of quality improvement, including examining their assessments and judgments for evidence of bias.[37] Chapter 16 provides a wealth of information to guide the creation, management, and continuous improvement of group process and CCCs.

Importance of Longitudinal Design Thinking in Programmatic Assessment

Given health professions education is an intensely developmental process that occurs over time and a continuum of a career, assessment programs must logically be longitudinal in design.[35] Van der Vleuten and colleagues nicely described this longitudinal process (Fig. 3.3).

There are several key concepts in this figure. First, the assessment activities are aligned with the curricular activities: assessment drives learning *and* learning drives the right type of assessment. For example, imagine a primary care physician trainee learning to care for patients with chronic conditions such as diabetes, hypertension, congestive heart

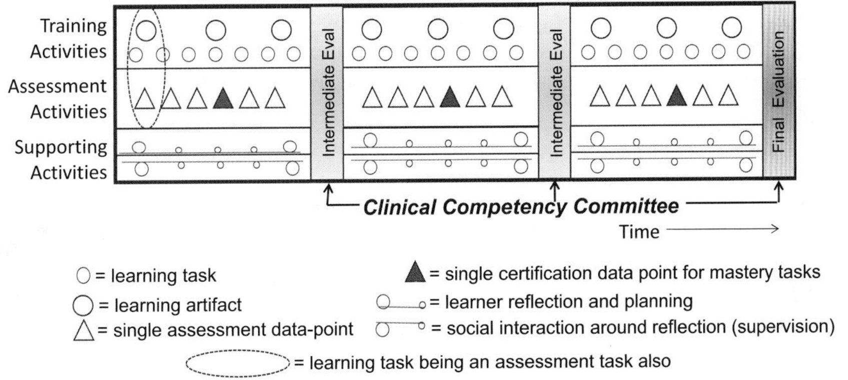

• **Fig. 3.3** Model for programmatic assessment. (From van der Vleuten CP, Schuwirth LW, Driessen EW, et al. A model for programmatic assessment fit for purpose. *Med Teach*. 2012;34(3):205-214. doi: 10.3109/0142159X.2012.652239.)

failure, and so forth. We now know from years of research that effective care of chronic conditions requires a coordinated effort among multiple health professionals (e.g., nurse case managers, pharmacists, social work, etc.) working as an interprofessional team.[39] In addition, informed decision-making and coproduction with patients and families is essential.[39] Thus the clinical curriculum ("learning") must include all of these elements and clinical experiences. The assessments should target these competencies, and the best assessment approaches in this example would include multiple-source feedback for interprofessional abilities (see Chapter 12) and direct observation for the informed decision-making abilities (see Chapter 5).

These assessments will accrue over time, especially direct observations that should occur multiple times with different patients and contexts. At some juncture, usually prespecified as part of the assessment program, all the assessment data are collated, analyzed, and reviewed by a group such as a CCC to judge the learner's developmental trajectory and create an individualized learning plan an advisor will use with the learner to plan (coproduce) the next cycle of learning.

If this longitudinal, integrated process works effectively, the final evaluation session will be mostly a quality assurance check to ensure that the learner is truly ready to graduate from their current program. As van der Vleuten points out, this final review is a "heavy," high-stakes summative entrustment decision (Fig. 3.4). This final judgment must have been preceded by many moments of feedback with a learning coach/mentor during the entire training program. An important principle is that the final decision should never come as a surprise to the learner.

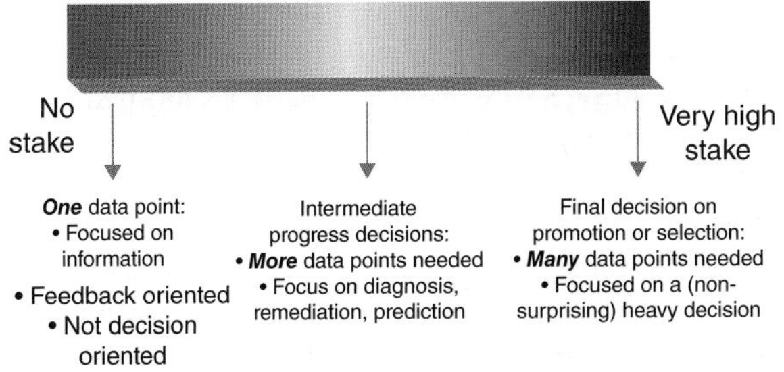

• **Fig. 3.4** Continuum of assessment stakes.

Specific Opportunities to Improve Programmatic Assessment

Gain Clarity Around the "Why" of Assessment

Multiple factors, including the profound impact of the COVID-19 pandemic on UME and GME around the globe, have led to a healthy reexamination of assessment practices. The medical education community is realizing that we need more developmentally focused assessment, grounded in clinical practice—especially toward the latter stages of training in the health professions (see Chapter 1). A developmental mindset requires significant rethinking of the purpose of assessment to better support professional development, feedback, and coaching.[8,9,40] This will require a greater focus on workplace-based assessment (WBA) because, unlike other assessments, WBAs can provide more timely, longitudinal feedback and occur at the point of care with patients and families. Technology is also enabling more efficient implementation of WBA with greater ability to capture narrative assessment using natural language processing (NLP) on smartphones.[41,42] Table 3.1 provides a list of the "W's" that programs should ask themselves about concerning their assessment program.

Ensure Comprehensive and Fair Coverage of All Core Competencies

No single assessment tool or approach can sufficiently judge and support a learner's professional development. Table 3.2 provides a matrix and combination of approaches that can assess all six general competencies currently used in the United States for GME and continuous professional development. This matrix applies equally well to other competency frameworks highlighted in Chapter 1. Ideally, competency frameworks

TABLE 3.1 The 6 W's of Assessment to Ensure Clarity of Purpose

The W	Description
Why	Why should the assessment be used? The purpose of the assessment tool should be connected to a meaningful educational outcome.
Who	Who should perform (e.g., observations) or administer the assessment (e.g., exams)?
What	What is the content or focus of the assessment tool (e.g., what knowledge or skills will be ascertained)?
Ho**w**	How will the assessment be conducted and completed? This should include details about assessor training.
When	When and how often should an assessment tool should be used?
Where	Where should the assessment be applied? This includes the setting where the assessment will be used (e.g., ambulatory clinic, operating room, etc.).

and programmatic assessment should better align across the UME–GME continuum.

To ensure comprehensive coverage, programs should complete an assessment map that includes where, when, and how the competency is being taught, experienced, and assessed (and must include more than one tool or method per competency). Assessment maps are a good way to ensure that all core competencies are being properly assessed (see Appendix 3.1 for an example using the US competency framework). The map also can help identify competencies receiving insufficient attention. In many locales around the world, that includes quality improvement and patient safety, interprofessional teamwork, care coordination such as daily handoffs and patient discharge, interpersonal communication skills, EBP, and systems thinking.[43,44]

Providing high-quality healthcare requires integrated contributions of all members of the interprofessional care team. Indeed, most care is provided by teams, not individuals acting in silos. However, the predominant lens for most assessment is attribution, not contribution. Attribution in assessment, meaning the results of an assessment can be clearly and predominantly attributed to the learner, may infer that the quality or safety of a clinical care process or outcome was only the direct result of a particular learner's clinical skills. Contribution, in contrast, implies that the quality or safety of clinical care is the result of the interdependent contributions from all healthcare professions involved with the patient's care. This creates a challenging situation where assessment is viewed as unfair if a specific patient care outcome cannot be predominantly attributed to the learner. Moving forward, assessment programs will have to pay greater attention to how the learner, in collaboration with the team, contributed to the patient's care and outcomes.[45] Even in competencies such as clinical reasoning, group involvement using distributed and situated cognition can lead to reductions in diagnostic and therapeutic errors (see Chapter 8).[46] Therefore, going forward, it will be important to discern not only the individual learner's contributions to care, but also how that learner contributes to the effectiveness of their teams.

Rebalance the Focus of Programmatic Assessment to Emphasize More Work-Based Assessments

As noted earlier, assessment programs overemphasize high-stakes assessments, such as clerkship grades, single-event tests, and end-of-rotation summative faculty evaluations, that can undermine timely formative assessments that better support professional development. As a learner progresses along the continuum, assessment programs should shift the balance of assessments to WBAs that trained groups (e.g., CCCs) can integrate and synthesize into developmental judgments, such as Accreditation Council for Graduate Medical Education (ACGME) Milestones, the Royal College of Physicians and Surgeons of Canada's (RCPSC's) Entrustable Professional Activities (EPAs), and the Association of American Medical Colleges' core Entrustable Professional Activities (EPAs).[47–51] There are in fact multiple specialties that have created EPAs worldwide that can be a good place to start in designing what and where assessment programs should target their efforts and ensure that the EPAs sufficiently cover all competencies (see Chapter 1).

Higher-stakes WBA and non-WBA assessments (e.g., clerkship grades or licensing examinations and objective structured clinical examinations) will continue to have a role in holistic programmatic assessment. Use of these higher-stakes assessments should be fit-for-purpose and support professional development. Govaerts and colleagues recommended using "both/and" polarity thinking when designing local and national assessment systems.[7] For example, assessment programs must properly balance standardization and authenticity, quantitative and qualitative data, and WBA and non-WBA assessments. Van der Vleuten also cautioned against making firm distinctions between formative and summative, describing a formative-summative spectrum of stakes based on assessment purpose.[35] For example, a single, direct observation–based assessment should primarily focus on gathering accurate information for feedback, for coaching, and to provide a data point to the program for aggregation and synthesis. In contrast, a CCC making a higher-stakes graduation decision must use multiple, aggregated, and longitudinally generated assessments.

Embrace Narrative Assessment to Make Entrustment Decisions

Entrustment is quickly becoming a predominant assessment construct in medical education. As noted in Chapter 1, ten Cate and colleagues extended Miller's pyramid, placing "entrusted with future care" as the ultimate assessment *decision*. Entrustment has been operationalized as EPAs, defined

TABLE 3.2 Examples of Minimal Required Competency-Based Assessments and Core Competencies

		Competencies (US General Competency Framework)					
	Explanation of Assessment	**Medical Knowledge**	**Patient Care**	**Interpersonal and Communication Skills**	**Professionalism**	**Practice-Based Learning and Improvement**	**Systems-Based Practice**
Faculty Assessments: • Observations of patient, family, procedures, and interprofessional team interactions • Work-based clinical reasoning	Observation with or without questions. Single-encounter work-based assessment tools (e.g., mini-clinical evaluation exercise) are primarily designed to guide the observation of a clinical encounter between learners and patients.	X	X	X	X	X	X
Multisource feedback (including interprofessional team and patients)	Combination of observations made by the assessor from interactions with the learner that are captured through a series of questions (i.e., survey items) using various types of rating scales with or without narrative comments.		X	X	X		X
In-training, licensing, and certification examination	Typically, MCQs and SAQs	X					
Medical record audit	Observation through an explicit (structured) or implicit (unstructured) interrogation of a medical record. Structured audits typically involve extraction of performance measures (an observation of whether a component of care was delivered or not) that are aggregated into a score. Unstructured audits typically involve judging the quality of medical record documentation and description of medical interviews, physical exam, counseling, etc.		X			X	X
Individualized learning plan (not technically an assessment, but crucial in development)	Reflective practice is now a codified subcompetency in GME under PBLIU and the ability to coconstruct an ILP should be a component of reflective practice.					X	
Mastery-based simulation for procedures, high-risk and rare clinical situations	An observational assessment that can be combined with questions (checklists) depending on the purpose of the assessment. SPs typically convert their observations to ratings using various types of scales with or without narrative comments.	X	X	X			

GME, Graduate medical education; *ILP*, Individualized learning plan; *MCQs*, multiple-choice questions; *PBLI*, Practice-based learning and improvement; *SAQs*, short-answer questions; *SPs*, Standardized patients.

as the routine *professional*-life activities of physicians based on their specialty and subspecialty, where entrustable means "a practitioner has demonstrated the necessary knowledge, skills, and attitudes to be trusted to perform this activity unsupervised"[49] (see Chapter 1). In transitioning to EPAs, medical educators have created entrustment scales. Entrustment rating scale anchors are defined by either the amount of supervision the rater believes the learner will require in future clinical encounters or the level of supervision and clinical care the rater (usually clinical faculty) contributed to the patient's care during learner–patient interactions or procedures. Faculty report more satisfaction using entrustment scales because the scales align more closely with how they think about the learner's ability, trustworthiness, and supervision needs[52] (see Chapter 4).

Despite faculty satisfaction with entrustment-based scales, they are no panacea for what ails more effective use of WBA. For decades, numbers, especially rating scales, have dominated faculty assessment approaches. However, numeric rating scales are nothing more than a code that requires translation by the rater (and learner).[53] Simply stopping the assessment process at assigning a rating is inadequate if the data informing the rating cannot be effectively communicated to the learner in a way that the learner finds credible, actionable, trustworthy, and free of bias.

While studies have found evidence for improved reliability of and satisfaction with entrustment scales, two recent studies have questioned their validity and accuracy.[54,55] For example, Schumacher and colleagues found no to little correlation between supervisors' entrustment ratings and the quality of care pediatric residents delivered in an emergency department.[56] Kogan and colleagues found that faculty entrustment ratings on scripted videos of learners at different entrustment levels were highly variable, with greater variation in ratings occurring at the lowest level of ability in medical interviewing and counseling.[57] In sum, there is nothing magical about scales. While they enable statistical and psychometric analysis, these analyses still depend on the quality of the ratings provided on the scale. If the codes are not an accurate and valid reflection of the learner's performance, the utility of the rating scale output (results) is greatly diminished. This is not meant to diminish the meaningful (i.e., warranted) variation seen between faculty raters.[58] As discussed extensively in Chapter 5, raters bring variable levels of ability in assessment and clinical skills. When variable interpretations of performance by faculty are grounded in strong educational *and* clinical science, that can be a good thing for both the learner and patient. When ratings and interpretations are not, both the learner and patient can be adversely affected.

Additionally, an overemphasis on scales can undermine the importance of narrative assessments, which capture rich descriptions of what happened in an encounter, particularly when the assessment is grounded in evidence-based clinical and educational practice. For example, faculty can provide feedback on medical interviewing by referencing specific behaviors (e.g., agenda setting, active listening with silence, etc.) instead of the generic "good bedside manner" comment. Ginsburg and colleagues found that narrative comments can possess high levels of reliability. They noted that "using written comments to discriminate between residents can be extremely reliable even after only several reports are collected. This suggests a way to identify residents early on who may require attention. These findings contribute evidence to support the validity argument for using qualitative data for assessment."[59,60] Prentice and colleagues in Australia found that flagging procedures (i.e., identifying learners at risk) using qualitative data was useful in identifying trainees in need of interventions to help them.[60] In addition, assessment programs can leverage robust and rigorous qualitative research methodologies designed to analyze qualitative data as part of group process such as CCCs.[61] The specific qualitative techniques and their correlates in assessment programs are provided in Table 3.3.

Take Seriously and Address Unwarranted Variation

Unwarranted variation is an underappreciated problem in programmatic assessment.[58] Some variation in assessments is good, such as when a faculty member leverages a particular strength or aspect of effective practice (i.e., warranted variation). However, assessments driven by idiosyncrasies or bias that is no evidence based represent unwarranted variation (see Chapter 5). Unwarranted variation can be harmful, can contribute to suboptimal and variable educational outcomes, and, by extension, risks graduates delivering suboptimal healthcare. Bias is a particularly unwelcome form of unwarranted variation. Faculty are often the primary sources of unwarranted variation, which we will address shortly, but poor group process is another source of unwarranted variation in programmatic assessment. There is abundant evidence that unwarranted variation at the program and institutional levels also can affect educational outcomes and the quality of care graduates deliver.[62–69]

Learners are nested within training programs (medical schools, residencies, fellowships, and other postgraduate training programs) that are nested within institutions that are nested within communities. These nested relationships are interdependent, and this interdependence impacts clinical and educational outcomes and can amplify competency deficiencies and structural biases with potentially profound effects. Warm and colleagues argued that optimizing assessment requires all participants within the system to clearly identify its assessment purpose, develop a deep and nuanced understanding of the variation occurring within the training program, and then use this information for improvement interventions.[30]

Programs can analyze a faculty member's rating patterns and provide feedback on suboptimal and counterproductive assessment behaviors, such as straight-lining (i.e., all assessment items are given the same rating), leniency, stringency, halo rating errors, and bias (see Chapter 5), as part

TABLE 3.3 A Model for Programmatic Assessment Fit for Purpose

Strategies to establish trustworthiness	Criteria	Potential assessment strategy
Credibility	Prolonged engagement	Train assessors
		People who know that the learner (coach, peers) best provides information for assessment
		Incorporate intermittent feedback cycles in the assessment procedure
	Triangulation	Involve many assessors and different credible groups
		Use multiple sources of assessment within or across methods
		Organize a sequential judgment procedure where conflicting information necessitates the gathering of more information
	Peer examination (sometimes called peer debriefing)	Assessors talk about benchmarking, the assessment process, and results before and at the halfway point during an activity
		Separate assessors' multiple roles by removing summative assessment decisions from the coaching role
	Member checking	Incorporate the learner's point of view in the assessment procedure (using coproduction)
		Incorporate longitudinal, intermittent feedback cycles
	Structural coherence	Assessment committee (e.g., clinical competency committee) discusses inconsistencies in the assessment data and looks for signs of bias
Transferability	Time sampling	Sample broadly over different contexts and patients over time
	Thick description (or dense description)	Assessment instruments facilitate inclusion of qualitative, narrative information
		Give narrative information a lot of weight in the assessment procedure
Dependability	Stepwise replication	Sample broadly over different assessors and over time
Dependability/ confirmability	Audit	Document the different steps in the assessment process (a formal assessment plan approved by an examination board, especially for high-stakes assessments; provide overviews of the results per phase)
		Quality assessment of procedures with external auditor
		Learners can appeal the assessment decision

From van der Vleuten CPM, Schuwirth LWT, Driessen EW, et al. A model for programmatic assessment fit for purpose. *Med Teach*. 2012;34(3):205-214. doi: 10.3109/0142159X.2012.652239.

of the assessment program's ongoing evaluation and continuous improvement efforts (see Chapter 18). All participants, including learners, should use all available data to identify and address the sources and causes of unwarranted variation in the training program, including the assessment program.[30]

Feedback loops across the continuum are also needed to support continuous quality improvement of assessment programs and reduce unwarranted variation and bias. As one example, UME programs should assess how their graduates perform in residency (postgraduate) training as feedback about the effectiveness of the medical school program. Similarly, GME programs will need to leverage clinical performance measures in early practice as feedback on the effectiveness of residency and/or fellowship programs. More work is needed on how to access, interpret, and carefully use such data on graduates for continuous improvement of training programs. Use of clinical performance measures should be a part of program evaluation (see Chapter 18) with a clear-eyed understanding of the limitations of such measures. Undergraduate and postgraduate training programs are not factories all producing the same product. Therefore abundant caution and humility is needed to ensure that the focus of the assessment program is directed toward using meaningful measurement-type data fit for purpose. Patients being cared for by recent graduates deserve high-quality care, and where we have information that can provide useful insights to improve care we should use it. Several recent studies examining the relationship between Milestone ratings and early clinical practice provide some optimism for how these feedback loops could be created leveraging different clinical data sets despite the challenges in using clinical data (see Chapter 11).[70–73]

Regardless, all training programs, especially postgraduate training programs, need to use more clinical performance data as part of their assessment programs (see Chapter 11).

As noted earlier, attribution of clinical performance, such as care for patients with chronic conditions or procedural complications, often cannot be directly or fully attributed to the actions and behaviors of the learner. Yet the learner contributed to the quality of care provided and the learner should leverage quality and safety measures for formative purposes as an important way to reduce unwarranted variation in clinical care provided by training programs.[56,74]

Use Learning Analytics and Big Data

Learning analytics using both local and national data (e.g., "big data") must be embedded in programs of assessment.[46] Learning analytics refers to "the interpretation of a wide range of data produced by and gathered on behalf of students in order to assess academic progress, predict future performance, and spot potential issues."[75] Programs must become more facile using all their available quantitative and qualitative assessment data to create a meaningful dashboard of professional development for program leaders and learners. Most learning management systems can create these dashboards, which provide both criterion and normative-referenced snapshots of learner development.[76] However, learning analytics and "big data" must account for issues of bias that can be unwittingly incorporated into assessment analytics.[75,76] This will be especially important in using artificial intelligence (AI), machine learning (ML), and large language machine learning (LLML) techniques. AI/ML/LLML holds tremendous promise if used wisely and thoughtfully within and across programs and will be the next frontier in assessment to identify patterns of learners' developmental trajectories more accurately. For example, locally collected GME assessment data can now be compared to national GME "big data." Residency programs can use Milestones' nationally based predictive probability values (PPVs) to identify specific subcompetencies where individual learners may be struggling.[72] However, the critical point is that the quality of the assessment is defined by the *interpretation* of the data. A PPV, for example, does not itself tell you what is actually happening with the learner. It is simply a quantitative "signal" that something concerning may be present. Proper interpretation of this "signal" requires further investigation and conversation with the learner and the educational team, using mostly qualitative (narrative) data. Chapter 16 provides an example of what a longitudinal dashboard can look like to guide programs; such a dashboard should contain both quantitative and qualitative data elements.

Explicitly Define Assessors' Roles and Responsibilities in the Assessment System

Thus far we have focused on the purpose and role of assessment at the program level. However, the majority of WBAs are performed by individual faculty focused on individual learners who are fed into programs of assessment. And here we define "faculty" more broadly to include any healthcare professional involved in the training of another healthcare professional. It is therefore imperative that everyone involved in the assessment program clearly understands their roles and responsibilities.

All frontline health professionals who contribute to learners' professional development are the backbone of any program of assessment. While physician faculty will likely perform most of the assessments for physician training, for example, training programs must also look to learners' interprofessional faculty colleagues as a rich source of education and assessment. The core assessment responsibilities for faculty are (1) perform direct observation of clinical skills; (2) provide rich narrative descriptions of performance and accurate ratings; (3) provide ongoing feedback and coaching; (4) provide robust assessment information to program leadership and the CCC to support the learner's professional development; and (5) ensure that all patients receive safe, effective, equitable, patient-centered care through appropriate learner supervision.

There are multiple issues in faculty assessment that must be considered. In addition to those already highlighted, other issues include poor reliability and accuracy, raters' own clinical abilities, and inaccurate use of inference[77] (see Chapters 1, 2, and 5). As a result, learners must, often independently, make sense of disparate assessments and feedback from faculty. What feedback should learners trust and prioritize? Is feedback grounded in EBP and based on sufficient interaction time to capture the learner's abilities? Are assessments affected by bias? The most frequently proposed solution to poor reliability and accuracy is ensuring that enough assessments are performed by multiple raters completing multiple assessments longitudinally. Obtaining multiple assessments leverages psychometric science and, from a programmatic perspective, supports better summative entrustment judgments of learners if multiple assessments are collected longitudinally. However, supervision decisions based on inaccurate and unreliable assessments by individual faculty may lead to poor patient care when faculty entrust a learner to function with less oversight when, in reality, more is needed. To ensure the probability that high-quality care is delivered as frequently as possible, faculty must make valid and accurate assessments. How can the current situation be improved?

Assessors, particularly faculty, need ongoing training in assessment. Unfortunately, a certain level of nihilism surrounds faculty development in assessment. Time, financial costs, and perceived ineffectiveness are often cited as the major barriers to assessment training. However, if assessors are not trained, what are the costs to patients and learners? Patients, followed next in line by learners, are the stakeholders most affected by poor assessment practices and unwarranted variation in assessments. Most clinical supervisors have to make judgments and provide feedback even if they don't like it. An investment in faculty training is an investment in efficiency and effectiveness in their educational role while concomitantly having to manage and provide patient care in busy clinical settings. One factor that hampers faculty

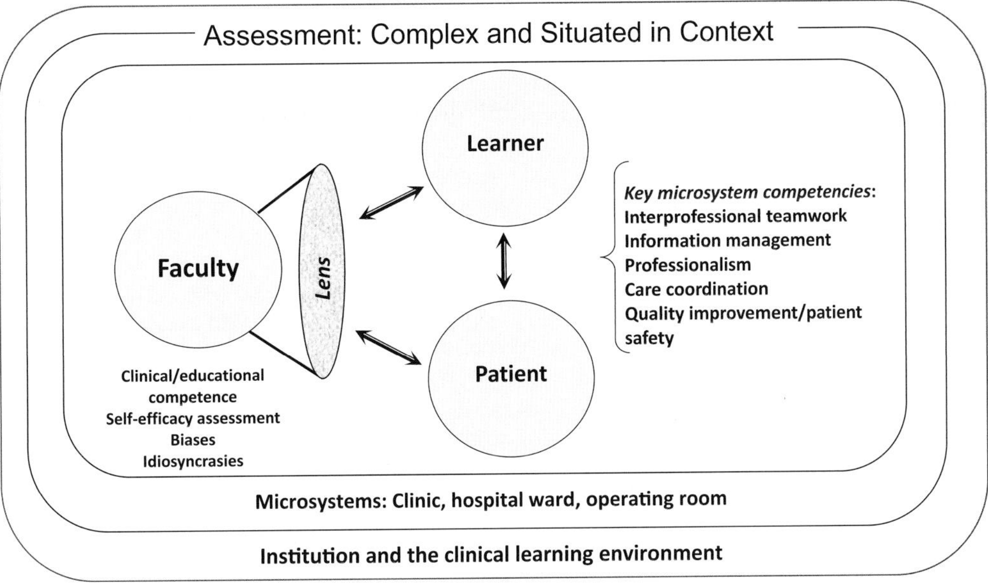

• **Fig. 3.5** Assessment: complex and situated in context.

development process even further is the experience faculty had with education when they were the learners themselves. This sometimes leads them to believe they understand education because they have experienced it and with the mindset, "I turned out OK, right?"

For example, a faculty member with years of experience reading the literature doesn't alone make them a clinician specialist, especially if that experience dates from decades ago and therefore runs the risk of being outdated. After all, we don't practice medicine like we did 25 years ago, so why would we think we should practice education like we did 25 years ago? The failure of faculty to recognize and acknowledge that things have changed, and will continue to change, requires an investment in faculty development to improve efficiency and effectiveness in both educational and clinical practice.

Faculty development in assessment is hard and requires sustained, ongoing effort. Much like the challenges of implicit bias, where patterns of behavior become subconscious, ingrained habits, faculty members' assessment habits can follow a similar pattern. Faculty very often use themselves as their primary frame of reference, or standard, when assessing learners' clinical skills[77] (see Chapter 5). However, faculty's abilities in the very clinical skills they assess are variable. Going forward, the primary frame of reference, or minimal standard, for WBAs should be whether the patient received safe, effective, equitable, and patient-centered care.[78]

Faculty development programs should also teach faculty how to account for contextual factors that affect a learner's ability to provide equitable, high-quality, safe care (Fig. 3.5). This does not mean there should always be an adjustment of an individual learner's assessment, as there will be times when the learner must adapt to the circumstances to provide effective, safe, equitable, and patient-centered care. For example, residents will need to adapt their counseling for patients with lower health literacy to meet those patients' needs, even if the healthcare setting lacks helpful resources. Assessors and programs should assess learner adaptability as a core competency. Chapter 5 provides a wealth of suggested faculty development approaches to improve assessment by faculty.

Similar to addressing bias in assessment, improving faculty development in assessment must also be treated as a translational activity. McGaghie adapted the clinical translation framework for medical education, and all training programs should keep the translational steps and goals in mind as it creates, implements, and continuously refines its program of assessment.[29] It is well past time to make a more sustained effort in faculty development, grounded in evidence, to concomitantly improve assessment for the purpose of improving professional development and clinical care.

Address Bias in Assessment

While I have previously described some specific issues regarding bias, I want to emphasize the urgent need to address the many facets of bias in medical education that threaten learners' professional development: bias and inequity in the learning environment, bias inherent in the assessment instruments, bias on the part of individual evaluators who assess learners, and bias on the part of CCCs or other groups that review assessments and make high-stakes decisions.[79] Going forward, as described earlier, assessment tools should include additional domains essential to the physician role, such as advocacy for at-risk populations. Furthermore, it will be important to ensure that the definition of competence is not biased. For example, there is increasing concern that the assessment of professionalism is predicated on gender- and race-normative constructs and definitions.[80]

Despite the current lack of robust evidence supporting interventions to reduce bias and prejudice, faculty development remains essential to address the multiple types and foci

TABLE 3.4 Five Possible Strategies Programs and Faculty Can Try to Reduce Bias in Assessment

Strategy	Description	Assessment Example
Stereotype replacement	Recognizing when a stereotype has been activated, thinking about why, and then actively substituting nonstereotypical thoughts	When completing a narrative assessment of a female learner, the assessor stops to consider if they may be using gender-laden language or uses an online tool to assess for gender bias. If bias is found, the assessor substitutes evidence-based behavioral skills that are more neutral.
Perspective taking	Considering what it would be like to be a member of the minoritized group	During rounds, faculty witness a difficult interaction between a learner from a URiM group with a discriminatory patient. Faculty should ask themselves: What must that be like for the learner? How will I intervene in this situation?
Individuation	Recognizing when you have stereotyped someone according to their group affiliation and instead thinking about what makes them an individual	A faculty member watches a learner from another country struggle to interview a patient with a possible sexually transmitted disease and initially stereotypes the learner as from a group "uncomfortable talking about sex." Instead, the faculty sees an individual learner struggling and seeks to understand why they are struggling as an individual.
Counter-stereotypic imaging	Imagining an individual or situation that counteracts a stereotypical reaction in detail	A faculty member starts with an assumption that women are not strong enough to perform orthopedic procedures and then instead thinks about successful women who are orthopedic surgeons
Increased opportunities for contact	Increasing opportunities for contact with members of a stereotyped group	Programs and faculty can spend meaningful time with URiM trainees to listen and learn more about their lived experiences and their path to the current training program.

Adapted from Holmboe ES, Osman NY, Murphy CM, Kogan JR. The urgency of now: rethinking and improving assessment practices in medical education programs. *Acad Med*. 2023 Apr 18. doi:10.1097/ACM.0000000000005251.

URiM, Underrepresented in medicine.

of bias.[81] Programs can attend to the individual or interpersonal effects of bias by offering faculty development about the history of bias and racism in medicine, writing bias-free narratives, and engaging in individual mindfulness practice to mitigate the effects of assessors' own bias. The scope and focus of bias (i.e., which URiM groups are most impacted by the bias) will vary by country.

Medical education should leverage existing literature around bias-reducing interventions, despite current limitations in the evidence within medical education, to build on and study the effectiveness of specific techniques from bias reduction research in patient care. Intervention procedures that induce threat or emotions in participants are minimally effective. A recent metaanalysis found that one-time, limited-focus interventions had little impact on reducing bias or prejudice.[55] This should not be surprising as implicit biases and prejudices often become personal habits that require repeated attention and practice to change.[82] Multifaceted and longitudinal interventions show more promise and should be studied in medical education.[83] Table 3.4 lists five promising strategies along with potential examples in medical education.[83]

Educators should also be aware of other cognitive biases that affect assessment. These include the well-known correlational and distributive type rating errors, cognitive load, and many more.[84] Correlational errors refer to the phenomenon where performance on one competency domain significantly influences the rating in other competency domains. An example of such an error is the halo effect, where everything is rated high based on perceived strong performance in one domain such as medical knowledge. Distributional errors involve raters using limited ranges of a scale such as leniency error (everything rated higher) or stringency error (everything rated lower). Cognitive load entails asking the assessor to judge too many items in a short period of time. Dickey and colleagues provide a nice overview of other cognitive biases, and Chapters 4 and 5 cover other cognitive biases in more detail.[84]

Research in reducing bias through faculty development and program evaluation (see Chapter 16) should use the translational science approach described earlier (i.e., bench to bedside). The first step is to identify whether there is bias in the assessment program. Programs can examine their assessment data (ratings and bias-laden narrative comments) looking for differences in learners by identity subgroups compared to the majority group. CCCs can ask nonparticipant observers to watch and listen for bias-laden terms, descriptions, or decisions. Once a needs assessment has occurred, T1 studies can be done to identify theory-supported strategies (Fig. 3.6) to reduce implicit bias among educators. Future efforts might specifically teach learning strategies to reduce implicit bias in direct observation assessments. Implicit prejudice toward patients, for example, manifests itself in verbal and nonverbal communication behaviors. The same may hold true between learners and faculty and is an opportunity to target communication-based interventions with faculty to reduce implicit bias. T2 studies target effectiveness among a larger group

Health Professions Education as Translational Science

	Translational Stages			
Focus	T1	T2	T3	T4
Increased or improved...	Knowledge, skill, attitudes, professionalism	Patient care practices	Patient outcomes	Collateral effects, e.g., skill retention, ROI, indirect outcomes
Target groups	Individuals and teams	Individuals and teams	Individuals and public health	Individuals, teams, and public health
Setting	Educational setting; e.g., simulation lab	Clinic and bedside	Clinic, bedside, and community	Clinic, bedside, and community

• **Fig. 3.6** Health professions education as translational science. (From McGaghie WC, Barsuk JH, Wayne DB, eds. Comprehensive Healthcare Simulation: Mastery Learning in Health Professions Education. Springer; 2020.)

of educators and other assessments. Finally, T3 studies target wider implementation as the new assessment practice designed to reduce implicit bias is embedded across the assessment program. We have much to learn about how to address bias most effectively in assessment, but early research in clinical practice provides a foundation to design faculty development around more effective communication strategies in assessment.

Recognize the Importance of Coproduction With Learners

For programmatic assessment to be fully effective, learners must be active participants with individual agency. Medical students, residents, fellows, and other health professionals learn in, and sit at, the center of bidirectional and mutually beneficial relationships with the leaders and faculty of their training programs. These relationships require a coproduction mindset. In a coproduction mindset, assessments take place in a psychologically safe environment in which assessments are predominantly done *with* learners instead of *to* them.[36]

Coproduction has gained a strong foothold in clinical care. Coproduction of healthcare is defined as "the ***interdependent*** work of users and professionals to design, create, develop, deliver, assess, and improve the relationships and actions that contribute to the health of individuals and populations."[39] Recently, Englander and colleagues laid out benefits of coproduction in medical education, noting: ". . . like the relationship between patients and providers, the relationship between learner and teacher requires the integrated expertise of each nested in the context of their system, community, and society to optimize outcomes."[85] Coproduction is a bidirectional interaction between the learner and the training program. Coproduction fuels a cyclical, ongoing process. Fig. 3.7 highlights how incorporating coproduction as part of learning cycles along a trajectory can empower learners to view their own professional development as an ongoing, coproduced, iterative assessment process. Fig. 3.8 brings together the key concepts of professional development learning curves, programmatic assessment, and iterative learning cycles using a coproduction approach.

Adapted from Englander and colleagues, Table 3.5 compares and contrasts traditional assessment approaches to one using coproduction. UME and GME programs can use this framework to improve their assessment programs and empower learners to strive for better outcomes.[85] However, medical education has struggled to create psychologically safe environments for learners. This is especially true for URiM learners who often must overcome stereotype threats and impostor syndrome. Partnering with learners to understand and attend to their lived experiences with current and past assessment activities will help programs improve assessment and confront and reduce bias in assessment. Program leaders will need to inform learners about coproduction, recognize and reward the learner role in coproduction, and create system changes to enable learners to receive more timely feedback and assessments through dashboards and rich information systems. Table 3.5 provides a summary of the key assessment roles of program leadership, faculty, and learners.

In summary, a robust program of assessment must be coproduced and include multiple, integrated assessment methods and tools performed as a series of learning-assessment cycles conducted longitudinally over the course of the entire training program. A coproduced assessment program should be guided by informed group judgment and decision-making, and actively involve the learner embracing the philosophy of coproduction across the medical education continuum.

Putting It All Together: Implementation Science and Programmatic Assessment

While developing new assessment approaches and tools remains necessary, we already possess multiple, useful assessment approaches and tools. Therefore, going forward medical education should focus primarily on *how* to better use our

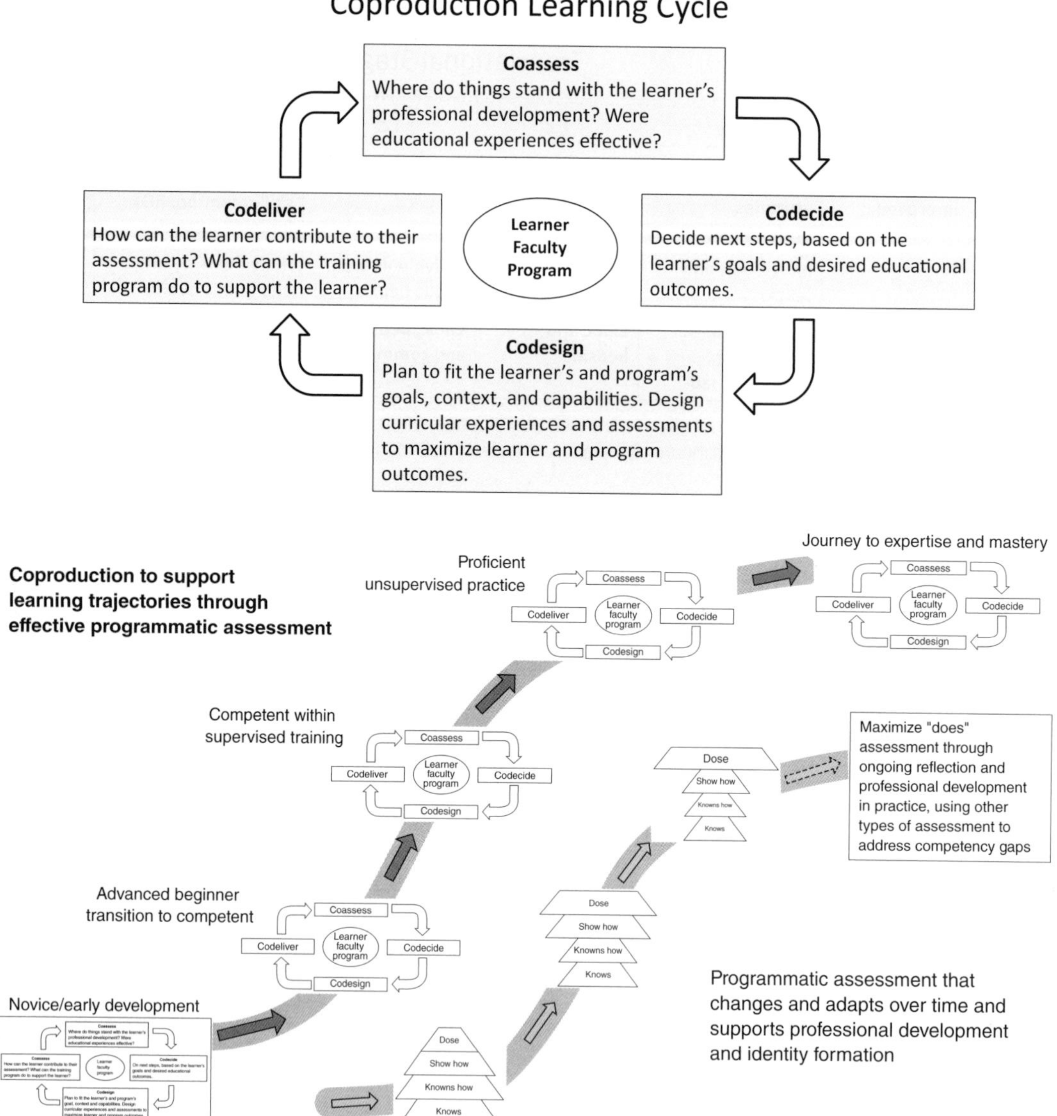

• **Figs.** 3.7 and 3.8. Medical training during the undergraduate medical education and graduate medical education years is an intensely developmental and iterative process. Each learner will experience different trajectories and must be an active partner with agency to coproduce their own educational experiences, including assessment. Fig. 3.7 displays key stages and questions in the coproduction cycle that must be iteratively implemented as part of the longitudinal growth curve shown in Fig. 3.8.

existing wealth of assessment approaches. As program leaders evolve their assessment approaches, lessons and tools from implementation science can help. Ultimately, designing and running training programs and their system of assessment is not about a destination, but rather an ongoing developmental journey to continuously improve educational approaches (e.g., learning environment, curriculum, and assessment programs as all are integrated) as biological, medical, health system, and educational sciences evolve. By default, change and continuous improvement is a messy process. Medical education must embrace implementation science to support transformation in assessment, including the elimination of harmful bias.

Medical education programs are embedded within complex educational and clinical systems. The hallmark of complex systems are the interdependencies and interactions between all the "parts and components" with people (i.e., health professions faculty, program directors, program coordinators, and learners) being the most important components of the system, as noted earlier. When implementing a change, or new interventions in an assessment program, training program leadership must attend to key aspects of implementation.

Lessons and tools from implementation science can help educational leaders determine *how* to implement assessment programs and specific assessments. For example, the Consolidated Framework for Implementation Research (CFIR) can guide implementation and continuous quality improvement efforts in assessment.[86] The CFIR explicitly calls attention to five components: the conditions and characteristics of the outer setting (e.g., institutional social contexts); the inner setting (e.g., training program administrative support); the

TABLE 3.5 **Traditional Versus Coproduction Models of Assessment in Medical Education**

System variable	Traditional/Hierarchical	Coproduction
Logic dominant model	"Goods" model. Learner viewed as "product" where assessment is done primarily to ensure that the "product" meets minimal standards for release to the next stage of a career.	"Service" model. Learner viewed as health professional ultimately providing service to others. A service model requires a coproduction mindset because services are, by definition, always coproduced between two parties.
Primary driver	Teacher is primary assessor.	Learner(s)–teacher partnership designs, performs, and interprets assessments.
Focus	Emphasis on summative, retrospective assessments using rating scales that "quantify" the learner (e.g., end-of-rotation evaluations or grades).	Increased emphasis on narratively rich assessments that demonstrate developmental improvement in which learner contributes to their assessments. Assessments deemphasize overreliance on quantitative rating scales.
Information "ownership"	Medical school, residency, or fellowship program owns and controls assessment information.	Learners own their assessment data that are transportable to new schools/programs. "Nothing about me without me." The institution is a trusted custodian of assessment data and uses the assessment data in aggregate (with consent from the learner) to improve curriculum and assessment.
Relationship between professionals	Each assessor provides assessment in isolation and assessment data from multiple professionals is often lacking, of poor quality, or not incorporated into a learning plan for improvement. Assessments from other health professionals mostly used to identify problems and "outliers."	Assessment data from multiple health professionals is integrated into a more holistic picture of abilities in all competencies using a developmental mindset.
Connections between aspects of the system	Abrupt transitions between phases of training (e.g., medical school to residency, to fellowship, to practice). No sharing ("feed-forward") of assessment data is performed, encouraged, or supported.	Clear transitions with systematic "warm handoffs." Sharing assessment data to support tailored learning for professional development across the continuum and variable time-based training based on competence and learner needs.
Improvement model	Limited system perspective—blame and punishment model. Focused on "weeding" out "bad" or underperforming learners.	Continuous improvement of the assessment program based on input from all stakeholders to support professional development.

Adapted from Englander R, Holmboe E, Batalden P, et al. Coproducing health professions education: A prerequisite to coproducing health care services? *Acad Med*. 2020;95(7):1006–1013. doi:10.1097/ACM.0000000000003137.

characteristics of the assessment approach (e.g., complexity in using the assessment, learner perceptions); the individuals involved (e.g., do they have agency and self-efficacy around the assessment; and the process (e.g., capacity of the program for change, presence of change agents and opinion leaders). Yaghmour and colleagues applied this framework to better understand the developmental change journey of residency programs implementing Milestones and uncovered at least three program-level stages.[40] In 2017, all residencies at Queens University Canada implemented an outcomes-based, time-variable approach and shared their early implementation results using rapid cycle evaluations. They uncovered several expected and unexpected challenges, a common phenomenon with major system changes.[87] Both of these studies highlight how using implementation frameworks to guide the evaluation of large-scale initiatives can produce deeper insights into programmatic change. Appendix 3.2 provides an example of a CFIR template for implementing the revised Milestones 2.0 (see Chapter 1) for specialty training in the United States.

Conclusion

Medical education training programs already possess a wealth of assessment approaches and tools. Now we must commit to using these tools and approaches more effectively within programs of assessment (i.e., programmatic assessment) using systems thinking to continuously improve. There is much we can do now to improve assessment practices (Box 3.2). This requires creating educational systems that allow the development, implementation, and sustainment of assessment programs. Assessment must be a high priority and not treated as an adjunct or afterthought in an educational program. Ideally, the purpose of assessment

• BOX 3.2 A (Partial) List of Actions Medical Education Programs Can Do Now to Improve Assessment

1. Ensure the majority of assessments are developmentally designed and focused.
2. Use assessment data to investigate, understand, and address sources of bias in the assessment program.
   a. Seek to understand the effects of program culture and the institutional learning environment on learners' professional development.
3. Develop and implement programmatic assessment.
   a. Emphasize workplace-based assessments for the purpose of supporting learners' professional development.
   b. Embrace narrative assessments.
   c. Use learning analytics to support learners' professional development and the continuous improvement of the assessment program.
4. Leverage existing technologies to improve assessments (e.g., natural language processing, smartphone apps, etc.).
5. Investigate, understand, and address sources of unwarranted variation in the assessment program.
6. Explicitly define the assessment roles of all faculty (physicians and other health professionals) and learners.
7. Invest in training of faculty and learners in assessment.
8. Leverage coproduction to support assessment practices and learners' professional development.
9. Use translational and implementation science to build, revise, and improve assessment programs and practices.
10. Honestly assess and confront inertia in changing assessment practices.

aligns with learning (assessment drives learning *and* learning drives the right type of assessments). Unfortunately, that is still not the situation in the majority of health professions education programs. Assessment is too often designed to incentivize competition where the quality of the assessment is defined by how well it can distinguish (discriminate) performance among learners (ranking and normative mindset) instead of ensuring that all learners attain a high level of performance (criterion and mastery mindset). The uncomfortable reality of the ranking type of assessment system finds its origins in psychological testing that had and still has the primary purpose of telling people apart: normal from abnormal, suited for the position versus unsuitable for the position, et cetera. But in education the purpose is not to tell whether Jane is better than Jim but to ensure that Jane and Jim become the best health professional they can be. When our predominant conceptualization of the role of assessment in education is one of measurement, grading, selection, and discrimination, its value proposition conflicts with the primary value proposition of education. Programmatic assessment must be viewed, using a systems lens, as an intrinsic and inseparable component of education and therefore as inseparable from medical education's core value proposition to improve health and healthcare.

Educational environments need to have the time and the resources and be designed so that learners and all faculty assessors have enough time working together to enable effective assessment and feedback to occur. This requires confronting the uncomfortable inertia that has persistently limited improvement and change in programmatic assessment, especially around issues of structural bias and racism. Change will require humility to recognize what is not working and concerted effort to address weaknesses and gaps within our assessment systems, including the regulatory components of professional assessment. Effective and efficient programmatic assessment is within reach of all health professions education.[88–92] We have strong assessment science to make a difference in the lives of our learners and patients through better assessment practices grounded in a developmental, coproduction mindset embedded in integrated, well-designed programs of assessment.

Acknowledgments

I wish to thank Dr. Lambert Schuwirth for his helpful review, suggestions, and edits.

Parts of this chapter were originally produced for a Macy Foundation white paper by E.S. Holmboe, N. Osman, C. Murphy, and J. Kogan.

References

1. Frank JR, Snell LS, ten Cate O. Competency-based medical education: theory to practice. *Med Teach.* 2010;32(8):638–645. doi: 10.3109/0142159X.2010.501190.
2. Nelson EC, Batalden PB, Godfrey MM. *Quality by Design: A Clinical Microsystems Approach.* Jossey-Bass; 2007.
3. Batalden P, Leach D, Swing S, Dreyfus H, Dreyfus S. General competencies and accreditation in graduate medical education. *Health Aff (Millwood).* 2002 Sep-Oct;21(5):103–111. doi:10.1377/hlthaff.21.5.103.
4. Association of American Medical Colleges. Learning objectives for medical student education—guidelines for medical schools: report I of the Medical School Objectives Project. *Acad Med.* 1999 Jan;74(1):13–18. doi:10.1097/00001888-199901000-00010.
5. Royal College of Physicians and Surgeons of Canada. CanMEDS: Better standards, better physicians, better care. Accessed March 19, 2023. at CanMEDS Framework:: The Royal College of Physicians and Surgeons of Canada
6. General Medical Council. 2019. Good Medical Practice. Accessed March 19, 2023. Available at: Good medical practice - ethical guidance - GMC (gmc-uk.org).
7. Govaerts MJB, van der Vleuten CPM, Holmboe ES. Managing tensions in assessment: moving beyond either-or thinking. *Med Educ.* 2019 Jan;53(1):64–75. doi:10.1111/medu.13656.
8. Dweck CS, Yeager DS. Mindsets: a view from two eras. *Perspect Psychol Sci.* 2019 May;14(3):481–496. doi:10.1177/1745691618804166.
9. Richardson D, Kinnear B, Hauer KE, et al. Growth mindset in competency-based medical education. *Med Teach.* 2021 Jul;43(7):751–757. doi:10.1080/0142159X.2021.1928036.
10. Pusic MV, Boutis K, Hatala R, Cook DA. Learning curves in health professions education. *Acad Med.* 2015 Aug;90(8):1034–1042. doi:10.1097/ACM.0000000000000681.
11. Ericsson KA. Acquisition and maintenance of medical expertise: a perspective from the expert-performance approach with deliberate practice. *Acad Med.* 2015 Nov;90(11):1471–1486. doi:10.1097/ACM.0000000000000939.

12. McGaghie WC. When I say . . . mastery learning. *Med Educ.* 2015 Jun;49(6):558–559. doi:10.1111/medu.12679.
13. Van Melle E, Frank JR, Holmboe ES, et al. A core components framework for evaluating implementation of competency-based medical education programs. *Acad Med.* 2019 Jul;94(7):1002–1009. doi:10.1097/ACM.0000000000002743.
14. Hagiwara N, Kron FW, Scerbo MW, Watson GS. A call for grounding implicit bias training in clinical and translational frameworks. *Lancet.* 2020;395(10234):1457–1460. doi:10.1016/S0140-6736(20)30846-1.
15. Onumah CM, Lai CJ, Levine D, Ismail N, Pincavage AT, Osman NY. Aiming for equity in clerkship grading: recommendations for reducing the effects of structural and individual bias. *Am J Med.* 2021 Sep;134(9):1175–1183.e4. doi:10.1016/j.amjmed.2021.06.001.
16. Jaffe RC, Bergin CR, Loo LK, et al. Nested domains: a global conceptual model for optimizing the clinical learning environment. *Am J Med.* 2019;132(7):886–891. doi:10.1016/j.amjmed.2019.03.019.
17. Boatright D, Ross D, O'Connor P, Moore E, Nunez-Smith M. Racial disparities in medical student membership in the Alpha Omega Alpha Honor Society. *JAMA Intern Med.* 2017;177(5):659–665. doi:10.1001/jamainternmed.2016.9623.
18. Lucey CR, Saguil A. The consequences of structural racism on MCAT scores and medical school admissions: the past is prologue. *Acad Med.* 2020;95(3):351–356. doi:10.1097/ACM.0000000000002939.
19. Wijesekera TP, Kim M, Moore EZ, Sorenson O, Ross DA. All other things being equal: exploring racial and gender disparities in medical school honor society induction. *Acad Med.* 2019;94(4):562–569. doi:10.1097/ACM.0000000000002463.
20. Teherani A, Hauer KE, Fernandez A, King Jr TE, Lucey C. How small differences in assessed clinical performance amplify to large differences in grades and awards: a cascade with serious consequences for students underrepresented in medicine. *Acad Med.* 2018 Sep;93(9):1286–1292. doi:10.1097/ACM.0000000000002323.
21. Bravata DM, Watts SA, Keefer AL, et al. Prevalence, predictors, and treatment of impostor syndrome: a systematic review. *J Gen Intern Med.* 2020;35(4):1252–1275. doi:10.1007/s11606-019-05364-1.
22. Osseo-Asare A, Balasuriya L, Huot SJ, et al. Minority resident physicians' views on the role of race/ethnicity in their training experiences in the workplace. *JAMA Netw Open.* 2018;1(5):e182723. doi:10.1001/jamanetworkopen.2018.2723.
23. Wheeler M, de Bourmont S, Paul-Emile K, et al. Physician and trainee experiences with patient bias. *JAMA Intern Med.* 2019;179(12):1678–1685. doi:10.1001/jamainternmed.2019.4122.
24. Bullock JL, Lai CJ, Lockspeiser T, et al. In pursuit of honors: a multi-institutional study of students' perceptions of clerkship evaluation and grading. *Acad Med.* 2019;94(11 suppl):S48–S56. doi:10.1097/ACM.0000000000002905.
25. Olsen LD. The conscripted curriculum and the reproduction of racial inequalities in contemporary US medical education. *J Health Soc Behav.* 2019;60(1):55–68. doi:10.1177/0022146518821388.
26. Valentine N, Shanahan EM, Durning SJ, Schuwirth L. Making it fair: learners' and assessors' perspectives of the attributes of fair judgement. *Med Educ.* 2021;55(9):1056–1066. doi:10.1111/medu.14574.
27. Valentine N, Durning SJ, Shanahan EM, van der Vleuten C, Schuwirth L. The pursuit of fairness in assessment: looking beyond the objective. *Med Teach.* 2022 Apr;44(4):353–359. doi:10.1080/0142159X.2022.2031943.
28. Valentine N, Durning S, Shanahan EM, Schuwirth L. Fairness in human judgement in assessment: a hermeneutic literature review and conceptual framework. *Adv Health Sci Educ Theory Pract.* 2021 May;26(2):713–738. doi:10.1007/s10459-020-10002-1.
29. McGaghie WC. Medical education research as translational science. *Sci Transl Med.* 2010 Feb 17;2(19):19cm8. doi:10.1126/scitranslmed.3000679.
30. Warm EJ, Kinnear B, Kelleher M, Sall D, Holmboe E. Transforming resident assessment: an analysis using Deming's System of Profound Knowledge. *Acad Med.* 2019;94(2):195–201. doi:10.1097/ACM.0000000000002499.
31. Edgar L, Jones MD Jr, Harsy B, Passiment M, Hauer KE. Better decision-making: shared mental models and the clinical competency committee. *J Grad Med Educ.* 2021;13(2 suppl):51–58. doi:10.4300/JGME-D-20-00850.1.
32. Moonen-van Loon JM, Overeem K, Donkers HH, van der Vleuten CP, Driessen EW. Composite reliability of a workplace-based assessment toolbox for postgraduate medical education. *Adv Health Sci Educ Theory Pract.* 2013;18(5):1087–1102. doi:10.1007/s10459-013-9450-z.
33. Hauer KE, O'Sullivan PS, Fitzhenry K, Boscardin C. Translating theory into practice: implementing a program of assessment. *Acad Med.* 2018 Mar;93(3):444–450. doi:10.1097/ACM.0000000000000199.
34. Schuwirth LW, van der Vleuten CP. Programmatic assessment: from assessment of learning to assessment for learning. *Med Teach.* 2011;33(6):478–485. doi:10.3109/0142159X.2011.565828.
35. Van der Vleuten CP, Schuwirth LW, Driessen EW. A model for programmatic assessment fit for purpose. *Med Teach.* 2012;34(3):205–214. doi:10.3109/0142159X.2012.65223.
36. Delbanco T, Berwick DM, Boufford JI, et al. Healthcare in a land called People Power: nothing about me without me. *Health Expect.* 2001 Sep;4(3):144–150. doi:10.1046/j.1369-6513.2001.00145.x.
37. Andolsek K, Padmore J, Hauer KE, Ekpenyong A, Edgar L, Holmboe E. *Clinical Competency Committees: A Guidebook for Programs.* 3rd ed.; January 2020. Accessed March 17, 2023. https://www.acgme.org/globalassets/acgmeclinicalcompetencycommitteeguidebook.pdf.
38. Kogan JR, Hauer KE, Holmboe ES. The dissolution of the Step 2 Clinical Skills Examination and the duty of medical educators to step up the effectiveness of clinical skills assessment. *Acad Med.* 2021;96(9):1242–1246. doi:10.1097/ACM.0000000000004216.
39. Batalden M, Batalden P, Margolis P, et al. Coproduction of healthcare service. *BMJ Qual Saf.* 2016 Jul;25(7):509–517. doi:10.1136/bmjqs-2015-004315.
40. Yaghmour NA, Poulin LJ, Bernabeo EC, et al. Stages of milestones implementation: a template analysis of 16 programs across 4 specialties. *J Grad Med Educ.* 2021;13(2 suppl):14–44. doi:10.4300/JGME-D-20-00900.1.
41. Bohnen JD, George BC, Williams RG, et al. The feasibility of real-time intraoperative performance assessment with SIMPL (System for Improving and Measuring Procedural Learning): early experience from a multi-institutional trial. *J Surg Educ.* 2016;73(6):e118–e130. doi:10.1016/j.jsurg.2016.08.010.
42. Marty AP, Linsenmeyer M, George B, Young JQ, Breckwoldt J, ten Cate O. Mobile technologies to support workplace-based assessment for entrustment decisions: guidelines for programs and educators: AMEE Guide No. 154. *Med Teach.* 2023;Jan 27;1–11. doi:10.1080/0142159X.2023.2168527.

43. Puscas L, Kogan JR, Holmboe ES. Assessing interpersonal and communication skills. *J Grad Med Educ.* 2021;13(2 suppl):91–95. doi:10.4300/JGME-D-20-00883.1.
44. Guralnick S, Fondahn E, Amin A, Bittner EA. Systems-based practice: time to finally adopt the orphan competency. *J Grad Med Educ.* 2021;13(2 suppl):96–101. doi:10.4300/JGME-D-20-00839.1.
45. Schumacher DJ, Dornoff E, Carraccio C, et al. The power of contribution and attribution in assessing educational outcomes for individuals, teams, and programs. *Acad Med.* 2020;95(7):1014–1019. doi:10.1097/ACM.0000000000003121.
46. Choi JJ, Durning SJ. Three learning concepts to improve diagnosis and enhance the practice of medicine. *Diagnosis (Berl).* 2021;9(1):140–142. doi:10.1515/dx-2021-0030.
47. Holmboe ES, Iobst WF. The Assessment Guidebook. Accessed July 14, 2022. at Toolbox of (acgme.org)
48. Edgar L, McLean S, Hogan SO, Hamstra S, Holmboe ES. The Milestones Guidebook. Version 2020. Accessed March 29, 2023. at Competency-Based Training (acgme.org)
49. ten Cate O, Balmer DF, Caretta-Weyer H, Hatala R, Hennus MP, West DC. Entrustable professional activities and entrustment decision making: a development and research agenda for the next decade. *Acad Med.* 2021;96(7S):S96–S104. doi:10.1097/ACM.0000000000004106.
50. Royal College of Physicians and Surgeons of Canada. EPAs and CanMEDS Milestones. Accessed March 29, 2023. at EPAs and CanMEDS Milestones:: The Royal College of Physicians and Surgeons of Canada
51. Association of American Medical Colleges. The Core Entrustable Professional Activities (EPAs) for Entering Residency. Accessed March 29, 2023. at The Core Entrustable Professional Activities (EPAs) for Entering Residency | AAMC
52. Rekman J, Gofton W, Dudek N, Gofton T, Hamstra SJ. Entrustability scales: outlining their usefulness for competency-based clinical assessment. *Acad Med.* 2016;91(2):186–190. doi:10.1097/ACM.0000000000001045.
53. Delandshere G, Petrosky AR. Assessment of complex performances: limitations of key measurement assumptions. *Educ Res.* 1998;27(2):14–24. doi:10.3102/0013189X027002014.
54. Weller JM, Castanelli DJ, Chen Y, Jolly B. Making robust assessments of specialist trainees' workplace performance. *Br J Anaesth.* 2017 Feb;118(2):207–214. doi:10.1093/bja/aew412.
55. Valentine N, Wignes J, Benson J, Clota S, Schuwirth LW. Entrustable professional activities for workplace assessment of general practice trainees. *Med J Aust.* 2019 May;210(8):354–359. doi:10.5694/mja2.50130.
56. Schumacher DJ, Holmboe E, Carraccio C, et al. Resident-sensitive quality measures in the pediatric emergency department: exploring relationships with supervisor entrustment and patient acuity and complexity. *Acad Med.* 2020;95(8):1256–1264. doi:10.1097/ACM.0000000000003242.
57. Kogan JR, Dine CJ, Conforti LN, Holmboe ES. Can rater training improve the quality and accuracy of workplace-based assessment narrative comments and entrustment ratings? A randomized controlled trial. *Acad Med.* 2023;98(2):237–247. doi:10.1097/ACM.0000000000004819.
58. Holmboe ES, Kogan JR. Will any road get you there? Examining warranted and unwarranted variation in medical education. *Acad Med.* 2022;97(8):1128–1136. doi:10.1097/ACM.0000000000004667.
59. Ginsburg S, van der Vleuten CPM, Eva KW. The hidden value of narrative comments for assessment: a quantitative reliability analysis of qualitative data. *Acad Med.* 2017;92(11):1617–1621. doi:10.1097/ACM.0000000000001669.
60. Prentice S, Benson J, Schuwirth L, Kirkpatrick E. A meta-analysis and qualitative analysis of flagging and exam performance in general practice training. *Aus J Primary Health.* 2019;25(3):XLIII. doi:10.1007/s10459-021-10031-4.
61. Driessen E, van der Vleuten CPM, Schuwirth LWT, Van Tartwijk J, Vermunt J. The use of qualitative research criteria for portfolio assessment as an alternative to reliability evaluation: a case study. *Med Educ.* 2005 Feb;39(2):214–220. doi:10.1111/j.1365-2929.2004.02059.x.
62. Asch DA, Nicholson S, Srinivas S, Herrin J, Epstein AJ. Evaluating obstetrical residency programs using patient outcomes. *JAMA.* 2009;302(12):1277–1283. doi:10.1001/jama.2009.1356.
63. Epstein AJ, Srinivas SK, Nicholson S, Herrin J, Asch DA. Association between physicians' experience after training and maternal obstetrical outcomes: cohort study. *BMJ.* 2013 Mar 28;346:f1596. doi:10.1136/bmj.f1596.
64. Epstein AJ, Nicholson S, Asch DA. The Production of and Market for New Physicians' Skill. National Bureau of Economic Research working paper 18678. January 2013. Accessed September 19, 2013. http://www.nber.org/papers/w18678.
65. Asch DA, Nicholson S, Srinivas SK, Herrin J, Epstein AJ. How do you deliver a good obstetrician? Outcome-based evaluation of medical education. *Acad Med.* 2014 Jan;89(1):24–26. doi:10.1097/ACM.0000000000000067.
66. Bansal N, Simmons KD, Epstein AJ, Morris JB, Kelz RR. Using patient outcomes to evaluate general surgery residency program performance. *JAMA Surg.* 2016 Feb;151(2):111–119. doi:10.1001/jamasurg.2015.3637.
67. Chen C, Petterson S, Phillips R, Bazemore A, Mullan F. Spending patterns in region of residency training and subsequent expenditures for care provided by practicing physicians for Medicare beneficiaries. *JAMA.* 2014 Dec 10;312(22):2385–2393. doi:10.1001/jama.2014.15973.
68. Sirovich BE, Lipner RS, Johnston M, Holmboe ES. The association between residency training and internists' ability to practice conservatively. *JAMA Intern Med.* 2014 Oct;174(10):1640–1648. doi:10.1001/jamainternmed.2014.3337.
69. Phillips RL Jr, Petterson SM, Bazemore AW, Wingrove P, Puffer JC. The effects of training institution practice costs, quality, and other characteristics on future practice. *Ann Fam Med.* 2017 Mar;15(2):140–148. doi:10.1370/afm.2044.
70. Kendrick DE, Thelen AE, Chen X, et al. Association of surgical resident competency ratings with patient outcomes. *Acad Med.* 2023 Jul 1;98(7):813–820. doi:10.1097/ACM.0000000000005157.
71. Smith BK, Hamstra SJ, Yamazaki K, et al. Expert consensus on the conceptual alignment of Accreditation Council for Graduate Medical Education competencies with patient outcomes after common vascular surgical procedures. *J Vasc Surg.* 2022 Nov;76(5):1388–1397. doi:10.1016/j.jvs.2022.06.091.
72. Holmboe ES, Yamazaki K, Nasca TJ, Hamstra SJ. Longitudinal milestones data and learning analytics to facilitate the professional development of residents: early lessons from three specialties. *Acad Med.* 2020 Jan;95(1):97–103. doi:10.1097/ACM.0000000000002899.
73. Han M, Hamstra SJ, Hogan SO, et al. Trainee physician milestone ratings and patient complaints in early post-training practice. *JAMA Netw Open.* 2023 Apr 3;6(4):e237588. doi: 10.1001/jamanetworkopen.2023.7588.
74. Kim JG, Rodriguez HP, Holmboe ES, et al. The reliability of graduate medical education quality of care clinical performance measures. *J Grad Med Educ.* 2022 Jun;14(3):281–288. doi:10.4300/JGME-D-21-00706.1.

75. US Department of Education, Office of Educational Technology Education. Enhancing teaching and learning through educational data mining and learning analytics: an issue brief. October 2012. Accessed September 16, 2022. https://tech.ed.gov/wp-content/uploads/2014/03/edm-la-brief.pdf.
76. Ellaway RH, Pusic MV, Galbraith RM, Cameron T. Developing the role of big data and analytics in health professional education. *Med Teach.* 2014;36(3):216–222. doi:10.3109/0142159X.2014.874553.
77. Kogan JR, Hess BJ, Conforti LN, Holmboe ES. What drives faculty ratings of residents' clinical skills? The impact of faculty's own clinical skills. *Acad Med.* 2010;85(10 suppl):S25–S28. doi:10.1097/ACM.0b013e3181ed1aa3.
78. Kogan JR, Conforti LN, Iobst WF, Holmboe ES. Reconceptualizing variable rater assessments as both an educational and clinical care problem. *Acad Med.* 2014;89(5):721–727. doi:10.1097/ACM.0000000000000221.
79. Lucey CR, Hauer KE, Boatright D, Fernandez A. Medical education's wicked problem: achieving equity in assessment for medical learners. *Acad Med.* 2020;95(12 suppl):S98–S108. doi:10.1097/ACM.0000000000003717.
80. Alexis DA, Kearney MD, Williams JC, Xu C, Higginbotham EJ, Aysola J. Assessment of perceptions of professionalism among faculty, trainees, staff, and students in a large university-based health system. *JAMA Netw Open.* 2020;3(11):e2021452. doi:10.1001/jamanetworkopen.2020.21452.
81. Forscher PS, Lai CK, Axt JR, et al. A meta-analysis of procedures to change implicit measures. *J Pers Soc Psychol.* 2019;117(3):522–559. doi:10.1037/pspa0000160.
82. Morsy L. Carnegie and Rockefeller's philanthropic legacy: exclusion of African Americans from medicine. *Acad Med.* 2023 Mar 1;98(3):313–316. doi:10.1097/ACM.0000000000005092.
83. Forscher PS, Mitamura C, Dix EL, Cox WTL, Devine PG. Breaking the prejudice habit: Mechanisms, time course, and longevity. *J Exp Soc Psychol.* 2017;72:133–146. doi:10.1016/j.jesp.2017.04.009.
84. Dickey CC, Thomas C, Feroze U, Nakshabandi F, Cannon B. Cognitive demands and bias: challenges facing clinical competency committees. *J Grad Med Educ.* 2017 Apr;9(2):162–164. doi:10.4300/JGME-D-16-00411.1.
85. Englander R, Holmboe E, Batalden P, et al. Coproducing health professions education: a prerequisite to coproducing health care services? *Acad Med.* 2020;95(7):1006–1013. doi:10.1097/ACM.0000000000003137.
86. Damschroder LJ, Aron DC, Keith RE, Kirsh SR, Alexander JA, Lowery JC. Fostering implementation of health services research findings into practice: a consolidated framework for advancing implementation science. *Implement Sci.* 2009;4:50. doi:10.1186/1748-5908-4-50.
87. Hall AK, Rich J, Dagnone JD, et al. It's a marathon, not a sprint: rapid evaluation of competency-based medical education program implementation. *Acad Med.* 2020;95(5):786–793. doi:10.1097/ACM.0000000000003040.
88. Rich JV, Luhanga U, Fostaty Young S, et al. Operationalizing programmatic assessment: The CBME Programmatic Assessment Practice Guidelines. *Acad Med.* 2022 May 1;97(5):674–678. doi:10.1097/ACM.0000000000004574.
89. Van Der Vleuten CPM, Schuwirth LWT, Driessen EW, Govaerts MJB, Heeneman S. Twelve tips for programmatic assessment. *Med Teach.* 2015 Jul;37(7):641–646. doi:10.3109/0142159X.2014.973388.
90. Schuwirth L, van der Vleuten C, Durning SJ. What programmatic assessment in medical education can learn from healthcare. *Perspect Med Educ.* 2017 Aug;6(4):211–215. doi:10.1007/s40037-017-0345-1.
91. Misra S, Iobst WF, Hauer KE, Holmboe ES. The importance of competency-based programmatic assessment in graduate medical education. *J Grad Med Educ.* 2021 Apr;13(2 Suppl):113–119. doi:10.4300/JGME-D-20-00856.1.
92. Iobst WF, Holmboe ES. Programmatic assessment: the secret sauce of effective CBME implementation. *J Grad Med Educ.* 2020 Aug;12(4):518–521. doi:10.4300/JGME-D-20-00702.1.
93. Holmboe ES, Osman NY, Murphy CM, Kogan JR. The urgency of now: rethinking and improving assessment practices in medical education programs. *Acad Med.* 2023 Apr 18. doi:10.1097/ACM.0000000000005251.

4

Evaluation Frameworks, Assessment Forms, and Rating Scales

LOUIS N. PANGARO, MD, MACP, STEVEN J. DURNING, MD, PHD, AND ERIC S. HOLMBOE, MD

CHAPTER OUTLINE

Introduction

As noted in earlier chapters, assessing trainee performance in the care of "real" patients in actual practice settings is critical to effective evaluation.* Central to this process is the faculty member who is the observer of the clinical care and of the specific interactions of the learner with a patient, the patient's family, and other members of the healthcare team. Central to the concept of "competency-based" education is that observations and the judgments made about a learner's progress and readiness for advancement are explicit, public, and demonstrable; further that they are applied with consistency and with sufficient sampling to ensure readiness for the next stage of professional development. This chapter concerns itself with how concepts of competence, rating scales, and other evaluation forms are intended to guide the observer in what to look for and how to interpret what is seen. It is now understood that the faculty observer is not a dispassionate servomechanism using the evaluation (assessment) rubric provided, but is engaged in a social judgment involving complex interactions[1] and emotions that can also be affected by various biases. In other words, the problem of assessing learners in the clinical setting to achieve accuracy and equity[2] is not simply cognitive (a choice of the rating rubric) but equally a social and emotional process for the teacher, as well as logistic in the time the faculty member has to observe the learner while at the same time ensuring the patient's well-being. Central to this chapter is the understanding that the program or clerkship director cannot simply provide the teacher-rater with an evaluation form or rating scale and expect that summative judgments (e.g., assessment of learning) with good validity evidence can be made. We hope that reviewing the premises and uses of frameworks and forms will give program directors confidence in their process of providing feedback and in making advancement decisions.

To achieve a summative judgment of readiness for advancement, these in vivo observations are combined with standardized and typically quantified in vitro assessments of knowledge and procedural and/or interpersonal skills. Educators may label this activity as in-training assessment[3] or, more recently, workplace-based assessment (WBA). Effective assessment of overall clinical performance requires a multidimensional approach using both descriptive and quantified tools to describe the ability to provide patient care, and these assessments may include input from both

*For this chapter we will use the words *assessment* and *evaluation* interchangeably.

faculty and nonphysician observers (Fig. 4.1).[4] Such evaluation or assessment involves judgment, often using a rating scale and narrative, about a learner's performance. This chapter will discuss the frameworks underlying evaluation, systems of descriptive assessment yielding narrative evaluation, rating systems yielding a quantified evaluation, and the use and pitfalls of rating scales. Evaluation forms and rating scales may initially be applied at the level of the interaction between the learner and a single patient, and the form provides the framework that allows teachers to convert their observations into information that can be used for feedback to the learner and to the program as part of its ongoing quality improvement efforts. To achieve an eventual decision about advancement of the learner to the next level of responsibility, there must be numerous observations in many contexts (i.e., clinical situations) by many observers that ultimately allow the process to achieve a level of confidence sufficient for a high-stakes ("summative") decision. To do this, the evaluation framework, the assessment form, and the rating scale must be robust; that is, have strong reliability and validity evidence in each use (see Chapter 2).

The most common method used by faculty for evaluating overall performance has been the global rating scale included as part of an evaluation form, in which the term *global* implies an all-inclusive synthesis of performance dimensions over some period of time; the term *scale* refers to a linear and ordinal analog (often a line with numbers) for distinguishing levels or steps of performance; and the term *rating* refers to the act of locating a person's performance on the continuum or at a specific level.[5,6] The rating scale is one component of an evaluation form, which typically also expects descriptive, written comments.[7] The intention is that the final evaluation documented on the form should be the aggregate of the scale rating(s) on specific competencies plus descriptive, written comments. The expectation is that the ratings on individual scales and the overall evaluation of the learner will reflect the institution's framework of assessment, and for graduate medical education (GME) will in turn reflect the expectations of the specialty's national organization, such as the Accreditation Council for Graduate Medical Education/American Board of Medical Specialties (ACGME/ABMS) Milestones in the United States. In other words, the premises about what successful performance looks like—the "construct" underlying the assessment—should be shared on the evaluation form in both the rating scale and the rater's observations; these are all aligned with a concept, construct, or mental model that is shared by the program, learners, and teachers.[8] As we will emphasize in this chapter, the more a rater accepts the premises of the rating scale—a process of construct alignment—the more successful the rating process will be.[9]

$$\text{Evaluation Form} = \text{Scale Rating}(s) + \text{Written Evaluation}$$

Where do evaluation forms fit into a medical education evaluation system? Comprehensive evaluation of a trainee is a multidimensional composite that is authored by the director of the academic program ("academic director"; i.e., fellowship director, program director, or clerkship director) and often includes both summary evaluations of learners by one or more teachers and a series of quantified measurements. Evaluations by individual teachers in turn may be their own syntheses of multiple observations over days or weeks, with or without direct observations of competence at individual tasks.

It is the role of academic managers[10] such as fellowship or residency program, clerkship, or course directors to achieve consistently credible evaluations of trainees, for the sake of both society and future patients (summative evaluation) and to enhance the improvement of trainees through feedback (formative evaluation) (see Chapter 1). Formative evaluation, "assessment for learning," is most important for professional development, feedback, and coaching. The design and systematic use of evaluation forms, with or without rating scales, is one strategy academic managers can use to foster credible evaluations that are valid and not arbitrary (i.e., the evaluations are based on societal, professional, and institutional goals and not on goals that may be idiosyncratic to the teacher); that are reliable and reproducible (i.e., the evaluation framework is applied consistently and not capriciously across observations by teachers; and in which formative evaluations can be relied upon by learners as anticipations of summative grading.[11] Faculty development in general is a quality improvement process in training teachers how to use evaluation forms and scales, and specifically is intended to minimize unacceptable variation[12,13]

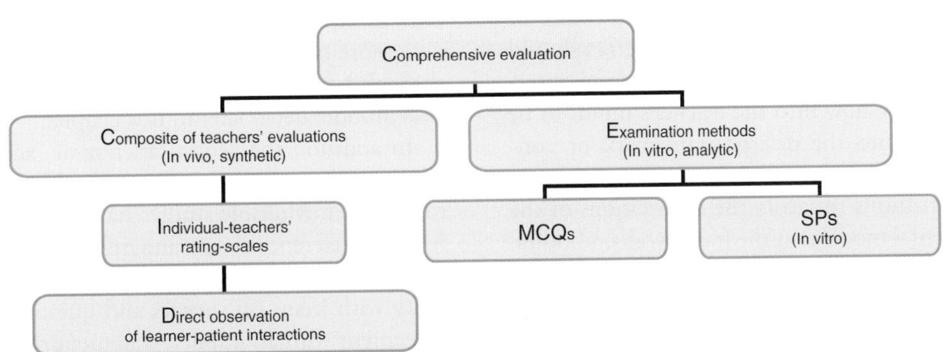

• **Fig. 4.1** Placing evaluation forms into a comprehensive system. *MCQs*, multiple-choice questions; *SPs*, standardized patient examinations.

between observers in which ratings would depend more upon teacher characteristics or teacher preferences than upon attributes of the trainee. It is important to understand that the teacher completing the rating scale is the actual assessment "instrument" and that the form provides a way to communicate and foster shared expectations and document performance.

Evaluation forms are in themselves, implicitly or explicitly, frameworks to guide teachers' observations and documentation of a learner's performance. Therefore they usually include an explicit statement of goals for the learners, or at least the criteria by which learners are to be judged. As an official and legal document of a program or institution, these forms publicly express curricular goals and are intended to avoid variance that is arbitrary due to having inconsistent goals and standards across teachers. However, they are not guarantees that teachers will not be capricious (inconsistent or idiosyncratic) in applying them to individual learners.[14] Indeed, the rating scale must make sense to the rater and foster construct alignment between the rater and institutional expectations.

We will begin this chapter by discussing the importance of evaluation frameworks to guide the user in their effective use. Next, we provide an outline of the advantages and disadvantages of rating scales and evaluation forms, including some important psychometric rating error issues that limit the effectiveness of evaluation forms. The chapter will close with practical suggestions on how to prepare faculty to use evaluation forms more effectively.

Evaluation Forms and Frameworks

In any evaluation form used in evaluating a trainee, there is an underlying set of assumptions about what we expect of the trainee (what are the educational goals?); and about the tasks that a trainee must complete successfully to demonstrate that the goals have been achieved (curricular objectives). This set of assumptions can be considered the underlying framework that encompasses ("frames") what the observer must compare the trainee to in order to decide whether the trainee is progressing. This side-to-side comparison between what the teacher *does* observe in this learner as distinct from what the teacher *expects* to see provides the "is-versus-ought" or "real-versus-ideal" that is the basis of most judgments that lead to assigning labels (i.e., codes) or classifications (e.g., rating scales). Program directors should not see this as a passive process in which meaningful observations will successfully flow into the teacher's mind, to be subsequently placed into the desired framework or construct. It should be seen as an active process in which the teacher seeks observations to satisfy the expectations of the evidence-based mental model that the framework embodies.

Just as in diagnosis of clinical syndromes, it is critical that the observer has an accurate and valid mental model against which to compare the trainee. Educational frameworks are ways to conceptualize expectations for the comparisons that underlie evaluations of trainees' success. Teachers commonly divide educational goals into the three familiar categories of knowledge, skills, and attitudes. We will describe this as well as other useful frameworks in the next section.

Analytic Frameworks

In the traditional framework used in education, including in elementary and secondary school, there are typically three domains: knowledge, skills, and attitudes (KSA). It is straightforward to place learning objectives for learners, especially in preclinical rotations, into the three KSA domains: for instance, *knowledge* of the structures within the chest cavity, *skill* in the physical examination of heart and lungs, and a proper *attitude* of respect for the patient's physical comfort and privacy.

The analytic approach to formulating educational goals provides a generic set of terms that can be applied to any curricular task in any field of education. The analytic approach is particularly useful when trying to measure discrete aspects of performance, and of course program directors are quite familiar with using a single multiple-choice test as a measure of knowledge and perhaps with using a checklist to rate skill in examining a patient's knee or in giving informed consent. By isolating one particular aspect of performance—for instance, the ability to interview the patient about an alcohol history or the ability to place a central venous catheter—the analytic method allows us to create a fairly detailed set of performance tasks that can be compiled into a checklist, which in turn can be placed on a rating form. Such a checklist can be as detailed as necessary to help the teacher document whether each aspect of a particular task can be performed separately, prior to the teacher combining them into a single (global) rating. Together, the checklist and overall global rating constitute the criterion description of what ultimate proficiency or competency looks like for this task. The analytic method requires an evaluation form to have at least three scales, with labels at the top of each gradation to distinguish levels of success (Fig. 4.2A). The scale is an example of using "quality of performance" as the ratings, and these scales continue to be used despite growing evidence that they suffer from a lack of construct alignment (discussed later in the chapter) and require a substantial amount of translation by the rater.[9] In the example given, the labels are rudimentary and require the user to infer what the terms mean. For the critical, central label of "Acceptable," the form might provide more concrete terms for or examples of what is meant through use of behaviorally anchored scales, which we discuss in more detail later in this chapter.

In addition the central anchor of "acceptability" is not made explicit and defers the applicable criterion or criteria to the rater. Multiple studies have shown that the primary frame of reference (i.e., standard) used by faculty is self (see Chapter 5). Rating scales on evaluation forms have similarity with items on surveys and questionnaires, asking for agreement with an implicit statement that the learner being evaluated meets, exceeds, or falls short of some criteria of acceptability. There are pitfalls that program directors can

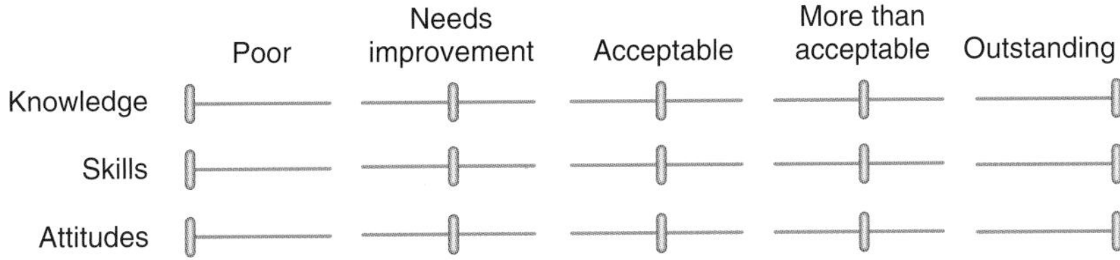

• **Fig. 4.2a** Rating scale in knowledge-skills-attitude framework with rudimentary anchors.

avoid in creating items for faculty to rate, such as not having anchors for each level or using both words and numbers for each level.[15]

It is also worth noting that other scale anchor types are still commonly used, and all suffer from the same issues noted earlier. The traditional mini clinical evaluation exercise (mini-CEX) uses a 9-point scale with the scale anchors of 1–3 (unsatisfactory), satisfactory,[4–6] and superior.[7–9] Others use normative scaling (i.e., assessed against the expected performance of others) with variable frames of reference for the expectations (i.e., compared to peer learner, graduating learner, or practicing physician). Such scales tend to range from "fails to meet expectations" to "exceeds expectations." Finally, some evaluations using an analytic framework will employ frequency scales (e.g., "rarely" to "almost always"), assuming a greater frequency of a behavior indicates higher levels of competence. While all of these types of analytic scales may have utility in specific circumstances, we do not recommend the routine use of these scales. Instead, we strongly recommend educators choose scales for their evaluation forms based on *developmental* frameworks.

Developmental Frameworks

The growth of human beings has often been used as a metaphor for the growth of trainees in an educational process. The pedigree of this approach is ancient, and Plato describes the growth of the individual from a preoccupation with surface, concrete details toward a perception of the true meaning and form underlying them. In the well-known *Taxonomy of Educational Objectives in the Cognitive Domain,* Bloom[16,17] provides a vocabulary for describing the progressively higher mental skills acquired by students in primary education: knowledge, comprehension, application, analysis, synthesis, and evaluation The developmental model of Dreyfus and Dreyfus,[18] revised for GME,[19] provides a generic vocabulary of educational progress for adult learners from novice to advanced beginner, competent performance, proficient performance, intuitive expert, and master. Developmental considerations are essential for medical school faculty because they reflect the facts that students grow, that not all learners are at the same level of performance, and that in the clinical setting there are often learners at several levels of training. The models of Bloom and Dreyfus typically focus on cognitive aspects of development, and personal and attitudinal characteristics are not always evident. Bloom, and to some extent Dreyfus, choose to treat the attitudinal ("affective") domain separately from the cognitive. However, one advantage of developmental over analytic models is that the recognition of growth and progress is explicit and does not have to be inferred by the teacher or the student. To this extent, any curriculum that has learners at different stages, like medical school, requires some explicitly developmental aspect. Using the Dreyfus model as an ordinal rating scale—similar to a Likert scale—could be constructed with the word *Novice* on the left and the word *Master* at the extreme right (see Fig. 4.2B).

The Dreyfus terms used as "anchors" on the linear scale shown in Fig. 4.2 are global (i.e., generic and nonspecific), and a more detailed, developmental scale could be devised for a specific domain within the analytic framework.

This can be made less vague, although still abstract, using Bloom's taxonomy for the growth of clinical reasoning. For example, Fig. 4.2C demonstrates how you might judge a resident's presentation of a patient.

In this example, the criterion against which the resident is to be rated is an idea or construct or what effective clinical

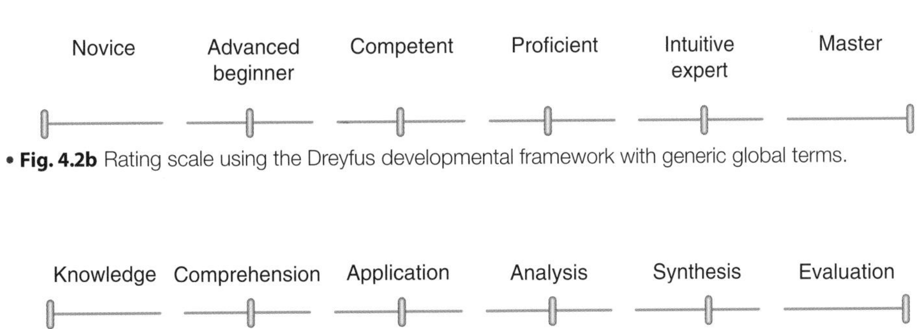

• **Fig. 4.2b** Rating scale using the Dreyfus developmental framework with generic global terms.

• **Fig. 4.2c** Rating scale using the developmental framework from Bloom's taxonomy in the cognitive domain.

reasoning looks like, and the program director should use the best available evidence of what effective clinical reasoning should look like (i.e., accurate diagnoses and treatment plans; see Chapter 7) as the expectation or standard of comparison.

Given the ACGME/ABMS framework of six competencies, in each of which a *finishing* resident is judged to be successful (or not), such static or pass/fail dichotomous ratings of competence must be modified for those earlier in their training. The faculty or program director must determine what is the standard to be met within the criterion for each level, and the program director must reframe each specific ACGME competency into a developmental model that can describe what the acceptable/passing standard of performance is for student, intern, resident, or fellow. To help in this process, more structured ways to describe and document progress have recently been introduced: Milestones and Entrustable Professional Activities (EPAs).[20] Milestones,[21,22] as described in Chapter 1, are observable behaviors or tasks that *combine or synthesize* knowledge, skill, and attitudes and therefore may be seen as synthetic to better define a competency in narrative terms. Using the concept of stages of development, the Milestones provide an explicit developmental scale for a resident's professional development across the competencies. The Royal College of Physicians and Surgeons of Canada (RCPSC) has also created Milestones for its competency-based medical education (CBME) initiatives.[23] These and EPAs are described in the next section. This combination of different domains into a single observation means Milestones are a synthetic approach.[24]

GME programs are now required to report residents' progress in a range of subcompetencies described in narrative Milestone levels (typically 20 to 25 subcompetencies per specialty), which represent progressive steps toward achieving mastery performance within an ACGME competency domain.[21] Milestones can allow faculty observers to focus on the task rather than the framework.[22] Milestones, although organized as a set of subcompetency domains, can be considered synthetic in that a number of the subcompetency domains, such as the subcompetency "System Navigation for Patient Care," do require the integration of knowledge, skills, and attitudes. Ultimately, however, a synthesis of all assessment information must be performed to answer the most important question of whether a learner is or is not ready for the next stage of their career, also satisfying the legal precept of looking at the "entirety" of the learner's record of performance.[10]

A Synthetic Model

As students and residents progress toward independence, we expect that they themselves will spontaneously bring whatever skills, knowledge, and attitudes are necessary to help a patient each day; the learner is responsible for deciding (either consciously or not) what the patient needs. This leads to a "synthetic" definition of competence as "the ability to bring to each patient seen in one's practice everything that that patient needs, and nothing else."[25] In other words, competence at the point of unsupervised (aka independent) practice requires that the resident decides what the task is, right at this moment, and summons up whatever skill, knowledge, or attitude is needed.[16] In rating performance, we might comment separately on a resident's fund of knowledge or "attitude," but in the end we have to judge whether residents have been able to master all the necessary attributes and—on their own—combine them successfully. A synthetic framework "puts things together" in a vocabulary that emphasizes progressively higher expectations as a student progresses through the clinical years and through residency. The underlying premise is that the goal of medical education is growing independence from supervision, understanding that medicine is a team activity and that no individual is ever truly independent when caring for patients. Interns are in supervised practice, but their level of responsibility is clearly higher than that of students. More importantly, when residents graduate and move into practice, their ability to function without supervision must be documented. These concepts of responsibility, entrustability, and function are all synthetic, in which a combination of knowledge, skills, and attitudes is required.

"Independence" does not mean a lack of accountability, or freedom to function outside the medical care system; in fact, the opposite is now taught in training programs under the "Systems-based Practice" competency of the ACGME. However, growing independence from supervision is one underlying premise of the synthetic model, and it has this in common with developmental models (differences will be discussed later in the chapter).

A useful synthetic framework for evaluating students and residents in their progress from understanding into action uses a descriptive, developmental vocabulary: Reporter-Interpreter-Manager-Educator (RIME)[11] (see Table 4.1 and Appendix 4.1).

The RIME framework can be used by itself as a tool for structuring observations of each learner–patient interaction, for categorizing an overall level achieved in a rotation, or as a larger framework for teachers to frame more granular systems such as Milestones, competencies, or EPAs. Since the underlying rhythm of RIME is observation-reflection-action, it corresponds to the History & Physical – assessment – plan sequence that all clinicians have used during their years of training (see Table 4.2).

TABLE 4.1 RIME Framework: Short Definitions

Reporter: learner takes ownership of collecting and communicating the patient's findings and priorities (symptoms, exam, labs, images, medications).

Interpreter: learner takes ownership of explaining new, abnormal, or important findings.

Manager: learner takes ownership of planning with patients (diagnostic, therapeutic, and patient education).

Educator: learner takes ownership of improving care through study.

(see Appendix 1 for fuller definitions)

TABLE 4.2 The Analogous Rhythm of the Scientific, Clinical, and RIME Processes

Classical Scientific Method	Clinical Process	RIME Scheme
Observation	History and physical	Reporter
Reflection	Diagnosis	Interpreter
Action	Therapy	Manager
Reflection/Further observations Follow-up		Educator

This supports the framework's acceptance as a shared mental model and helps achieve the desired construct alignment[9] of teachers and activities of learners. Each of the more granular ACGME subcompetencies can be mapped to the RIME framework (see Appendix 4.2).[26] The Patient Care Milestones of each specialty can be visualized in what Hemmer has termed "RIME-stones" (see Appendix 4.3) and the 13 Core Entrustable Professional Activities for Entering Residency (CEPAERs) proposed by the Association of American Medical Colleges (AAMC) can be implemented as ready-to-use dimensions of performance within the RIME framework[27] (see Table 4.3).

We can see that different frameworks provide degrees of granularity that are useful in different settings (Fig. 4.3).

The RIME framework uses these classifications (reporter, etc.) to describe the ability at which the trainee functions—either in a single patent encounter or globally. Each RIME step is a final "common pathway" that requires a synthesis of skills, knowledge, and attitude. This can be used for setting minimal expectations for learners in each year of training, or for describing the level of activity for which the learner is judged or trusted to be consistent. The RIME framework does not set the upper bound of what a student or resident is allowed to do, but rather the minimal standard of acceptable performance for the learner's level of training. In this respect RIME is a "razor," helping teachers set a clear-cut point below which the learner is classified as not yet ready for higher responsibility.

In rating an individual learner–patient encounter, the RIME method can be applied directly to the level of performance just observed. On the other hand, for an end-of-rotation evaluation form, it is up to the teacher to be sure that the overall rating reflects the level the learner has achieved with consistency, and with the common, core medical issues that are likely to be encountered at the next level of training or practice.

Learners may be quite proficient at interpreting chest pain in a hospitalized patient but complete novices in dealing with nodular goiter in an outpatient clinic. This content- and context-based expertise has been demonstrated in both students and residents. The RIME framework describes how

TABLE 4.3 EPAs within the RIME Framework

Core Entrustable Professional Activity (EPA) Pregraduation	EPA #
Reporter	
Gather a history and perform a physical exam.	1
Document a clinical encounter in the patient record.	5
Provide an oral presentation of a clinical encounter.	6
Collaborate as a member of an interprofessional team.	9
Interpreter	
Prioritize a differential diagnosis following a clinical encounter.	2
Recognize a patient requiring urgent or emergent care.	10
Recommend and interpret common diagnostic and screening tests.	3
Manager	
Enter and discuss orders and prescriptions.	4
Give or receive a patient handover to transition care responsibility.	8
Obtain informed consent for tests and/or procedures.	11
Perform the general procedures of a physician.	12
Educator	
Form clinical questions and retrieve evidence to advance patient care.	7
Identify system failures and contribute to a culture of safety and improvement.	13

The EPAs and the associated numbers are from the *Core Entrustable Professional Activities for Entering Residency*, Association of American Medical Colleges, 2014.

a learner interacts with a particular patient, and it is up to the teacher to make a judgment about their overall level of performance with common, core problems that are expected to be seen within each educational experience.

The RIME framework is not developmental in the sense that learners do not sequentially drop prior functions. Residents and faculty, for instance, continue to perform their roles as reporter. Advanced learners do not typically separate the tasks of reporting and interpreting or reporting and managing. For an expert, the fundamentals of differential diagnosis underlie the way patients are interviewed and examined; in other words, the task of interpretation is contained within the gathering of data, and a good oral case presentation typically contains an implicit interpretation. Like other approaches that describe function, the level of performance does depend upon context and the patient's problem. Learners may be quite proficient at interpreting chest pain in a hospitalized patient, but complete novices in dealing with nodular goiter in a referral clinic.

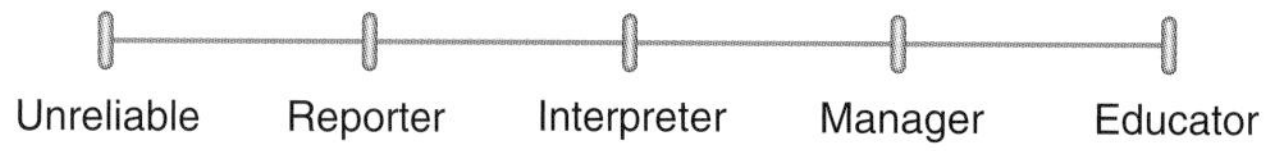

Unreliable Reporter Interpreter Manager Educator

• **Fig. 4.2d** "Distances" between performance levels on any scale may not be equal, as illustrated in RIME.

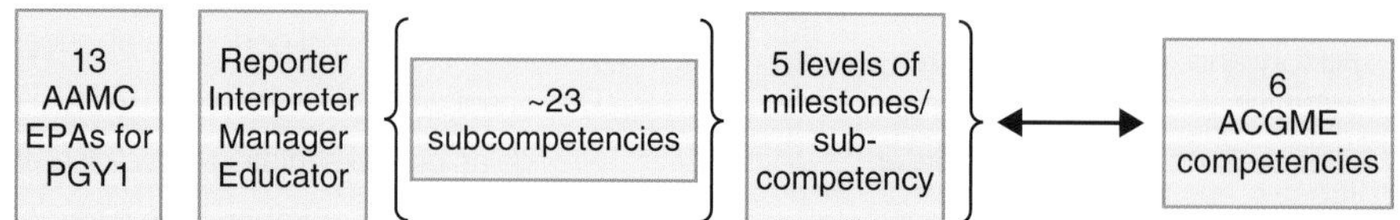

• **Fig. 4.3 Relationships and degree of granularity in assessment frameworks used in graduate medical education in the United States.** *AAMC*, Association of American Medical Colleges; *ACGME*, Accreditation Council for Graduate Medical Education; *EPAs*, Entrustable Professional Activities; *PGY1*, postgraduate year 1.

However, a resident ready for independent practice is not simply a manger for pneumonia, but also reports and interprets successfully. In other words, the RIME synthetic framework has an explicit developmental aspect but is not, strictly speaking, developmental.

The RIME scheme guides teachers' observations in looking for the signs of interpretation or management within the trainee's act of reporting. Perhaps more importantly, the apparent stages of the RIME scheme can be used to establish a minimally acceptable level of performance for learners at each level. A clinical clerk must always be an acceptable reporter, even though interpreting is not yet proficient. A resident, on the other hand, must always be successful as reporter, interpreter, and manager.

In the global rating scale (Fig. 4.2D), interpreter is depicted as a higher level of performance than reporter and manager is higher than interpreter. Are the distances between the three equal? There are no empirical data to support this, and since being an educator is part of the action phase of the process, it is difficult to assign a visual distance between them (Fig. 4.2D).

EPAs have emerged in both graduate medical education and undergraduate medical education (UGME). Originally defined by Olle ten Cate, EPAs represent the routine professional-life activities of physicians based on their specialty and subspecialty (see Chapter 1). Entrustable means a physician has demonstrated the necessary knowledge, skills, and attitudes (or competencies) to be trusted to ultimately perform the activity unsupervised. EPAs logically have led to the development of entrustment scales that are focused on levels of learner ability and defined by the actions of the rater regarding supervision of those actions, as opposed to inference of the competence of the individual trainee.[28]

A central concept of EPAs is that *trust* is an internal construct in the teacher that can be relied upon for consistent assessment of learners. Per ten Cate and colleagues, "Trust involves the confident expectation that a person (i.e., student or learner) can be relied on to honour implied or established commitments to an individual (i.e., *faculty and patient*) and to protect [the individual's] interest. It renders the individual (i.e., *faculty and patient*) vulnerable to the extent (s)he cannot oversee or control the actions of the other, on whose expertise or integrity (s)he may depend."[29]

Teachers decide when and for what tasks they trust trainees to assume clinical responsibilities. As units or domains of entrustment, EPAs are believed to represent the critical activities of the profession that the learner should be able to achieve unsupervised (i.e., earned independence) prior to graduation. EPAs are synthetic as they require multiple knowledge, skills, and attitudes and encompass multiple competency milestones (see Chapter 1). Like RIME, EPAs enable better construct alignment of the evaluation task and the activity being assessed and thus may improve evaluation[9,30] (also see Chapter 9).

For example, managing an upper gastrointestinal hemorrhage is an EPA. Doing so requires knowledge (e.g., anatomy and causes of bleeding), skills (e.g., performing endoscopy), and attitude/behavior (e.g., confidence to perform the task in an unstable patient). Like Milestones, it also encompasses multiple subcompetencies in the ACGME framework and thus represents a synthetic product.

Two main types of entrustment scales are currently in use. The first type often uses a 1–5 rating scale based on improving performance and the nature of supervision required. Supervision-based entrustment scales are sometimes referred to as "prospective entrustment scales" as the rater is judging the performance or encounter in relation to the amount of supervision that will be required moving forward. For supervision-based scales, a resident at Level 1 either can only observe others perform the task or cannot perform the EPA without direct assistance from a teacher. Level 2 embodies a learner who can perform the EPA under direct supervision while at Level 3 the learner can perform the procedure with the teacher standing outside the room or at a distance (indirect supervision). At Levels 4 and 5 the learner can perform the task independent of the teacher (they are entrusted to perform the activity without direct or indirect supervision). Tables 4.4 and 4.5 provide several examples of supervision-type entrustment scales directed at GME and at UME.

The other version of entrustment rating is the coactivity scale, which defines the level of entrustment by the amount of input and contribution required on the part of supervising faculty. The surgical O-SCORE is a commonly used coactivity scale (see Fig. 4.4).

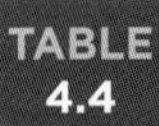

TABLE 4.4 **Entrustment in Postgraduate Education**

Based on this single observation, please provide an overall judgment of this learner.

Level

1. Learner can be present but only as an **observer**. I would not let the learner perform this skill the next time.
2. Learner can practice skill with **direct supervision** (supervisor in room). I (or someone else) would need to watch the learner perform the skill in real time.
3. Learner can practice skill with **indirect supervision** (supervision available within minutes). I (or someone else) do not need to watch the learner in the room but will need to reassess the patient/confirm findings with the patient.
4. **Unsupervised practice** allowed (distant oversight). I (or someone else) do not need to watch the learner but I (or someone else) am available if the learner comes for help or to provide feedback.

From Kogan JR, Dine CJ, Conforti LN, Holmboe ES. can rater training improve the quality and accuracy of workplace-based assessment narrative comments and entrustment ratings? A randomized controlled trial. *Acad Med*. 2023 Feb 1;98(2):237-247. doi:10.1097/ACM.0000000000004819.

TABLE 4.5 **Entrustment in Medical School Education**

Proposed UME scale

1. Not allowed to practice
   a. Inadequate knowledge/skill (e.g., does not know how to preserve sterile field); not allowed to observe
   b. Adequate knowledge, some skill; allowed to observe
2. Allowed to practice only under proactive, full supervision
   a. As coactivity with supervisor
   b. With supervisor in room ready to step in as needed
3. Allowed to practice only under reactive/on-demand supervision
   a. With supervisor immediately available, all findings double-checked
   b. With supervisor immediately available, key findings double-checked
   c. With supervisor distantly available (e.g., by phone), findings reviewed
4. Allowed to practice EPA unsupervised
5. Allowed to supervise others in practice

From Chen C, Sjoukje van den Broek WE, ten Cate O. The case for use of Entrustable Professional Activities in undergraduate medical education. *Acad Med*. 2015 Apr; 90(4):431-436. doi:10.1097/ACM.0000000000000586.

EPA, Entrustable Professional Activity; *UME*, undergraduate medical education.

The Ottawa Surgical Competency Operating Room (O-SCORE) Scale[a]: An Entrustability-Aligned Anchor Scale

Level	Descriptor
1	"I had to do" (i.e., requires complete hands on guidance, did not do, or as not given the opportunity to do)
2	"I had to talk them through" (i.e., able to perform tasks but requires constant direction)
3	"I had to prompt them from time to time" (i.e., demonstrates some independence, but requires intermittent direction)
4	"I needed to be there in the room just in case" Table (i.e., independence but unaware of risks and still requires supervision for safe practice)
5	"I did not need to be there" (i.e., complete independence, understands risks and performs safely, practice ready)

[a]The authors addoted the scale 'rom Gof:on W, Dudek N, Wood T, Balaa F, Hamstra S. The Ottawa surgical competency operaTing room evaluation (0-SCORE): A tool to assess surgical competence. Acad Med. 2012;87:1401-407.

• **Fig. 4.4** The Ottawa Surgical Competency Operating Room (O-Score) Scale: an entrustability-aligned anchor scale.

Finally, the Zwisch scale (Fig. 4.5) has also gained a following in the procedural community (see Chapter 9) and contains a 4-level scale: level 1 = show and tell; level 2 = active help ("smart help"); level 3 = passive help ("dumb help"); and level 4 = supervision only ("no help").[33]

Achieving Construct Alignment Through Simplicity

One way to enhance the construct alignment of newer, more granular assessment methods is to locate them within the rhythm of observation-reflection-action also seen in the Subjective-Objective-Assessment-Plan (SOAP) format and in RIME. In this way the RIME framework can function as an organizer that allows assimilation or subsumption of more elaborate structures under something already familiar. One example of this locates the 13 EPAs recently proposed by the AAMC as a set of tasks in which all students should be minimally proficient before beginning graduate medical education.[34] As seen in Table 4.3, the items in the CEPAERs list align well with the RIME framework and allow the teacher to use prior knowledge of RIME to remember and use the longer list of newer terms. In a report of 10 pilot schools using EPAs to establish readiness for GME, 66% of students met reporter EPAs, 36% met interpreter EPAs, and 17% met manager/educator EPAs.[35] A similar

TABLE 1. Zwisch Proposed Model for Teaching and Assessment in the Operating Room (Level Designated Based on Supervision Provided for the Majority of the Key Portions of the Case)

Zwisch Stage of Supervision	Attending Behaviors	Resident Behaviors Commensurate with This Level of Supervision
Show and Tell	Does majority of key portions as the surgeon Narrates the case (i.e., thinks out loud) Demonstrates key concepts, anatomy, and skills	Opens and closes First assists and observes
Cues to advancement		When first assisting, begins to actively assist (i.e., anticipates surgeons needs)
Smart Help	Shifts between surgeon and first assist roles When first assisting, leads the resident in surgeon role (active assist) Optimizes the field/exposure Demonstrates the plane or structure Coaches for specific techinal skills Coaches regarding the next steps Continues to identify anatomical landmarks for the resident	The above, plus: Shifts between surgeon and first assist roles Knowns all the component technical skills perform different key parts of the operation with attending assistance
Cues to advancement		Can execute the majority steps of procedure with active assistance
Dumb Help	Assists and follows the lead of the resident (passive assist) Coaching regarding polishing and refinement of skills Follows the resident's lead throught the operation	The above, plus: Can "set up" and accomplish the next step for the entire case with increasing efficiency Recognizes critical transition point issues
Cues to advancement		Can transition between all steps with passive assist from faculty
No Help	Largely provides no unsolicited advice Assisted by a junior resident or an attending acting like a junior resident Monitors progress and patient saftey*	The above plus: Can work with inexperienced first assistant Can saftely complete a case without faculty Can recover most errors Recognizes when to seek help/advice

• **Fig. 4.5** The Zwisch Proposed Model for Teaching and Assessment in the Operating Room.

correspondence exists between the six ACGME competences and, for instance, the 22 subcompetencies in internal medicine[26] and may also allow teachers to manage the more granular system of competencies.

Descriptive Terminology for Narratives in Evaluation

Why is it necessary to have a vocabulary of descriptive evaluation for use by teachers in the clinical setting? Such evaluations are often felt to be subjective and susceptible to biases of the individual teacher.[36] Objective assessment tools, such as multiple-choice tests or an objective structured clinical examination (OSCE) using standardized patients, have been considered to be more reliable. However, such highly structured examinations are resource intensive, are under the control of program and clerkship directors rather than everyday teachers, and are difficult to arrange frequently enough to provide ongoing feedback. Moreover, they often assess only one dimension or competency at a time. The ability to "put it all together" and bring it to the current specific clinical situation usually requires an expert to make the judgment; that is, a faculty member who is trained or calibrated to make such determinations. In any case, clinical teachers spend so much time with learners that a descriptive vocabulary and framework are very helpful if their observations are to be used for formative evaluation (feedback) or summative evaluation (grading). We hope to persuade our teachers that their descriptions of a student's behavior are not inevitably inferior to computerized tests and high-fidelity simulations using mannequins; in fact, because of its feasibility and easy application, we would argue that "low-tech is good tech."

The RIME scheme is one attempt to help teachers make their observations more structured and more consistent, by providing a useful description of what success looks like for each trainee. In fact, using the RIME scheme it is possible to achieve the level of reliability that is sufficient for pass/fail decisions,[37] that has predictive validity for identifying poor performance during internship,[38,39] and that helps achieve a high degree of intersite consistency in a multisite curriculum.[40] In other words, evaluations using words can be both reliable and valid, if they are part of a system of regular *frame of reference* training for teachers (see Chapter 5).[41–43] It may be more appropriate to refer to such evaluations by teachers as *descriptive*, avoiding the term *subjective*, which carries a pejorative connotation for those trained in sciences. Teachers are more reluctant to offer comments on personal behaviors, which they or students might consider hard to measure (subjective); yet these are exactly what we must capture if we are to give feedback on professional growth.[44,45] The RIME descriptive vocabulary has been reported to be feasible and fair by students and faculty at multiple institutions.[46–48] Perhaps more importantly, several studies by Hemmer et al. have shown what would probably seem intuitive: that teachers will tell you what they will not write down on evaluation forms, and that this information is more sensitive in detecting students who have deficiencies of general knowledge on multiple-choice final examination scores and in detecting students with professionalism problems.[45,49] In other words, the "low-tech" method of asking teachers what they think about students can be helpful in providing students with interim information about their progress that can help them anticipate summative evaluations. The work of Hemmer also highlights the importance of group process (i.e., asking faculty for an evaluation using a framework like RIME) combined with the evaluation forms to obtain a more complete picture of performance (see Chapter 16).

The synthetic RIME framework provides a way for teachers and trainees to visualize what success looks like. The RIME terms are more concrete and are more behavioral than the generic terms of the analytic models (*knowledge, skills,* and *attitudes*) or the developmental model of Dreyfus (*novice, beginner, expert,* etc., when used without narrative descriptors). RIME takes advantage of clinicians' ability to make diagnoses from sets of observations and to classify learners as reporting, interpreting, et cetera. Since its "rhythm" (observation-reflection-action) parallels the day-to-day activities of clinicians and scientists, it has an intuitive value and acceptance by teachers, as noted in Table 4.2.

There is probably not an intern in the United States who has not written a "SOAP" note in which that classic rhythm of observation-reflection-action is reproduced, with observations recorded as "Subjective, Objective" and reflection-action as "Assessment and Plan." In other words, the rhythm within the RIME scheme captures what physicians and scientists do every day. It is simple without being simplistic.

Complementary Frameworks: ACGME General Competencies and RIME

It is helpful to explain the how frameworks can be complementary and not mutually exclusive. Three of the ACGME/ABMS general competencies are the traditional knowledge, skills, and attitudes of the analytic approach and are implicit, not explicit, in the RIME framework. In other words, if after a night on call the resident can successfully propose an evidence-based management plan that incorporates patient preferences, it follows that they have the needed medical knowledge and the reasoning, interpersonal, and communication skills and have accepted professional ownership of the need to do so. The ACGME term *Patient Care* is the primary competency and essentially a synthetic term that is encompassed in the four terms of the RIME scheme. Systems-based Practice is contained in the term *Manager*, and Practice-based Learning and Improvement is an advanced form of being an Educator.

The approaches used to assess development also have alignment across competency milestones and EPAs, as shown in Table 4.6.

Frameworks: Concluding Thoughts

Frameworks are not inherently right or wrong. They are mental constructs that reflect goals and help structure instruction and assessment. Frameworks are useful in their different ways to help teachers assess trainees' progress toward independence. Synthetic models are strongest in structuring observations made of learners in their actual care of patients (in vivo), since these involve complex tasks that require multiple attributes. Analytic models are best at looking at discrete tasks whether in the care of patients (in vivo) or under testing conditions (in vitro).

We wish to stress two principles of assessment in the clinical setting. First, the framework must be accepted by the teacher rating the learner, which we discussed earlier as construct alignment. If the framework appears arbitrary to teachers, they will feel free to use their own intuitive and potentially less effective frameworks. Second, the framework must be applied consistently across teachers and across students; otherwise, the process is capricious. We should not assume that any form or framework is so intuitively valid and easy to use that teachers will apply it with consistency. Therefore there must be ongoing training and feedback about the framework and the use of the rating scale (we will discuss faculty development later in this chapter).

To some extent the integrity of the assessment process for trainees depends on teachers using it and using it consistently. Many educators understand that an evaluation form,

TABLE 4.6 Milestone Levels Related to Dreyfus Stages and Expected Behaviors

Milestone Level	Dreyfus Stage	Learner Behavior	Transition to Practitioner	Level of Supervision
1	Novice	Doing what is told, rules driven	Intro to clinical practice	Observation, no entrustment
2	Advanced beginner	Comprehension	Guided clinical practice	Act under direct supervision
3	Competent	Application to common practice	Early independence	Act under indirect supervision
4	Proficient	Application to uncommon practice	Full unsupervised practice	Clinical oversight
5	Expert	Experienced, up-to-date clinician	Aspirational growth	Supervise others

checklist, or other form is not an evaluation tool, but a way of communicating expectations to the teacher, who is in fact the instrument ("tool") of evaluation. This in turn may depend on its ease of use, its portability from one trainee or location to another, and its ability to be remembered. While the primary effect of a framework is to structure learning and assessment, its secondary effects involve the feasibility of implementation and the faculty development resources needed for use across a large faculty.[50] Our strategy is that simplicity leads to acceptance; acceptance leads to use; use leads to consistency; and consistency is an important element of fairness.

Rating Scales

Rating scales arose from a need to evaluate areas of performance not captured by standard knowledge-based instruments, such as multiple-choice tests. Such scales are still used now in the form of developmental Milestones for assessment in GME and of entrustment scales for the abilities of residents and students. This section will review both classic and newer rating scales, with an emphasis on the latter. It should be understood that while a scale tries to distinguish levels of ability in a way corresponding to arithmetical, ordinal integers, there is a continuum of ability not just across learners but within a learner across patients seen even in the same month of training and in how the observations documented on the scale are used for formative or summative purposes or for both.[51] Furthermore, by definition all rating scales of human performance are ordinal, meaning the "distance" between interval on the scale does not necessarily equate to a linear, equal gain (or loss) in ability.

Impetus for the development of rating scales came from two sources in the early 1900s: psychologists looking to measure human attitudes, and the Armed Forces who wanted to better evaluate their trainees who were using new technologies.[3,5] In 1932 Likert developed the well-recognized scale employing equal intervals and adding descriptors at each point along the scale (i.e., Strongly Agree, Agree, Undecided, Disagree, Strongly Disagree). Over the past 70 years many scales have been developed with better psychometric properties, including specific rating scales and evaluation forms for medical education. These forms were developed with the goal of evaluating such important competencies as clinical skills, clinical judgment and decision-making, interpersonal and communication skills, and professionalism.

Rating Scales: Basic Design

Most evaluation forms in medicine training currently use a *behaviorally anchored rating scale* (*BARS*). A BARS form provides descriptors of performance at various points along the scale. The major evolution of BARS in medical education has been the transition to greater use of developmental behavioral descriptors like the competency milestones and RIME synthetic framework. Older forms typically only provided brief adjectival descriptors

• BOX 4.1 Various Types of Anchors for Scales, Both Preferred and Cautiously Usable

Rating scales: Types of anchors

A. Still in use but should be used cautiously based on assessment purpose:
- Performance "quality"
- E.g., unsatisfactory-satisfactory-superior
- Frequency
- Rarely–always
- Normative
- Level of comparative performance (e.g., peers; stage of training, etc.)

B. Preferred and recommended whenever possible:
- Developmental
- Entrustment/supervision
- Narrative

These can overlap depending on purpose and construction of the scales. For example the Internal Medicine subcompetencies include a developmental scale (levels) where Level 4 is designated as "Ready for Unsupervised Practice" (entrustment/supervision) using narrative (Milestones as a format of a behaviorally anchored rating scale) to describe each level.

at the terminal ends of the scale and we discourage their use moving forward. (An example of a discontinued older version is shown in Appendix 4.3.)

It is becoming more apparent that the choice of scale anchors is important. Box 4.1 describes various types of anchors for scales. These are not mutually exclusive, but when choosing a scale several considerations are paramount:

1. Returning to the earlier part of the chapter, the scale anchors must align with the purpose of the assessment and the framework chosen. "Quality" anchors such as superior, excellent, and unsatisfactory align poorly with developmental and synthetic frameworks. Even when using an analytic framework (see Fig. 4.2A) these type of anchors require the additional work of translation on the part of the rater. In essence, these types of scales represent a strange form of encryption that is often not accessible to the rater or the learners. Evaluation forms and scales, as noted earlier, signal what is important and should guide judgment. When additional, nebulous steps are added some translation is required and ineffective use of the scales results. Chapter 5 covers in greater detail issues around the frame of reference faculty use when providing ratings.
2. Scales have to be aligned with the assessment task and purpose.
3. Faculty development is absolutely crucial. Evaluation forms are not the measurement instrument; the rater is the true instrument and they need training to develop shared mental models around the evaluation framework, task, and purpose (see Chapter 5).
4. Where possible, criterion-referenced scales and forms (such as RIME and the Milestones) are preferable.

Appendix 4.2 shows an example of a BARS form for medical students from the Uniformed Services University

Patient Care 1: History				
Level 1	Level 2	Level 3	Level 4	Level 5
Elicits and reports a comprehensive history for common patient presentations, with guidance	Elicits and concisely reports a hypothesis-driven patient history for common patient presentations	Elicits and concisely reports a hypothesis-driven patient history for complex patient presentations	Efficiently elicits and concisely reports a patient history, incorporating pertinent psychosocial and other determinants of health	Efficiently and effectively tailors the history taking, including relevant historical subtleties, based on patient, family, and system needs
Seeks data from secondary sources, with guidance	Independently obtains data from secondary sources	Reconciles current data with secondary sources	Uses history and secondary data to guide the need for further diagnostic testing	Models effective use of history to guide the need for further diagnostic testing
Comments:				Not Yet Complete Level 1 ☐ Not Yet Assessable ☐

• **Fig. 4.6** Internal Medicine Milestone Patient Care 1: History. There are transitional zones between levels.

of the Health Sciences containing detailed descriptors (incorporating "RIME" terms) at each level of performance on a 5-point scale. This is a better example of a construct-aligned scale.

The optimal range of a numeric scale is debated, but most experts recommend a scale contain between four and nine gradations depending on purpose, and these ranges have been retained in both Milestones and EPAs. A 9-point scale can be helpful when comparing a large population of trainees. The best example is the validity studies of the US Milestones that use a five-level developmental scale with transition zones between levels, resulting in a 9-point scale. As seen in Fig. 4.6, the Internal Medicine Milestone for taking a Medical History within the Patient Care Milestone, there are five levels of ability but the 9-point scale is retained. More importantly, the behavioral anchors in the BARS form provide verbal descriptions to be used by the teacher in classifying a resident's ability along the entire scale.

As stated before, the Milestones of most specialties use a 5-level system in which 1 = novice or advanced beginner and 5 = "aspirational" for a trainee (but might be expected of someone in practice). One specialty, general surgery, decided to label the first level "critical deficiencies" to signify significant deficiencies needing urgent intervention. In Fig. 4.6, the 5 levels show a level of progression that is similar to the levels of entrustment in EPAs (Table 4.5). One very important caveat should be noted about the Milestones used in the United States. Milestones are designed to guide the judgment of clinical competency committees (CCCs) reviewing 4 to 6 months of resident performance and assessment data (discussed later in the chapter) and are *not recommended* for use as an evaluation form for short rotations. However, some GME programs have used the Milestones in their specialty as an "item bank" to construct more focused and meaningful assessment forms for specific curricular experiences. Much more work is needed in this area, but some early work suggests this may be a useful approach for programs.[52–54]

Purposes and Advantages of Evaluation Forms

Relative to other evaluation tools, evaluation forms can be relatively time efficient for the program or clerkship director. To supplement forms using Milestones, programs can modify or develop evaluation forms to suit specific needs. However, several additional caveats should be noted if you choose to develop a new evaluation form with a rating scale. First, the training program should assess, at a minimum, the reliability if not also the validity of the forms (see Chapter 2). Second, development of "new" forms, independent of efforts to teach faculty how to effectively use the new forms, does not necessarily lead to more reliable or valid assessments of the resident.[55] In fact, attention has shifted away from developing "better" forms because most performance appraisal experts believe that more focus is needed on how to train raters to use the form more effectively.[56,57] This is why awareness of the evaluation framework discussed earlier is so important,[45] and we will provide suggestions for faculty training later in the chapter (also see Chapter 5). We should emphasize that reliability can be increased by increasing the number of observers and/or the observations in a composite evaluation (see Chapters 2 and 5).

Evaluation forms, if used consistently by teachers, can provide a longitudinal "composite" assessment. Other tools, such as standardized patients, while very valuable, usually only provide a cross-sectional assessment at a single point in time. Evaluation forms have the potential to prompt and document judgments of individual faculty, based on multiple observations, conducted over time. The first task of rating forms should be to structure the observations of faculty so that their "findings" (analogous to a patient's symptoms or vital signs) are focused to the goals of the program and are not idiosyncratic to the observer. Observations must then be interpreted and placed in an evidence-based framework being used by the program (e.g., RIME, Milestones, and/or EPAs), and a conclusion reached as to whether this learner is meeting the expectations or values of the program and profession; this interpretation of the observations is called evaluation. After the teacher has observed one or a few interactions with patients the evaluation yields information that may be used to provide feedback to the learner about their progress. However, conversion of the evaluations into a grade or an advancement decision is an administrative action rather than simply an educational one.[14] This conversion of information into knowledge requires more certainty achieved through sufficient and reliable sampling and documentation of information across enough observers and important skills (e.g., information gathering, clinical reasoning, procedures) across a variety of clinical problems (trauma, infection, cardiac, etc.) in the settings in which the learner will practice (e.g., outpatient, emergency, inpatient). It also requires that the decision-making group (promotions committee or competency committee) understand the uses and limitations of the rating forms and assessment techniques that provide the material for a decision.

Evaluation forms can also help minimize the potential bias of the Hawthorne effect: when the process of measurement itself affects what is being measured by collecting observations and judgments over a period of time. However, the impact of the Hawthorne effect is actually quite modest and tends to minimize with habituations over time. Evaluation forms should serve as an important template for feedback. Since evaluation forms usually include the competencies of interest, reviewing the form with the trainee will help them gain knowledge about the content and characteristics of the clinical competencies and understand the framework used for evaluation. Reviewing with trainees their evaluation forms using Milestones, EPAs RIME, or Canadian Medical Education Directives for Specialists (CanMEDS) roles can allow discussion of the specifics of the task or activity involved, and even the competencies that are required to do the task successfully.

The trainee should be able to review completed evaluation forms as part of a comprehensive evaluation program; for instance, as part of a portfolio approach to comprehensive assessment (see Chapter 15). It is important to remember that one of the evaluation form's major purposes is to document the professional development of the trainee at their current stage of training. Ideally, the evaluation record, whether paper or electronic, should provide space for the trainee to react and respond to the evaluation. And the trainee should be encouraged to provide in writing their reactions and subsequent plans for personal development based on the evaluation. In this respect, a portfolio may be more than a tool for documentation or assessment and may move into a curricular device for stimulating reflection (see Chapter 15). However, to be most effective, faculty must take responsibility for completing and returning evaluation forms in a timely fashion and review the evaluation form with the trainee prior to the end of an educational or training experience.

Narrative-Based Assessment

Until recently, less attention has been given to the written comments often provided on the rating forms, and as noted earlier, descriptive evaluation is a crucial aspect of trainee evaluation.[58] Narratives, which describe a resident's progress in the six ACGME competencies in terms of meeting Milestones, are expected as part of the residency program's report on each resident's progress toward independence.[54] As discussed earlier, BARS such as RIME and competency milestones *provide* exemplar narratives. The revision of the US Milestones for each specialty now comes with a supplemental guide that provides specific examples for each Milestone level Table 4.7.

The other significantly important form of narrative is what is provided by teachers from their own verbal or written observations about their residents. However, educators have often found the quality of written comments to be of little help; written comments tend to be brief, cryptic comments such as "works hard" or "should read more." Obviously, such comments would not be sufficiently helpful for the trainee if the goal is to guide improvement by specific direction. An older study, involving two internal medicine residency programs using the low-tech approach, investigated the effectiveness of a brief, multifaceted educational intervention with faculty to improve their written evaluation of residents on inpatient ward rotations.[59] The intervention was quite simple: a 15-minute review of evaluation and feedback prior to the start of the rotation and a folded 5 × 7–inch card that contained educational reminders and space to record observations. The main goals of that study were to improve the specificity of the comments with regard to the areas of competence being evaluated (e.g., medical knowledge versus clinical judgment) and to encourage faculty to provide behavioral examples in support of any low or high rating.

The investigators found a modest increase in the number of category-specific written comments and comments related to the clinical skills (e.g., history taking, physical exam) categories in the intervention group compared to the control group. However, residents in the intervention group also reported two important effects: residents were more likely to change their medical management based on feedback from the attending, and they rated the feedback from the attending significantly higher than residents in the control group. The study suggests that a fairly simple, brief faculty intervention may lead to changes in faculty-written evaluations. Given the increasingly busy nature of academic clinical practice, training programs clearly need educational interventions that are both brief and effective. Technology appears to hold some promise in this area. For example, surgery programs are using a smartphone application to complete a Zwisch scale immediately after a procedure, linked to Milestones.[33] This smartphone app also uses natural language processing (NLP) that

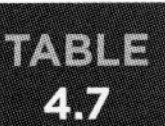

TABLE 4.7 Examples of Narrative Text for the Levels of the Patient Care History Milestone for Internal Medicine

Patient Care 1: History

Overall intent: To competently interact with patients from diverse backgrounds and consistently use all available resources to obtain a comprehensive patient history

Milestones	Examples
Level 1 *Elicits and reports a comprehensive history for common patient presentations, with guidance* *Seeks data from secondary sources, with guidance*	• Obtains accurate, patient-centered history from a 30-year-old patient with a red swollen joint using open-ended and directed questions but without exploring clear underlying hypotheses • Presents oral and written report that is organized but not focused on the chief complaint • Needs prompting to seek data from family members, ancillary staff members, outside pharmacy, outside labs, and databases for controlled substances
Level 2 *Elicits and concisely reports a hypothesis-driven patient history for common patient presentations* *Independently obtains data from secondary sources*	• Interviews a patient with no past medical history with a chief complaint of a red swollen joint, asking the patient about recent alcohol use, diet, trauma, sexual history, and other pertinent questions; reports history limited to pertinent positive and negative facts • Respectfully uses the pronouns that a transgender patient identifies with and asks pertinent sexual orientation and activity questions to provide high-quality care in primary care clinic • Without prompting, reviews and presents relevant data from previous medical records, including past labs and primary care physician notes, family members, ancillary staff members, outside pharmacy, outside labs, and databases for controlled substances • Proactively reviews prescription history from available databases and calls the patient's pharmacy for recent prescriptions that note allopurinol has not been refilled in months
Level 3 *Elicits and concisely reports a hypothesis-driven patient history for complex patient presentations* *Reconciles current data with secondary sources*	• Presents an 85-year-old with a history of congestive heart failure, coronary artery disease, chronic obstructive pulmonary disease, and diabetes with a chief complaint of several weeks of shortness of breath, asking about medication and dietary adherence; reports on the presence of angina or heart failure symptoms, recent upper respiratory infection, and allergen exposure • Completes accurate medication reconciliation using multiple sources and clarifies history based on new information as it becomes available from caregivers who note recent weight gain
Level 4 *Efficiently elicits and concisely reports a patient history, incorporating pertinent psychosocial and other determinants of health* *Uses history and secondary data to guide the need for further diagnostic testing*	(Note: Example uses same patient from Level 3) • Discovers the patient has not filled recent prescriptions and determines it was due to an insurance lapse, and that the patient does not have reliable transportation to a pharmacy • Determines patient has no reliable prescription plan coverage • Determines patient recently had cardiac work-up at another hospital 1 month ago and does not order echocardiogram based on previous results
Level 5 *Efficiently and effectively tailors the history taking, including relevant historical subtleties, based on patient, family, and system needs* *Models effective use of history to guide the need for further diagnostic testing*	• Obtains a history from a patient presenting with macrocytosis, gout, and liver function test abnormalities, building trust to explore relevant history and learns that the patient consumes alcohol despite initial denial • Takes a history from an injured patient and realizes that the boyfriend answers all the questions; identifies that the patient may be a victim of intimate partner violence based on nonverbal cues • Obtains history of medication prescription plan and recognizes that patient may not have Medicare Part D or is in the coverage gap (i.e., "donut hole") • Evaluates a patient with a complaint of headache and illustrates to the more junior learners the elements of the history that preclude the need for additional testing

enables faculty to dictate part of the evaluation form feedback that is instantly available to the resident. The ACGME has made available an assessment app called Direct Observation of Clinical Care (DOCC) that leverages the NLP software embedded within smartphones to capture narrative from the teacher.[60] More work is needed to see whether repeated interventions would produce sustained or greater improvement in written evaluations.

Unfortunately, many forms do not provide enough space for written comments and the form is meant to provide a summative rather than formative evaluation. Perhaps more importantly, descriptive comments written down by teachers are often characterized with the pejorative term *subjective*, since they are neither quantified nor consistently anchored in specific behaviors observed by all teachers. It is possible that research into the use of descriptive terminology has been inappropriately retarded by the "subjective–objective" terminology, and we should refer to numerical methods (such as multiple-choice examinations) more appropriately as "quantified" or "objectified" rather than "objective."[61] Kogan and colleagues tested a new design for the mini-CEX by placing the narrative questions first and asking for an entrustment rating as the last assessment activity. The DOCC app uses this same approach (see Chapter 5).

While we believe technology will make it more feasible to collect narrative assessment from teachers, limitations of written comments on evaluation forms will likely remain a challenge. What can educators do to enhance the utility of teachers' evaluations of trainees in longitudinal educational experiences?

Evaluation Sessions

Evaluation sessions, in which the program, clerkship, or course director sits down with teachers to discuss performance of their residents or students, can be a powerful adjunct to evaluation forms. After the introduction of formal evaluation sessions—regularly scheduled meetings of clerkship directors with teachers[45,47–49]—studies documented the intuitive expectation that teachers would report in conversations what they had not initially written down on their forms.[25,31] These sessions do not need to be long; 10 to 15 minutes is sufficient to explore professionalism issues and additional detail about the trainee's performance during the educational rotation. All programs should consider using in-person evaluation meetings with faculty. In all US residency and fellowship programs, a CCC is required as part of the assessment program. CCCs assess residents and fellows twice a year using the Milestones framework to provide feedback, guide individual learning plans, and hopefully identify learners in difficulty earlier[62] (see Bloom [1956] to learn more about effective group process). It is helpful to develop a systems approach to evaluation in which observations about learners' progress are made by teachers who have been calibrated by organizational educators who in turn calibrate themselves and make the eventual advancement decisions.[63]

Psychometric Issues

Use of any rating scales must possess sufficient reliability and validity to provide useful information about clinical competence. Furthermore, the quality and process of data collection used for the ratings are critically important (see Chapter 2). We will examine some of the psychometric challenges in using evaluation forms. The paper by Gray provides a helpful and basic review of the psychometric issues in rating scales.[7] The article by Rekman and colleagues (cf. Annotated Bibliography) provides a more recent overview of entrustment scales.[64]

A brief review of some key psychometric issues is provided in the following subsections.

Reliability

Reliability refers to the consistency of assessment measurements when repeated[65] (see Chapter 2). Scoring information that is consistent and confirmable is a true score or signal; the remainder is considered an error score or noise. And of course the closer the rating is to the true score the better or more reliable the assessment method is. Reliability estimates (i.e., coefficients) of greater than 0.8 are considered necessary for higher-stakes decisions. High interrater agreement is a desirable property for rating scales, especially if the forms are completed by more than one evaluator during a similar time period. Results from older studies are conflicting. Older studies found highly variable reliability using mostly quality-type scale anchors. In 2011, Crossley and colleagues, using a newly designed construct-aligned scale based on expectations for stage of training in the UK Foundation program, found much higher reliabilities on the mini-CEX.[9] More recently, Park and colleagues found that Milestone-based trajectories in a family medicine residency reliably differentiated individual longitudinal patterns for formative purposes using growth rate and growth curve reliability analysis.[66] Weller and colleagues have found that entrustment scales also possessed better reliability than older scales such as the 9-point quality-based mini-CEX.[67] This work could inform the redesign of typical evaluation scales moving forward. The most straightforward solution to improve reliability is simply to increase the number of evaluations. Reliability is a measure of reproducibility, and the more one does anything the more stable the measurement becomes (e.g., the error around the mean narrows). Increased reliability may result from asking teachers to decide in their day-to-day activities whether they trust a trainee to do a particular task, rather than comparing the trainee to a rating scale based on abstract domains.[64,68]

Validity

Validity is confidence that we measured what we wanted to measure. Modern validity frameworks now regard all validity as construct validity (see Chapter 2) where validity is of an argument or inference from the available data and not something an assessment tool possesses.[69,70] Usually a gold standard is required to adequately assess validity (e.g., relationship with other variables in the Kane or Messick validity framework). Unfortunately, no definitive standard exists for important areas of interest such as professionalism, attitudes, and clinical judgment, to name a just a few.

Performance on multiple-choice examinations has long been used as a comparison variable for correlation studies of evaluation forms. For instance, a study with family practice residents found that the ability to correctly predict scores on the In-Training Exam (ITE) was dependent on the faculty's years of teaching experience. A study using the ITE as the gold standard in family medicine showed that an online tool could be used to improve teachers' ratings.[71] Conversely, a study of surgery residents found no correlation between the American Board of Surgery ITE and a 12-item 7-point ward evaluation rating form.[72] Finally, an older study at a military internal medicine residency found that faculty were unable to predict in which tertile of performance residents would score on their ITE despite having worked closely with the residents.[73] More recently, multiple studies have found a correlation between competency milestone ratings and performance on board certification exams in the United States.[74–76]

Thus use of knowledge-based examinations may serve as a reasonable reference standard for knowledge ratings, but little has been done to study the relationship of other important domains on the rating scales such as professionalism, humanism, and physical exam skills. One prior study did find modest correlations between a 25-item rating scale for interns completed by residency program directors and their interns' performance in medical school. These authors identified 5 factors from the rating scale that accounted for most of the variance: interpersonal communication, clinical skills, population-based health, recordkeeping skills, and critical appraisal skills.[77] Thus ratings from medical school appear to have some predictive validity when compared to program director ratings.[78] Another study of internal medicine residents found that low ratings in professionalism and other competencies at graduation were associated with a higher odds ratio of adverse state licensing board actions in practice, but the absolute rate was still quite modest.[79,80]

Early outcomes research with the competency milestones provides some hope that use of developmental scales in combination with group-based evaluation sessions may provide better predictive value as a feedback mechanism to help learners while in training based on graduate performance in practice. Heath and colleagues found that low professionalism ratings during internal medicine residency training predicted subsequent low ratings in pulmonary fellowship.[81] Han and colleagues found that ratings in professionalism and communication competencies were significantly associated with receipt of impactful patient complaints in early practice.[82] Smith and colleagues found that a composite rating of Milestones (akin to an EPA) of vascular surgeons during training was significantly associated with surgeons' serious complication rate in endovascular aneurysm repair (EVAR) in early practice.[83]

Rating Errors

Errors in rating the performance of an individual may result from issues in the raters (e.g., their memory of their observations and their expectations and standards of comparison); from issues in the measurement scale (e.g., terms or categories that do not make sense to the rater); or from issues in the context of the rating (e.g., practical aspects such as time to observe, interruptions, or behaviors of the trainee or a patient). Most problems with rating scales are due primarily to how faculty use them and not necessarily to major defects in the scales themselves.

Medical educators commit the same types of *rating errors* noted in all types of performance appraisals. There are two main categories of rater errors: distributional errors and correlational errors.[56]

1. Distributional errors

   Two common distributional errors are range restriction and leniency:

   Range restriction: failure to utilize the entire range of the scale. A "central tendency" error is a subtype of a range restriction error where the rater uses just the middle portion of the scale. However, in medicine, attendings usually restrict the marks to the upper ends of the scale (discussed later in the chapter). An exception to this was seen by Battistone and colleagues who reported a shift of the grading curve to the left (away from the inflation) when the behavioral terms based on the RIME scheme (observer, reporter, interpreter, manager, educator) were substituted for numerical ratings.[46]

   Leniency/severity error: a type of distributional error where the faculty is being either too kind (a "dove") or too harsh (a "hawk"), respectively. Many would argue there are currently few "hawks" in medicine.

2. Correlational errors

   An important goal of ratings is to accurately discriminate between levels of ability, whether using an analytic, developmental, or synthetic framework. For example, one resident may possess substandard knowledge as evidenced by other measures (e.g., the ITE) but display extraordinary humanistic skill. Such a resident should receive high marks under humanistic qualities but should receive a lower rating for medical knowledge if the attending has effectively evaluated the resident. Unfortunately, most raters have difficulty discriminating between dimensions of competence and tend to use a limited range on the rating scale.

Correlational error is where faculty give similar ratings to each aspect of a trainee's performance regardless of what dimension of competence is being assessed, even when the dimensions are clearly separate;[56] as Murphy and Cleveland note, "the result is an inflation of the inter-correlations among the dimensions." When rating inflation occurs, the result is commonly known as a halo error. This is a very common problem in medical education where everyone is always above average or better. Having the entire list of desirable attributes of the candidate present, synoptically, at one time, is intended to minimize the chance that teachers will confuse the different domains of evaluation, but caution is needed. The increasing length and complexity of forms may in themselves make the teachers less able or willing to use it as intended by the form's author(s); a problem known as cognitive load. Therefore increasing the number of domains, rating criteria, or items on a form may aggravate the halo effect.

A number of older studies within a single or limited number of programs, using factor analysis, found that evaluation forms containing multiple items or competencies could be reduced to just two factors, typically cognitive skills and interpersonal skills.[84,85] However, a more recent study using national competency milestone data found that in fact the six competency domains held up very well, and two other validity studies found that the nonmedical knowledge competency milestones either did not or only weakly correlate with performance on a high-stakes medical knowledge certification exam.[74,75,86] What these Milestone studies suggest is again that more developmental frameworks combined with group process may provide more discriminating evaluations of learners.

A few notes of caution are warranted in interpreting factor analytic studies. First, factor analysis is a statistical technique that attempts to reduce a data set to the fewest number of factors using large correlational matrices.[87] Second, factor analysis assumes each category is independent of the other and that the relationship between two or more factors is linear. For example, items that load onto more than one factor are typically eliminated from the final factor model. In medicine we know that is illogical. For example, you cannot perform a high-quality history and physical without robust medical knowledge, and it is hard to be professional and have excellent interpersonal and communication skills. It is important that competencies mostly serve as frameworks, as described earlier. Using factor analysis to determine whether faculty can discriminate between categories of competence may fail to uncover modest differences between ratings. While faculty may not make major distinctions among the competencies in their ratings for reasons listed earlier, they still can help signal what is important. Finally, certain approaches to factor analysis used in studies fail to address or account for clustering within programs (i.e., residents are nested within programs).

What are the reasons for halo error when it occurs? For one, raters may rely more on their global impressions when rating trainees on specific dimensions of competence. Two, and one we all recognize, is the unwillingness of so many faculty to give lower ratings on any dimension of competence. This is often called the "there goes my teaching award syndrome." Other possible causes of halo error include confirmation bias (self as frame of reference: "that's how I would do it, so it must be right"), ignoring discordant or inconsistent information or observations about the trainee, the simple lack of enough observation or information about performance, and bias.[68,88] Box 4.2 provides a list of possible reasons for halo error.

• BOX 4.2 Possible Reasons for the Halo Error

1. Global impression drives the rating for all dimensions of competence
2. Unwillingness or inability to discriminate among different dimensions
3. Reluctant to give negative evaluations
4. Insufficient observation and/or information about a trainee's performance
5. Implicit and/or confirmation bias
6. Discounting conflicting or discordant information, observations
7. Level of familiarity with trainee
8. Level of familiarity with the medical knowledge, skills, and attitudes
9. Dimensions of competence are interdependent

Rater Accuracy

Rater accuracy answers the question: How well does the rating match the actual performance? There are two distinct types of accuracy measures. The first are behavioral-based measures. These types of measures allow the rater to specifically focus on whether the behavior did or did not occur. Checklists are the most common type of rating scale used on evaluation forms for behaviorally based measures. The level of ability may be included in a checklist, but typically the rater is expected only to provide "credit" for behaviors performed properly based on a standard. They are particularly useful for structured, controlled assessments such as standardized patients. However, checklists, like other evaluation forms, can ask too much of faculty and create a situation known as cognitive load. The more items we ask faculty to rate (judge) in shorter periods of time, the greater the cognitive load that leads to less effective evaluations. As one example, Byrne and colleagues compared the cognitive load between completing a 21-item checklist for an OSCE station versus inducing anesthesia for routine surgery.[89] The same principle applies to evaluation forms. The more straightforward synthetic RIME framework can classify and document observations of the behaviors observed in an individual trainee's care of each in a series of patients as consistent with reporting, interpreting, managing, and educating.

The other type of accuracy involves judgmental measures. As the name implies, the rater must apply judgment when providing a rating. Accuracy in judgment is particularly important for rating scales and evaluation forms used in longitudinal educational experiences. There are several types of judgmental accuracy measures: accuracy in whether a trainee has attained a level of performance (criterion accuracy); accuracy in distinguishing among trainees (differential or normative accuracy); and accuracy in discriminating between specific performance or competence dimensions (stereotype accuracy). For evaluation in medical education, accuracy measures are important because defining key behaviors at various levels of competence facilitates better judgment and helps support better patient care.

Another caution is that the concept of trust may be too complicated a social judgment to reduce to a rating scale. Gingerich argued that assessment involves some degree of social judgment and that some idiosyncrasy is to be expected because all teachers have strengths and weaknesses in their own clinical and teaching practices.[90] These idiosyncrasies can benefit the learner when they represent excellence or clinical mastery. However, they can be harmful when they do not represent an evidence-based practice (EBP; see Chapter 5). Gingerich and colleagues also described that in a study of faculty rating a resident's performance there was a tendency for subgroups of physicians who had described similar social judgments to have also given more similar performance ratings.[91] Faculty development may be an important process to articulate shared assumptions among teachers.

Finally, an important note of caution about entrustment scales and accuracy. Two recent studies uncovered serious problems in entrustment ratings against an outcomes-based standard. First, Schumacher and colleagues examined the correlation between supervisor ratings of the clinical encounters of pediatric residents in the emergency department and the quality of care delivered to the child assessed through quality performance measures. The results were sobering: there was little to no correlation with the quality for care for asthma, bronchiolitis, and closed head injury and the entrustment ratings.[92] Kogan and colleagues compared the entrustment ratings of primary care residency faculty as part of a randomized trial on a series of videos rigorously scripted to depict a specific entrustment level. While the accuracy of entrustment ratings was good when the performer depicted a resident "ready for unsupervised practice (Level 4)," accuracy was less than 50% when the performer was Level 2 or 3 on the entrustment, with leniency error most common.[31] Thus entrustment scales are no panacea for all the challenges described in this chapter, highlighting the critical need for ongoing faculty development (discussed next; see also Chapter 5).

Faculty Development and Evaluation Forms

The quality of the information on evaluation forms depends mostly on the individual completing the form, not the form itself. For too long medical educators have been looking for the holy grail of the ideal evaluation form. Landy and Farr in 1980 called for a moratorium on this quest, arguing instead for an increased emphasis on training the evaluators.[55] As noted earlier, even simple approaches to faculty development such as observation cards can modestly improve the quality of information on evaluation forms, and the growing availability of smartphone apps offers even more promise around improving faculty development efforts. However, to realize the full potential of evaluation forms, more structured faculty training is still needed.

Throughout this chapter we have highlighted the importance of an evaluation framework to guide the evaluation process. This is a critical first step to ensure that faculty possess shared mental models and an understanding of the goals of outcomes of evaluation, Studies have shown specific types of training can improve interrater agreement using a simple four-step process[25] (see also Chapter 9):

1. Standardize the observation of the behavior of interest.
2. Reach agreement on common nomenclature for the desired expectations of interest through conversation and dialogue.
3. Agree on the relative importance of the different components of behavior being assessed.
4. Practice assessment skills longitudinally and with feedback about potential rating errors and bias.

Steps 1 and 2 in this process are called performance dimension training (PDT). PDT provides raters with the expected performance standards for each level of performance. Many have argued that such agreement about performance dimension standards is lacking in GME. Step 3 is known as frame of reference training (FoRT). These techniques have been applied in training faculty to use the RIME framework (see Chapter 5 for guidance on how to perform PDT and FoRT).[31]

Performance Dimension Training and RIME

The Uniformed Services University of the Health Sciences (USUHS) has incorporated PDT and FoRT as part of the evaluation for medical students rotating on an internal medicine clerkship for over 30 years.[11,24,38,40] Raters participate in evaluation sessions with clerkship directors where descriptive evaluations are collected. Clerkship directors use these evaluation sessions to train preceptors about expected levels of performance for each category of rating and how the student's performance should be documented on the rating scale form. The evaluation system goes one step further by incorporating the student's performance in multiple domains of competence into an overall performance level. Goals for each level of performance are divided into performance categories with defined expectations. Since "reporter" skills are introduced in the first year (see Appendix 4.2), it is felt that achieving proficiency in them is a reasonable, nonnegotiable level for advancing to the next level of responsibility, yielding this conversion of observations into grades:

Reporter (Pass):
Interpreter (High Pass):
Manager/Educator (Honors):

The Appendix 4.2 provides a more comprehensive description of the model and a copy of the performance matrix used at USUHS. The descriptions and criteria are more applicable for residents than for students, since no accommodation distinguishing "Reasonable" (student level) from "Accurate " (resident level) needs to be made.

Murphy and Cleveland in 1995[56] made several important points about performance appraisal training pertinent to the use of rating scales that still hold today:

1. Define performance dimensions in behavioral terms (e.g., use RIME and Milestones narrative descriptions) and be sure to communicate these terms to the resident and the faculty. It may even be helpful to use a blank evaluation form at the beginning of a rotation as a template to discuss goals and expectations before the evaluation process actually starts.

2. Ratings will more likely correspond with actual rater judgment if training programs support distinctions between house staff on the basis of *performance*, the raters perceive a strong link between the rating they give and specific outcomes, and the raters believe that outcomes should be based on *present* performance.
3. What the rater chooses to communicate through the form depends heavily on the rater's goals and contextual factors, such as the individual resident's relationship with the teachers and the perceived purpose of the evaluation at hand. Therefore raters need to communicate goals directly to the residents, and raters must be cognizant of both internal and external environmental factors affecting the context of the evaluation. Chapter 5 provides greater detail and suggestions for running PDT and FoRT faculty development exercises.

Conclusions

Directors of academic programs should not presume that an evaluation form, even one with behaviorally anchored rating scales, will do the work of getting faculty on the same page. Evaluation forms should possess several desirable properties: be user friendly, be unobtrusive, be flexible, capture important narrative descriptions of performance, and if needed, be quantifiable. The quantification to a rating scale should be an accurate translation of level of performance. Forms that are not well understood and/or are too elaborate may pose a challenge in cognitive load that can only be met with additional faculty development and training. As importantly, teachers' acceptance of the scale and its educational framework are prerequisites of consistent use. To some extent, there is an emotional barrier for teachers that has to be bridged—they often see themselves (and certainly describe themselves) as "giving" the student or resident a grade, rather than making a diagnosis that reflects their observations (something they would never do with a serious medical condition). Therefore the teacher's emotional difficulty in "giving" a grade is contaminated by their acceptance of "subjective-objective" distinctions, and by an intuitive, clinical fear of inadequate sampling of the student's abilities. The teacher may see each observation of a trainee with a patient as not just evaluation but grading with premature or incomplete data.

While reasonable questions remain regarding reliability, validity, and the ability to discriminate among different aspects of clinical competence, most notably "soft areas" such as humanism, attitudes, professionalism, and judgment, recent research supports the use of synthetic and developmental scales such as RIME, Milestones, and entrustment over older types of scales. However, despite the improved operating characteristics of these scales, such as improved acceptance by faculty and reliability, they alone do not "fix" lingering problems around other elements of validity and accuracy. It is crucial to remember that the actual assessment instrument is the individual using the evaluation form, not the form itself. Teacher training in assessment is crucial to the effective use of even the newer rating scales. While the optimal approach to rater training in medical education remains to be defined, a growing body of research[57] and the general principles discussed throughout this chapter and in Chapter 5 are an excellent and evidence-based place to begin.

Annotated Bibliography

1. Rekman J, Gofton W, Dudek N, Gofton T, Hamstra SJ. Entrustability scales: outlining their usefulness for competency-based clinical assessment. *Acad Med.* 2016 Feb;91(2):186–190. doi:10.1097/ACM.0000000000001045.
   As the abstract nicely summarizes, the paper "outlines how 'entrustability scales' may help bridge the gap between the assessment judgments of clinical supervisors and WBA instruments. Entrustment-based assessment evaluates trainees against what they will actually do when independent; thus 'entrustability scales'—defined as behaviorally anchored ordinal scales based on progression to competence—reflect a judgment that has clinical meaning for assessors. Rather than asking raters to assess trainees against abstract scales, entrustability scales provide raters with an assessment measure structured around the way evaluators already make day-to-day clinical entrustment decisions, which results in increased reliability."
2. Pangaro LN. Evaluating professional growth: a new vocabulary and other innovations for improving the descriptive evaluation of students. *Acad Med.* 1999 Nov;74(11):1203–1207. doi:10.1097/00001888-199911000-00012.
   a. *This article provides additional background and detail about the RIME framework. This is a very useful paper to give to all faculty involved in evaluating trainees in any setting.*
3. Battistone MJ, Milne C, Sande MA, Pangaro LN, Hemmer PA, Shomaker TS. The feasibility and acceptability of implementing formal evaluation sessions and using descriptive vocabulary to assess student performance on a clinical clerkship. *Teach Learn Med.* 2002 Winter;14(1):5–10. doi:10.1207/S15328015TLM1401_3.
4. Hemmer P, Hawkins R, Jackson J, Pangaro L. Assessing how well three evaluation methods detect deficiencies in medical students' professionalism in two settings of an internal medicine clerkship. *Acad Med.* 2000 Feb;75(2):167–173. doi:10.1097/00001888-200002000-00016.
5. Hemmer PA, Pangaro L. Using formal evaluation sessions for case-based faculty development during clinical clerkships. *Acad Med.* 2000 Dec;75(12):1216–1221. doi:10.1097/00001888-200012000-00021.
   These three articles provide valuable data and insight into the value of using formal evaluation sessions to enhance the evaluation process and improve the consistency of the evaluation process by providing ongoing, longitudinal faculty development. The fourth article provides specific guidance on how to use evaluation sessions for ongoing faculty development. This is a very important concept: the need to embed faculty development into ongoing educational activities and to move away from using only the workshop approach to faculty development.
6. Pangaro L, ten Cate O. Frameworks for learner assessment in medicine (Theories in Medical Education series). *Med Teach.* 2013;35:524–537.
   This AMEE Guide from the Association for Medical Education in Europe reviews the premises underlying common frameworks used in educational assessment.
7. Gingerich A, Kogan J, Yeates P, Govaerts M, Holmboe E. Seeing the 'black box' differently: assessor cognition from three research perspectives. *Med Educ.* 2014 Nov;48(11):1055–1068. doi:10.1111/medu.12546.

This article explores the process of rater cognition through three perspectives: (1) the assessor as trainable—assessors vary because they do not apply assessment criteria correctly, use varied and at times frames of reference that are not evidence based, and make unjustified inferences; (2) the assessor as fallible—variations arise as a result of fundamental limitations in human cognition that mean assessors are readily and haphazardly influenced by their immediate context, and (3) the assessor as meaningfully idiosyncratic—experts are capable of making sense of highly complex and nuanced scenarios through inference and contextual sensitivity, which suggests assessor differences may represent legitimate experience-based interpretations.

References

1. Govaerts M, VandeWiel MWJ, Schuwirth LWT, Van der Vleuten CPM, Muijtjens AMM. Workplace-based assessment: raters' performance theories and constructs. *Adv in Health Sci Educ.* 2013 Aug;18(3):375–396. doi:10.1007/s10459-012-9376-x.
2. Lucey CR, Hauer KE, Boatright D, Fernandez A. Education's wicked problem: achieving equity in assessment for medical learners. *Acad Med.* 2020 Dec;95(12S Addressing Harmful Bias and Eliminating Discrimination in Health Professions Learning Environments):S98–S108. doi:10.1097/ACM.0000000000003717.
3. Turnbull J, van Barnveld C. Assessment of clinical performance: in-training evaluation. In: Norman GR, van der Vleuten CPM, Newble DI, eds. *International Handbook of Research in Medical Education.* Kluwer Academic; 2002.
4. Lockyer J. Multi source feedback in the assessment of physician competencies. *J Contin Educ Health Prof.* 2003 Winter;23(1):4–12. doi:10.1002/chp.1340230103.
5. Streiner DL. Global rating scales. In: Neufeld VR, Norman GR, eds. *Assessing Clinical Competence.* Springer; 1985.
6. Devellis RF. *Scale Development: Theory and Applications.* Sage Publications; 1991.
7. Gray JD. Global rating scales in residency education. *Acad Med.* 1996 Jan;71(1 Suppl):S55. doi:10.1097/00001888-199601000-00043.
8. Edgar L, Jones MD Jr, Harsy B, Passiment M, Hauer KE. Better decision-making: shared mental models and the clinical competency committee. *J Grad Med Educ.* 2021 Apr;13(2 Suppl):51–58. doi:10.4300/JGME-D-20-00850.1.
9. Crossley J, Johnson G, Booth J, Wade W. Good questions, good answers: construct alignment improves the performance of workplace-based assessment scales. *Med Educ.* 2011 Jun;45(6):560–569. doi:10.1111/j.1365-2923.2010.03913.x.
10. Schuster B, Pangaro L. Understanding systems of education: what to expect of, and for, each faculty member. In: Pangaro L, ed. *Leadership Careers in Medical Education.* American College of Physicians; 2010:51–71.
11. Pangaro L. A new vocabulary and other innovations for improving the descriptive evaluation of students. *Acad Med.* 1999 Nov;74(11):1203–1207. doi:10.1097/00001888-199911000-00012.
12. Wennberg JE. Unwarranted variations in healthcare delivery: implications for academic medical centers. *BMJ.* 2002 Oct 26;325(7370):961–964. doi:10.1136/bmj.325.7370.961.
13. Holmboe ES, Kogan JR. Will any road get you there? Examining warranted and unwarranted variation in medical education. *Acad Med.* 2022 Aug 1;97(8):1128–1136. doi:10.1097/ACM.0000000000004667.
14. Jamieson T, Hemmer P, Pangaro L. Legal aspects of failing grades. In: Pangaro LN, McGaghie WC, eds. *Handbook on Medical Student Evaluation and Assessment.* Gegensatz Press; 2015.
15. Artino AR Jr, Gehlbach H. AM last page. Avoiding four visual-design pitfalls in survey development. *Acad Med.* 2012 Oct;87(10):1452. doi:10.1097/ACM.0b013e31826a06b2.
16. Bloom BS. *Taxonomy of Educational Objectives, Handbook I, Cognitive Domain.* Longman; 1956.
17. Krathwohl DR. A revision of bloom's taxonomy: an overview. *Theory Pract.* 2002;41(4):212–218. doi:10.1207/s15430421tip4104_2.
18. Dreyfus SE, Dreyfus HL. *Mind Over Machine.* Macmillan: Free Press; 1986:16–51.
19. Carraccio CL, Benson BJ, Nixon LJ, Derstine PL. From the educational bench to the clinical bedside: translating the Dreyfus developmental model to the learning of clinical skills. *Acad Med.* 2008 Aug;83(8):761–767. doi:10.1097/ACM.0b013e31817eb632.
20. ten Cate O. Nuts and bolts of entrustable professional activities. *J Grad Med Educ.* 2013 Mar;5(1):157–158. doi:10.4300/JGME-D-12-00380.1.
21. Nasca TJ, Philibert I, Brigham T, Flynn TC. The next GME Accreditation System—rationale and benefits. *N Engl J Med.* 2012 Mar 15;366(11):1051–1056. doi:10.1056/NEJMsr1200117.
22. Edgar L, McLean S, Hogan S, Hamstra S, Holmboe ES. The Milestones Guidebook. Accessed November 7, 2023. https://www.acgme.org/globalassets/milestonesguidebook.pdfining
23. Royal College of Physicians and Surgeons of Canada. CanMEDS: Better standards, better physicians, better care. Accessed March 19, 2023. at CanMEDS Framework: The Royal College of Physicians and Surgeons of Canada. https://www.royalcollege.ca/en/canmeds/canmeds-framework.html.
24. Pangaro L. A primer of evaluation terminology: definition and important distinctions. In: Pangaro LN, McGaghie WC, eds. *Handbook on Medicine Student Evaluation and Assessment.* Gegensatz Press; 2015:13–26.
25. Pangaro L. Investing in descriptive evaluation: a vision for the future of assessment. *Med Teach.* 2000;22(5):478–481. doi:10.1080/01421590050110740.
26. Rodriguez RG, Pangaro LN. AM last page: mapping the ACGME competencies to the RIME framework. *Acad Med.* 2012 Dec;87(12):1781. doi:10.1097/ACM.0b013e318271eb61.
27. Meyer EG, Kelly WF, Hemmer PA, Pangaro LN. The RIME model provides a context for Entrustable Professional Activities across undergraduate medical education. *Acad Med.* 2018 Jun;93(6):954. doi:10.1097/ACM.0000000000002211.
28. ten Cate. Entrustable professional activities versus competencies and skills: exploring why different concepts are often conflated. *Adv Health Sci Educ Theory Pract.* 2022;27(2):491–499. doi:10.1007/s10459-022-10098-7.
29. ten Cate O, Hart D, Ankel F, et al. Entrustment decision making in clinical training. *Acad Med.* 2016 Feb;91(2):191–198. doi:10.1097/ACM.0000000000001044.
30. Rekman J, Gofton W, Dudek N, Gofton T, Hamstra SJ. Entrustability scales: outlining their usefulness for competency-based clinical assessment. *Acad Med.* 2016 Feb;91(2):186–190. doi:10.1097/ACM.0000000000001045.
31. Kogan JR, Dine CJ, Conforti LN, Holmboe ES. can rater training improve the quality and accuracy of workplace-based assessment narrative comments and entrustment ratings? A randomized controlled trial. *Acad Med.* 2023 Feb 1;98(2):237–247. doi:10.1097/ACM.0000000000004819.
32. Chen C, Sjoukje van den Broek WE, ten Cate O. The case for use of Entrustable Professional Activities in undergraduate medical education. *Acad Med.* 2015 Apr; 90(4):431–436. doi:10.1097/ACM.0000000000000586.

33. DaRosa DA, Zwischenberger JB, Meyerson SL, et al. A theory-based model for teaching and assessing residents in the operating room. *J Surg Educ.* 2013 Jan-Feb;70(1):24–30. doi:10.1016/j.jsurg.2012.07.007.
34. Association of American Medical Colleges (AAMC). Core Entrustable Professional Activities for Entering Residency, Curriculum Development Guide, Association of American Medical Colleges, 2014.
35. Association of American Medical Colleges (AAMC). Core Entrustable Professional Activities for Entering Residency. Summary of the 10-School Pilot 2014-2021. Association of American Medical Colleges, 2022.
36. Williams RG, Klamen DA, McGaghie WC. Cognitive, social and environmental sources of bias in clinical performance ratings. *Teach Learn Med.* 2003 Fall;15(4):270–292. doi:10.1207/S15328015TLM1504_11.
37. Roop S, Pangaro L. Measuring the impact of clinical teaching on student performance during a third year medicine clerkship. *Am J Med.* 2001 Feb 15;110(3):205–209. doi:10.1016/s0002-9343(00)00672-0.
38. Lavin B, Pangaro L. Internship ratings as a validity outcome measure for an evaluation system to identify inadequate clerkship performance. *Acad Med.* 1998;73:998–1002. doi:10.1097/00001888-199809000-00021.
39. Hemann BA, Durning SJ, Kelly WF, Dong T, Pangaro LN, Hemmer PA. The association of students requiring remediation in the internal medicine clerkship with poor performance during internship. *Mil Med.* 2015 Apr;180(4 Suppl):47–53. doi:10.7205/MILMED-D-14-00567.
40. Durning S, Pangaro L, Denton GD, et al. Inter-site consistency as a standard of programmatic evaluation in a clerkship with multiple, geographically separated sites. *Acad Med.* 2003 Oct;78 (10 Suppl):S36–S38. doi:10.1097/00001888-200310001-00012.
41. Noel G. A system for evaluating and counseling marginal students during clinical clerkships. *J Med Educ.* 1987 Apr;62(4):353–355. doi:10.1097/00001888-198704000-00010.
42. Hemmer PA, Pangaro L. Using formal evaluation sessions for case-based faculty development during clinical clerkships. *Acad Med.* 2000 Dec;75(12):1216–1221. doi:10.1097/00001888-200012000-00021.
43. Ginsburg S, Van der Vleuten CPM, Eva KW. The hidden value of narrative comments for assessment: a quantitative reliability analysis of qualitative data. *Acad Med.* 2017 Nov;92(11):1617–1621. doi:10.1097/ACM.0000000000001669.
44. Epstein RM, Hundert EM. Defining and assessing professional competence. *JAMA.* 2002 Jan 9;287(2):226–235. doi:10.1001/jama.287.2.226.
45. Hemmer P, Hawkins R, Jackson J, Pangaro L. Assessing how well three evaluation methods detect deficiencies in medical students' professionalism in two settings of an internal medicine clerkship. *Acad Med.* 2000 Feb;75(2):167–173. doi:10.1097/00001888-200002000-00016.
46. Battistone MJ, Pendleton B, Milne C, et al. Global descriptive evaluations are more responsive than global numeric ratings in detecting students' progress during the inpatient portion of an internal medicine clerkship. *Acad Med.* 2001 Oct;76 (10 Suppl):S105–S107. doi:10.1097/00001888-200110001-00035.
47. Battistone MJ, Milne C, Sande MA, Pangaro LN, Hemmer PA, Shomaker TS. The feasibility and acceptability of implementing formal evaluation sessions and using descriptive vocabulary to assess student performance on a clinical clerkship. *Teach Learn Med.* 2002 Winter;14(1):5–10. doi:10.1207/S15328015TLM1401_3.
48. Ogburn T, Espey E. The R-I-M-E method for evaluation of medical students on an obstetrics and gynecology clerkship. *Am J Obstet Gynecol.* 2003 Sep;189(3):666–669. doi:10.1067/s0002-9378(03)00885-8.
49. Hemmer P, Pangaro LN. The effectiveness of formal evaluation sessions during clinical clerkships in better identifying students with marginal funds of knowledge. *Acad Med.* 1997 Jul;72(7):641–643. doi:10.1097/00001888-199707000-00018.
50. Pangaro L, ten Cate O. AMEE Guide—Frameworks for learner assessment in medicine (Theories in Medical Education series). *Med Teach.* 2013;35:524–537. doi:10.3109/0142159X.2013.788789.
51. Kinnear B, Warm EJ, Caretta-Weyer H, et al. Entrustment unpacked: aligning purposes, stakes, and processes to enhance learner assessment. *Acad Med.* 2021 Jul 1;96(7S):S56–S63. doi:10.1097/ACM.0000000000004108.
52. Nabors C, Peterson SJ, Forman L, et al. Operationalizing the internal medicine milestones—an early status report. *J Grad Med Educ.* 2013 Mar;5(1):130–137. doi:10.4300/JGME-D-12-00130.1.
53. Warm EJ, Mathis BR, Held JD, et al. Entrustment and mapping of observable practice activities for resident assessment. *J Gen Intern Med.* 2014 Aug;29(8):1177–1182. doi:10.1007/s11606-014-2801-5.
54. Edgar L, McLean S, Hogan SO, Hamstra S, Holmboe ES. The Milestones Guidebook. Accessed March 19, 2023. at Competency-Based Training (acgme.org)
55. Landy FJ, Farr JL. Performance rating. *Psychol Bull.* 1980;87:72–107. doi:10.1037/0033-2909.87.1.72.
56. Murphy KR, Cleveland JN. *Understanding Performance Appraisal.* Sage Publications; 1995.
57. Hauenstein NMA. Training raters to increase the accuracy of appraisals and the usefulness of feedback. In: Smither JW, ed. *Performance Appraisal.* Jossey Bass; 1998.
58. Rodriguez RG, Hemmer PA. Descriptive evaluations and clinical performance evaluations in the workplace. In: Pangaro LN, McGaghie WC, eds. *Handbook on Medical Student Evaluation and Assessment.* Gegensatz Press; 2015:77–96.
59. Holmboe ES, Fiebach NF, Galaty L, Huot S. The effectiveness of a focused educational intervention on resident evaluations from faculty: a randomized controlled trial. *J Gen Intern Med.* 2001 Jul;16(7):1–6. doi:10.1046/j.1525-1497.2001.016007427.x.
60. Direct observation of clinical care (DOCC) assessment tool. Accessed April 7, 2023. https://dl.acgme.org/pages/assessment.
61. Norman GR, Van der Vleuten CP, De Graaff E. Pitfalls in the pursuit of objectivity: issues of validity, efficiency and acceptability. *Med Educ.* 1991 Mar;25(2):119–126. doi:10.1111/j.1365-2923.1991.tb00037.x.
62. Andolsek K, Padmore J, Hauer KE, Ekpenyong A, Edgar L, Holmboe ES. Clinical Competency Committees: A Guidebook for Programs. Accessed March 26, 2023. www.acgme.org.
63. Pangaro LN. System approaches to student assessment. In: Pangaro LN, McGaghie WC, eds. *Handbook of Medical Student Assessment and Evaluation.* Gegensatz Press; 2015.
64. Rekman J, Gofton W, Dudek N, Gifton T, Hamstra SJ. Entrustability scales: outlining their usefulness for competency-based clinical assessment. *Acad Med.* 2016 Feb;91(2):186–190. doi:10.1097/ACM.0000000000001045.
65. Downing SM. Reliability: on the reproducibility of assessment data. *Med Educ.* 2004 Sep;38(9):1006–1012. doi:10.1111/j.1365-2929.2004.01932.x.

66. Park YS, Hamstra SJ, Yamazaki K, Holmboe E. Longitudinal reliability of milestones-based learning trajectories in family medicine residents. *JAMA Netw Open*. 2021 Dec 1;4(12):e2137179. doi:10.1001/jamanetworkopen.2021.37179.
67. Weller JM, Misur M, Nicolson S, et al. Can I leave the theatre? A key to more reliable workplace-based assessment. *Br J Anaesth*. 2014 Jun;112(6):1083–1091. doi:10.1093/bja/aeu052.
68. Gingerich A, Kogan J, Yeates P, Govaerts M, Holmboe E. Seeing the 'black box' differently: assessor cognition from three research perspectives. *Med Educ*. 2014 Nov;48(11):1055–1068. doi:10.1111/medu.12546.
69. Downing SM, Haladyna TM. Validity threats: overcoming interference with proposed interpretations of assessment data. *Med Educ*. 2004 Mar;38(3):327–333. doi:10.1046/j.1365-2923.2004.01777.x.
70. Downing SM. Validity: on meaningful interpretation of assessment data. *Med Educ*. 2003 Sep;37(9):830–837. doi:10.1046/j.1365-2923.2003.01594.x.
71. Post RE, Jamena GP, Gamble JD. Using Precept-Assist to predict performance on the American Board of Family Medicine on In-Training Examination. *Fam Med*. 2014 Sep;46(8):603–607.
72. Schwartz RW, Donnelly MB, Sloan DA, Johnson SB, Strodel WE. The relationship between faculty ward evaluations, OSCE and ABSITE as measures of surgical intern performance. *Am J Surg*. 1995 Apr;169(4):414–417. doi:10.1016/s0002-9610(99)80187-1.
73. Hawkins RE, Sumption KF, Gaglione M, Holmboe ES. The In-training Examination (ITE) in internal medicine: resident perceptions and correlation between resident ITE scores and faculty predictions of resident performance. *Am J Med*. 1999 Feb;106(2):206–210. doi:10.1016/s0002-9343(98)00392-1.
74. Bienstock JL, Shivraj P, Yamazaki K, et al. Correlations between Accreditation Council for Graduate Medical Education Obstetrics and Gynecology Milestones and American Board of Obstetrics and Gynecology qualifying examination scores: an initial validity study. *Am J Obstet Gynecol*. 2021 Mar;224(3):308.e1–308.e25. doi:10.1016/j.ajog.2020.10.029.
75. Francisco GE, Yamazaki K, Raddatz M, et al. Do milestone ratings predict physical medicine and rehabilitation (PM&R) board certification examination scores? *Am J Phys Med Rehabil*. 2021 Feb 1;100(2S Suppl 1):S34–S39. doi:10.1097/PHM.0000000000001613.
76. Hauer KE, Vandergrift J, Lipner RS, Holmboe ES, Hood S, McDonald FS. National internal medicine milestone ratings: validity evidence from longitudinal three-year follow-up. *Acad Med*. 2018 Aug;93(8):1189–1204. doi:10.1097/ACM.0000000000002234.
77. Paolo AM, Bonaminio GA. Measuring outcomes of undergraduate medical education: residency directors' ratings of first year residents. *Acad Med*. 2003 Jan;78(1):90–95. doi:10.1097/00001888-200301000-00017.
78. Durning SJ, Pangaro LN, Lawrence LL, Waechter D, McManigle J, Jackson JL. The feasibility, reliability, and validity of a program director's (supervisor's) evaluation form for medical school graduates. *Acad Med*. 2005 Oct;80(10):964–968. doi:10.1097/00001888-200510000-00018.
79. Papadakis MA, Teherani A, Banach MA, et al. Disciplinary action by medical boards and prior behavior in medical school. *N Engl J Med*. 2005 Dec 22;353(25):2673–2682. doi:10.1056/NEJMsa052596.
80. Papadakis MA, Arnold GK, Blank LL, Holmboe ES, Lipner RS. Performance during internal medicine residency training and subsequent disciplinary action by state licensing boards. *Ann Intern Med*. 2008 Jun 3;148(11):869–876. doi:10.7326/0003-4819-148-11-200806030-00009.
81. Heath JK, Wang T, Santhosh L, et al. Longitudinal milestone assessment extending through subspecialty training: the relationship between ACGME internal medicine residency milestones and subsequent pulmonary and critical care fellowship milestones. *Acad Med*. 2021 Nov 1;96(11):1603–1608. doi:10.1097/ACM.0000000000004165.
82. Han M, Hamstra SJ, Hogan SO, et al. *JAMA Netw Open*. 2023 Apr 3;6(4):e237588. doi:10.1001/jamanetworkopen.2023.7588.
83. Smith B, Yamazaki K, Tekian A, et al. ACGME milestone ratings of surgeon competence during training predict early career patient outcomes. Submitted 2023.
84. Thompson WG, Lipkin M Jr, Gilbert DA, Guzzo RA, Roberson L. Evaluation: assessment of the American Board of Internal Medicine resident evaluation form. *J Gen Intern Med*. 1990 May-Jun;5(3):214. doi:10.1007/BF02600537.
85. Silber CG, Nasca TJ, Paskin DL, Eiger G, Robeson M, Veloski JJ. Do global rating forms enable program directors to assess the ACGME competencies? *Acad Med*. 2004 Jun;79(6):549–556. doi:10.1097/00001888-200406000-00010.
86. Yamazaki K, Holmboe ES, Hamstra SJ. An empirical investigation into milestones factor structure using national data derived from clinical competency committees. *Acad Med*. 2022 Apr 1;97(4):569–576. doi:10.1097/ACM.0000000000004218.
87. Feinstein A. *Principles of Medical Statistics*. Chapman and Hall/CRC; 2002.
88. Holmboe ES. The importance of faculty observation of trainees' clinical skills. *Acad Med*. 2004 Jan;79(1):16–22. doi:10.1097/00001888-200401000-00006.
89. Byrne A, Soskova T, Dawkins J, Coombes L. A pilot study of marking accuracy and mental workload as measures of OSCE examiner performance. *BMC Med Educ*. 2016 Jul 25;16:191. doi:10.1186/s12909-016-0708-z.
90. Gingerich A. What if the 'trust' in entrustable were a social judgement? *Med Educ*. 2015 Aug;49(8):750–752. doi:10.1111/medu.12772.
91. Gingerich A, Regehr G, Eva KW. Rater-based assessments as social judgments: rethinking the etiology of rater errors. *Acad Med*. 2011 Oct;86(10 Suppl):S1–S7. doi:10.1097/ACM.0b013e31822a6cf8.
92. Schumacher DJ, Holmboe E, Carraccio C, et al. Resident-sensitive quality measures in the pediatric emergency department: exploring relationships with supervisor entrustment and patient complexity and acuity. *Acad Med*. 2020 Aug;95(8):1256–1264. doi:10.1097/ACM.0000000000003242.

5

Direct Observation

JENNIFER R. KOGAN, MD, AND ERIC S. HOLMBOE, MD

CHAPTER OUTLINE

Introduction

Medical educators are responsible for evaluating the clinical skills of learners and providing learners with timely, useful feedback to ensure continued growth and development of competence. Despite advances in diagnostic technology, the basic clinical skills of taking a medical history, doing a physical examination, and counseling remain essential to successful patient care. In the United States, for example, the Association of American Medical Colleges (AAMC), the Liaison Committee of Medical Education (LCME), the Accreditation Council for Graduate Medical Education (ACGME), and the American Board of Medical Specialties (ABMS) strongly endorse the evaluation of students, residents, and fellows in these clinical skills.[1–4] Furthermore, the Institute of Medicine (now the National Academy of Medicine; NAM) placed *patient-centered care* at the heart of its five core competencies for all health professionals, including physicians, in its 2003 competency framework.[5] Direct observation of learners performing a medical interview, physical examination, and counseling is mandatory to assess these skills with reliability and validity. This chapter focuses on direct observation of clinical skills (history, physical exam, and counseling), an assessment strategy that is foundational to competency-based medical education.[6] Direct observation of procedural skills is discussed in Chapter 9.

In this chapter we contextualize direct observation of clinical skills as a form of workplace-based assessment (WBA). We review four reasons why direct observation is important: to ensure assessment of clinical skills that are essential to patient care; to facilitate deliberate practice, coaching, and feedback; to inform assessment in competency-based education; and to promote high-quality supervision. Next, we review assessment tool formats and factors that explain the poor reliability and validity of direct observation assessments. We discuss how poor reliability and validity can undermine assessment quality and negatively impact patient care. The remainder of the chapter focuses on how to improve direct observation assessments. We describe rater training faculty development approaches that can improve assessment quality. We conclude by describing strategies that can be used to implement direct observation at the programmatic level. We describe barriers to frequent direct observation and strategies to increase direct observation frequency. We discuss how to engage learners and create systems for direct observation that consider the institutional culture, the healthcare delivery system, and the educational system in which direct observation is occurring. Faculty development materials are provided throughout the chapter and in the appendices.

Direct Observation as Workplace-Based Assessment

Direct observation of clinical skills is defined as observing a learner (i.e., medical student, resident, fellow) interacting with a patient taking a history, doing a physical exam, or counseling for the purpose of learner assessment. Direct observation also includes observation of physician–physician interactions (e.g., observing a learner doing a patient handoff to another learner, observing a learner calling a consult), physician–interprofessional team interactions (e.g., observing a learner interacting with a nurse or social worker), leadership activities (e.g., observing a resident leading a team), or teaching (e.g., observing a resident teaching a medical student). This chapter focuses on direct observation of learners with patients, but many of the principles discussed pertain to the other types of direct observation.

Direct observation is a workplace-based assessment (WBA). WBA is the assessment of day-to-day practice in the clinical environment; direct observation is assessment of what doctors actually do in practice.[7,8] Therefore direct observation captures what a learner "does" with patients (the top of George Miller's assessment pyramid),[9] recognizing observation may change learner behaviors (i.e., known as the Hawthorne effect) (Fig. 5.1). An extended version of Miller's pyramid was recently proposed in which being trusted for future care sits at the top of the pyramid (Fig. 5.1).[10]

As discussed in Chapter 6, standardized patients (SPs) are a valuable assessment methodology to teach and evaluate clinical skills. However, SP-based evaluation methods have limitations. SPs are optimally used for clinical skills teaching and assessment to supplement similar activities in the real clinical setting. SP assessments cannot replace physician educators routinely observing learners with actual patients.[11–14] SPs may have less validity with more advanced learners because assessment instruments used for SP exercises, depending upon case development and standard setting approaches, may favor completeness over efficiency and the use of sophisticated illness scripts.[14–16] Direct observation is an important assessment approach that more closely replicates practice, particularly for more advanced learners.

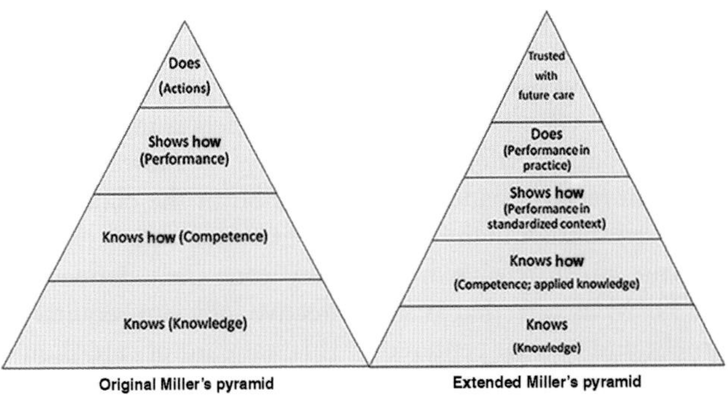

• **Fig. 5.1** Miller's pyramid and the extended Miller's pyramid.

Rationale for Direct Observation

Direct observation is required by medical education accrediting bodies such as the LCME, the ACGME, and the UK Foundation Program.[2,3,17] There are multiple reasons direct observation of clinical skills is important and relevant (Box 5.1). First, history taking, physical exam, and counseling remain important to high-quality care but are often deficient among physicians. Given the importance of these skills in patient care, these skills must be assessed. Second, direct observation is necessary to provide feedback and coach learners as part of deliberate practice. Third, direct observation is a key assessment strategy in competency-based education. Fourth, direct observation helps ensure high-quality supervision. In the remainder of this section we describe these reasons in more detail.

Importance of and State of Core Clinical Skills

It has long been recognized that students and residents have variable skills, and sometimes substantial deficiencies, in medical interviewing (e.g., history), physical examination, and counseling.[18–25] For example, there have been longstanding deficiencies in learners' auscultatory skills,[26,27] and poor clinical skills continue to plague US students and residents today.[28–30]

Furthermore, clinical skills do not necessarily improve after training. In a study using unannounced standardized patients (USPs), Ramsey and colleagues found that a group of primary care physicians only asked 59% of essential history items.[31] Braddock and colleagues found that only 9% of primary care physicians' and surgeons' counseling encounters met basic criteria for effective informed decision-making.[32] Physicians frequently fail to elicit over half

• BOX 5.1 Rationale for Direct Observation of Clinical Skills

- History taking, physical exam, and counseling are fundamental to quality care but often deficient in learners and physicians.
- Observation is necessary for deliberate practice and feedback.
- Workplace-based assessment is essential in competency-based education.
- Medical education accrediting bodies require direct observation.
- Observation is necessary to inform high-quality supervision to ensure that patients receive, at a minimum, safe, effective, patient-centered care.

of patients' complaints, and many of the public's complaints about physicians relate to communication problems.[33–41]

Because accurate data collection remains physicians' most potent diagnostic tool (even in the current era of diagnostic technology), inadequate history and physical exam skills are problematic.[42–44] The medical interview alone can lead to the correct diagnosis in nearly 80% of patients presenting to an ambulatory care clinic with a previously undiagnosed condition.[42,43] Excellent history and physical exam skills are necessary to provide high-value, cost-conscious care that avoids unnecessary expensive diagnostic tests. The 2015 NAM report, "Improving Diagnosis in Medicine," highlighted the persistent and pernicious problem of diagnostic error. This report found that data collection errors are one of the principal factors causing physician diagnostic errors.[45] In fact, diagnostic error may be the third most common cause of death in the United States.[46] In 2012, national organizations representing medical specialties in the United States asked their members to identify commonly ordered tests or performed procedures whose necessity should be questioned and discussed as part of the Choosing Wisely Campaign. The Choosing Wisely Campaign, now in multiple countries including Canada, helps physicians provide care that is supported by evidence, free of harm, and truly necessary.[47,48]

In addition to data collection and diagnostic evaluation and management, effective physician–patient communication improves patient outcomes. Improved outcomes include patients' involvement in their care, self-efficacy, adherence, and well-being while decreasing costs.[49–52] Furthermore, most patients want an active role in decision-making.[53,54] These findings reemphasize the importance of teaching and evaluating physician–patient communication.[55] Assessing history taking, physical exam, and counseling via direct observation legitimizes the importance of these skills while simultaneously assessing clinical skills that are important for high-quality care.

Direct Observation as an Educational Tool for Feedback and Deliberate Practice

Medical educators must ensure the professional development of their learners who begin training as novices and must graduate competent to practice unsupervised (in the case of residents and fellows). The goal, however, is not for learners to just be competent. Rather, medical educators should strive for learners to achieve proficiency, expertise, and mastery. Achieving expertise requires deliberate practice, and receiving feedback and coaching from others is a key component of deliberate practice.[56] Feedback from others is important because physicians often self-assess inaccurately, especially when self-assessment occurs without external guidance and data.[57–59] Feedback from others provides the external data that helps learners calibrate their self-assessments.[60,61] Direct observation of clinical skills is an important source of this meaningful external data. Just as an athletics coach could not give effective feedback to their players if they did not observe them on the field during a game, medical educators cannot effectively provide meaningful feedback to learners if they have not observed the skills about which they are providing feedback. Direct observation is important to generate the firsthand observations that become the feedback that learners can use to calibrate their self-assessments. Learners can then work with a faculty coach to define an action plan, and set new learning goals[62] (see Chapter 14).

Direct Observation as an Assessment Method in Competency-Based Medical Education

In competency-based medical education medical educators must ensure that all graduates are competent, at a minimum, in the essential domains needed for modern clinical practice (see Chapter 1).[63,64] Training programs/specialties, depending on the locale, are expected to implement and assess required competencies, competency components, developmental milestones, Entrustable Professional Activities (EPAs), and performance levels. As discussed in Chapter 1, the competency Milestones currently used in the United States are demonstrable abilities that can be observed and assessed. Direct observation assessment tools should measure progress along the milestones.[65,66]

To effectively assess the milestones, learners must be observed engaged in real patient care/clinical activities.[6] Historically, knowledge examinations, oral patient presentations, and written notes have served as proxy measures of history taking, physical exam, and counseling skills. In competency-based medical education, the predominant evaluation setting should be "in the trenches" rather than a setting removed from practice (e.g., conference room or hallway).[6] The only way to determine whether graduating residents and fellows are clinically competent is by having skilled clinicians repeatedly observe them providing care for the kinds of patients (in the appropriate practice settings) whom they will encounter when they enter practice.[67] Both the ACGME and the LCME, the accrediting bodies in the United States for graduate and undergraduate medical education, respectively, have emphasized the importance of direct observation as a key assessment strategy.[2,3]

Direct Observation as a Method to Guide Supervision

A learner's skills directly affect patient experience and outcomes, and effective supervision of learners is important to improve patient safety and care quality.[68–70] However, leaners often receive inadequate supervision in the clinical setting even though many learners want better supervision![69,71] Patients must receive high-quality care (i.e., defined by the NAM as care that is safe, effective, efficient, equitable, timely, and patient centered).[5] This standard of care should not be compromised because a patient is cared for by a team that includes learners.

Learners' competence is influenced by content and context. For example, a learner may be competent caring for a patient with pneumonia but not a patient with an acute myocardial infarction (case specificity). A learner might be less competent working in a new hospital where they are unfamiliar with the electronic health record or EHR (context specificity). Clinical supervisors are expected to fill in the gap between what a learner can do and what a patient needs to receive safe, effective patient-centered care.

Supervisors must observe learners to know what they can and cannot do. Inferring history, physical exam, and counseling skills indirectly (e.g., how well the learner presents and/or writes notes) may result in erroneous conclusions about a learner's competence and the amount of supervision they require. Ideally, direct observation assessment tools focus on evidence-based skills that help assessors identify what a learner has done well and what should be improved, increasing the likelihood of high-quality care. Therefore direct observation of clinical encounters serves the dual purpose of assessing learners and ensuring that patients receive, at a minimum, safe, effective, and patient-centered care. The Assessment for Accountable Care and Quality Supervision (AACQS) equation illustrates this idea[72] (Fig. 5.2). The AACQS equation states the product of a learner's competence (which is a function of their competence in context) and the faculty's competence (which is a function of their competence in context) should result in safe, effective, patient-centered care. In sum appropriate supervision decisions require accurate knowledge of a learner's skills. This requires direct observation.

Assessment Tools for Direct Observation

Multiple assessment tools are available to assess learners taking a history, doing a physical exam, and counseling patients.[73–75] These assessment tools serve multiple purposes. First, they can guide faculty in their observations of the learner (what behaviors/skills faculty should attend to). Second, they can be used to document the observation. Third, they can be used to provide the learner with feedback.

High-quality direct observation requires using assessment tools with validity evidence. It is important to appreciate that in WBA, the assessment instrument is the faculty, not the tool (see Chapter 2). Two systematic reviews have summarized the validity evidence for direct observation assessment tools.[73,74] The mini clinical evaluation exercise (mini-CEX) is one of the most commonly used WBA tools and has robust validity evidence.[73,74,76] The mini-CEX was designed to evaluate residents doing a *focused* history, physical examination, or counseling on the inpatient wards, intensive care units, outpatient clinics, and emergency department.[77] It also has been used with medical students and fellows.[76] On the original mini-CEX, faculty complete a 9-point rating scale evaluating specific skills and overall competency and provide immediate feedback to the learner (Fig. 5.3). Multiple assessors making multiple observations over time improves both the reliability and validity of the evaluations. Just four mini-CEXs per resident can be acceptable for pass/fail determinations or to determine whether a learner is significantly struggling.[76,77] Use of the original mini-CEX has declined substantially as multiple new iterations of the mini-CEX have been developed with new scale descriptors and anchors (see Figs. 5.3 and 5.4 and Chapter 4).

Assessment Tool Format

Direct observation assessment tools have different formats, and formats have evolved over time. Some direct observation assessment tools have global ratings; other assessment forms are checklists. Forms also have different anchors (e.g., ordinal, normative, entrustment). In the following subsections we describe some of these differences.

Global Ratings Versus Checklists

Some direct observation assessment tools ask evaluators to select global ratings (i.e., giving a rating for history-taking skills, physical exam skills, or overall clinical skills). The mini-CEX is an example of a global rating scale. Other direct observation tools are checklists (i.e., items are behaviors/skills that comprise history taking or physical exam). The SEGUE and Calgary-Cambridge instruments are examples of checklists for medical interviewing.[78,79] The choice of instruments depends primarily on the objectives of the assessment.

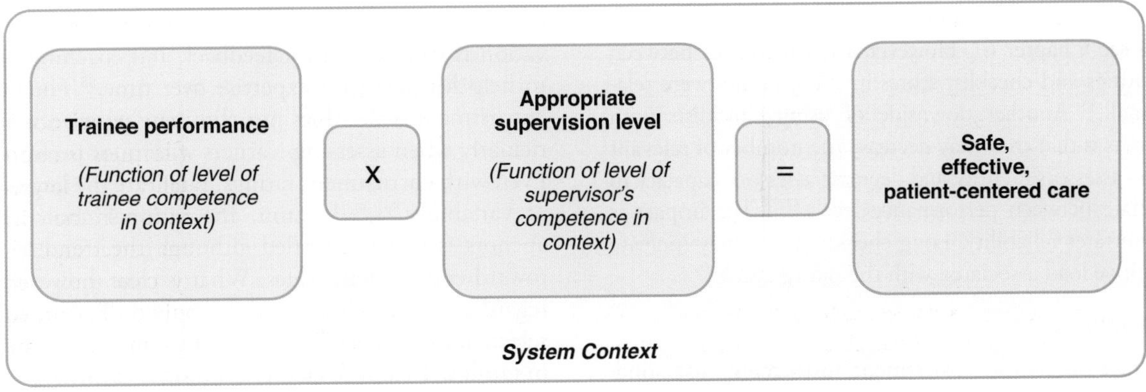

• **Fig. 5.2** Assessment for Accountable Care and Quality Supervision equation.

Mini-Clinical Evaluation Exercise (CEX)

Evaluator: ______ **Date:** ______

Resident: ______ ❍ R-1 ❍ R-2 ❍ R-3

Patient Problem/Dx: ______

Setting: ❍ Ambulatory ❍ In-patient ❍ ED ❍ Other ______

Patient: Age: ______ Sex: ______ ❍ New ❍ Follow-up

Complexity: ❍ Low ❍ Moderate ❍ High

Focus: ❍ Data Gathering ❍ Diagnosis ❍ Therapy ❍ Counseling

1. **Medical Interviewing Skills** (❍ Not observed)
1 2 3 UNSATISFACTORY | 4 5 6 SATISFACTORY | 7 8 9 SUPERIOR

2. **Physical Examination Skills** (❍ Not observed)
1 2 3 UNSATISFACTORY | 4 5 6 SATISFACTORY | 7 8 9 SUPERIOR

3. **Humanistic Qualities/Professionalism**
1 2 3 UNSATISFACTORY | 4 5 6 SATISFACTORY | 7 8 9 SUPERIOR

4. **Clinical Judgment** (❍ Not observed)
1 2 3 UNSATISFACTORY | 4 5 6 SATISFACTORY | 7 8 9 SUPERIOR

5. **Counseling Skills** (❍ Not observed)
1 2 3 UNSATISFACTORY | 4 5 6 SATISFACTORY | 7 8 9 SUPERIOR

6. **Organization/Efficiency** (❍ Not observed)
1 2 3 UNSATISFACTORY | 4 5 6 SATISFACTORY | 7 8 9 SUPERIOR

7. **Overall Clinical Competence** (❍ Not observed)
1 2 3 UNSATISFACTORY | 4 5 6 SATISFACTORY | 7 8 9 SUPERIOR

Mini-CEX Time: Observing ______ **Mins** **Providing Feedback:** ______ **Mins**

Evaluator Satisfaction with Mini-CEX
LOW 1 2 3 4 5 6 7 8 9 HIGH

Resident Satisfaction with Mini-CEX
LOW 1 2 3 4 5 6 7 8 9 HIGH

Comments: ______

______ Resident Signature ______ Evaluator Signature

• **Fig. 5.3** The mini-CEX.

Checklists can improve faculty observation quality by increasing detection of specific errors.[80] Checklists can help faculty identify whether critical data-gathering actions are completed and help them provide specific feedback to learners. However, it is not feasible to develop highly detailed checklists for every type of patient encounter. Some degree of faculty interpretation of behavior and skills is required when working in clinical settings. Additionally, the SP literature has raised concerns about the validity of highly structured checklists[15–81] (see Chapter 6). However, the differences between global ratings and checklist scores in these studies were relatively small.[82] Another downside of using checklists with many items is that they may decrease the number of relevant behaviors assessors identify and decrease assessors' capacity to differentiate between performance levels.[83,84] The impact is lower interrater reliability. Long checklists also may increase the cognitive load associated with the rating task.[85,86]

Scale Anchors

Most direct observation assessment instruments use some type of ordinal scale. Some numerical scales have adjectival anchors such as unsatisfactory, satisfactory, and superior (e.g., the original mini-CEX). Other tools have normative anchors (below expectations, at expectations, exceeds expectations). Some tools have behavioral anchors (descriptions of the behaviors) associated with each rating scale number. The Minicard is a direct observation tool with behavioral anchors[87,88] (Fig. 5.4). Behavioral anchors represent best practices that cue observers in each domain and for each of the scoring levels. Behavioral anchors may help assessors more accurately detect unsatisfactory performance, identify specific behaviors, identify struggling residents, and generate more action-oriented feedback.[87,88]

Increasingly, direct observation assessment tools use entrustment scales.[89–93] Entrustment scales can be retrospective or prospective.[93,94] Retrospective entrustment scales ask the rater to indicate how much supervision a learner needed (e.g., 1 = I had to do, 2 = I had to talk them through, 3 = I had to prompt them from time to time, 4 = I needed to be in the room just in case, 5 = I did not need to be there). Prospective supervision scales ask the rater to indicate how much supervision a learner is expected to need in the future (e.g., 1 = Can be observer only, 2 = Direct supervision, 3 = Indirect supervision, 4 = Unsupervised practice, 5 = Able to supervise others). Faculty often perceive entrustment scales as more cognitively aligned with their experience and supervision tasks.[89] Early research suggested that using entrustment anchors rather than conventional scoring systems increased discrimination, improved reliability, minimized assessor leniency, and better identified learners performing below expectations.[89,92] Entrustment scales were found to reduce the number of mini-CEXs needed from six to three and the number of ratings for a surgical assessment from 50 to 7 (to get a reliability coefficient of 0.7). In practical terms, this means decreased assessor workload.[92] Entrustment anchors can make WBA ratings more concrete, justifiable, and transparent as they convey learner progress and can align with training outcomes to improve feedback.[91]

However, more recently, educators have started to describe problems with entrustment scales.[95–97] First, reliability does not necessarily ultimately equate to validity as discussed in Chapter 2. Entrustment decisions may differ depending on whether assessors prioritize patient safety, efficiency, learner welfare, or learner autonomy. Second, even if a learner is deemed "entrustable," ongoing observation is still needed for feedback and coaching purposes to help learners gain expertise over time.[98] Finally, using entrustment scales does not eliminate poor accuracy, particularly when assessing learners with poor performance.[99] Even with entrustment ratings, raters are the largest source of variability.[94,100] In sum, the optimal choice of scale anchors is still not settled although the trend is moving toward entrustment scales. What is clear, however, is that regardless of which assessment tool and scale anchors are selected, the assessor will account for much of the variance in ratings. Therefore faculty training is essential to successfully implement WBA.

Reading Hospital Mini-CEX Rating Instrument **Date___/___/___**
Student:_____________________________ **Observer**:_____________________________
Case description:

Directions: **circle features done CORRECTLY, place "X" over ERRORS noted**

History

Interpersonal/Communication skills

1 Greeting Set agenda, "*anything else*?" Uses open-ended , non-leading questions
Gives /responds to patient's non-verbal cues Uses summarizing/clarifying/reflective statements
Demonstrates empathy "*that must have been upsetting*" Avoids medical jargon Attentive

Excellent	**Good**	**Marginal**	**Poor**
Demonstrated all of above, outstanding interaction	missed 1-2 items without egregious mistake	missed >2 or borderline egregious mistake; marginal connection	offended patient, obviously negative interaction

Comments:

Data Collection: Medical Knowledge

2 Elicits focused chief complaint General-to-specific questioning Got relevant PMH/SH
Asked discriminatory questions that prioritized differential

Excellent	**Good**	**Marginal**	**Poor**
understands historical nuances; no irrelevant data collected;	collected enough to correctly rank ddx, rarely tangential	Missed 1 or more vital data points; failed to discriminate Ddx or prioritize complaints	tangential data collector; missed major topics; "lost" in data
Senior resident/staff	**Resident/Intern**	**Intern/Med student**	

Comments:

Professional Conduct

3 Non-judgmental Does not make pt. "prove" illness Respectful to person/privacy/spirituality

Excellent/Good	**Marginal /Poor**
Patient pleased with the interaction	any above feature

Comments:

Physical Exam

Medical knowledge: physical diagnosis skills

4 Technically proficient at exam maneuvers Avoided irrelevant exam portions
Did not omit necessary elements of exam Used tools/positioning appropriately

Excellent	**Good**	**Marginal**	**Poor**
No omissions	1-2 less important omissions or 1 irrelevant exam feature	missed or botched major item or non-focused exam	appeared not to understand relevant exam

Comments:

• **Fig. 5.4** The MiniCard. (From Donato AA, Park YS, George DL, Schwartz A, Yudkowsky R. Validity and feasibility of the minicard direct observation tool in 1 training program. *J Grad Med Educ*. 2015 Jun;7(2):225-229. doi:10.4300/JGME-D-14-00532.1.)

5

Medical reasoning/exam interpretation
Understood extenuating circumstances that limit exam's usefulness (e.g. steroids/peritonitis)
Understood general sensitivity and specificity of findings

Excellent	Good	Marginal	Poor
Can use findings to effectively rank Ddx; aware of limitations Of exam findings	understands relation between disease suspected and test performed	did general physical of that organ system; omitted/did not comprehend discriminators	not able to use exam to refine historical inquiry
Senior res. / staff	**Res./Intern**	**Med student**	

Comments:

6

Professional Conduct
Asked permission/ explained exam   Respects comfort/modesty   Washes hands

Excellent/Good	Marginal /Poor
No or minor omissions	any major infraction

Comments:

Assessment of findings

7

Oral case presentation
Could logically organize all relevant data   Omitted irrelevant data
Incorporated pertinent pos/neg data   Data given aids listener in assembling/ranking ddx

Excellent	Good	Marginal	Poor
Flowing, relevant presentation; top and next ddx items obvious from data given	minor ddx item or finding neglected; major ddx captured poss. out of order	rambling presentation, all data captured; major ddx item missed but organ system correct	student lost or unfamiliar with relevant features; dangerous misses
Sr. res/staff	**Res./Intern**	**Med student**	

Comments:

8

Data synthesis/reasoning (medical knowledge components)
Logic, prioritization of differential is consistent, accurate   Values datapoints appropriately
Analysis of prevalence of disease, test sensitivity/specificity obvious in discussion
Not reliant on single data point   No omission of relevant data points that may refute diagnosis
Recognizes knowledge gaps, formulates appropriate clinical questions   Avoids early closure

Excellent	Good	Marginal	Poor
No omissions, Clear, accurate logic for ddx, formulates approp. clin ?'s	correct ddx, possibly miss or omit data, did not use/understand prev/sens/spec	Got major ddx item and correct organ system but 1 or greater major error; or can't see error	unable to synthesize data or faulty reliance on bad data point
Sr. res/staff	**Res./Intern**	**Intern/Med student**	

Comments:

• Fig. 5.4 cont'd

9 **Plan: systems-based practice**
Able to incorporate comorbid conditions into test/ treat. choices
Cost-conscious, ethical approach to testing Correctly identifies level of urgency of evaluation
Understands what to do with (pos or neg) test results Uses ancillary staff/resources appropriately
Understands limitations of tests chosen (sens/spec/ risks of false pos results)

Excellent	**Good**	**Marginal**	**Poor**
Mature, forward-thinking decisions consideration of patient's unique circumstances	Orders correct tests relevant to disorder without considering comorbidities, cost	"shotguns" tests, not aware of dz history, fails to use anc. staff, fail to consider pt issues	Makes 2 or more major mistakes
Sr. res/staff	**Res./Intern**	**Intern/Med student**	

Comments:

<u>Presentation of plan to patient/Counseling/Behavioral Change</u>

10 **Interpersonal/Communication Skills**
Defines issue Shared decisionmaking "*Let's do this together*" Good pace
Common ground/patient education/understanding evaluated "*what do you understand about..*"
Avoids medical jargon Explores variables that would affect pt's choice
Pauses for/invites questions Respects pt. opinions and preferences Summarizes
Gives and responds to patient's non-verbal cues

Excellent	**Good**	**Marginal**	**Poor**
Found common ground, shared decision/uncertainty comfortably	missed some minor (defining/shaping discussion) issues overall positive	missed 1 major (defining "where pt is", stud. not aware they are not understood)	dictatorial; patient with negative experience

Comments:

11 **Medical Knowledge components**
Addresses uncertainties with choice (limitations of testing/therapy/varied patient response to tx)
Discussion of pros/cons of options (incl. nothing) Conveys risk in testing/treating
Demonstrates understanding of limitations in test/tx

Excellent	**Good**	**Marginal**	**Poor**
Thorough understanding of all diagnostic and therapeutic options; comfort with uncertainty	knows major options may miss minor nuances of tx/ less important side fx	can name 1-2 options and basic dz course; unaware of major alternatives	makes >2 major errors
Sr. Res/Staff	**Res./Intern**	**Med Student**	

Comments:

12 **Professionalism**
Demonstrated bias Condescending Ignored pt's preferences Disrespectful

Excellent/Good	**Marginal /Poor**
No or minor omissions	any major infraction

Comments:

Total time observed____ **Feedback given? Y / N**

ACTION PLAN____

• **Fig. 5.4 cont'd**

Narrative Comments

Narrative assessment is becoming an increasingly important component of WBA.[101,102] Many WBA instruments have space for narrative comments. WBA that includes a space for narrative comments or prompts verbal feedback provides learners with rich information about how they can improve (more so than numbers). Narrative comments can both explain and elaborate checklist scores, contextualize the assessment, and convey unique content. Work by Ginsberg and colleagues has described the reliability and validity of narrative assessments.[103] Learners too describe how narrative feedback is more helpful than receiving a rating.[104,105] Fig. 5.5 shows an example of a narrative assessment form that also includes an entrustment rating. We recommend that narrative assessments are made before selecting a numeric rating so that the rating can be informed by the narrative (Fig. 5.6; see Chapter 3 for more detail on managing bias).

Rater Assessment Form

Instructions
Thinking about the encounter that you just watched, please answer the following questions.

1. What, if anything, did you observe the resident do well (i.e., behavior that enables safe, effective, patient-centered care) and what deficiencies/errors did the resident commit (i.e., behavior that impedes or hinders safe, effective, patient-centered care)? Be as complete as possible.

Did Well	Errors/Deficiencies

2. Of the observations in #1, place a checkmark next to those that you think are most important to share with the resident if you had to give prioritized feedback.

• **Fig. 5.5** Revised rater assessment form.

3. In a few words or phrases, how would you summarize/synthesize the big picture of this resident's skills in this scenario?

4. Based on this single observation, provide an overall judgment of the resident.

    - The resident can be present, but only as an **observer**. I would not let the resident perform this skill the next time.
    - The resident can practice skill with **direct supervision** (supervisor in room). I (or someone else) would need to watch the resident perform the skill in real time.
    - The resident can practice skill with **indirect supervision** (supervision available within minutes). I (or someone else) do not need to watch the resident in the room, but will need to reassess the patient/confirm findings with the patient.
    - **Unsupervised practice** allowed (distant oversight). I (or someone else) do not need to watch the resident, but I (or someone else) am available if the resident comes for help or to provide feedback.

5. What is your individual learning/action plan (next steps) for this resident?

• **Fig. 5.5 cont'd**

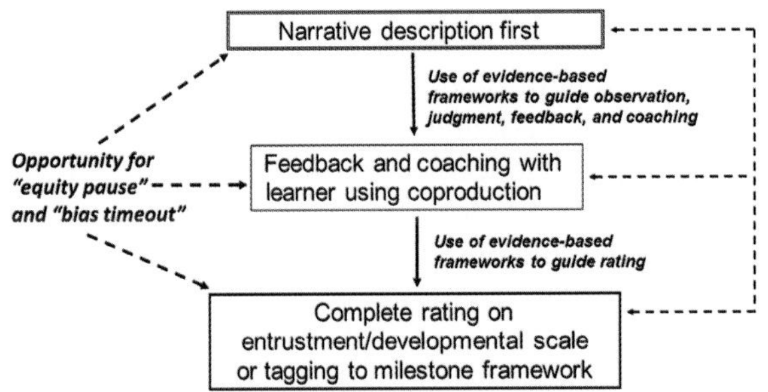

• **Fig. 5.6** Rethinking the assessment process.

Issues With Reliability and Validity

Despite the importance of WBA, the quality of assessment remains challenged by the reliability and validity issues described in the following subsections.

Accuracy

A significant problem with WBA is poor accuracy of faculty ratings. For example, faculty do not detect up to 68% of errors committed by a resident scripted to depict marginal performance on a training video.[80,99,106] Use of specific checklists that prompt faculty to look for certain skills can increase error detection accuracy nearly twofold but do not produce more accurate overall ratings of competence.[80] Nearly 70% of faculty may still rate a resident depicting marginal performance as satisfactory or superior.[80] Kalet and colleagues examined the reliability and validity of faculty observations using videos of student performance on an objective structured clinical examination (OSCE) evaluating interviewing skills.[107] Faculty inconsistently identified the use of open-ended questions and empathy, and the positive predictive value of faculty ratings for "adequate" interviewing skills was only 12%. Another study found that faculty members could not reliably evaluate 32% of the physical examination skills assessed and had the most difficulty with examination of the head, neck, and abdomen.[108]

Variable Assessment Standards

There is an increasing body of literature exploring rater cognition: how faculty observe, synthesize their observations, and make assessment judgments.[109,110] The rater cognition literature has shown that faculty use variable standards against which they compare the learner. Furthermore, assessors often develop their assessment criteria experientially and idiosyncratically and interpret scale anchors variably.[111,112] Different faculty subsequently focus on different aspects of performance and have variable definitions of quality and competence.[111–113] When assessors use different standards to assess learners, they rate learners differently, decreasing interrater reliability.

Common standards are normative, self, and use of gestalt. Some faculty use a normative standard and compare the learner to learners at a similar level of training. However, faculty are often uncertain about what skills are expected at a given stage of training.[111,112,114] More commonly, faculty use themselves as the standard when evaluating a learner.[111] This can be problematic given the robust literature describing the shortcomings practicing physicians can have in their clinical skills.[28,31–33,38–41,115] Medical educators with clinical skill deficiencies may be less likely to detect those skill deficits in learners. This is supported by a small study showing that faculty who were more complete in their history taking and had better interpersonal skills, as rated by a standardized patient, were more likely to be stringent when evaluating residents.[116] An important limitation to the study was the use of standardized patients to assess faculty skills since standardized patient assessments often reward completeness over the use of sophisticated illness scripts and efficiency.[14] Nevertheless, another study found that assessors often feel they lack content expertise in the skills they are being asked to assess.[114] Another standard used in WBA is the use of gestalt. Many faculty say that their assessment decisions are based on gestalt and they are unable to articulate how they arrived at their assessment decision(s).[111] While gestalt assessments can be accurate, they are problematic when faculty cannot deconstruct their gestalt to provide the learner with specific, constructive feedback. In contrast to the common use of normative standards, self as standard, and gestalt, faculty rarely use a criterion-referenced standard. When faculty use a criterion-referenced standard, they compare what the learner has done to the evidence-based best practice components for that particular skill.[111] An example of using a criterion-referenced approach would be assessing which of nine shared decision-making behaviors a resident performed when counseling a patient about starting a new medication.

Role of Inference

Another source of WBA error is when faculty make inferences during observation. Inference occurs when observers derive what seems to be logical conclusions from premises that are assumed to be true rather than assessing observable behaviors.[111,117] For example, imagine a resident standing with their arms crossed breaking bad news to a patient. Rather than note that the resident had their arms crossed (the observable behavior), some faculty may conclude the resident does not know how to break bad news (inference). Other faculty may believe the resident lacks empathy and humanism or might assume the resident is uncomfortable having never broken bad news before (also inference). Assessors make inferences about learners' knowledge, skills (competence), and attitudes (work ethic, emotions, intentions, personality).[111,117] Assessors often do not recognize when they are making inferences and rarely validate the accuracy of their inferences.[111] Unchecked inferences risk "distorting" accurate assessment of the learner because the assessor's inferences cannot be observed and measured; this leads to greater interassessor variability and ultimately faulty assessment.

Impact of Educational Culture

While some faculty embrace their roles and responsibilities as assessors and coaches and do not shy away from giving low ratings,[111] others modify their assessments to avoid unpleasant repercussions (both for themselves and their learners). This is another source of interrater variability.[111] Medicine has a "failure to fail" culture. As a result, some faculty inflate ratings to avoid discussing a marginal rating with a learner.[118,119] Other faculty may inflate assessments to be seen as a popular, likable teacher.[111] Some faculty avoid stringent assessments so that they will not have to defend their assessments with institutional leaders.[111,120,121]

Rater Limitations and Bias

Limitations in human cognition may also explain variability in WBA.[85] For example, contrast effects occur when the scores faculty give to learners are influenced by their recent observations of other learners. Faculty may rate a learner with borderline skills lower if they are observed after a learner with excellent skills; conversely, the same learner with borderline skills may be rated higher if the faculty observed them after a learner who is less skilled.[122,123] These biases affect both numerical ratings and narrative feedback.[124,125]

In addition to contrast effects and recency bias, there is an urgent need to confront and address the persistent and pernicious effects of bias in assessment. Explicit bias refers to conscious beliefs and attitudes one possesses about another person or group. Implicit bias refers to an individual's "prejudicial attitudes toward and stereotypical beliefs about a particular social group or members therein."[126] These individual attitudes are often subconscious. A growing body of literature describes the factors contributing to, and the harmful effects of, implicit bias and educational inequity on learners who are underrepresented in medicine (URiM) or otherwise at risk for marginalization in assessment practices. Multiple studies have found that learners from groups historically URiM receive lower assessment ratings from faculty.[127–129] In addition, gender-based differences have repeatedly been demonstrated in faculty assessments of medical trainees.[130–135] These differences have been observed in quantitative measurements where women residents receive lower competency ratings despite no differences in performance.[136–138] Narrative assessments often include linguistic differences and describe personality traits that differ by gender and URiM status.[134,135,139–141] Conflicting priorities, time constraints, and burnout can lower the threshold for faculty to unconsciously apply their activated biases when they assess learners. Fig. 5.6 provides suggestions on where raters can use self-awareness and self-assessment for bias in the observation and rating process.

Conceptual Model Summarizing Rater Cognition

Fig. 5.7 is a conceptual model of the factors that influence faculty's WBA.[111] This model highlights the complexity of direct observation and WBA. Letter labels direct you to the corresponding part of the figure. When faculty observe, they bring their attitudes and emotions about observation and feedback, clinical competence (i.e., their own clinical skills in the domain they are assessing the learner), educational competence (i.e., their skills in observation, assessment, and feedback as well as their biases), and traits (e.g., age, gender, clinical, and teaching experience) (A). Faculty observe learner–patient interactions through two lenses (B). While observing, they make inferences and use variable frames of reference (normative, self, criterion-referenced, gestalt). After the observation, faculty must interpret and synthesize their observations (C) to select a numerical rating or create a narrative assessment (D). Sometimes faculty modify their assessments in anticipation of the feedback they need to give (E). For example, faculty may select a higher rating to avoid discussing a low rating with the learner. Experiential modifiers can further influence faculty's observations and their interpretation and synthesis of observations and feedback (F). For example, prior experiences working with a learner (e.g., learner's prior performance, receptivity to feedback, etc.) can influence faculty assessment and feedback. Finally, observations are influenced by the clinical system (G) (e.g., familiarity with the patient, patient complexity, system factors such as multiple patients waiting to be seen) and the institution's educational culture (e.g., assessment culture, culture of oversight/supervision) (H).

Improving the Quality of Direct Observation Assessments

In this section of the chapter, we describe the need for faculty development to address some of the aforementioned factors that negatively influence WBA. Before doing so, we

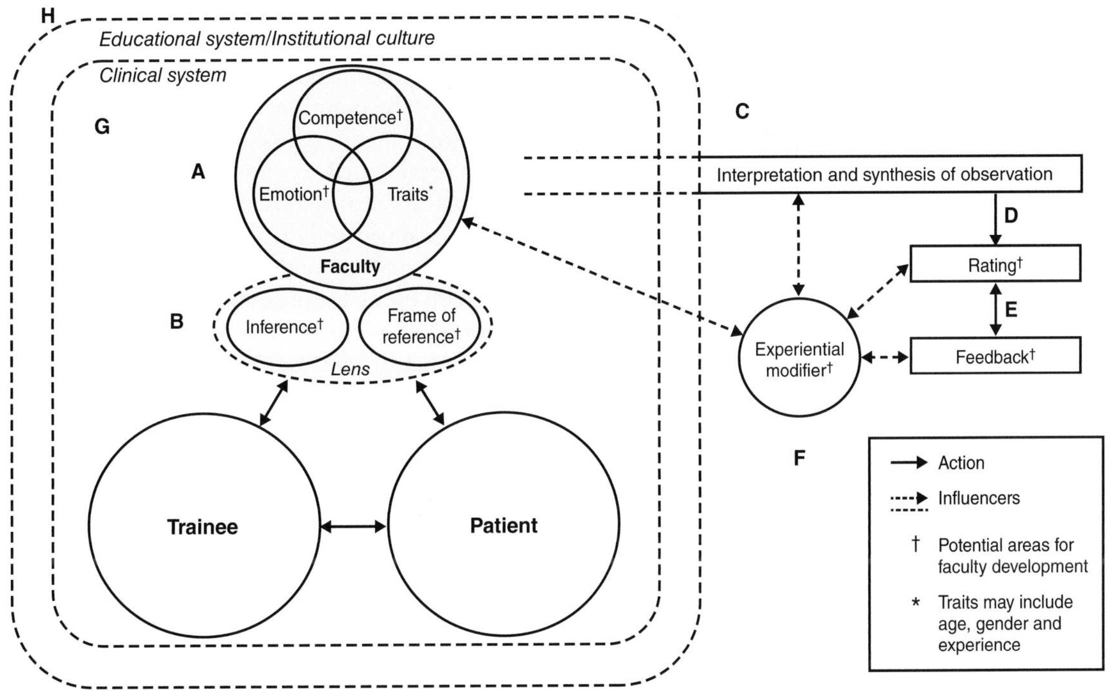

• **Fig. 5.7** Conceptual model: process of direct observation (see text for details).

recognize that some educators do not believe interrater variability is problematic and embrace the variable perspectives of multiple raters.[7,110,142,143] Educators holding this perspective believe that assessment is enriched by the unique perspectives of multiple evaluators whose assessments, when taken together, can provide meaningful information about the learner. While multiple perspectives can be valuable, we believe that acceptable medical care is bounded, and as such, not all assessments are of equal quality. In other words, there are important limits for what is acceptable patient care based on the *patient's* specific context, needs and desires and not that of the *learner*.

Some variation in assessments is beneficial, such as when an assessor leverages one of their areas of expertise associated with effective practice (i.e., warranted variation). In contrast, assessments driven by idiosyncrasies or bias that is not evidence based represent unwarranted variation. Unwarranted variation is an underappreciated problem in assessment.[144] Unwarranted variation can be harmful and can contribute to suboptimal and variable educational outcomes. Unwarranted variation at the program and institutional levels also can affect educational outcomes and, ultimately, the quality of care graduates deliver.[145]

The impact of unwarranted variation in assessment is depicted in Fig. 5.8.[144] Care delivered to patients can either be acceptable (represented in turquoise), questionable (light blue), or unacceptable (white). A much smaller amount of acceptable care is supported by best evidence (purple). Imagine there are two faculty (Faculty 1 and Faculty 2) who observe and assess the same learner with a patient. The care the learner provides to the patient is shown in yellow. In this example, the learner provided some best-evidence care, some acceptable care, and some unacceptable care. Faculty 1 observed some, but not all, of the learner's best-evidence care and some, but not all, of the acceptable care. Faculty 1 missed the learner's unacceptable care. In contrast, Faculty 2 identified some of the learner's best-evidence care but also believe they observed best-evidence care and acceptable care that was not actually done by the learner. However,

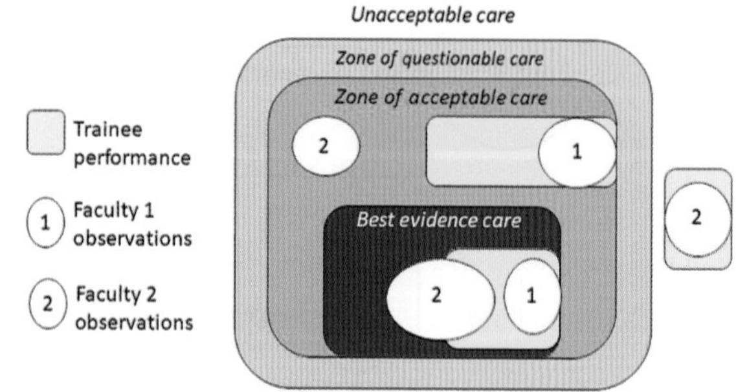

• **Fig. 5.8** Warranted and unwarranted variation in clinical skills assessment (see text for details).

Faculty 2 did pick up on the learner's unacceptable care. This example shows how faculty can make errors of omission and commission. This diagram also underscores that poor accuracy in assessment is not just an educational issue but a patient quality of care issue as well, as the patient potentially receives unacceptable care that is not identified.

Overview of Faculty Development Approaches to Improve Assessment Quality

Being a good clinician and teacher does not necessarily equate to skill completing WBA. The quality of WBA is primarily dependent on faculty's ability to make and document high-quality observations of the learner and provide the learner with feedback. As mentioned previously, faculty are the assessment instrument in WBA. Therefore time developing faculty is paramount to ensure effective observation and assessment of clinical skills.[71,146–148] Said another way, improving WBA quality requires faculty development.[147]

There are only a few studies that have explored the effectiveness of rater training to improve WBA.[99,149–152] Therefore there is not an extensive body of "evidence" to guide approaches to rater training faculty development. Additionally, rater training studies have showed mixed effects. For example, a randomized controlled trial (RCT) of an 8-hour faculty development intervention that included live practice with standardized residents and patients led to meaningful changes in faculty ratings.[149] Another RCT of two 3-hour workshops followed by three asynchronous online spaced learning modules improved rating accuracy and the accuracy and quality of narrative assessment.[99] However, a study with a briefer 2-hour training intervention and no hands-on practice failed to show meaningful change.[150]

One-time faculty development interventions are less robust than longitudinal interventions.[153] Too often, faculty development occurs as a one-time event where participants are taught information. However, without reinforcement, acquired skills diminish with time. For rater training faculty development to be effective over time, assessors need to be "recalibrated."[154] Longitudinal faculty development also enables participants to share successes, discuss challenges, learn new skills, and refresh previously learned skills. Another benefit of longitudinal faculty development is that it can also create learning communities or "communities of practice."[155]

The goal of rater training is to improve the quality of WBA. The rater training approaches described in this chapter are informed by our qualitative and quantitative research studies and our experience running faculty development programs.[99,111,116,151] In the next part of this chapter, we will describe eight parts of rater training: (1) motivating faculty to participate in rater training, (2) performance dimension training, (3) frame of reference training, (4) recognizing inference, (5) prioritizing observations and creating a summary statement, (6) mitigating bias, (7) creating opportunities for additional practice, and (8) practicing feedback after direct observation. Appendix 5.1 has examples of 1.5-hour,

3-hour, and full-day rater training workshops, and examples of longitudinal training.

Motivating Faculty to Participate in Rater Training

It is sometimes necessary to motivate faculty to participate in rater training. It can be helpful to review the importance of assessing clinical skills before starting rater training. While discussing the importance of assessing clinical skills may encourage direct observation, it is unlikely to motivate faculty to improve the quality of their assessments. Many faculty erroneously believe they effectively and accurately assess learners and, as a result, may not be motivated to participate in rater training. To motivate faculty to participate in rater training, we describe the problems with WBA accuracy, reliability, and validity. However, "showing" the need to improve assessment is more effective than "telling." Therefore we show faculty a video of a standardized resident performing a history or counseling a standardized patient. In the video the resident demonstrates "intermediate/satisfactory" clinical skills. (See Appendix 5.2 on the Expert Consult website; video scenarios for medical interviewing [Videos 5.1–5.3]; physical examination [Videos 5.4–5.6], and counseling [Videos 5.7–5.9]). Participants are not told how the resident is scripted. Participants watch the video, identify the resident's strengths and weaknesses, circle a mini-CEX rating, and indicate how they arrived at their overall rating (normative standard, self as standard, gestalt, etc.). Next, we poll faculty on the rating they selected. Inevitably, there is a range of ratings (for example, rating scores ranging from 2–8), which demonstrates low interrater reliability. Participants are usually surprised by the degree of rating variability (particularly when participants are more experienced educators) and are interested in hearing how other faculty selected their ratings. This nicely sets the stage for performance dimension training.

Performance Dimension Training

Performance dimension training (PDT) is a critical element for all rater training programs.[156–158] The overarching goal of PDT is to ensure that faculty understand the definitions and criteria for the competency of interest and build shared mental models of competence. The steps of PDT are summarized in Appendix 5.3. PDT starts with the facilitator asking participants to define, for a specific skill (e.g., starting a new medication), all the criteria and learner behaviors that constitute superior skills (i.e., expertise and mastery) from the perspective of patient outcomes. Faculty can use the video they just watched to help them with PDT. For example, faculty list the verbal and nonverbal behaviors necessary for effective counseling. All items should be observable. That is, if empathy is important, faculty should identify the behaviors that demonstrate empathy. PDT exercises should be performed in small groups of five to eight individuals. Small groups can share their results with the larger group. Group differences lead to productive discussions about what are the criteria for competence in counseling. After groups generate their list of behaviors, we distribute evidence-based standards of the skill (frameworks) (Appendix 5.3). Examples include the SEGUE model for medical interviewing, Braddock's elements or the Agency for Healthcare Research and Quality's (AHRQ) SHARE framework for shared decision-making, and the SPIKES model for breaking bad news.[32,78,159,160] Faculty compare their list of behaviors to those listed on the framework. This step further standardizes and calibrates faculty on the criteria associated with that skill. Faculty feel validated when they identify the same skills that have been published.[151] When faculty identify a list of behaviors before seeing the framework, they will consider skills on the distributed frameworks they had not identified on their own.[151] Faculty then rewatch the video encounter using the new criteria (the behavioral framework) to guide their observations. The PDT exercise takes approximately 30 minutes for a single clinical skill. Interactive group conservations during PDT help create a "shared mental model" for assessment that faculty buy into.[151] Although the group process takes time, faculty prefer creating their list of skills before being handed a list of behaviors constituting the skill.[151] Faculty are skeptical of assessment frameworks they have not developed.[151] The video scenarios (Appendix 5.2, Videos 5.1–5.9) on the Expert Consult website can be used for PDT for history taking, physical exam, and counseling.

There are several benefits of PDT[151] (Box 5.2). When faculty agree on assessment criteria using a group process, it validates the skills they believe are important. Sometimes

• BOX 5.2 Benefits of Performance Dimension Training and Frame of Reference Training

- Creates a shared mental model for important assessment criteria
- Validates skills that faculty believe are required for competence
- Creates buy-in for skills originally not considered to be important
- Enables more standardized, systematic approach to direct observation
- Encourages attention to broader array of skills during direct observation
- Facilitates assessment of skills underpinning high-quality patient care
- Improves accuracy of entrustment supervision rating
- Improves accuracy and specificity of narrative comments
- Increases breadth of skills discussed during feedback
- Provides more granular vocabulary for feedback
- Increases self-efficacy giving specific, constructive feedback
- Helps deconstruct holistic assessments for feedback
- Helps faculty learn new skills or refresh previously learned skills
- Increases faculty mindfulness during patient care
- Helps faculty identify gaps in the care they provide to patients

faculty question whether they are the only one who believes a particular skill is essential for competence. Group process during PDT often reveals that their peers also believe the skill is essential. Additionally, faculty find it helpful to create and use the list of behaviors as a guideline to inform their holistic judgment and guide feedback content. Faculty describe how PDT helps them approach direct observation in a more standardized, systematic way, paying attention to a broader array of skills, including interpersonal and communication skills.[151] PDT also helps faculty assess skills underpinning high-quality patient care that they might not have focused on prior to training.[151] Faculty believe PDT helps them give more effective feedback after direct observation by increasing the breadth of skills they can discuss. PDT can also provide them more granular vocabulary which helps them give more specific, constructive feedback.[151] PDT can help faculty deconstruct their holistic assessments to provide more specific feedback.[151] The goal of PDT is not to create a checklist that is used as a reductionistic, mindless tool. Rather, the value lies in the process of creating the framework to understand the components of a skill and develop a shared mental model around a patient-focused entrustment outcome.

Earlier in this chapter we described how direct observation quality may be limited by deficiencies in faculty's clinical skills. PDT can improve assessment while also allowing faculty to reflect on their own clinical skills. PDT can help faculty improve their clinical skills, either through learning new skills, identifying gaps in their own skills, reviewing previously learned skills, or simply becoming more reflective and mindful in their clinical care.[151] For example, faculty may learn important skills about motivational interviewing that they had not been taught prior to PDT. PDT creates potential economies of scale by simultaneously developing faculty's own skills as clinicians and as assessors. This is particularly appealing given the pressures to justify the cost of medical education.[161–163] There is a profound lack of this type of professional development for faculty.

Frame of Reference Training

Frame of reference training (FoRT) targets rating accuracy.[156,157] FoRT is an extension of PDT. Using the results of PDT, the main goal of FoRT' is to have faculty consistently apply the performance criteria to distinguish between skill *levels*. FoRT supports the developmental model of competency-based medical education by helping faculty distinguish between skill levels and identify where a learner is on the "developmental spectrum." Appendix 5.4 provides an overview of the FoRT process.

Through FoRT, faculty define the minimal criteria for *satisfactory* skills. We recommend faculty define satisfactory as what is needed for safe, effective, patient-centered care unsupervised.[72] This definition of satisfactory is consistent with the Institute of Medicine's (now NAM) definition of high-quality care and practices associated with improved patient outcomes.[5,50–52] Alternatively, satisfactory can be defined as the learner being able to competently perform the skill unsupervised.[164] These criteria for competence then anchor marginal and unsatisfactory performance. Once the group defines marginal criteria, by default any lesser performance is ineffective, not patient centered, and/or unsafe (i.e., "unsatisfactory"). The next steps in FoRT are to show additional videos of learners demonstrating different levels of skill. Participants are asked to write their observations (narrative assessment) and select an entrustment rating. Participants share their observation and ratings, and the facilitator provides the group with feedback on the expert rating (and rationale) and narrative assessment. Participants discuss differences between their observations, narrative assessments, and ratings with those of the facilitator or expert. This exercise helps faculty differentiate learners with different skill levels.

There are multiple benefits of FoRT (Box 5.2). FoRT promotes deliberate practice of assessment skills.[165] Watching a clinical encounter performed at three learner skill levels helps faculty discriminate between performance levels. This is beneficial because assessors have difficulty distinguishing between unsatisfactory and satisfactory performance (calling for direct and indirect supervision, respectively) or between satisfactory and aspirational performance (no supervision needed).[165] Comparing and contrasting learners across a video series helps faculty better understand the range of behaviors for or variable execution of a given skill.[165] For example, across the video series, participants can see a range of how much and how well a resident explores the physical, psychological, and emotional impact of a symptom on a patient. Watching a three-video series can also help faculty gain clarity about the importance of specific clinical skills.[165] For example, after initially doubting that agenda setting is necessary for safe, effective, patient-centered care, participants see why agenda setting is beneficial and important after watching a video where the resident starts the encounter with agenda setting (see Video 5.3).[165] Furthermore, seeing aspirational performance highlights the value and importance of certain clinical behaviors that may have initially been dismissed as unimportant or minimally important.[165]

Watching a three-video series emphasizes the importance of direct observation.[165] Participants often have an "ah ha" moment when they realize that a resident's oral case presentation might be identical after all three video encounters and not represent what occurred during the patient visit. As such, FoRT underscores how a learner's patient presentation is an incomplete and inadequate proxy for what occurred during an office visit (in turn impacting what a patient does after the visit). This realization reinforces the value of direct observation. Together PDT and FoRT can increase the quality and specificity of narrative assessment, although at the expense of increased stringency.[99]

Recognizing Inference

As described earlier, during direct observation faculty frequently and unknowingly make inferences about learners.[110,111,151]

During rater training workshops, workshop facilitators (and participants) should point out when inferences are made. When an inference is made, the group should discuss the behavior that was observed and discuss the potential explanations for that behavior. The "cause" of the behavior can then be explored during feedback. For example, imagine after watching a video, a faculty member says, "The resident was uncomfortable addressing the patient's substance use." This is an inference. Whomever notices the inference should name it as such. The individual who made the inference should describe what they observed. For example, perhaps the resident had a halting speech pattern, started to fidget in their chair, and quickly changed topics. Rather than assuming the learner was uncomfortable, these behaviors should be discussed during feedback. During feedback the preceptor can determine the drivers of the behaviors (e.g., the resident's inadequate knowledge about how to address substance use disorder versus adequate knowledge about what to ask the patient or concern about how questions will be received by the patient versus the resident having a close friend recently hospitalized with substance use disorder, etc.).

Prioritizing Observations and Creating a Summary Statement

Given the importance of narrative assessment in competency-based assessment[101–103] and the importance of providing learners with feedback following direct observation,[105] faculty should learn how to prioritize and synthesize their observations. After each video, faculty should identify and discuss which of their observations they would prioritize during feedback. Prioritized observations should include what was done well and what could be improved. Prioritized feedback could focus on (1) skills the learner identified as a learning goal; (2) skills that were performed exceptionally well or that are often not seen in an encounter; (3) skills that are most in need of attention; or (4) skills that would most help a future patient receive high-quality care.

While faculty make multiple observations during direct observation, many observations have a similar theme. It is helpful, prior to providing feedback, to consider how individual observations relate to each other. For example, imagine a learner appropriately recognizes the need to prescribe a cholesterol-lowering medication but chooses a statin with an inappropriate potency, fails to mention the most common side effects, discusses uncommon side effects, selects an inappropriate dose of the medication, and recommends the wrong follow-up interval. In addition, the learner does not address the patient's hesitance in starting a medication. While these are six unique observations, they can be summarized: *The resident appropriately identified the patient qualified for a statin but did not demonstrate adequate knowledge about prescribing the medication and did not engage the patient in a shared decision-making conversation.* Summary statements do not need to be shared with the learner but creating one can help faculty organize and synthesize their observations prior to feedback. The skill can be practiced by asking several faculty to share their summary statement after watching and discussing a training video.

Mitigating Bias

Similar to identifying inference, it is helpful to discuss the role of bias in assessment and discuss strategies to mitigate the bias. At a minimum, assessors should do a "bias check" after making their observations and selecting their rating (Fig. 5.6). Additionally, assessors should review their narrative comments for biased language. Given bias is often unconscious, program directors and educational systems should ensure a programmatic approach to identifying bias in assessments. While mitigating bias in assessment is beyond the scope of this chapter, Box 5.3 provides examples of some strategies that can be used to mitigate bias that are drawn from the patient communication literature.[166]

Opportunities for Additional Practice

As we alluded to earlier, most faculty development occurs as a single workshop. However, like any skill, improving observation and feedback requires practice. Therefore effective faculty development courses have opportunities for longitudinal practice.[153] There are several options for longitudinal practice. Faculty can apply their PDT frameworks to new videos. Ideally practice should include viewing, assessing, and discussing trigger videos in groups and comparing narrative assessments and ratings to an expert. Practice sessions can be brief and can occur either during a preexisting conference or at a standalone meeting. Faculty can practice "virtually" through video meetings or asynchronous online modules. Longitudinal training can also include PDT and FoRT for new skill domains.

Repeated practice helps faculty refresh their skills in direct observation while bringing intervening real-world experience to practice.[165] Faculty who participate in ongoing practice describe how it mitigates losing previously acquired skills and promotes longer-term learning.[165] Practice helps reinforce the frameworks, thereby building an "internal model" for the competency being observed.[165] With repeated practice over time, applying the frameworks starts to become "second nature." With time, faculty describe being better able to identify the more subtle differences in learner skill.[165] FoRT spaced learning also serves as a reminder that learner presentations are a poor proxy for what a learner does in the room with a patient.[165]

Practicing Skills in Feedback After Direct Observation

It is beneficial to provide faculty with opportunities to practice their WBA and feedback skills with live standardized residents and standardized patients. Since direct observation is most valuable when it is followed by feedback, we recommend pairing a rating training workshop with a workshop on providing effective feedback. This is then followed by practice giving feedback in which faculty,

• BOX 5.3 Strategies to Mitigate Bias in Assessment

Strategy	Description	Assessment example
Stereotype replacement	Recognizing when a stereotype has been activated, thinking about why, and then actively substituting nonstereotypical thoughts	When writing a narrative after direct observation of a woman learner, the assessor stops to consider if they may be using gender-laden language or uses an online tool to assess for gender bias. If bias is found, the assessor substitutes evidence-based behavioral skills that are more neutral.
Perspective taking	Considering what it would be like to be a member of the minoritized group	During bedside rounds faculty witness a difficult interaction between a learner from a URiM group with a discriminatory patient. Faculty should ask themselves: What must that be like for the learner? How will I intervene in this situation?
Individuation	Recognizing when you have stereotyped someone according to their group affiliation and instead thinking about what makes them an individual	A faculty member watches a learner from another country struggle to interview a patient with a possible sexually transmitted disease and initially stereotypes the learner as from a group "uncomfortable talking about sex." Instead, the faculty sees an individual learner struggling and seeks to understand why they are struggling as an individual.
Counterstereotypic imaging	Imagining an individual or situation that counteracts a stereotypical reaction in detail	A faculty member starts with an assumption that women are not strong enough to perform orthopedic procedures and then instead thinks about successful women who are orthopedic surgeons.
Increased opportunities for contact	Increasing opportunities for contact with members of a stereotyped group	Programs and faculty can spend meaningful time with URiM trainees to listen and learn more about their lived experiences and their path to the current training program.

URiM, Underrepresented in medicine.

in groups of four to six, rotate through four or five different "stations." Each station focuses on direct observation of a different clinical skill (e.g., history taking, physical exam, counseling, breaking bad news, motivational interviewing, etc.). A facilitator leads faculty in a brief PDT exercise for that station (e.g., breaking bad news). The facilitator then distributes an evidence-based framework for breaking bad news.[130] Next, one participant is designated the "preceptor." The group watches a standardized resident (trained to perform the skill at different levels of competence) deliver bad news to a standardized patient. After the encounter, the standardized patient and resident step out of the room and the preceptor discusses their observations and entrustment rating. The rest of the participants share their observations and ratings, and the group tries to reach consensus about the assessment.

The standardized resident (who has been trained to respond to feedback in different ways) returns to the room and the preceptor gives them feedback. The other participants observe the feedback. The preceptor self-assesses the quality of their feedback; the group then provides the preceptor with feedback. The standardized resident can also provide feedback to the preceptor. The standardized residents frequently have valuable feedback from their experiences as learners. The session trainer facilitates the feedback and provides suggestions for improving the observation and feedback. The activity repeats itself across the different stations so that each faculty member has a turn to practice observation and feedback. Each station can focus on a different skill or on the same skill performed at different levels. Residents' responses to feedback can differ across the stations. We typically start with feedback that is easier to give (i.e., giving feedback to a resident who is skilled, has insight, and is receptive to feedback). Subsequent stations are progressively more difficult (a resident who is unskilled, has insight, and is receptive to feedback; a resident who is unskilled, lacks insight, and is not receptive to feedback). The stations can be recorded so that faculty can review their videos at a later point in time.

Faculty describe how one of the most useful components of rater training is observing standardized resident-standardized patient encounters and providing the standardized resident with feedback. Practice observing residents, comparing observations with other faculty, synthesizing observations into a judgment, and providing feedback to different "types" of learners is relevant to faculty's day-to-day practice. For many faculty, this is the first time they have been observed giving feedback, and for most it is the first time they have gotten feedback about their feedback.

It is helpful to have access to a simulation center and a standardized patient trainer/coordinator for this activity. However, if a simulation center is not available, this activity also can be done with standardized patients and residents in conference rooms or open rooms in available clinics. Chief residents and junior faculty are excellent standardized residents and can easily be trained using tip sheets that describe varying resident skill levels. Training materials for faculty development facilitators and standardized residents is provided in Appendix 5.5 on the Expert Consult website. The live standardized patient/resident session can be performed the afternoon of the PDT and FoRT training or can be done on a separate day.

If there is not access to a simulation center, standardized residents and/or standardized patients and facilitators can do a modified version of this activity using videos of a resident performing a skill (see Appendices 5.2 and 5.6). Faculty assess the resident in the video and discuss their ratings and observations as mentioned earlier. Then faculty role-play feedback. One faculty participant gives feedback to another faculty who plays the resident. The individual role-playing the resident can be given a brief vignette that describes the resident's insight and receptivity to feedback (i.e., insightful/not insightful; receptive/not receptive). After the role-play, the group can debrief the feedback as previously described.

Implementing Workplace-Based Assessment

Medical student, residency, and fellowship program directors are responsible for creating or improving systems for direct observation. This section covers how to implement direct observation at the programmatic level and how to think about institutional culture and the educational system in which direct observation occurs. Successful WBA implementation requires consideration of work structures (ensuring sufficient time), organizational culture, instruments (previously discussed), and users.[147,148] Attention to implementation strategies can help address WBA enablers and barriers, leading to more successful uptake of WBA.[167–169]

There are several barriers to direct observation including lack of faculty buy-in about the importance of direct observation, perceived or real lack of time for direct observation, limited comfort doing direct observation, and concerns about interfering with the learner–patient relationship. Barriers also include learner buy-in to direct observation. Finally, there are practical challenges such as assigning responsibility for direct observations and tracking observations. For each of these challenges, we offer practical methods to help faculty improve and increase observation.

Increasing Faculty Buy-In for Direct Observation

Getting faculty to observe learners is challenging. For decades faculty have taken at face value the veracity of the history and physical examination presented on rounds without ever watching the learner perform these skills. Furthermore, observation may only happen once or twice during a clinical rotation. Faculty observing students on electives, residents, and fellows occurs even less frequently. It is therefore important to convince faculty that direct observation is important and worthwhile. You can share the evidence about the importance of direct observation described in the beginning of the chapter (Box 5.1).

It is beneficial to explore faculty's attitudes about direct observation at the start of faculty development workshops. Ask faculty to recall a time when they were observed as a learner with a patient for the purpose of getting feedback. Have faculty reflect about that experience and whether it was or was not helpful. Faculty can share their reflections in pairs and then as a larger group. Some faculty will describe how they were never observed. These faculty might describe how the lack of observation and feedback left them uncertain about their level of competence. Others may describe that the lack of observation did not jeopardize their skill development. These faculty may not believe direct observation is necessary in clinical training (which is important to know at the outset of faculty development). Other faculty will describe being infrequently observed as a student and even less frequently as a resident or fellow. Many faculty recall these experiences as anxiety provoking or as a checkbox activity.[170] Rarely, faculty will remember being observed and finding it helpful. The point is that asking faculty about their experiences being observed can shed light on their perspectives about direct observation and their potential willingness to do direct observation.

A second, related activity is asking faculty to recall a time when they observed a learner with a patient for the purpose of feedback. Have faculty share how it felt to be the observer and what, if anything, was useful. This exercise can highlight how faculty learned something new about the learner's skills they otherwise would not have known (e.g., a learner who gives excellent patient presentations but has poor interpersonal skills at the bedside). Other faculty may describe their discomfort doing direct observation and their uncertainty about what behaviors they should focus on. Some faculty might describe how observing learners was required but was not educationally beneficial for the learner. Again, these conversations enable you to understand the attitudes of faculty prior to faculty development or the implementation of direct observation programs.

To increase faculty motivation for direct observation, ask faculty to share their "*You will never believe what I observed today*" experiences. That is, a time when they learned something about their learner's skills that they never would have discovered had they not observed the learner with the patient. We share an experience where one of us observed a learner evaluating a patient with probable endocarditis. The learner did the fundoscopic exam holding the ophthalmoscope backward (so that the light was shining in the learner's, not the patient's, eye). Without direct observation we would not have realized that the statement "the fundi were not well visualized" was because of poor examination technique, not miotic pupils. We also share an example where direct observation helped us appreciate what a learner was doing well. One of us observed a learner who appeared to have poor interpersonal skills and a negative attitude toward patient care in the precepting room but who was highly skilled at empathic patient-centered interviewing during the clinical encounter. Asking faculty to identify these "surprise" experiences allows faculty to share unexpected insights into learners' clinical skills through direct observation. Doing so helps build buy-in for direct observation.

Finding Time for Direct Observation

One of the greatest barriers to direct observation is faculty's real or perceived lack of time.[167] It is helpful to emphasize that direct observation does not require watching a patient encounter from start to finish. While observing an entire encounter may be valuable, there is rarely time for this. It is perfectly acceptable to watch *part* of a patient encounter, a so-called observation snapshot. Observation snapshots improve the feasibility of direct observation. Furthermore, multiple observation snapshots across various contents and contexts by multiple faculty and other health professionals improves the validity of the assessments and the inferences that are made from them.[146,171] Since faculty may be used to watching full patient encounters, have them brainstorm potential observation snapshots.

It is important to make direct observation meaningful for the learner. There is low value in observing a learner begin a patient encounter if you already know the learner is highly skilled in agenda setting. It would be more valuable to focus observation on an area in which the learner is less skilled; for example, taking a history from a nonnative language–speaking patient using an in-person or telephone interpreter. Additionally, direct observation should focus on observing skills that the learner wants and needs to develop. Encourage faculty to work with their learners to identify learner-centered snapshots (a skill the learner would like to work on and receive feedback about). When learners perceive that WBA is being used for learning, they are more likely to seek out corrective feedback rather than "play to the test."[172]

Faculty should be encouraged to identify snapshots that are also meaningful for the patient (a skill that could improve the care a patient receives). An example snapshot is watching a resident counsel a patient with poorly controlled type 2 diabetes about the need to initiate insulin. In this scenario, the faculty can observe the resident and provide feedback about the resident's counseling skills while assisting the learner in the conversation with the patient.

Observation snapshots should be aligned with the competency milestones or EPAs, depending on the educational system being used. Faculty and/or program directors should identify observations that will inform the milestones. For example, if a competency milestone is "the ability to identify and incorporate patient preference in shared decision-making," faculty might observe a learner discussing a controversial screening decision (e.g., screening mammography between 40 and 50), starting a cholesterol-lowering medication, or engaging in a goals of care discussion.

It is beneficial to help faculty identify observation snapshots that can save time. For example, faculty can save time by watching a learner do a shoulder exam rather than having the learner present the shoulder exam and then going back to see the patient and repeat the exam. This approach benefits the patient who then does not need two exams on their painful shoulder. In the ambulatory setting, encourage faculty to observe one of the residents seeing their "first patient" of the day. This strategy works well because residents are not yet running behind or waiting to present a patient. Observation snapshots may not simultaneously meet all these goals of helping the learner, helping the patient, and saving time. However, some snapshots can accomplish many of these goals simultaneously. An observation snapshot tip sheet is provided in Appendix 5.6.

Most importantly, observation snapshots are more likely to happen when there is an educational culture that values and supports direct observation and feedback.[173] Support includes sufficient time to do direct observation. Programs need to determine whether their current resident:faculty staffing models permit WBA. If not, institutions should consider reducing faculty:resident precepting ratios.

Preparing Learners for Direct Observation

Program directors and faculty must prepare learners for direct observation.[167] Program or course directors should orient learners to the purpose of direct observation and feedback and introduce learners to the concepts of deliberate practice, feedback, and coaching. Program directors should teach their learners how to be proactive identifying the skills they want/need to develop since feedback is most effective when the learner has a self-directed agenda. Program directors should explain to learners how self-assessment guided by external assessments can inform personal learning goals about which learners can then seek feedback. Learners can identify goals/skills independently or in a group. For example, learners can brainstorm lists of skills that are PGY specific (intern vs. PGY 3) or rotation specific (ambulatory vs. critical care skills, etc.).

Learners also benefit from being taught how to elicit effective feedback that is specific and includes an action plan.[174] Learners can then "mentor-up" by eliciting useful feedback from a teacher who otherwise may not have provided effective feedback. Program directors can demonstrate the difference between nonspecific, open-ended questions to elicit feedback (e.g., "How am I doing?") and more specific questions (e.g., "How are my counseling skills?") and even more specific questions (e.g., "What aspects of shared decision-making could I work on?"). Additionally, program directors can teach learners how to elicit a specific action plan (e.g., "What suggestions do you have for how I can be even more patient centered when I am counseling patients?").

While some learners readily accept direct observation and find WBA valuable, many learners do not see WBA as a meaningful assessment activity for their professional growth.[175–177] Learners often find direct observation anxiety provoking and try to actively avoid it.[178] To address this, direct observation and the feedback that follows are most effective when situated in longitudinal learner and assessor relationships.[174,179] These longitudinal relationships promote the formative intent of WBA. Longitudinal relationships also increase the likelihood learners will find feedback credible and trustworthy (and therefore act on it). It is therefore important that program directors maximize longitudinal relationships when planning educational rotations.

Preparing Faculty for Performing the Observation

Faculty often describe feeling uncomfortable doing direct observation.[114] They worry that their presence will interfere with and/or undermine the learner–patient therapeutic relationship. This can be addressed by reviewing how faculty can prepare themselves, the learner, and the patient for observation (Box 5.4). Preparation for observation is often overlooked or absent in faculty training.

Prior to observation, faculty should explain to the learner what will happen during observation. As noted earlier, faculty should ask what the learner would like the focus of the observation to be. This helps faculty determine the goals of the observation before entering the patient's room. For example, if the goal of the observation is to observe a learner's physical examination skills, faculty should consider what physical examination components are relevant to the patient's chief complaint or medical condition. This usually requires hearing the patient's history prior to observation. Bedside presentations are an efficient way to hear about the patient's history and patients appreciate such presentations.[180] Faculty can also prepare for observation by identifying how and when they will confirm (if deemed necessary) the learner's findings.

When preparing the learner, faculty should encourage the learner to "do what they would normally do," recognizing the presence of an observer changes the context of the encounter. If doing an observation snapshot, faculty should remind the learner they will not be observing the entire encounter. If faculty plan to take notes during the observation, faculty should inform the learner they are noting both strengths and areas for improvement. Otherwise, the learner may erroneously assume that every time the faculty is writing, the learner is making a mistake.

It is valuable to teach faculty where to position themselves in the room when observing. Correct positioning minimizes interfering in the learner–patient relationship while simultaneously ensuring that faculty can see both the learner and the patient. Faculty observers should not be distracting and should safeguard the learner–patient relationship whenever possible. Fig. 5.9 demonstrates the principle of triangulation. Triangulation maximizes faculty's ability to observe while minimizing visual interference. Faculty should also prepare the patient for the observation. Either the learner or faculty should explain to the patient why the faculty will be present during the encounter. Faculty should inform patients if they do not plan to stay for the entire encounter.

Faculty can practice their observation skills by watching a video of a faculty observing a learner (Video 5.10, Scenario: Conducting an Observation). After watching the video, faculty can discuss the following questions in a group: What did the faculty do well during the observation? What didn't they do well? How could the faculty be more effective doing direct observation? How could the faculty better prepare the learner and patient? How could the faculty better position themselves? How could the faculty minimize distractions and interruptions?

Assigning Responsibility for Direct Observation

Early in training, direct observation should be used to identify learners who have outlier performance. Program directors and faculty should "frontload" observation as part of learners' baseline needs assessment. This is especially

• BOX 5.4 Preparing for and Performing Direct Observation

- Prepare learner for direct observation
  - Set expectations with the learner about what will happen during direct observation.
  - Ask the learner what the observation focus should be (i.e., what does the learner want feedback about).
- Faculty preparation for direct observation
  - Determine goals of observation.
  - Consider using observational aids.
  - Consider positioning in the room (triangulation).
  - Consider how findings will be confirmed.
  - Minimize external interruptions (e.g., avoid taking routine calls).
- Patient preparation for direct observation
  - Explain the presence of the assessor in the room.
  - Explain that the assessor may leave the room before the encounter ends.
- Avoiding intrusions
  - Avoid interjecting or interrupting.
  - Do interject to correct misinformation.
  - Do interject if something egregious is occurring.

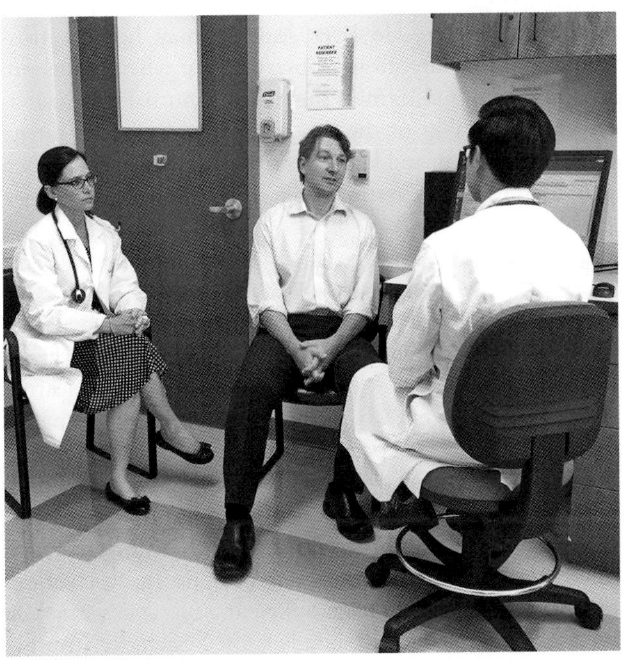

• Fig. 5.9 Triangulation.

important when learners transition to new roles and responsibilities (i.e., July in the United States and Canada, which is the start of the academic year). Early observation can identify learners who need additional support, coaching, and remediation. Just four observations can detect outlier performance.[77] Over time, the focus of direct observation can shift to assessment and feedback for ongoing skill development. Most importantly, learners should be evaluated multiple times, in multiple contexts, across multiple evaluators, and longitudinally over time. Although rater training can improve the quality of assessments, the best validity evidence occurs when there is broad sampling of skills.

At the programmatic level, it is helpful to identify how the responsibility for direct observation snapshots can be shared. Consider adopting a "divide and conquer" approach. Parse out what skills will be observed and assessed on what rotations. For example, faculty attending on the geriatric service might be responsible for observing the geriatric functional assessment. Faculty in the intensive care unit might be responsible for assessing breaking bad news and goals of care discussions. Outpatient preceptors could be responsible for assessing agenda setting and the musculoskeletal exam. Consider asking core faculty to identify the skills that should be prioritized for direct observation in their specialty. Including core faculty in this way promotes buy-in to WBA because faculty then observe skills that they believe are important. As previously discussed, observations should be aligned with or inform milestones or EPAs.

Program directors should decide who is responsible for initiating observation snapshots: learners or faculty. There are pros and cons to each approach. Placing the responsibility for direct observation on faculty emphasizes that direct observation is valued by the program. However, learners may then feel that direct observation is happening "to them," not "for them" or "with them." Placing the responsibility on learners can give learners control and ownership of their skill development. However, learners may become frustrated when faculty do not observe them when requested. Ideally faculty and learners should take mutual responsibility and ownership of the process. That is, faculty initiate direct observation and learners also ask to be observed when they need feedback to further develop a clinical skill.[181]

Tracking Observations

Programs should create a plan to monitor and track whether observation is happening. Online evaluation systems facilitate tracking and allow data to be aggregated by learner and evaluator. If observations are still recorded on paper, a process to tally observations is needed. A simple strategy is posting a piece of paper in the rounding or precepting room that lists all learners, the minimum number of snapshots required for each learner, and a place for faculty to initial and date each time they have done an observation. Smartphone apps or forms linked to QR codes can also track observations. One example is the System for Improving and Measuring Procedural Learning (SIMPL) app that is designed for observation of surgical procedures using an entrustment type scale.[182,183] This tool has a significant amount of research behind it and is currently being widely piloted in the United States. The ACGME also hosts the Direct Observation of Clinical Care (DOCC) app.[184]

Key Messages About Faculty Development and Implementation

Direct observation/WBA, which has always been important in medical education, is a key assessment approach in competency-based education. Direct observation of clinical skills followed by feedback is necessary for deliberate practice and for high-quality supervision. Because there are multiple threats to frequent, high-quality, valid assessments, programs need to invest in faculty development to maximize the effectiveness of direct observation. Faculty development should utilize rater training techniques that help faculty develop a shared mental model of clinical skills that is aligned with high-quality patient-centered care. To improve direct observation frequency, faculty development should help faculty identify observation snapshots that are meaningful for the learner and could improve patient care quality. Programs need to discuss the importance of direct observation and feedback with learners. Finally, faculty development programs should include longitudinal training and practice since direct observation, assessment, and feedback are complex skills that require ongoing practice.

Annotated Bibliography

1. Anderson HL, Kurtz J, Kirkpatrick E. Implementation and use of workplace-based assessment in clinical learning environments: a scoping review. *Acad Med.* 2021 Nov 1;96(11S):S164–S174. doi:10.1097/ACM.0000000000004366.
   This is a scoping review of the barriers and enablers of WBA. Identified themes include lack of trainee and assessor engagement in design, time constraints of the clinical environment, and distilling the complex language of competency-based assessments into terms and parameters assessors and trainees can easily use. This article discusses the importance of technology solutions and areas for future research and innovation.
2. Gingerich A, Kogan J, Yeates P, Govaerts M, Holmboe E. Seeing the 'black box' differently: assessor cognition from three research perspectives. *Med Educ.* 2014 Nov;48(11):1055–1068. doi:10.1111/medu.12546.
   This perspective piece from an international group of researchers presents key findings in assessor cognition research focused on WBA. The piece explores different perspectives for variability in assessment judgments. Three prevailing approaches to assessor cognition research are reviewed: assessor as trainable, assessor as fallible, and assessor as meaningfully idiosyncratic. The implications for assessor training/faculty development are addressed.
3. Kogan JR, Conforti L, Bernabeo E, Iobst W, Holmboe E. Opening the black box of clinical skills assessment via observation: a conceptual model. *Med Educ.* 2011 Oct;45(10):1048–1060. doi:10.1111/j.1365-2923.2011.04025.x.
   This is a qualitative study using a grounded theory approach that was designed to create a conceptual framework identifying the factors impacting faculty's judgments and ratings of residents after direct observation

with patients. Participants were 44 internal medicine faculty outpatient preceptors from 16 internal medicine residency programs in the United States. Four factors were identified that explained variability of faculty's ratings of residents: variable frames of reference, high levels of inference, variable approaches to translating observations to numerical ratings, and institutional/cultural factors. This article summarizes the findings in a conceptual model that describes factors influencing the variability of observations and judgment during workplace-based assessment.

4. Kogan JR, Dine CJ, Conforti LN, Holmboe ES. Can rater training improve the quality and accuracy of workplace-based assessment narrative comments and entrustment ratings? A randomized controlled trial. *Acad Med.* 2023 Feb 1;98(2):237–247. doi:10.1097/ACM.0000000000004819.
   This is a multiinstitution, single blind RCT of a rater training intervention using the techniques of performance dimension training, frame of reference training, and spaced learning. The purpose of this study was to determine whether rater training could improve WBA narrative comment quality and accuracy. A secondary aim was to assess impact on entrustment rating accuracy. The quality and specificity of narrative comments improved with rater training; the effect was mitigated by inappropriate stringency. Training improved accuracy of prospective entrustment-supervision ratings but the effect was more limited.
5. Kogan JR, Hatala R, Hauer KE, Holmboe E. Guidelines: the do's, don'ts and don't knows of direct observation of clinical skills in medical education. *Perspect Med Educ.* 2017 Oct;6(5):286–305. doi:10.1007/s40037-017-0376-7.
   This evidence-informed guideline outlines approaches faculty, programs, and learners can take to improve the frequency and quality of direct observation. The article includes factors that undermine WBA and areas for future research.
6. Pelgrim EA, Kramer AW, Mokkink HG, van den Elsen L, Grol RPTM, van der Vleuten CPM. In-training assessment using direct observation of single-patient encounters: a literature review. *Adv Health Sci Educ Theory Pract.* 2011 Mar;16(1):131–142. doi:10.1007/s10459-010-9235-6.
   This is a systematic review that describes the feasibility, reliability, validity, and educational effect of workplace-based assessment instruments and describes validity evidence of the mini-CEX. The review also highlights the lack of research on educational effects of direct observation tools.
7. Ten Cate O, Carraccio C, Damodaran A, et al. Entrustment decision making: extending Miller's pyramid. *Acad Med.* 2021 Feb 1;96(2):199–204. doi:10.1097/ACM.0000000000003800.
   In this perspective the authors discuss how assessing is important in competency-based medical education and discuss adding "trusted" to the apex of Miller's pyramid.
8. Ten Cate O, Schwartz A, Chen HC. Assessing trainees and making entrustment decisions: on the nature and use of entrustment-supervision scales. *Acad Med.* 2020 Nov;95(11):1662–1669. doi:10.1097/ACM.0000000000003427.
   In this perspective the authors describe entrustment scales and use of entrustment as a component of WBA. The authors describe the distinction between ad hoc entrustment decisions and summative entrustment decisions. The authors discuss prospective and retrospective entrustment-supervision scales.
9. Young JQ, Sugarman R, Schwartz J, O'Sullivan PS. Faculty and resident engagement with workplace-based assessment tool: use of implementation science to explore enablers and barriers. *Acad Med.* 2020 Dec;95(12):1937–1944. doi:10.1097/ACM.0000000000003543.
   This qualitative study explores faculty and resident enablers and barriers to the use of a direct observation tool. Enabling factors include the need for ongoing training, design features of the assessment tool, predisposing beliefs, and dedicated faculty time. Barriers include length of the assessment form, discomfort with feedback, and variability in the quality of delivered feedback.

References

1. American Association of Medical Colleges. Core Entrustable Professional Activities for Entering Residency. Accessed January 16, 2023. https://store.aamc.org/downloadable/download/sample/sample_id/63.
2. Liaison Committee of Medical Education. Functions and Structure of a Medical School. Accessed January 16, 2023. http://lcme.org.
3. Accreditation Council for Graduate Medical Education. Common Program Requirements. Accessed January 16, 2023. http://www.acgme.org.
4. American Board of Medical Specialties. Accessed January 16, 2023. http://www.abms.org.
5. Institute of Medicine. *Crossing the Quality Chasm: A New Health System for the 21st Century*. National Academy Press; 1999.
6. Carraccio C, Wolfsthal SD, Englander R, Ferentz K, Martin C. Shifting paradigms: from Flexner to competencies. *Acad Med.* 2002 May;77(5):361–367. doi:10.1097/00001888-200205000-00003.
7. Govaerts MJB, van der Vleuten CPM, Schuwirth LWT, Muijtjens AMM. Broadening perspectives on clinical performance assessment: rethinking the nature of in-training assessment. *Adv Health Sci Educ Theory Pract.* 2007 May;12(2):239–260. doi:10.1007/s10459-006-9043-1.
8. Swanwick T, Chana N. Workplace-based assessment. *Br J Hosp Med.* 2009 May;70(5):290–293. doi:10.12968/hmed.2009.70.5.42235.
9. Miller GE. The assessment of clinical skills/competence/performance. *Acad Med.* 1990 Sep;65(9 Suppl):S63–S67. doi:10.1097/00001888-199009000-00045.
10. Ten Cate O, Carraccio C, Damodaran A, et al. Entrustment decision making: extending Miller's pyramid. *Acad Med.* 2021 Feb 1;96(2):199–204. doi:10.1097/ACM.0000000000003800.
11. Ram P, van der Vleuten C, Rethans JJ, Grol R, Aretz K. Assessment of practicing family physicians: comparison of observation in a multiple-station examination using standardized patients with observation of consultations in daily practice. *Acad Med.* 1999 Jan;74(1):62–69. doi:10.1097/00001888-199901000-00020.
12. Kopelow ML, Schnabl GK, Hassard TH, et al. Assessing practicing physicians in two settings using standardized patients. *Acad Med.* 1992 Oct;67(10 Suppl):S19–S21. doi:10.1097/00001888-199210000-00026.
13. Rethans JJ, Sturmans F, Drop R, van der Vleuten C, Hobus P. Does competence of general practitioners predict their performance? Comparison between examination setting and actual practice. *BMJ.* 1991 Nov 30;303(6814):1377–1380. doi:10.1136/bmj.303.6814.1377.
14. Hodges B, Regehr G, McNaughton N, Tiberius R, Hanson M. OSCE checklists do not capture increasing levels of expertise. *Acad Med.* 1999 Oct;74(10):1129–1134. doi:10.1097/00001888-199910000-00017.
15. Regehr G, MacRae H, Reznick RK, Szalay D. Comparing the psychometric properties of checklists and global rating scales for assessing performance on an OSCE-format examination.

Acad Med. 1998 Sep;73(9):993–997. doi:10.1097/00001888-199809000-00020.
16. Hawkins R, MacKrell Gaglione M, LaDuca T, et al. Assessment of patient management skills and clinical skills of practising doctors using computer-based case simulations and standardised patients. *Med Educ.* 2004 Sep;38(9):958–968. doi:10.1111/j.1365-2929.2004.01907.x.
17. Royal College of Physicians. Assessment and CPD | RCP London. Accessed October 1, 2023. https://www.rcplondon.ac.uk/education-practice/assessment-and-cpd.
18. Lypson ML, Frohna JG, Gruppen LD, Woolliscroft JO. Assessing residents' competencies at baseline: identifying the gaps. *Acad Med.* 2004 Jun;79(6):564–570. doi:10.1097/00001888-200406000-00013.
19. Sachdeva AK, Loiacono LA, Amiel GE, Blair PG, Friedman M, Roslyn JJ. Variability in the clinical skills of residents entering training programs in surgery. *Surgery.* 1995 Aug;118(2):300–308. doi:10.1016/s0039-6060(05)80338-1.
20. Pfeiffer C, Madray H, Ardolino A, Willms J. The rise and fall of students' skill in obtaining a medical history. *Med Educ.* 1998 May;32(3):283–288. doi:10.1046/j.1365-2923.1998.00222.x.
21. Mangione S, Nieman LZ. Cardiac auscultatory skills of internal medicine and family practice trainees. A comparison of diagnostic proficiency. *JAMA.* 1997 Sep 3;278(9):717–722.
22. Mangione S, Burdick WP, Peitzman S. Physical diagnosis skills of physicians in training: a focused assessment. *Acad Emerg Med.* 1995 Jul;2(7):622–629. doi:10.1111/j.1553-2712.1995.tb03601.x.
23. Li JT. Assessment of basic physical examination skills of internal medicine residents. *Acad Med.* 1994 Apr;69(4):296–299. doi:10.1097/00001888-199404000-00013.
24. Wilson BE. Performance-based assessment of internal medicine interns: evaluation of baseline clinical and communication skills. *Acad Med.* 2002 Nov;77(11):1158. doi:10.1097/00001888-200211000-00023.
25. Fox RA, Ingham Clark CL, Scotland AD, Dacre JE. A study of pre-registration house officers' clinical skills. *Med Educ.* 2000 Dec;34(12):1007–1012. doi:10.1046/j.1365-2923.2000.00729.x.
26. Butterworth JS, Reppert EH. Auscultatory acumen in the general medical population. *JAMA.* 1960;174(10):32–34.
27. Raferty EB, Holland WW. Examination of the heart: an investigation into variation. *Am J Epidemiol.* 1967 May;85(3):438–444. doi:10.1093/oxfordjournals.aje.a120705.
28. Vukanovic-Criley JM, Criley S, Warde CM, et al. Competency in cardiac examination skills in medical students, trainees, physicians, and faculty: a multicenter study. *Arch Intern Med.* 2006 Mar 27;166(6):610–616. doi:10.1001/archinte.166.6.610.
29. Hauer KE, Teherani A, Kerr KM, O'Sullivan PS, Irby DM. Student performance problems in medical school clinical skills assessments. *Acad Med.* 2007 Oct;82(10 Suppl):S69–S72. doi:10.1097/ACM.0b013e31814003e8.
30. Feddock CA. The lost art of clinical skills. *Am J Med.* 2007 Apr;120(4):374–378. doi:10.1016/j.amjmed.2007.01.023.
31. Ramsey PG, Curtis JR, Paauw DS, Carline JD, Wenrich MD. History-taking and preventive medicine skills among primary care physicians: an assessment using standardized patients. *Am J Med.* 1998 Feb;104(2):152–158. doi:10.1016/s0002-9343(97)00310-0.
32. Braddock 3rd CH, Edwards KA, Hasenberg NM, Laidley TL, Levinson W. Informed decision making in outpatient practice: time to get back to basics. *JAMA.* 1999 Dec;282(24):2313–2320. doi:10.1001/jama.282.24.2313.
33. Marvel MK, Epstein RM, Flowers K, Beckman HB. Soliciting the patient's agenda: have we improved. *JAMA.* 1999 Jan 20;281(3):283–287. doi:10.1001/jama.281.3.283.
34. Rao JK, Weinberger M, Kroenke K. Visit-specific expectations and patient-centered outcomes: a literature review. *Arch Fam Med.* 2009 Nov-Dec;9(10):1148–1155. doi:10.1001/archfami.9.10.1148.
35. Bernabeo E, Holmboe ES. Patients, providers, and systems need to acquire a specific set of competencies to achieve truly patient-centered care. *Health Aff.* 2013 Feb;32(2):250–258. doi:10.1377/hlthaff.2012.1120.
36. Levinson W, Roter DL, Mullooly JP, Dull VT, Frankel RM. Physician-patient communication: the relationship with malpractice claims among primary care physicians and surgeons. *JAMA.* 1997 Feb 19;277(7):553–559. doi:10.1001/jama.277.7.553.
37. Levinson W, Lesser CS, Epstein RM. Developing physician communication skills for patient-centered care. *Health Aff.* 2010 Jul;29(7):1310–1318. doi:10.1377/hlthaff.2009.0450.
38. Wofford MM, Wofford JL, Bothra J, Bryant Kendrick S, Smith A, Lichstein PR. Patient complaints about physician behaviors: a qualitative study. *Acad Med.* 2004 Feb;79(2):134–138. doi:10.1097/00001888-200402000-00008.
39. Kee JWY, Khoo HS, Lim I, Koh MYH. Communication skills in patient-doctor interactions: learning from patient complaints. *Health Prof Educ.* 2018 Jun;4(2):97–106. doi:10.1016/j.hpe.2017.03.006.
40. Liu J, Hou S, Evans R, Xia C, Xia W, Ma J. What do patients complain about online: a systematic review and taxonomy framework based on patient centeredness. *J Med Internet Res.* 2019 Aug 7;21(8):e14634. doi:10.2196/14634.
41. Raberus A, Holmstrom IK, Galvin K, Sundler AJ. The nature of patient complaints: a resource for healthcare improvements. *Int J Qual Health Care.* 2019 Aug 1;31(7):556–562. doi:10.1093/intqhc/mzy215.
42. Hampton JR, Harrison MJ, Mitchell JR, Prichard JS, Seymour C. Relative contributions of history-taking, physical examination, and laboratory investigation to diagnosis and management of medical outpatients. *Br Med J.* 1975 May 31;2(5969):486–489. doi:10.1136/bmj.2.5969.486.
43. Peterson MC, Holbrook JH, Von Hales D, et al. Contributions of the history, physical examination, and laboratory investigation in making medical diagnoses. *West J Med.* 1992 Feb;156(2):163–165.
44. Kirch W, Schafii C. Misdiagnosis at a university hospital in 4 medical eras. *Medicine.* 1996 Jan;75(1):29–40. doi:10.1097/00005792-199601000-00004.
45. National Academy of Medicine. *Improving Diagnosis in Medicine.* National Academy Press; 2015.
46. Makary MA, Daniel M. Medical error—the third leading cause of death in the US. *BMJ.* 2016 May 3;353:i2139. doi:10.1136/bmj.i2139.
47. Choosing Wisely US. Accessed January 16, 2023. https://www.choosingwisely.org
48. Choosing Wisely Canada. Accessed January 16, 2023. https://choosingwiselycanada.org
49. Dimatteo MR. The role of effective communication with children and their families in fostering adherence to pediatric regimens. *Patient Educ Couns.* 2004 Dec;55(3):339–344. doi:10.1016/j.pec.2003.04.003.
50. Belasen A, Belasen AT. Doctor-patient communication: a review and a rationale for using an assessment framework. *J Health Organ Manag.* 2018 Oct 8;32(7):891–907. doi:10.1108/JHOM-10-2017-0262.

51. Vermeir P, Vandijck D, Degroote S, et al. Communication in healthcare: a narrative review of the literature and practical recommendations. *Int J Clin Pract.* 2015 Nov;69(11):1257–1267. doi:10.1111/ijcp.12686.
52. Zolnierek KB, Dimatteo MR. Physician communication and patient adherence to treatment: a meta-analysis. *Med Care.* 2009 Aug;47(8):826–834. doi:10.1097/MLR.0b013e31819a5acc.
53. Benbassat J, Pilpel D, Tidhar M. Patients' preferences for participation in clinical decision making: a review of published surveys. *Behav Med.* 1998 Summer;24(2):81–88. doi:10.1080/08964289809596384.
54. Guadagnoli E, Ward P. Patient participation in decision-making. *Soc Sci Med.* 1998 Aug;47(3):329–339. doi:10.1016/s0277-9536(98)00059-8.
55. Carraccio CL, Englander R. From Flexner to competencies: reflections on a decade and the journey ahead. *Acad Med.* 2013 Aug;88(8):1067–1073. doi:10.1097/ACM.0b013e318299396f.
56. Ericsson KA. Deliberate practice and the acquisition and maintenance of expert performance in medicine and related domains. *Acad Med.* 2004 Oct;79(10 Suppl):S70–S81. doi:10.1097/00001888-200410001-00022.
57. Davis DA, Mazmanian PE, Fordis M, et al. Accuracy of physician self-assessment compared to observed measures of competence: a systematic review. *JAMA.* 2006 Sep 6;296(9):1094–1102. doi:10.1001/jama.296.9.1094.
58. Yates N, Gough S, Brazil V. Self-assessment: with all its limitations why are we still measuring and teaching it? Lessons from a scoping review. *Med Teach.* 2022 Nov;44(11):1296–1302. doi: 10.1080/0142159X.2022.2093704.
59. Eva KW, Regehr G. Exploring the divergence between self-assessment and self-monitoring. *Adv Health Sci Educ Theory Pract.* 2011 Aug;16(3):311–329. doi:10.1007/s10459-010-9263-2.
60. Sargeant J, Eva KW, Armson H, et al. Features of assessment learners use to make informed self-assessments of clinical performance. *Med Educ.* 2011 Jun;45(6):636–647. doi:10.1111/j.1365-2923.2010.03888.x.
61. Sargeant J, Armson H, Chesluk B, et al. The processes and dimensions of informed self-assessment: a conceptual model. *Acad Med.* 2010 Jul;85(7):1212–1220. doi:10.1097/ACM.0b013e3181d85a4e.
62. Armson H, Lockyer JM, Zetkulic M, Könings KD, Sargeant J. Identifying coaching skills to improve feedback use in postgraduate medical education. *Med Educ.* 2019 May;53(5):477–493. doi:10.1111/medu.13818.
63. Frank JR, Snell LS, Cate OT, et al. Competency-based medical education: theory to practice. *Med Teach.* 2010;32(8):638–645. doi:10.3109/0142159X.2010.501190.
64. Frank JR, Mungroo R, Ahmad Y, Wang M, De Rossi S, Horsley T. Toward a definition of competency-based education in medicine: a systematic review of published definitions. *Med Teach.* 2010;32(8):631–637. doi:10.3109/01421 59X.2010.500898.
65. Iobst WF, Sherbino J, Cate OT, et al. Competency-based medical education in postgraduate medical education. *Med Teach.* 2010;32(8):651–656. doi:10.3109/0142159X.2010.500709.
66. Holmboe ES, Sherbino J, Long DM, Swing SR, Frank JR. The role of assessment in competency-based medical education. *Med Teach.* 2010;32(8):676–682. doi:10.3109/014215 9X.2010.500704.
67. Whitcomb ME. Redirecting the assessment of clinical competence. *Acad Med.* 2007 Jun;82(6):527–528. doi:10.1097/ACM.0b013e31805556f8.
68. Institute of Medicine. Resident duty hours: enhancing sleep, supervision and safety. 2008. Accessed January 16, 2023. http://iom.nationalacademies.org/Reports/2008/Resident-Duty-Hours-Enhancing-Sleep-Supervision-and-Safety.aspx
69. Kilminster SM, Jolly BC. Effective supervision in clinical practice settings: a literature review. *Med Educ.* 2000 Oct;34(10):827–840. doi:10.1046/j.1365-2923.2000.00758.x.
70. Kilminster S, Cottrell D, Grant J, Jolly B. AMEE guide No.27: Effective educational and clinical supervision. *Med Teach.* 2007 Feb;29(1):2–19. doi:10.1080/01421590701210907.
71. Holmboe ES. Faculty and the observation of trainees' clinical skills: problems and opportunities. *Acad Med.* 2004 Jan;79(1):16–22. doi:10.1097/00001888-200401000-00006.
72. Kogan JR, Conforti LN, Iobst WF, Holmboe ES. Reconceptualizing variable rater assessments as both an educational and clinical care problem. *Acad Med.* 2014 May;89(5):721–727. doi:10.1097/ACM.0000000000000221.
73. Kogan JR, Holmboe ES, Hauer KE. Tools for direct observation and assessment of clinical skills of medical trainees: a systematic review. *JAMA.* 2009 Sep 23;302(12):1316–1326. doi:10.1001/jama.2009.1365.
74. Pelgrim EA, Kramer AW, Mokkink HG, van den Elsen L, Grol RPTM, van der Vleuten CPM. In-training assessment using direct observation of single-patient encounters: a literature review. *Adv Health Sci Educ Theory Pract.* 2011 Mar;16(1):131–142. doi:10.1007/s10459-010-9235-6.
75. Weller JM, Coomber T, Chen Y, Castanelli DJ. Key dimensions of innovations in workplace-based assessments for postgraduate medical education. a scoping review. *Br J Anaesth.* 2021 Nov;127(5):689–703. doi:10.1016/j.bja.2021.06.038.
76. Mortaz Hejri S, Jalili M, Masoomi R, Shirazi M, Nedjat S, Norcini J. The utility of mini-CEX evaluation exercise in undergraduate and postgraduate medical education: a BEME review. BEME Guide No. 59. *Med Teach.* 2020 Feb;42(2):125–142. doi: 10.1080/0142159X.2019.1652732.
77. Norcini JJ, Blank LL, Arnold GK, Kimball HR. The mini-CEX (clinical evaluation exercise): a preliminary investigation. *Ann Intern Med.* 1995 Nov 15;123(10):795–799. doi:10.7326/0003-4819-123-10-199511150-00008.
78. Makoul G. The SEGUE framework for teaching and assessing communication skills. *Patient Educ Couns.* 2001 Oct;45(1): 23–34. doi:10.1016/s0738-3991(01)00136-7.
79. Kurtz SM, Silverman JD. The Calgary-Cambridge referenced observation guides: an aid to defining the curriculum and organizing the teaching in communication training programmes. *Med Educ.* 1996 Mar;30(2):83–89. doi:10.1111/j.1365-2923.1996.tb00724.x.
80. Noel GL, Herbers JE, Caplow MP, Cooper GS, Pangaro LN, Harvey J. How well do internal medicine faculty members evaluate the clinical skills of residents? *Ann Intern Med.* 1992 Nov 1; 117(9):757–765. doi:10.7326/0003-4819-117-9-757.
81. Regehr G, Freeman R, Robb A, Missiha N, Heisey R. OSCE performance evaluations made by standardized patients: comparing checklist and global rating scores. *Acad Med.* 1999 Oct;74 (10 Suppl):S135–S137. doi:10.1097/00001888-199910000-00064.
82. Norcini J, Boulet J. Methodological issues in the use of standardized patients for assessment. *Teach Learn Med.* 2003 Fall;15(4):293–297. doi:10.1207/S15328015TLM1504_12.
83. Tavares W, Eva KW. Impact of rating demands on rater-based assessments of clinical competence. *Educ Prim Care.* 2014 Nov;25(6):308–318. doi:10.1080/14739879.2014.11730760.

84. Tavares W, Ginsburg S, Eva KW. Selecting and simplifying: rater performance and behavior when considering multiple competencies. *Teach Learn Med.* 2016;28(1):41–51. doi:10.1080/10401334.2015.1107489.
85. Tavares W, Eva KW. Exploring the impact of mental workload on rater-based assessments. *Adv Health Sci Educ Theory Pract.* 2013 May;18(2):291–303. doi:10.1007/s10459-012-9370-3.
86. Paravattil H, Wilby KJ. Optimizing assessors' mental workload in rater-based assessment: a critical narrative review. *Perspect Med Educ.* 2019 Dec;8(6):339–345. doi:10.1007/s40037-019-00535-6.
87. Donato AA, Pangaro L, Smith C, et al. Evaluation of a novel assessment form for observing medical residents: a randomised, controlled trial. *Med Educ.* 2008 Dec;42(12):1234–1242. doi:10.1111/j.1365-2923.2008.03230.x.
88. Donato AA, Park YS, George DL, Schwartz A, Yudkowsky R. Validity and feasibility of the minicard direct observation tool in 1 training program. *J Grad Med Educ.* 2015 Jun;7(2):225–229. doi:10.4300/JGME-D-14-00532.1.
89. Weller JM, Misur M, Nicolson S, et al. Can I leave the theatre? A key to more reliable workplace-based assessment. *Br J Anaesth.* 2014 Jun;112(6):1083–1091. doi:10.1093/bja/aeu052.
90. Duijn CCMA, van Dijk EJ, Mandoki M, Bok HGJ, Cate OTJT. Assessment tools for feedback and entrustment decisions in the clinical workplace: a systematic review. *J Vet Med Educ.* 2019 Fall;46(3):340–352. doi:10.3138/jvme.0917-123r.
91. Rekman J, Gofton W, Dudek N, Gofton T, Hamstra SJ. Entrustability scales: outlining their usefulness for competency-based clinical assessment. *Acad Med.* 2015 Feb;91(2):186–190. doi:10.1097/ACM.0000000000001045.
92. Crossley J, Johnson G, Booth J, Wade W. Good questions, good answers: construct alignment improves the performance of workplace-based assessment scales. *Med Educ.* 2011 Jun;45(6):560–569. doi:10.1111/j.1365-2923.2010.03913.x.
93. Ten Cate O, Schwartz A, Chen HC. Assessing trainees and making entrustment decisions: on the nature and use of entrustment-supervision scales. *Acad Med.* 2020 Nov;95(11):1662–1669. doi:10.1097/ACM.0000000000003427.
94. Kelleher M, Kinnear B, Sall D, et al. A reliability analysis of entrustment-derived workplace-based assessments. *Acad Med.* 2020 Apr;95(4):616–622. doi:10.1097/ACM.0000000000002997.
95. Dudek N, Gofton W, Rekman J, McDougall A. Faculty and resident perspectives on using entrustment anchors for workplace-based assessment. *J Grad Med Educ.* 2019 Jun;11(3):287–294. doi:10.4300/JGME-D-18-01003.1.
96. Hatala R, Ginsburg S, Hauer KE, Gingerich A. Entrustment ratings in internal medicine training: capturing meaningful supervision decisions or just another rating? *J Gen Intern Med.* 2019 May;34(5):740–743. doi:10.1007/s11606-019-04878-y.
97. Kinnear B, Warm E, Caretta-Eyer H, et al. Entrustment unpacked: aligning purposes, stakes, and processes to enhance learner assessment. *Acad Med.* 2021 Jul 1;96(7S):S56–S63. doi:10.1097/ACM.0000000000004108.
98. Gingerich A, Daniels V, Farrell L, Olsen SR, Kennedy T, Hatala R. Beyond hands-on and hands-off: supervisory approaches and entrustment on the inpatient ward. *Med Educ.* 2018 Oct;52(10):1028–1040. doi:10.1111/medu.13621.
99. Kogan JR, Dine CJ, Conforti LN, et al. Can rater training improve the quality and accuracy of workplace-based assessment narrative comments and entrustment ratings? A randomized controlled trial. *Acad Med.* 2023 Feb 1;98(2):237–247. doi:10.1097/ACM.0000000000004819.
100. Ryan MS, Khamishon R, Richards A, Perera R, Garber A, Santen SA. A question of scale? Generalizability of the Ottawa and Chen scales to render entrustment decisions for the core EPAs in the workplace. *Acad Med.* 2022 Apr 1;97(4):552–561. doi:10.1097/ACM.0000000000004189.
101. Hatala R, Sawatsky AP, Dudek N, Ginsburg S, Cook DA. Using in-training evaluation report ITER) qualitative comments to assess medical students and residents: a systematic review. *Acad Med.* 2017 Jun;92(6):868–879. doi:10.1097/ACM.0000000000001506.
102. Young JQ, Sugarman R, Holmboe E, O'Sullivan PS. Advancing our understanding of narrative comments generated by direct observation tools: lessons from psychopharmacology-structured clinical observation. *J Grad Med Educ.* 2019 Oct;11(5):570–579. doi:10.4300/JGME-D-19-00207.1.
103. Ginsberg S, Watling CJ, Schumacher DJ, Gingerich A, Hatala R. Numbers encapsulate, words elaborate: towards the best use of comments for assessment and feedback on entrustment ratings. *Acad Med.* 2021 Jul 1;96(7S):S81–S86. doi:10.1097/ACM.0000000000004089.
104. Martin L, Sibbald M, Vegas DB, Russell D, Govaerts M. The impact of entrustment assessments on feedback and learning: trainee perspectives. *Med Educ.* 2020 Apr;54(4):328–336. doi:10.1111/medu.14047.
105. Scarff CE, Bearman M, Chiavaroli N, Trumble S. Trainees' perceptions of assessment messages: a narrative systematic review. *Med Educ.* 2019 Mar;53(3):221–233. doi:10.1111/medu.13775.
106. Herbers JE, Noel GL, Cooper GS, Harvey J, Pangaro LN, Weaver MJ. How accurate are faculty evaluations of clinical competence? *J Gen Intern Med.* 1989 May-Jun;4(3):202–208. doi:10.1007/BF02599524.
107. Kalet A, Earp JA, Kowlowitz V. How well do faculty evaluate the interviewing skills of medical students? *J Gen Intern Med.* 1992 Sep-Oct;7(5):499–505. doi:10.1007/BF02599452.
108. Elliot DL, Hickam DH. Evaluation of physical examination skills. Reliability of faculty observers and patient instructors. *JAMA.* 1987 Dec 18;258(23):3405–3408.
109. Gauthier G, St-Onge C, Tavares W. Rater cognition: review and integration of research findings. *Med Educ.* 2016 May;50(5):511–522. doi:10.1111/medu.12973.
110. Gingerich A, Kogan J, Yeates P, Govaerts M, Holmboe E. Seeing the 'black box' differently: assessor cognition from three research perspectives. *Med Educ.* 2014 Nov;48(11):1055–1068. doi:10.1111/medu.12546.
111. Kogan JR, Conforti L, Bernabeo E, Iobst W, Holmboe E. Opening the black box of clinical skills assessment via observation: a conceptual model. *Med Educ.* 2011 Oct;45(10):1048–1060. doi:10.1111/j.1365-2923.2011.04025.x.
112. Yeates P, O'Neill P, Mann K, Eva K. Seeing the same thing differently: mechanisms that contribute to assessor differences in directly-observed performance assessment. *Adv Health Sci Educ Theory Pract.* 2013 Aug;18(3):325–341. doi:10.1007/s10459-012-9372-1.
113. Govaerts MJ, Van de Wiel MW, Schuwirth LW, Van der Vleuten CPM, Muijtjens AMM. Workplace-based assessment: raters' performance theories and constructs. *Adv Health Sci Educ Theory Pract.* 2013 Aug;18(3):375–396. doi:10.1007/s10459-012-9376-x.
114. Berendonk C, Stalmeijer RE, Schuwirth LW. Expertise in performance assessment: assessors' perspectives. *Adv Health Sci Educ Theory Pract.* 2013 Oct;18(4):559–571. doi:10.1007/s10459-012-9392-x.

115. Paauw DS, Wenrich MD, Curtis JR, Carline JD, Ramsey PG. Ability of primary care physicians to recognize physical findings associated with HIV infection. *JAMA*. 1995 Nov 1; 274(17):1380–1382.
116. Kogan JR, Hess BJ, Conforti LN, Holmboe ES. What drives faculty ratings of residents' clinical skills? The impact of faculty's own clinical skills. *Acad Med*. 2010 Oct;85(S10):S25–S28. doi:10.1097/ACM.0b013e3181ed1aa3.
117. Govaerts MJ, Schuwirth LW, van der Vleuten CP, Muijtjens AM. Workplace-based assessment: effects of rater expertise. *Adv Health Sci Educ Theory Pract*. 2011 May;16(2):151–165. doi:10.1007/s10459-010-9250-7.
118. Friedman Z, Bould MD, Matava C, Alam H. Investigating faculty assessment of anesthesia trainees and the failing-to-fail phenomenon: a randomized controlled trial. *Can J Anaesth*. 2021 Jul;68(7):1000–1007. doi:10.1007/s12630-021-01971-x.
119. Swails JL, Gadgil MA, Goodrum H, Gupta R, Rahbar MH, Bernstam EV. Role of faculty characteristics in failing to fail in clinical clerkships. *Med Educ*. 2022 Jun;56(6):634–640. doi:10.1111/medu.14725.
120. Dudek NL, Marks MB, Regehr G. Failure to fail: the perspectives of clinical supervisors. *Acad Med*. 2005 Oct;80(10 Suppl):S84–S87. doi:10.1097/00001888-200510001-00023.
121. Cleland JA, Knight LV, Rees CE, Tracey S, Bond CM. Is it me or is it them? Factors that influence the passing of underperforming students. *Med Educ*. 2008 Aug;42(8):800–809. doi:10.1111/j.1365-2923.2008.03113.x.
122. Yeates P, O'Neill P, Mann K, Eva KW. Effect of exposure to good vs poor medical trainee performance on attending physician ratings of subsequent performances. *JAMA*. 2012 Dec 5;308(21):2226–2232. doi:10.1001/jama.2012.36515.
123. Yeates P, O'Neill P, Mann K, Eva K. 'You're certainly relatively competent': assessor bias due to recent experiences. *Med Educ*. 2013 Sep;47(9):910–922. doi:10.1111/medu.12254.
124. Yeates P, Cardell J, Byrne G, Eva KW. Relatively speaking: contrast effects influence assessors' scores and narrative feedback. *Med Educ*. 2015 Sep;49(9):909–919. doi:10.1111/medu.12777.
125. Gingerich A, Schokking E, Yeates P. Comparatively salient: examining the influence of preceding performances on assessors' focus and interpretations in written assessment comments. *Adv Heath Sci Educ Theory Pract*. 2018 Dec;23(5):937–959. doi:10.1007/s10459-018-9841-2.
126. Hagiwara N, Kron FW, Scerbo MW, Watson GS. A call for grounding implicit bias training in clinical and translational frameworks. *Lancet*. 2020 May 2;395(10234):1457–1460. doi:10.1016/S0140-6736(20)30846-1.
127. Teherani A, Hauer KE, Fernandez A, King Jr TE, Lucey C. How small differences in assessed clinical performance amplify to large differences in grades and awards: a cascade with serious consequences for students underrepresented in medicine. *Acad Med*. 2018 Sep;93(9):1286–1292. doi:10.1097/ACM.0000000000002323.
128. Klein R, Ufere NN, Schaeffer S, et al. Association between resident race and ethnicity and clinical performance assessment scores in graduate medical education. *Acad Med*. 2022 Sep 1;97(9):1351–1359. doi:10.1097/ACM.0000000000004743.
129. Low D, Pollack SW, Liao ZC, et al. Racial/ethnic disparities in clinical grading in medical school. *Teach Learn Med*. 2019 Oct-Dec;31(5):487–496. doi:10.1080/10401334.2019.1597724.
130. Arkin N, Lai C, Kiwakyou LM, et al. What's in a word? Qualitative and quantitative analysis of leadership language in anesthesiology resident feedback. *J Grad Med Educ*. 2019 Feb;11(1):44–52. doi:10.4300/JGME-D-18-00377.1.
131. Mueller AS, Jenkins TM, Osborne M, Dayal A, O'Connor DM, Arora VM. Gender differences in attending physicians' feedback to residents: a qualitative analysis. *J Grad Med Educ*. 2017 Oct;9(5):577–585. doi:10.4300/JGME-D-17-00126.1.
132. Klein R, Julian KA, Snyder ED, et al. Gender bias in resident assessment in graduate medical education: review of the literature. *J Gen Intern Med*. 2019 May;34(5):712–719. doi:10.1007/s11606-019-04884-0.
133. Li S, Fant AL, McCarthy DM, Miller D, Craig J, Kontrick A. Gender differences in language of standardized letter of evaluation narratives for emergency medicine residency applicants. *AEM Educ Train*. 2017 Sep 19;1(4):334–339. doi:10.1002/aet2.10057.
134. Chen S, Beck Dallaghan GL, Shaheen A. Implicit gender bias in third-year surgery clerkship MSPE narratives. *J Surg Educ*. 2021 Jul-Aug;78(4):1136–1143. doi:10.1016/j.jsurg.2020.10.011.
135. Khan S, Kirubarajan A, Shamsheri T, Clayton A, Mehta G. Gender bias in reference letters for residency and academic medicine: a systematic review. *Postgrad Med J*. 2023 May 22;99(1170):272–278. doi:10.1136/postgradmedj-2021-140045.
136. Berthold HK, Gouni-Berthold I, Bestehorn KP, Böhm M, Krone W. Physician gender is associated with the quality of type 2 diabetes care. *J Intern Med*. 2008 Oct;264(4):340–350. doi:10.1111/j.1365-2796.2008.01967.x.
137. Baumhäkel M, Müller U, Böhm M. Influence of gender of physicians and patients on guideline-recommended treatment of chronic heart failure in a cross-sectional study. *Eur J Heart Fail*. 2009 Mar;11(3):299–303. doi:10.1093/eurjhf/hfn041.
138. Tsugawa Y, Jena AB, Figueroa JF, Orav EJ, Blumenthal DM, Jha AK. Comparison of hospital mortality and readmission rates for Medicare patients treated by male vs female physicians. *JAMA Intern Med*. 2017 Feb 1;177(2):206–213. doi:10.1001/jamainternmed.2016.7875.
139. Dayal A, O'Connor DM, Qadri U, Arora VM. Comparison of male vs female resident milestone evaluations by faculty during emergency medicine residency training. *JAMA Intern Med*. 2017 May 1;177(5):651–657. doi:10.1001/jamainternmed.2016.9616.
140. Rojek A, Khanna R, Yim JWL, et al. Differences in narrative language in evaluations of medical students by gender and under-represented minority status. *J Gen Intern Med*. 2019 May;34(5):684–691. doi:10.1007/s11606-019-04889-9.
141. Ross DA, Boatright D, Nunez-Smith M, Jordan A, Chekroud A, Moore EZ. Differences in words used to describe racial and gender groups in medical student performance evaluations. *PLoS One*. 2017 Aug 9;12(8):e0181659. doi:10.1371/journal.pone.0181659.
142. Gingerich A, van der Vleuten CP, Eva KW, Regehr G. More consensus than idiosyncrasy: categorizing social judgments to examine variability in Mini-CEX ratings. *Acad Med*. 2014 Nov;89(11):1510–1519. doi:10.1097/ACM.0000000000000486.
143. Ten Cate O, Regehr G. The power of subjectivity in the assessment of medical trainees. *Acad Med*. 2019 Mar;94(3):333–337. doi:10.1097/ACM.0000000000002495.

144. Holmboe ES, Kogan JR. Will any road get you there? Examining warranted and unwarranted variation in medical education. *Acad Med.* 2022 Aug 1;97(8):1128–1131. doi:10.1097/ACM.0000000000004667.
145. Asch DA, Nicholson S, Srinivas S, Herrin J, Epstein AJ. Evaluating obstetrical residency programs using patient outcomes. *JAMA.* 2009 Sep 23;302(12):1277–1283. doi:10.1001/jama.2009.1356.
146. van der Vleuten CP, Schuwirth LW, Scheele F, Driessen EW, Hodges B. The assessment of professional competence: building blocks for theory development. *Best Pract Res Clin Obstet Gynaecol.* 2010 Dec;24(6):703–719. doi:10.1016/j.bpobgyn.2010.04.001.
147. Massie J, Ali JM. Workplace-based assessment: a review of user perception and strategies to address identified shortcomings. *Adv Health Sci Educ Theory Pract.* 2016 May;21(2):455–473. doi:10.1007/s10459-015-9614-0.
148. Lorwald A, Lahner FM, Mooser B, et al. Influences of the implementation of mini-CEX and DOPS for postgraduate medical trainees' learning: a grounded theory study. *Med Teach.* 2019 Apr;41(4):448–456. doi:10.1080/0142159X.2018.1497784.
149. Holmboe ES, Hawkins RE, Huot SJ. Effects of training in direct observation of medical residents' clinical competence: a randomized trial. *Ann Intern Med.* 2004 Jun 1;140(11):874–881. doi:10.7326/0003-4819-140-11-200406010-00008.
150. Cook DA, Dupras DM, Beckman TJ, Thomas KG, Pankratz VS. Effect of rater training on reliability and accuracy of mini-CEX scores: a randomized, controlled trial. *J Gen Intern Med.* 2009 Jan;24(1):74–79. doi:10.1007/s11606-008-0842-3.
151. Kogan JR, Conforti LN, Bernabeo E, Iobst W, Holmboe E. How faculty members experience workplace-based assessment rater training: a qualitative study. *Med Educ.* 2015 Jul;49(7):692–708. doi:10.1111/medu.12733.
152. George BC, Teitelbaum EN, DaRosa DA, et al. Duration of faculty training needed to ensure reliable OR performance ratings. *J Surg Educ.* 2013 Nov-Dec;70(6):703–708. doi:10.1016/j.jsurg.2013.06.015.
153. Steinert Y, Mann K, Centeno A, et al. A systematic review of faculty development initiatives designed to improve teaching effectiveness in medical education: BEME Guide No. 8. *Med Teach.* 2006 Sep;28(6):497–526. doi:10.1080/01421590600902976.
154. Hemmer PA, Dadekian GA, Terndrup C, et al. Regular formal evaluation sessions are effective as frame-of-reference training for faculty evaluators of clerkship medical students. *J Gen Intern Med.* 2015 Sep;30(9):1313–1318. doi:10.1007/s11606-015-3294-6.
155. Steinert Y. Perspective on faculty development: aiming for 6/6 by 2020. *Perspect Med Educ.* 2012 Mar;1(1):31–42. doi:10.1007/s40037-012-0006-3.
156. Woehr DJ, Huffcutt AI. Rater training for performance appraisal: a quantitative review. *J Occup Org Psychol.* 1994;67:189–205. doi:10.1111/j.2044-8325.1994.tb00562.x.
157. Hauenstein NMA, Smither JW. Training raters to increase the accuracy of appraisals and the usefulness of feedback. *Performance Appraisal.* Jossey-Bass; 1998:404–442.
158. Stamoulis DT, Hauenstein NMA. Rater training and rating accuracy: training for dimensional accuracy versus training for rater differentiation. *J Appl Psychol.* 1993;78:994–1003.
159. Kaplan M. SPIKES: a framework for breaking bad news to patients with cancer. *Clin J Oncol Nurs.* 2010 Aug;14(4):514–516. doi:10.1188/10.CJON.514-516.
160. Agency for Healthcare Research and Quality. The SHARE Approach. Accessed January 16, 2023. www.ahrq.gov/professionals/education/curriculum-tools/shareddecisionmaking/index.html
161. Iglehart JK. The uncertain future of Medicare and graduate medical education. *N Engl J Med.* 2011 Oct 6;365(14):1340–1345. doi:10.1056/NEJMhpr1107519.
162. Chandra A, Khullar D, Wilensky GR. The economics of graduate medical education. *N Engl J Med.* 2014 Jun 19;370(25):2357–2360. doi:10.1056/NEJMp1402468.
163. Institute of Medicine of the National Academies. Graduate medical education that meets the nation's health needs. 2014. Accessed January 16, 2023. www.iom.edu/Reports/2014/Graduate-Medical-Education-That-Meets-the-Nations-Health-Needs.aspx
164. ten Cate O. AM last page: what entrustable professional activities add to a competency-based curriculum. *Acad Med.* 2014 Apr;89(4):691. doi:10.1097/ACM.0000000000000161.
165. Kogan JR, Conforti LN, Holmboe ES. Faculty perceptions of frame of reference training to improve workplace-based assessment. *J Grad Med Educ.* 2023 Feb;15(1):81–91. doi: 10.4300/JGME-D-22-00287.1.
166. Holmboe ES, Osman NY, Murphy CM, Kogan JR, The urgency of now: rethinking and improving assessment practices in medical education programs. *Acad Med.* 2023 Apr 18. doi: 10.1097/ACM.0000000000005251.
167. Young JQ, Sugarman R, Schwartz J, O'Sullivan P. Faculty and resident engagement with WBA tool: use of implementation science to explore enablers and barriers. *Acad Med.* 2020 Dec;95(12):1937–1944. doi:10.1097/ACM.0000000000003543.
168. Prentice S, Benson J, Kirkpatrick E, Schuwirth L. Workplace-based assessments in postgraduate medical education: a hermeneutic review. *Med Educ.* 2020 Nov;54(11):981–992. doi:10.1111/medu.14221.
169. Anderson HL, Kurtz J, West DC. Implementation and use of workplace-based assessment in clinical learning environments: a scoping review. *Acad Med.* 2021 Nov 1;96(11S):S164–S174. doi:10.1097/ACM.0000000000004366.
170. Barrett A, Galvin R, Scherpbier AJJA, Teunissen PW, O'Shaughnessy A, Horgan M. Is the learning value of workplace-based assessment being realized? A qualitative study of trainer and trainee perceptions and experiences. *Postgrad Med J.* 2017 Mar;93(1097):138–142. doi:10.1136/postgradmedj-2015-133917.
171. van der Vleuten C, Verhoeven B. In-training assessment developments in postgraduate education in Europe. *ANZ J Surg.* 2013 Jun;83(6):454–459. doi:10.1111/ans.12190.
172. Gaunt A, Patel A, Rusius V, Royle TJ, Markham DH, Pawlikowska T. Playing the game': how do surgical trainees seek feedback using workplace-based assessment? *Med Educ.* 2017 Sep;51(9):953–962. doi:10.1111/medu.13380.
173. Fokkema JP, Teunissen PW, Westerman M, et al. Exploration of perceived effects of innovations in postgraduate medical education. *Med Educ.* 2013 Mar;47(3):271–281. doi:10.1111/medu.12081.
174. Lefroy J, Watling C, Teunissen PW, Brand P. Guidelines: the do's, don'ts and don't knows of feedback in clinical education. *Perspect Med Educ.* 2015 Dec;4(6):2840289. doi:10.1007/s40037-015-0231-7.
175. Alves de Lima, Henquin R, Thiere HR, et al. A qualitative study of the impact on learning of the mini clinical evaluation exercise in postgraduate training. *Med Teach.* 2005 Jan;27(1):46–52. doi:10.1080/01421590400013529.

176. Ali JM. Getting lost in translation? Workplace based assessments in surgical training. *Surgeon*. 2013 Oct;11(15):286–289. doi:10.1016/j.surge.2013.03.001.
177. Fokkema JP, Scheele F, Westerman M, et al. Perceived effects of innovations in postgraduate medical education: a Q study focusing on workplace-based assessment. *Acad Med*. 2014 Sep;89(9):1259–1266. doi:10.1097/ACM.0000000000000394.
178. Malhotra S, Hatala R, Courneya CA. Internal medicine residents' perceptions of the mini-clinical evaluation exercise. *Med Teach*. 2008;30(4):414–419. doi:10.1080/01421590801946962.
179. Kogan JR, Hatala R, Hauer KE, Holmboe E. Guidelines: the do's, don'ts and don't knows of direct observation of clinical skills in medical education. *Perspect Med Educ*. 2017 Oct;6(5):286–305. doi:10.1007/s40037-017-0376-7.
180. Rogers HD, Carline JD, Paauw DS. Examination room presentations in general internal medicine clinic: patients' and students' perceptions. *Acad Med*. 2003 Sep;78(9):945–949. doi:10.1097/00001888-200309000-00023.
181. Englander R, Holmboe E, Batalden P, et al. Coproducing health professions education: a prerequisite to coproducing health care services? *Acad Med*. 2020 Jul;95(7):1006–1013. doi:10.1097/ACM.0000000000003137.
182. PLS Collaborative. Accessed January 16, 2023. www.proceduralllearning.org.
183. George BC, Teitelbaum EN, Meyerson SL, et al. Reliability, validity, and feasibility of the Zwisch scale for the assessment of intraoperative performance. *J Surg Educ*. 2014 Nov-Dec;71(6):e90–e96. doi:10.1016/j.jsurg.2014.06.018.
184. Accreditation Council of Graduate Medical Education Direct Observation of Clinical Care. Accessed January 20, 2023. Assessment (acgme.org). https://dl.acgme.org/pages/assessment.

6

Standardized Patients

TOSHIKO UCHIDA, MD, AND SUSANNAH CORNES, MD

CHAPTER OUTLINE

Introduction

Direct observation of a learner interacting with patients is essential for the assessment of clinical competence and may be accomplished with actual patients in the clinical environment as described in the preceding chapter or with simulated patients, commonly referred to as standardized patients (SPs). SPs are laypeople trained to portray patients, family members, healthcare professionals, or others in a realistic way for medical education and/or assessment purposes. Using SPs for assessment overcomes many of the challenges faced when working with actual patients, including providing a consistent, accessible, safe clinical encounter while still allowing learners to demonstrate the way they perform with real people. Through SP-based assessments, learners can "show" their clinical skills, as represented by the third level of Miller's pyramid, in comparison to the lower levels that focus solely on knowledge (see Chapter 1).

The methodology for SP-based assessments has been refined to the point[1,2] where this strategy is used for high-stakes decisions regarding promotion of learners to the next academic level[3] and even physician licensure.[4–8] In the United States, from 2004 to 2020 the National Board of Medical Examiners (NBME) and the Federation of State Medical Boards (FSMB) required all medical students to pass Step 2 Clinical Skills (Step 2 CS) of the United States Medical Licensing Examination (USMLE) to qualify for licensure in the United States.[9,10] Since Step 2 CS was officially discontinued in 2021,[11] individual medical schools and consortia of medical schools are now taking responsibility for assessing students' clinical skills, often still using SP-based assessments.[12]

This chapter focuses on assessments that involve SPs, beginning with an overview of SPs in performance-based examinations followed by the strengths and challenges of utilizing SPs in assessment and factors to consider when incorporating SP-based assessments within an overall program of assessment. Next, the chapter includes a practical guide for the development and implementation of SP assessments from blueprinting to case development, to training of SPs and raters. Consideration is then given to scoring and evaluating the psychometric properties of SP-based assessments before concluding with a discussion of the expansion of opportunities and future directions for the use of SPs in health professions education and assessment.

Overview of SPs in Education and Assessment

The use of SPs in medical education was first described by Barrows and Abrahamson in the 1960s[13,14] and has now expanded across the globe to include many disciplines of health professions education and assessment from podiatry to pharmacy to traditional East Asian medicine and beyond.[15–18] Some authors make a distinction between the term *simulated patient*, which is a broad term used whenever a layperson portrays a patient, and the term *standardized patient*, where the emphasis is on the consistency of portrayal.[19] Earlier work found that educators in Asia and Europe tend to use the term *simulated patient*, while those in North America more commonly use *standardized patient*.[19] More recently, the simple abbreviation *SP* has been used as an umbrella term, encompassing both "simulated" and "standardized" patients, as in the Association of SP Educators.[20] SPs come from many backgrounds, and some programs prefer professionally trained actors while others employ a wide range of laypeople or even recruit volunteers. SPs can be used for straightforward tasks such as serving as a model for a cardiovascular exam, or re-creating complex clinical behaviors such as a patient with psychosis or complex neurologic findings. SPs are also frequently trained to score learners in a consistent way and to provide individualized feedback on clinical skills including communication, history taking, physical examination, procedures, and other clinical tasks.

Depending on the purpose of the assessment, scenarios involving SPs may be carried out singly or in a sequence of several encounters run back-to-back. In 1975, Harden et al. described the process of linking together multiple stations assessing clinical skills into an assessment now known as an objective structured clinical examination (OSCE).[21] While many OSCEs include stations with SPs there are plenty of OSCE stations—such as suturing using a task trainer—that do not involve SPs.[22] Similarly, not all SP-based assessments would be considered an OSCE. For example, a single SP station used as a formative assessment of a comprehensive physical examination would typically not be referred to as an OSCE. The opportunities for utilizing SPs in education and assessment are very broad and wide open for innovation.

Strengths of Standardized Patient-Based Assessments

SP-based assessments have several strengths relative to other assessment modalities, including the ability to anchor the assessment around the clinical encounter while ensuring the experience is standardized and aligned with curricular aims. Assessments with SPs can be designed to enable timely and meaningful feedback to guide learning or to inform high-stakes assessment decisions as part of competency-based medical education (CBME). In addition, data from SP-based assessments provide valuable insights as a part of program evaluation and quality improvement.

Direct Observation of Skills

First and foremost, the use of SPs for teaching and assessing clinical skills enables direct observation of the interaction between the student, or resident, and the SP and focuses the curriculum, learners, and faculty on the patient encounter. The well-known influence of assessment on learning results in renewed interest in clinical medicine and focuses attention on developing patient-centered skills when SP-based assessments are introduced.[23–25] Regardless of whether the observer is a trained SP, faculty member, peer, or other party, the assessment of skills is not inferred from case presentations, preceptor sessions, or review of the medical record. The incorporation of some form of direct observation in medical education is essential to identify areas for improvement, target subsequent teaching, and certify competence at the time of high-stakes assessments. The last of these is essential to ensure patient safety before skills are applied in the clinical setting.[26]

Standardization and Curricular Alignment

SP-based assessments additionally allow the program, course, or clerkship director to control the instructional and assessment activities and align goals in a manner that is not possible in clinical care. Encounters with SPs can be scheduled to coincide with, or complement, other relevant educational or assessment activities. This is quite different from education in actual clinical settings where a particular learning experience depends on patient availability. The SP exercise can be designed to assess appropriate milestones for learner level or to serve specific individual or programmatic needs. For example, a case for an early learner may focus on communication skills and hypothesis-driven data collection for a common syndrome. Adding a patient note as a post-encounter exercise for a later learner then changes the focus from assessment of data gathering to evaluation of diagnostic management and documentation (see Chapter 7). In addition to modifying SP cases to focus on different aspects of clinical competence, examination blueprinting (see "Examination Content and Blueprinting") ensures that an appropriate range of clinically relevant syndromes, patient populations, and levels of acuity are represented within the program of assessment. Having a centrally coordinated assessment program that relies on a competency framework with developmental milestones ensures that SP-based assessments are used appropriately relative to other assessment tools[27,28] (see Chapter 3 and Fig. 6.1).

Timely and Meaningful Feedback

From the student and resident perspectives, the use of SPs within curricular sessions or low-stakes assessments allows

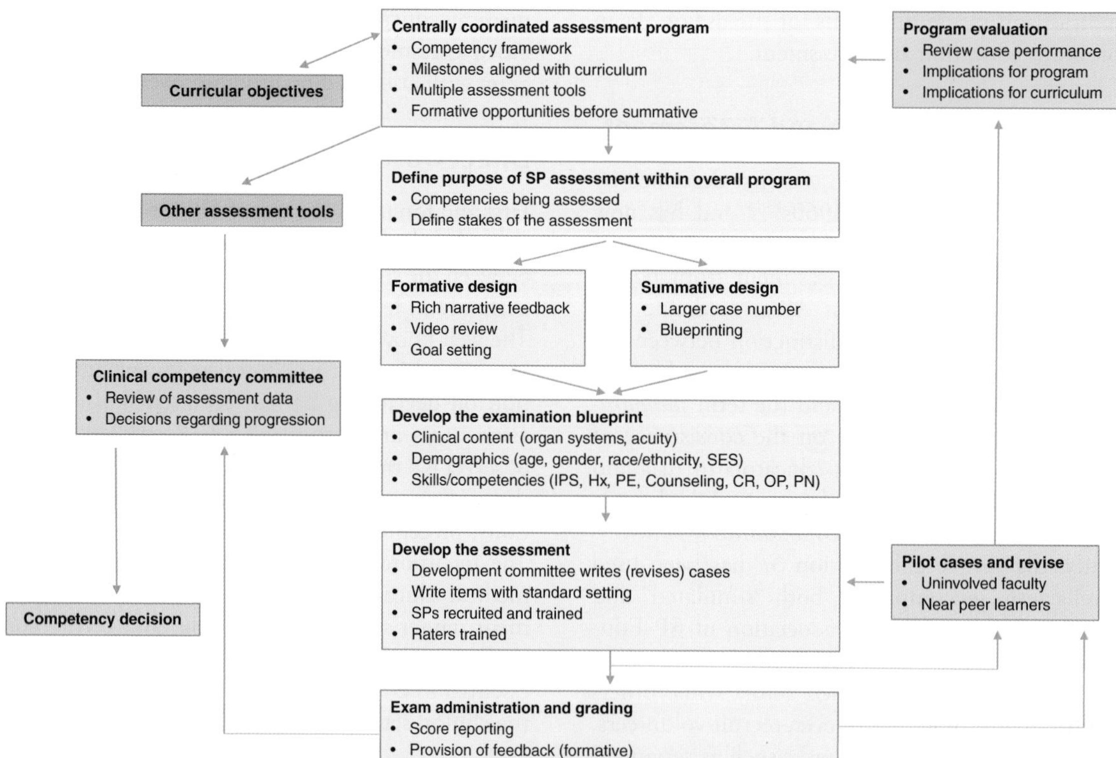

• **Fig. 6.1** Development of a standardized patient-based assessment. *CR*, Clinical reasoning; *Hx*, history; *IPS*, interpersonal skills; *OP*, oral presentation; *PE*, physical exam; *PN*, patient note; *SES*, socioeconomic status.

learners to practice clinical skills and receive feedback in a safe environment that also avoids the risk of harm to real patients. The lower stakes for such exercises make the use of SPs an ideal method for teaching and assessing difficult or sensitive communication or physical examination challenges before students attempt these skills with real patients. In particular, SPs have proven to be a valuable resource for teaching and assessment of an examinee's ability to deliver bad news to a patient, to discuss preferences for end-of-life care, to engage in patient counseling or education, and in teaching and assessing breast, rectal, and genitourinary examinations.[29–31] The use of SPs for these challenging communication and examination skills importantly enables feedback on the patient experience prior to application of these skills in genuine clinical settings. In addition, allowing for a "timeout" in which the SP encounter is interrupted to provide formative feedback allows the trainee to make adjustments or develop alternative approaches to difficult clinical situations in real time.

To ensure high-quality feedback, programs should consider feedback skills in SP recruitment, training, and oversight for SP performance.[19,32] SPs can provide valuable patient perspectives regarding trainee skills and behaviors, commenting on how they felt from the perspective of their character during various portions of the interaction. For curricular sessions occurring in small groups, peer observers and faculty can also provide immediate feedback to learners, focusing on discrete skills and behaviors. Alternatively, videotaped encounters can be rated by faculty, peers, SPs, or the trainees themselves. Review of videotapes allows evaluators to gather important diagnostic information such as when errors of commission or omission occur, and video review with struggling learners is invaluable during the development of remediation plans or when there is a need to build insight regarding areas of challenge (see Chapter 17).

High-Stakes Assessment Decisions

While allowing for flexibility in tailoring instruction and formative assessment to the level and needs of the learner and program, SP-based assessments can also be designed to enable higher-stakes assessment of competence.[33–35] As discussed in Chapter 1, the shift in educational philosophy over the past century from cognitive to behaviorist or outcomes-focused approaches aims to improve our ability to measure how the learner integrates communication, knowledge, technical skills, clinical reasoning, emotion, values, and reflection to demonstrate competence for practice.[36,37] This complex integration of behaviors is impossible to assess by any single instrument and almost certainly will require the thoughtful inclusion of SP-based assessments. Through standardization of individual cases, examinees are each exposed to the same clinical problem presented uniformly, which cannot be replicated in the workplace. By methods such as exam blueprinting, increasing the number of SP encounters within a single assessment, and ensuring inter-rater reliability, SP assessments can be designed to provide reliability and validity evidence to inform decisions regarding advancement, promotion, or even graduation.[38]

Program Evaluation

The use of SPs, either individually or as part of multiple-station OSCEs, not only allows clerkship and program directors to obtain valuable feedback concerning individual trainees but can also be used to evaluate whether the program as a whole has been successful in achieving important curricular objectives (see Chapter 18).[39,40] Using SP-based methods for program evaluation is ideal in that it identifies the patient encounter as a critical event in which learning should occur and on which individual assessment will focus. A poor performance on information sharing in a case of newly diagnosed diabetes, the omission of questions about cardiac risk factors in a case of angina, or the lack of assessment for volume overload in a case of dyspnea provides both information on individual performance and, when reviewed as part of program evaluation, on areas in the curriculum in need of improvement. Since a sound educational program is dependent upon the alignment of objectives, curriculum, and assessments, using SP-based assessment outcomes for evaluation encourages course and program directors to make improvements that impact patient care.

Challenges of Standardized Patient-Based Assessments

Challenges of SP-based assessments should also be considered when integrating SPs into an assessment program and include direct and indirect costs, the need for robust SP and faculty development, and the limits of simulation. The additional need to assess for validity evidence is discussed separately (see "Applying Kane's Validity Framework").

Expense of Standardized Patient Programs

Concerns regarding the expense of SP-based assessments understandably and appropriately curtail their use.[19,22,41] Research suggests that it may be difficult to capture the full range of direct and indirect costs associated with OSCEs, and that higher-stakes exams and initial administrations are more expensive than subsequent ones.[41] Costs may include faculty, staff, and center time as well as access to testing infrastructure, software platforms, and simulation equipment. Hiring SP trainers and SPs can be expensive and, depending upon the location of the program, recruitment may be challenging.

Logistic Complexity and Indirect Costs

Likewise, finding the time and space to conduct SP-based teaching and assessment activities may be difficult for programs that do not have clinical skills centers or are not affiliated with institutions where such centers are located. Program directors must also consider the logistic complexity of the assessment. Multistation OSCES are likely to require several days or weeks to administer, depending on the number of participants and stations, necessitating that small cohorts of students be made available on a rotating basis and impacting other curricular experiences during the test period. One potential remedy to resource limitations is collaboration among programs and institutions to combine resources and expertise, minimizing financial and other resource commitments and ensuring the availability of SPs, case material, and trained personnel. The development of regional consortia focusing on the use of SPs (and other simulation methods) in education and assessment is one such approach that is well described.[12,42]

Rater Training and Bias

The balance of faculty and SPs for observation and feedback highlights the need to consider how raters are assigned and trained within the assessment program to best advantage. Implementation of SP-based teaching and assessment in educational programs may decrease the need for faculty to participate in the more routine aspects of assessment and may better prepare SPs for their teaching and assessment roles.[19,40] Well-trained SPs can provide reliable assessment and feedback on interviewing and physical examination skills at the time of the assessment, allowing faculty to focus on developing and maintaining the case bank, standard setting, and quality assurance and on grading diagnostic or therapeutic management, case presentations, and problem-solving.[40] Faculty development efforts should ensure that faculty are familiar with expectations for observation and rating skills and not assume that faculty familiarity with workplace-based assessments (WBAs) will transfer to the simulation center or clinical skills laboratory. Faculty require training to ensure that ratings are reliable, and program quality assurance should include assessments of inter-rater reliability and bias, which has the potential to impact scoring based on gender, race/ethnicity, and primary spoken language other than English.[43,44] Rater training is discussed in more detail later in this chapter.

Limitations of the Simulation Environment

While the simulated encounter approximates a true clinical encounter, it is important to acknowledge its limitations, including the challenges in simulating certain findings, the effect of observation on the demonstration of skills, and uncertainty regarding how the learner would interpret pathologic findings in a real patient encounter. While task trainers offer opportunities to include an increasing array of findings (such as acute or chronic papilledema represented alongside an SP portrayal of a patient presenting with headache), the inclusion of the simulated finding prompts the student to anticipate the abnormal finding and does not necessarily measure the ability to recognize pathologic findings when present in real patients.[45] In addition, other physical examination findings (such as an anterior drawer sign in a patient with a knee injury) cannot be simulated and may undermine the ability to assess certain competencies using SPs. In this respect, SPs should be considered a supplement to rather than a replacement for assessing competence with real patients. Indeed, to ensure that a broad spectrum of physical findings are assessed within an educational program, a combination of real and simulated findings would be ideal,[19] keeping in mind that a high volume of "real" patient contact is still required for a trainee to appreciate the diversity of clinical presentations. The multilayered nature and social implications of real patient encounters may contribute to a learning effect not captured during encounters with simulated patients.[46]

Following on this theme, it is important to remember that the performance of students and residents in assessment environments may not define their capacity to perform in real clinical settings. In fact, data describing the use of SPs in assessing practicing physician competence suggest that there may be a significant difference between demonstrated capacity to perform (competence) and actual performance in practice, particularly when challenges with efficiency are not taken into account.[47,48] There is clearly an observation ("Hawthorne") effect operating under such simulated conditions, and a station that invites the student to demonstrate focused, discrete tasks risks encouraging learners to compartmentalize skills to perform well on the assessment rather than well in the clinical setting. For example, the ability to interpret an ECG could be better assessed using a written assessment, but the ability to elicit a relevant history for chest pain, perform a cardiac examination, and explain the need for an ECG to a patient better approximates clinical experiences. Conversely, asking too much of a learner in a time-limited OSCE station risks creating a cognitive load that is unrealistically challenging and may undermine the validity of the assessment.

Ultimately, the demonstration of competence in simulation should not be taken as final, absolute evidence that such abilities will be exercised in real clinical settings. Data on the correlation between OSCE scores and other clinical skills performance measures are variable and ultimately challenging to collect.[49,50] Still, assessment programs should monitor alignment with future exam and real-world performance and incorporate WBAs that ensure that relevant knowledge, skills, and behaviors are manifest in the day-to-day environment of the future physician, as well (see discussion of validity later in this chapter).[34,35]

The implications of the strengths and weaknesses for SP-based assessments is that, ultimately, SP assessments should be reserved to assess only those skills that cannot be better assessed in other ways.[22] Creating a program of SP-based assessments with appropriate scope, breadth, and depth requires an understanding of the purpose of each assessment and how it fits into the broader assessment program.

Planning for Standardized Patient-Based Assessments

When planning an SP assessment it is essential to know how it functions within the broader program of assessment (see Fig. 6.1). Principles guiding the development of an assessment program are well described elsewhere (see Chapter 3), but should begin with a centrally coordinated vision guided by a competency framework in which each assessment functions as "a tool fit for a purpose."[27,51–57] A well-designed program will include a range of instruments, a range of stakes to enhance learning while enabling decisions about progression, and the collection of data to inform program evaluation.[58] For SP-based assessments, considerations include (1) how SP-based assessments are mapped to a competency framework, (2) which competencies to assess using SPs, and (3) the impact of assessment for and of learning on the design.

Mapping to a Competency Framework

Mapping SP-based assessments within the program of assessment benefits from the adoption of a competency framework, of which there are several to consider (see Chapter 1, Table 1.3), including the Accreditation Council of Graduate Medical Education/American Board of Medical Specialties (ACGME/ABMS) core competencies,[59,60] Canadian Medical Education Directives for Specialists (CanMEDS) physician competency framework,[61] and United Kingdom General Medical Council's Outcomes for Graduates.[62] Institutions may also choose to create their own milestone or competency framework, or supplement an existing competency framework—for example, by adding relevant subcompetencies (e.g., components within patient care that are specific to the clinical skills of history and physical examination or that highlight which competencies relate to knowledge and comprehension versus application, analysis, synthesis, and evaluation).[28,63,64]

With the competency framework chosen, programs can embed longitudinal milestones divided into progressively advancing skill levels (proficiency levels) as described by the Dreyfus model of skill acquisition: novice, advanced beginner, competent, proficient, expert[65] (see Chapter 1, Table 1.4). Educators are then challenged to develop SP-based assessments to inform learner progress in milestones achievement, which may have implications for item development as well as the complexity of the case design.[64] For example, in terms of item development, an early learner being assessed for medical history (within the competency of patient care) may function as an "advanced beginner" by inquiring about the core characteristics of the chief concern (e.g., asked about the time course, what makes it better, what makes it worse, etc.) and may demonstrate a higher level of "competence" by also asking about pertinent positives and negatives to guide diagnostic reasoning. To assess for a higher degree of competence in the medical history, one could include a more challenging syndrome in a subsequent

SP-based assessment that requires consideration for special patient populations, or introduce a communication challenge. Mapping each subcompetency to the longitudinal milestones framework helps ensure that each assessment is appropriate for the learner level.[28,66] SP-based assessment should not be relied upon as the sole assessment method to inform a judgment on a particular milestone. When used as one component in a multifaceted assessment program, however, SP scenarios may be useful to determine where learners are at in terms of knowledge, skills, and attitudes prior to entering a new phase of training such as internship.[63]

Which Competencies to Assess With Standardized Patients

With a competency framework in place, assessment tools can be combined to create a well-rounded and robust program taking factors such as cost-effectiveness, acceptability, reliability, validity, and educational impact into account when choosing which tools to deploy.[56] Using the ACGME competencies as an example, assessment of Interpersonal and Communication Skills and the patient-centered elements (eliciting patient information, gathering essential and accurate information from patients, and counseling and educating patients) within the Patient Care domain will necessarily rely more heavily on assessments that include observation of the clinical encounter, both in simulation and in clinical care. Standardized patients may also be used to assess behaviors intrinsic to the Professionalism domain, including responsiveness to patients' culture, age, gender, health literacy, spiritual beliefs, and intellectual and physical disabilities.[67–70]

The flexibility of SP-based methods also facilitates development of assessment exercises to measure competence in Practice-based Learning and Improvement and Systems-based Practice, which are notoriously challenging to measure. Faculty, clerkship, and program directors can work with SP training staff to develop cases to assess trainees' abilities to search, appraise, and apply scientific evidence in patient management; use information technology in managing patient information and online resources; elicit patient preferences in making informed decisions; and provide appropriate care for selected conditions and health maintenance (see Chapter 10).[2] Over the past decade, health professions educators have focused their attention on the development of SP-based methods that measure competencies essential for achieving current healthcare priorities, particularly those related to patient safety, transitions of care, interprofessionalism, and working in teams.[71,72] SP-based assessment scenarios may also be created to assess the sociocultural dimensions of the patient safety competency including "near-miss" management and medical error disclosure.[73–75]

Standardized patients in the role of a standardized healthcare professional may be trained to receive a patient handoff,[76–78] or participate in an interdisciplinary team meeting designed to measure collaborative skills when developing a patient care plan.[79–81] Simulated interprofessional teams can also be created to assess performance of team-oriented behaviors including ability to manage conflict, advocate for the patient, and speak up against a power gradient.[82] A tool with high-quality validity evidence is available for assessment of these collaborative practice competency domains.[83] Using SP-based methodology to assess competency in these more complex health systems science constructs can be a challenge, as case scenarios by nature of their complexity may be more difficult to standardize, require the development of additional rating scales, and require additional resources including more than one SP involved in the station.

Assessment tools for the Medical Knowledge domain are likely to include paper- or online-based assessments that allow learners to describe their thinking outside the clinical encounter (see Chapter 7 for a discussion of other methods). While SP-based methods are not particularly efficient when applied to the evaluation of Medical Knowledge, they may be used to measure the application of knowledge in simulated patient care situations (see Chapter 7). The SP encounter can be supplemented with structured global ratings such as the mini clinical evaluation exercise (mini-CEX),[84] or, to tap other important skills, combined with a patient note or some form of chart stimulated recall process. Since these types of evaluation approaches model those currently used in real clinical settings, they are more readily accepted, both by those who are responsible for the assessment and those who are being assessed. Here, program or clerkship directors may also decide to employ SPs for assessment of knowledge application in important medical cases that are infrequently or inconsistently encountered during clinical rotations.

Implications of High- and Low-Stakes Assessments

SP-based assessment methods may be used for the purpose of summative assessment, in which the goal is to determine the proficiency of a learner against established standards, and their readiness to graduate or to move on to the next level of training; or formative assessment, in which the emphasis is on monitoring student learning and providing feedback (see Fig. 6.1). Summative assessment, which usually occurs at the conclusion of a phase of training, has been termed *assessment of learning*, whereas formative assessment typically is embedded within the instructional cycle and referred to as *assessment for learning*.[52] *Programmatic assessment* (see Chapter 3) describes an approach to assessment that takes advantage of multiple assessment tools and data points to optimize both learning and the development of competence. Assessments should occur longitudinally with assessment for learning opportunities placed at higher frequency within the instructional cycle and higher-stakes summative assessments based on a larger number of assessment data points.[51]

SP assessments generate a variety of assessment data, all of which may be used for assessment purposes but may be more or less appropriate depending on the stakes of the assessment. For example, within SP methodology, feedback can include face-to-face or written narrative feedback from faculty and/or SPs, or as part of a group debriefing session. Case-specific content checklists can be used to determine whether the trainee met expected performance standards for data gathering. The same checklist can serve as a discussion template for providing feedback to trainees regarding their success in meeting education or clinical objectives. Rating scales can be used to provide feedback regarding a student's communication and interpersonal skills or humanistic or professional behaviors and may be combined with narrative comments from SPs that provide specific critical or reinforcing feedback. Scores from the clinical interview, patient note, or other activities associated with individual patient encounters may be combined to obtain a final score that best meets the purpose of the educational assessment or exercise.

If the purpose is primarily to support learning, then the assessment data collected should enable high-quality, timely, and individualized feedback to guide student learning. It may be useful to support learning with faculty observers, scheduled opportunities for video review, inclusion of "timeouts" for immediate input, and postsession coaching to identify subsequent learning goals. If the purpose is summative in scope, the focus of data collection should be on ensuring adequate reliability (consistency of assessment results) and valid inferences about the clinical skill(s) being assessed (i.e., the assessment measures what it intends to measure).

Implications for summative OSCE designs include a lesser emphasis on feedback, the need for a larger number of cases, oversight for SP and faculty training, and greater attention to examination security, among other considerations. While a well-designed approach to score reporting could yield valuable and actionable information from high-stakes assessments, combining the roles of an assessment of and for learning is problematic for learners who are less able to engage effectively in reflection and goal setting when the assessment is perceived as high stakes.[85,86] In addition, when determining clinical competency, the OSCE data should be assembled along with adequate additional sources of assessment data and reviewed by a competency committee to enable informed decisions regarding progression.

The use of SP assessments for summative purposes is shifting with the USMLE decision to discontinue the Step 2 CS examination. While numerous studies conducted by both medical schools and licensing or certification bodies over the past 50 years have provided evidence that, with sufficient numbers of simulation encounters, properly sampled from the practice domain, reliable and valid assessment decisions could be made,[87] these examinations are expensive and complex to administer and maintain.[11] In addition, while some data exist from individual institutions, it has been challenging to demonstrate the predictive validity of SP assessments for clinical performance in the next stage of training or practice.[49] Many medical schools have developed mandatory SP-based clinical skills assessments required for graduation[88] and designed to prepare learners for high-stakes licensing examinations. Without licensing examinations in place to certify clinical competence, the responsibility for this final high-stakes decision lies with the institution and makes the responsibility all the greater for the development of high-quality summative SP-based exams.[12,89–91]

Developing Standardized Patient-Based Assessments

Examination Content and Blueprinting

Once the purpose of the SP assessment is clearly delineated, the content of the assessment can be defined (see Fig. 6.1). Sometimes SPs will be employed for a session regarding one particular topic such as breaking difficult news or practicing a trauma-informed physical exam. Often, however, multiple SP stations are compiled into an OSCE format to assess a broader range of skills that students may have acquired over the course of a block or clerkship. Regardless of whether the assessment focuses on one specific topic or a range of skills, it is essential to start with the learning objectives for the course of study and then to blueprint the content of the OSCE based on those objectives.[92] Blueprinting has been defined as "the process by which content experts ensure that constructs of interest are adequately represented."[38,93] Learners should be familiar with the learning objectives so that they know what is expected of them in the assessment. When learners are aware of the educational objectives and understand that these objectives will be tested, they are motivated to focus on the content that is most important.

Like all assessments, SP-based assessments are not able to test every possible disease in every possible patient in every possible clinical context. Instead, OSCEs employ systematic sampling across a range of patients and content areas to test a range of skills in a range of contexts.[33,38] One technique for blueprinting an OSCE involves mapping patient characteristics against diseases or clinical topics,[40,94] as shown in Table 6.1. For a more comprehensive OSCE, the blueprint may be built off both relevant content areas and common patient presentations. For example, an OSCE for a surgery clerkship may include a case from each subspecialty including general surgery, orthopedics, urology, and thoracic surgery. In addition, cases could be based on common chief concerns including abdominal pain, leg pain, flank pain, and trauma. Referencing local, regional, or national statistics on the prevalence of diseases and the primary reasons for presenting to medical attention will support the validity of the blueprinting.[95] In addition to topic areas, it may be important to sample across multiple contexts and patient characteristics. For example, an OSCE may include a range of clinical settings from the emergency department to the ambulatory clinic to the intensive care unit. Developers will also want to be mindful to include a diverse range of patients based on age, race, ethnicity, gender, socioeconomic status, and other characteristics.

TABLE 6.1 Blueprint for a Standardized Patient-Based Assessment

	Chief Concern				
	Cardiovascular/ Respiratory	Gastrointestinal/ Genitourinary	Neurologic/ Psychologic	General Symptoms	Other: Eyes, Ears, Integument, Musculoskeletal
Age: *at least* 2 >64 2 = 40–64 2 = 15–39					
Gender: *at least* 3 men 3 women 1 nonbinary					
Acuity: *at least* 2 acute 2 subacute 2 chronic					
Physical Exam: *at least* 1 system and 1 abnormality per case					

Alternatively, a blueprint could be generated by identifying competencies of interest such as communication and interpersonal skills, history taking, physical examination, counseling, clinical reasoning, oral presentations, and patient notes. In the end, a comprehensive blueprint will likely include a multidimensional matrix that selects content using several of these techniques. Regardless of the method, purposeful blueprinting reflecting important educational goals and objectives is essential for providing validity evidence for an SP-based assessment.[38,92] A common pitfall of SP-based assessments is to choose cases based on convenience, such as the availability of SPs, or to create cases based on the expertise of the lead faculty instead of sampling learning objectives in an intentional way. Obviously, the extent of the blueprint must also be balanced with the feasibility and cost of developing and administering the assessment.

Components of a Typical Standardized Patient Encounter

While the format of an SP encounter has great flexibility and is wide open to innovation, a typical session often includes the components as described in the following subsections. The learner and SP have separate tasks before and after their encounter, as shown in Fig. 6.2.

Orientation

Before the exercise, learners should be oriented to the format and goals of the session. Students are typically instructed to interact with SPs in the same way they would interact with real patients with the acknowledgment that this requires a "willing suspension of disbelief."[96] The process whereby all participants agree to behave as if they are acting in real life is known as the "fiction contract."[96] Instructions must be clear about any circumstances where the encounter would deviate from actual clinical practice such as: "Do not perform a breast, genital, or rectal exam. If you feel any of these exams are warranted based on the clinical scenario, please note it in your postencounter write-up." The orientation may include information about time limitations, personal protective and other equipment available, and how to handle student questions that might arise during the encounter. It should be clear to learners whether the exercise is formative or summative, whether the encounter will be video recorded, and who will have access to viewing the encounter and the data generated from it.[97] In the case of summative assessments that will be administered to other learners at a different time, participants should be reminded of expectations of professional behavior and keeping case content confidential.

Introduction to the Patient Scenario

The introduction to the patient scenario is called the stem. It often includes details that would be available when seeing a patient in a clinical encounter, such as the patient's name and basic demographic information, the setting for the encounter, the reason for the patient's visit, and the task assigned to the learner[98] (see Box 6.1).

The amount of detail provided in the introduction depends on the level of the learner and the goal of the

• **BOX 6.1 The Stem: Example of the Introduction to the Patient Scenario**

Name:	Julia Aguilar
Age:	58 years old
Gender/pronouns:	Woman, she/her/hers
Setting:	Urgent care clinic
Presenting concern:	Shortness of breath
Your task:	Elicit a focused history, perform a focused physical exam, and share your initial impression and initial plan with the patient.

exercise. For example, for novice students, the task may specifically list the physical exam maneuvers to be performed, whereas a more advanced student may be expected to identify which portions of the physical exam are relevant based on the clinical situation. As a practical matter, it is often easiest to create a scenario where the learner is meeting the patient for the first time so that the need for extensive background information is minimized.[98]

Standardized Patient Encounter

The encounter between the learner and SP will vary widely depending on the learning objectives. Students may be asked to elicit a history, perform a physical exam, and share information, all while conveying empathy and respect for the patient and family. A case may be focused on one particular topic such as eliciting a sexual history, performing a neurologic exam, or working with an interpreter. The SP may simulate physical exam findings such as tenderness or weakness, and moulage makeup or prosthetics may be used to simulate wounds or other physical findings. The case may include a standardized question from the SP such as "Can I get a refill on my sleeping pill?" to evaluate the learner's communication skills and clinical judgment. The scope of the encounter will be tailored to the skills being assessed.

Postencounter Activities (Interstation Exercises)

Often the SP encounter will be followed by a postencounter activity such as writing a clinical note or answering questions about the case. If there are multiple SP cases back-to-back, as in an OSCE, these postencounter activities are often referred to as interstations. Again, the format and tasks for the postencounter exercise will be based on the goals of the session and provide an additional opportunity to assess a wide array of clinical skills. Learners may be asked to list and justify a differential diagnosis, develop a diagnostic plan, or use a literature search to answer a clinical question related to the case. There is room for a great deal of creativity when developing interstations, but they should be carefully crafted to fit into the overall program of assessment described previously. From a logistical standpoint, the time while learners are completing an interstation exercise also allows time for the SP to score the student's performance

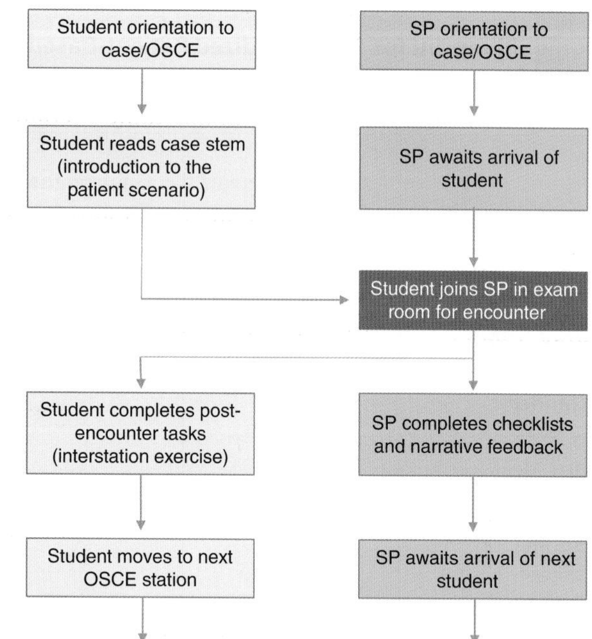

• **Fig. 6.2** Flow of a typical standardized patient encounter. *OSCE*, Objective structured clinical examination *SP*, standardized patient.

and provide written feedback before moving on to the next student, as shown in Fig. 6.2.

Case Development

Scripting a Case

Writing SP cases often requires close collaboration between clinicians who are the content experts and professional SP educators who have an in-depth understanding of the case formats that are most useful for SPs.[40,99] While clinicians usually have a clear idea of how a patient with a particular disease presents, they often do not have experience converting that mental image into a script that can be used by a layperson to portray a patient scenario. Furthermore, including patients, who may sometimes be the SPs themselves, in case development can ensure incorporation of the patient's perspective into the case.[19] Some clinicians like to base SP cases on real patients they have cared for, which can increase the authenticity of the case. Basing an SP case on a real patient, however, can sometimes lead to superfluous or idiosyncratic detail that can distract from the main goals of the case, or increase the cognitive load for the SP. In some circumstances, it may be more important to create a representative "textbook" case, particularly for high-stakes exams or novice learners.[100] MedEdPORTAL is an open-access journal of peer-reviewed medical education modules that includes many excellent SP cases that may be used as examples when constructing a new SP case.[101]

SP educators are essential in helping faculty translate a patient presentation into a written SP case. Having a standard template for a case will ensure that all important information is captured in a way that makes it easy for SPs to understand and recall.[40,102] Even though these cases are standardized, it is advisable to include only a very few direct quotes that the SP will recite verbatim. Including too many scripted lines can make the interaction stilted and unrealistic while preventing the SP from responding in a natural way to conversation with the learner. Scripted lines are often used only for the opening line, such as "I've been having this terrible headache, and I'm really getting worried," or for standardized questions asked of the learner, such as "Can we postpone some of these vaccines for my baby?" Cases may also need to include information about the patient's inner life, such as what emotions the patient is experiencing and what the patient's goals are for the encounter.[98,99]

As outlined in the Medical Council of Canada Guidelines for the Development of Objective Structured Clinical Examination (OSCE) Cases, an SP script will commonly include the content listed in Box 6.2.[98] For low-stakes assessments, SPs may be asked to use a simplified version of their own family or social history. When asked nonpertinent questions about the past medical history, social history, or family history, the standard reply can be either "No" or "I don't know," as appropriate.

Case Tasks

As noted earlier, the case stem includes the patient information that is provided to the learner at the start of the SP encounter along with a description of the task to be performed. Even when the task is general, such as "Elicit a focused history and perform a focused physical exam," it must be clearly stated.[38] SP cases typically have a time limit that can range from as short as 5 minutes for a specific skill such as examining the cranial nerves, to 20 minutes or longer for cases that include a history, physical exam, and sharing a diagnosis or diagnostic plan with the patient.[98] A committee of both content experts and educational experts should participate in the development of SP cases to ensure that there is sufficient time to perform the required tasks and that the level of difficulty is appropriate for the learners[38] (see Fig. 6.1).

Pilot Testing

Pilot testing is extremely helpful since it can be difficult to estimate both the time required for a case and how students will respond to case material. Providing insufficient time may encourage inappropriate test-taking behaviors, such as rapid-fire questioning, which may not support the overall goals of the assessment.[103] Finding representative learners to participate in a pilot can be a challenge since educators often do not want to allow students to see case materials ahead of an assessment. In this situation, slightly more advanced students can be used as proxies for pilot testing. For example, fourth-year medical students could be asked to try out cases that will be used in an OSCE created for third-year students. Alternatively, for high-stakes exams, new cases can be incorporated in an established OSCE but not included in the final scores to pilot-test the cases. This technique was utilized for the USMLE-Step 2 CS exam.[104]

• BOX 6.2 Components of a Standardized Patient Script from the Medical Council of Canada Guidelines for the Development of Objective Structured Clinical Examination (OSCE) Cases

- Room setup and props
- Demographic data: age, gender
- Standardized patient starting position: sitting, lying on a gurney, etc.
- Appearance: dress, hair, make-up/moulage
- Behavior, affect, and mannerisms
- Opening statement
- Questions the standardized patient must ask
- Physical findings
- History of presenting problem
- Relevant past medical history
- Relevant social history
- Relevant family history
- Critical review of systems

Checklists and Rating Scales

The most common means of evaluating performance during SP-based assessments is via the use of checklists and rating scales. Checklists are used for skills that can be scored categorically and often dichotomously such as "yes/no" or "done/not done." Rating scales are used for skills that have a more continuous and wider range of performance such as communication skills, which may be scored using a tiered scale and may also include behavioral anchors. Many cases include a combination of checklists and rating scales as described in more detail later in the chapter.

Content-based checklists are used to record whether specific actions are taken by the examinee and are commonly used to score history taking and the physical exam.[10] Examinee actions are scored in a categorical fashion such as "Elicited smoking history: done/not done." While many checklist items are dichotomous, they may also be polytomous.[105] In the preceding example, a student who asks the SP if they have a history of smoking but does not inquire further about the duration and intensity of smoking may be marked as "partially done." This example also illustrates the importance of clearly defining the criteria for "done," "partially done," and "not done," particularly in a high-stakes assessment. Physical exam maneuvers are often scored as "done/done incorrectly/not done." With this scoring system, a learner who at least attempts a maneuver (such as auscultating the heart for a patient with shortness of breath) but does it incorrectly (perhaps by listening over the gown) may still be awarded partial credit if deemed appropriate.

History and physical examination checklists are typically created during the initial case development and must be consistent with the learning objectives being assessed. Checklists are often developed by content experts through panels or written protocols.[106] Alternatively, checklists may be developed by having experts participate in the case, and then using the behaviors that the experts employ—such as which history questions they ask and which physical exam maneuvers they perform—to create a checklist.[107] When possible, checklists should include evidence-based, clinically discriminating items.[108,109] Clinically discriminating items are those that help distinguish one diagnosis from another. For example, examining jugular venous pressure will help distinguish heart failure from pneumonia for a patient with shortness of breath. Discriminating items stand in contrast to checklist items, which are included for the sake of thoroughness.[109] Case writers should be careful to avoid the natural tendency to include too many checklist items, which can negatively impact the reliability of the scores since the cognitive load for the SPs becomes excessive.[110,111] In addition given relatively frequent changes in clinical practice, checklists must be regularly reviewed and updated since checklist items considered important today may not be as relevant in the future.[112]

The content of the checklist will also depend on the experience and needs of the learner. If the goal is to assess the physical exam skills of a novice student in an introductory clinical skills curriculum, then the checklist may include specific items for inspection, palpation, percussion, and auscultation and may perhaps include several checklist items under each of those categories. This sort of detailed checklist will allow course directors to explicitly define and communicate the proper steps and techniques for each skill to the students. More experienced physicians, however, score less well on checklists that emphasize thoroughness.[113] For higher-level learners, or when making high-stakes decisions, checklists should instead reflect only the most essential actions or maneuvers required for an appropriate evaluation of a patient with a particular clinical presentation. More advanced examinees can use heuristics, or mental shortcuts, which minimizes the amount of analytic data they need to collect to formulate a reasonable differential diagnosis.[114] Therefore the case development team should be attentive to the potential for rewarding thoroughness or inappropriate test-taking behaviors rather than true clinical competence. That is, more capable examinees that arrive at the appropriate diagnostic or management decision via a more efficient, or alternative, data gathering approach should not be penalized.

Typically, the SP will complete a checklist immediately after the encounter, which sets practical limits on the lengths of checklists due to the cognitive load placed on the SPs.[111] Checklists longer than 15 to 20 items can exceed the ability of most SPs to accurately recall specific elements of examinee performance,[115] and raters have been shown to fatigue over the course of an exam.[116] On the other hand, in specific circumstances well-trained SPs have been shown to have acceptable accuracy on much longer checklists such as a head-to-toe physical exam.[117] Other strategies include checklist scoring by an observer either in the room or watching remotely from a control room, or scoring asynchronously by watching a video recording later on,[118,119] although these approaches require additional human resources.

In addition, faculty should work with SP educators to ensure that individual checklist items represent specific, observable behaviors that are amenable to categorical scoring. Broad or complex checklist items that require SPs to interpret examinee intentions or recall multiple actions are more likely to result in inaccurate scoring.[115] For example, instead of "The student asked about factors that precipitated my chest pain," the checklist should include several separate items such as:

The student asked if physical exertion caused my chest pain: Y/N
The student asked if taking a deep breath caused my chest pain: Y/N
The student asked if lying down caused my chest pain: Y/N

Additional methods for scoring SP-based encounters employ various types of rating scales.[120] Rating scales are often used when the skill or behavior being assessed requires some multifaceted judgment of examinee performance that is not amenable to dichotomous scoring. Rating scales are commonly used for measuring communication and interpersonal skills and for assessing humanistic or professional behaviors.[121,122] Rating scales may assess specific behaviors such as eye contact, or may be more global assessments of a student's performance.[123] For example, a global rating scale may ask an SP to rate the student's overall interpersonal skills as poor, below average, average, above average, or excellent. These sorts of global ratings may result in similar scores as more specific behaviorally anchored ratings and may correlate with assessments of actual clinical performance.[124] In contrast, rating scales may be used to assess multiple specific communication tasks, such as "Make a personal connection during visit (e.g., go beyond medical issues)" and "Explain rationale for diagnostic procedures (e.g., exam, tests)," which are from Makoul's SEGUE Framework.[125] A number of these communication frameworks are available in the literature.[126–133] These sorts of frameworks can then be further defined with a behaviorally anchored rating scale (BARS) as described in Chapter 4. A BARS assessment includes specific descriptions of the behaviors that define each point along the scale. See Appendix 6.1 for an example of a communication skills checklist that uses a BARS. The BARS format is particularly well suited to CBME since the criteria for meeting competence can be spelled out in the anchors.

When developing both checklists and rating scales, faculty often consider weighting the most important items more heavily. Many history and physical exam checklist items, however, are interdependent, and it can be difficult to determine the relative importance of various items. In the end, weighting of items does not have a significant impact on reliability or pass/fail determinations.[134] Therefore items should typically only be weighted to signal the relative importance of certain skills when assessment is used *for* learning as described earlier.

Standardized Patient Selection and Training

SPs come from a very wide range of backgrounds. Recruiting a diverse group of SPs is essential to the success of the overall SP program and should take into account as many characteristics as possible including age, gender, race, ethnicity, size, disability, and others. SPs should be motivated to contribute to the educational mission of the institution. SPs who are hostile or bitter toward the medical profession, or have a strong personal agenda, will often not create the best educational experiences for learners.[40] SPs are usually asked about scars or other observable physical findings that may influence their portrayal of a case. A clinician should also examine the SP to uncover any previously unknown physical examination findings that may impact a case, such as a thyroid nodule or a heart murmur.

Training SPs is a profession unto itself, and whenever possible SP educators should be employed to ensure that SPs are trained in a clear and consistent way. The Association of SP Educators (ASPE) is a tremendous resource for information on training SPs, particularly through the ASPE Center for SP Methodology.[135] Numerous strategies are used to train SPs including written scripts, videos of real patients with the target condition, videos of SPs portraying the same case, and virtual and in-person role-play. With careful training and feedback, multiple SPs can portray and score the same case with accuracy and consistency.[136] While most of the training can be accomplished by SP educators, clinical staff and faculty must observe and provide feedback to SPs to ensure a realistic portrayal of the clinical scenario. Clinician expertise is also required to provide training on proper physical exam technique. The intensity of training and the degree of standardization required depends on the stakes and the purpose of the assessment. For low-stakes formative assessments, training may be brief and SPs may be asked to ad lib or use some of their personal history—for instance, a general family history, which will be easier for the SP to remember than a fictional family history. For high-stakes summative assessments, the degree of standardization may be quite detailed, such as counting the number of seconds the student takes to wash their hands or counting the number of times the student says "um" or "ah."

SPs are also frequently trained to provide narrative feedback to learners—either verbally or in writing—particularly regarding communication and interpersonal skills.[137,138] One great advantage of working with SPs is that they can provide honest, individualized feedback to learners in a way that real patients typically cannot (except perhaps anonymously online) due to power dynamics and cultural expectations. SPs should be trained to follow the general principles of providing high-quality feedback, including referring to specific details that focus on behaviors and not on personal characteristics, and being clear that the feedback is based on the SP's own point of view. SPs have been found to provide a different perspective from physicians when providing feedback on communication skills, and this complementary viewpoint is often considered a strength of working with SPs.[139]

Not surprisingly, while not all studies are concordant, there is concern that SP biases based on race, ethnicity, and gender may influence the way SPs assess students' clinical skills.[43,44,140] SPs should routinely be included in the same implicit bias and cultural humility training that is required of all staff members at the institution where the SPs are working. Moreover, recruiting a wide diversity of SPs can greatly enhance the feedback provided to learners. Instead of trying to standardize the feedback SPs provide to learners, embracing a variety of opinions is likely to be of even greater benefit to the student and may also help the student recognize some of their own implicit biases.[92,141] When used for higher-stakes assessments, reliability can be improved by employing multiple observations from multiple examiners.[92]

Curriculum developers should also be keenly aware of the potential impact of case portrayal on SPs. In particular, SPs who are members of historically marginalized groups may be subject to stereotyping or tokenism. Cases must be developed, trained, and utilized in a way that attends to psychological safety for both the learner and the SP.[141,142]

Rater Training

Rater training is necessary to produce accurate and reliable scores.[143] With proper training and effective quality assurance procedures, SPs and other assessors can be trained to provide reproducible scores that are similar to the scores produced by clinicians.[144–146] For the history taking and physical examination checklist, the SP, or any other person who documents the data gathering activities, must be trained to understand variations in candidate questioning and discern between correct and incorrect physical exam maneuvers. For any rating scales employed, the assessors must be taught to differentiate performance along some relevant continuum. Performance dimension training (PDT) and frame of reference training (FoRT), discussed in Chapter 5, are rigorous techniques for standardizing the raters. PDT is a method by which faculty build a shared mental model and come to agreement on assessment criteria as a group. Next, through FoRT, faculty define the criteria for superior, satisfactory, and marginal performance, or better yet, performance criteria may be based on a developmental scale. For example, Entrustable Professional Activities (EPAs) rank the entrustment of learners along a continuum of permissions ranging from the learner who requires direct, proactive supervision to the learner who is entrusted to act with supervision not readily available.[147] Raters then score videos of learners (or other learner work products like a written note) at the varying levels of performance. A facilitator provides feedback on the "true" ratings, and the group discusses any discrepancies between individual raters' scores and the "true" score. Usually only faculty will participate in PDT and the first few steps of FoRT to define the criteria for levels of performance, but when SPs participate as raters of performance they must also participate in scoring videos, or notes, et cetera, and get feedback on their ratings. If this training is not done properly, a candidate's score may simply reflect the preferences of the rater (who may be a "hawk" or a "dove") as opposed to the learner's true ability.

Implementation of Standardized Patient Assessments

The logistical complexity of implementing an SP-based assessment should not be underestimated.[40,94,148] Large-scale, high-stakes assessments obviously require meticulous planning with a large interdependent team.[5] Several types of commercial software exist for recording, storing, and analyzing the often very large volume of data that is generated by an SP assessment like an OSCE.

Exam security must be taken very seriously during high-stakes SP assessments, especially since the same OSCE cases must often be administered multiple times over a number of days—or even months in the case of a licensing exam—to test all candidates sequentially. Some argue that because an OSCE requires examinees to demonstrate what they can do, knowing the tasks ahead of time may not provide much of an advantage.[92] In support of this argument, some studies show that while on average, examinees who retake high-stakes SP assessments do improve, being exposed to repeat cases or SPs does not give examinees an advantage.[149,150] Of course, examinee "cheating" is not really a concern for skills such as communication and interpersonal skills. In fact, it is often advisable to let candidates know the frameworks by which they will be assessed in advance. This practice allows students to work toward defined standards and also ensures that everyone starts on a level playing field.[9] On the other hand, students who know something about an OSCE's case content beforehand have been shown to score higher, with access to larger amounts of test material resulting in even higher scores.[151] Similarly, students who take the same cases later during the run of an OSCE have been shown to perform better.[152] This is a phenomenon known as the grapevine effect, and it is attributed to students sharing case information with one another despite pledges not to do so. Strategies to try to minimize cheating include grouping portions of the OSCE so that all examinees take the same cases in a shorter period of time and quarantining examinees for the duration of the OSCE.[152] For lower-stakes assessments, multiple versions of a case with key differences may be created. For example, one version of a vaginal discharge case may be a diagnosis of bacterial vaginosis, another may be trichomoniasis, and a third may be vaginal candidiasis. When similar cases yield systematic differences in scores, a score-equating strategy may be employed to make the scores comparable.[153,154]

Scoring and Psychometrics

Applying Kane's Validity Framework

The psychometric properties of SP-based assessments have been studied in depth for decades.[84,87,153] This sort of rigorous study allowed for the development of SP-based assessments used to make the highest-stakes determinations of medical certification and licensure.[9] Yet even low-stakes assessments utilizing SPs should be based on some degree of validity evidence. As discussed in Chapter 2 of this text, the concept of validity has evolved over time, and based on frameworks articulated by Messick[155] and Kane,[156] validity is now viewed not as a property of an assessment but as an argument with evidence to support the purpose of the assessment. In particular, Kane's framework includes four key inferences: scoring, generalization, extrapolation, and implication, which can be considered in a stepwise manner to move from the observation of performance to a final decision about the examinee. Several scholars have detailed how Kane's validity framework can be applied to performance-based assessments.[34,35,38]

Scoring

In Kane's framework, support for *scoring* includes evidence that the assessment data accurately reflect how well the examinees performed on the assessment. In SP-based assessments some practices that will support the scoring argument include:[38]

- Engaging content experts to develop scoring rubrics based on evidence and key features
- Developing rubrics with behavioral anchors to reduce rater bias
- Training SPs in a standard and stringent way to portray cases accurately
- Training raters in a rigorous way—such as through PDT and FoRT as noted earlier—so that rubrics are applied as intended
- Monitoring outcomes for learners from backgrounds underrepresented in medicine to assess for bias

Generalization

Generalization in Kane's framework focuses on how well the observed scores reflect unbiased, reliable scores across all possible performances. The classic concept of reliability, or reproducibility, falls under the generalization inference. While all the techniques listed in this section are important to consider when building the validity argument for an SP-based assessment, one of the greatest threats to validity for most OSCEs is the limited number of cases and/or the limited number of items assessed in each case.[33,157,158] Performance on SP encounters is quite case specific. For example, a student who is able to perform well on a case of chest pain may not be able to perform equally well on a case of headache, so there is limited generalizability from one clinical scenario to another.[159] Often the most important factor in improving reliability, and hence generalizability, of an OSCE is to include an adequate number of cases sampling an adequate range of skills.[40,160,161] Broadly speaking, about 4 to 8 hours of testing time[162] or 8 to 10 cases[33] are required to result in a reasonable degree of reliability. Specific actions that will support the generalizability argument for an OSCE include:

- Blueprinting the assessment in a systematic way to purposefully sample an appropriate breadth and depth of the defined content area[38]
- Maximizing the number of cases seen by each examinee as noted earlier[33,38]
- Limiting the number of raters for each case, and possibly having just one rater per case to reduce rater variance[33]
- Monitoring rater reliability[34]

Extrapolation

Evidence for extrapolation links performance on an assessment to performance in the real world. One strength of SP-based assessments is that they more closely reflect actual clinical performance than, for example, a multiple-choice exam. Stronger evidence for extrapolation, however, often results in a weaker argument for generalization. While OSCEs are much closer to real-life performance than multiple-choice exams, OSCEs are only able to assess a limited amount of content. Multiple-choice exams can sample a very broad range of topics, which supports the generalizability argument. Even the most rigorous OSCEs, however, will only include approximately 10 to 12 stations, and therefore 10 to 12 clinical topics. In this way, OSCEs support the argument for extrapolation at the expense of generalization.[34] Strategies for building an extrapolation argument include:

- Constructing cases that authentically represent the clinical situation of interest.[38] This may sometimes be accomplished by basing SP cases on real patient cases.
- Piloting cases to determine that there is sufficient time and that the level of difficulty is appropriate to the learners.[38]
- Correlating performance with experience of the examinee, by showing that experts score higher than novice examinees.[34]
- Demonstrating that OSCE scores are correlated with external assessments, such as real-world observation[163] or a national licensing exam.[50]

Implication

The final inference in Kane's framework requires evidence that the implications, or decisions made based on the test score, lead to appropriate consequences for the examinees and other stakeholders. Some scholars have found that it can be a challenge to find suitable evidence for the implication argument for performance-based assessments,[34,35] but some approaches may include:

- Beginning with the end in mind by stipulating what decisions will be made based on the results of the assessment[38]
- Employing defensible standard-setting techniques when choosing cut scores[38]
- Showing that students who participate in remediation have differential improvement or are more likely to succeed in future assessments if they participate in remediation (see Chapter 2)

In the end, it is not possible to say that an SP-based assessment has been "validated," but the more evidence that is gathered to support the assumptions in the preceding lists, the stronger the validity argument will be.

Standard Setting

For many SP-based assessments, namely those employed to support learning, there is little need to develop or apply specific performance standards. If competency or proficiency decisions are not being made, setting specific performance standards is usually not necessary. Instead, norm-referenced scores, such as percentiles or Z-scores, can be used to provide formative feedback to the examinees. These scores can be augmented with narrative comments from SPs or faculty. While normative scores are simple to calculate, a major drawback is that learners are presented with their performance relative to others in the assessment cohort instead of relative to a criterion standard. Unless learners have a clear understanding of optimal performance, the benefit of assessment for learning will be limited.[52] In contrast to normative scoring, when an assessment is being used for summative purposes (e.g., promotion, graduation, licensure), there is a need to determine the score, or scores, that delimit those who possess adequate skills from those who do not. In these circumstances, absolute, or criterion-referenced, standards must be set.

Standard-setting methods either focus on examination materials and are considered "test centered," or focus on examinee performance and are considered "examinee centered."[164] The most common test-centered method used for performance-based assessments is the modified Angoff, while the most common examinee-centered methods are the borderline group and borderline regression methods.[165,166] In the modified Angoff method, a group of experts are asked to review each checklist item for an SP case and to estimate the percentage of minimally competent students (i.e., students who would just meet the passing standard) who would get that item correct. Disagreements in scores are discussed and if a consensus is not reached, the item may be thrown out. Scores chosen by the experts are then averaged across all experts and all checklist items, and the average becomes the passing standard. Instead of reviewing individual checklist items, experts may also be asked to estimate a borderline student's score for a whole OSCE case. This may be preferable since checklist items are rarely completely independent of one another.[165] An advantage of the modified Angoff is that the students know the passing standard before they take the exam, while a disadvantage is the time and effort required of several experts to set the cut score.[166]

In the borderline group method, examinee performance is reviewed by experts and categorized as unsatisfactory, borderline, or satisfactory. The cut score is simply the mean score of the borderline students. This method is easy to implement, but it requires a larger cohort of students to have enough students who fall into the borderline category.[166]

The borderline regression method begins the same way as the borderline group method with experts categorizing students' scores as unsatisfactory, borderline, or satisfactory. Often for borderline regression, the students' scores will be divided into a larger number of categories such as inferior, poor, borderline unsatisfactory, borderline satisfactory, good, and excellent, which is the scale that has been used by the Medical Council of Canada.[167] Linear regression is then applied with the students' scores as the dependent variable and the grades as the independent variable. The passing score is then the score corresponding to the borderline grade.[165,166] The borderline regression method can be used with a much smaller cohort of examinees and a smaller number of borderline examinees. It also provides a wider array of metrics that can be used when evaluating the quality of the OSCE later on.[154] Any of these criterion-referenced methods may be applied to an individual case or may be applied to particular competencies such as communication skills, history taking, or physical exam skills across multiple cases. Some scholars emphasize that there is no one "best" standard setting method, and instead that the method chosen should be based on the goals of the assessment and the resources available for standard setting.[38,165] Other scholars note that the borderline regression method has the best validity evidence for OSCE standard setting.[92,166]

Regardless of which criterion-referenced method is used, the experts participating in the standard setting must be very familiar with the OSCE format, the exam content, and the level of learners being assessed.[165,166] Data show that experts tend to have unrealistically high performance expectations for OSCE examinees.[168] Therefore when embarking upon the standard setting process for SP-based examinations, it is particularly important that the standard setting panelists (usually clinicians) have a common definition of the purpose of the assessment and are intimately aware of the complexities and nuances of the evaluation method. Often, in addition to a thorough orientation, standard setting panelists are invited to partake in part of the assessment (e.g., be an examinee for a few cases) as a means to align their expectations with reality.[165]

Once standards are set for individual cases or individual skills, often a passing score needs to be determined for the examination as a whole. In this case the scoring can be either *compensatory* or conjunctive.[38,165] In compensatory scoring, the overall score is simply the average of each case or component score. In this way, low performance on one case or one skill is *compensated for* by higher performance on other cases or other skills. This approach may be appropriate when students may have had variable access to learning opportunities or when trying to reward students with a diverse array of strengths. In contrast, in conjunctive scoring, examinees must pass a predetermined number of cases, or reach the passing standard on certain skills. In some circumstances it may be reasonable to apply compensatory scoring across cases (e.g., chest pain, shortness of breath, abdominal pain, back pain) but still require students to pass each skill (e.g., history taking, physical examination, communication skills) using conjunctive scoring.[165]

Evaluation and Quality Assurance

For summative, high-stakes assessments with SPs, it is critical to evaluate the quality of the assessment itself. The same way a learner cannot be assessed by a single exam, the program of assessment cannot be evaluated with a single metric, but instead requires systematic and continuous evaluation.[38,154] Quantitative analysis of the performance of an OSCE typically requires the expertise of a psychometrician,[154,169] but there are also many straightforward analyses that can be completed without an advanced knowledge of statistics.

Simple steps include scanning checklists to be sure items were not left blank and systematic errors were not made in scoring. If an OSCE is conducted over multiple sites or at several different time points, then scores should be compared across sites or times to ensure that they are aligned.[154] Cases and individual items should be reviewed to identify outliers such as items or cases with very low scores, which may provide valuable feedback to the curriculum developers.[38] If a large group of students perform at a low level on a particular case, then the curriculum would need to be adjusted to ensure that students are being given the opportunity to learn that particular material before the exam. In addition, soliciting feedback from any faculty involved in administering or scoring an OSCE can be extremely helpful for refining cases.[40] Soliciting feedback from students themselves can also provide useful feedback for the curriculum and can help elucidate the impact of the OSCE itself on learning.[169]

SP performance should also be periodically monitored either live or via recorded encounters to ensure fidelity of case portrayal. If an SP is not performing a case as expected (e.g., if the SP's affect is not consistent with the case), then the examinee may be less likely to ask certain questions and/or perform related physical examination maneuvers. As a result, the data gathering score for the examinee will be error-prone. Quality assurance should include periodic observation, with feedback provided to the SP.

Also, despite efforts to develop high-quality checklist items and limit checklist length to avoid excessive cognitive load for SPs, it is likely that recording errors will occur.[170,171] SPs tend to commit more errors of commission than omission, giving examinees credit for action not taken about two or three times more often than failing to record actual examinee actions.[115,172] Nevertheless efforts to ensure that SPs are optimally prepared for their simulation roles, combined with the implementation of quality assurance programs that provide for periodic observation and monitoring of SP portrayal and scoring accuracy, can significantly reduce SP errors in these areas.[173] For any scores that are obtained, some subset should be verified, usually through the use of a second rater—either an SP, a trainer, or a content expert. While this second score will likely do little to enhance the overall reliability of the assessment being conducted, provided that a proper sampling framework is utilized, these data can be used to identify SPs who may not be scoring accurately and/or other assessors who are not using the rating scales as intended. As noted earlier, however, if additional SPs are available and enhanced overall reliability is the goal it makes more sense to add an extra case rather than provide additional scorers for existing cases.[33,158]

New Directions in Standardized Patient Assessments

Over the past 50 years, the use of SP-based education and assessments has expanded immensely, becoming part of standard education practice for healthcare professionals both within and outside medicine. Technologic innovations have enabled increasingly complex multifaceted simulation stations, expanding the skills that can be reasonably evaluated by incorporation of mannequins, task trainers, and virtual reality. In addition, with cost and logistic feasibility the major limiting factors for SP assessments, the future of automated grading and improved software platforms promises to fuel expansion in the coming decades by bringing down potential barriers for implementation and sustainability. Here we discuss these areas of expansion and innovation.

Innovation Highlights

There have been several recent highlights within SP innovations. One key advantage of simulation is the ability to practice an array of specific or challenging communication skills in a lower-stakes environment prior to applications in clinical care. Recently, SPs have been used to assess communication relevant to specific patient populations experiencing structural risk or oppression, including assessing gender affirming language in transgender health–related encounters[174,175] and approaching conversations about physical disabilities.[176] SPs can be used to assess communication regarding other difficult topics, such as the discussion of vaccine hesitancy,[177] application of value-based care,[178] or relaying pertinent handoff information via a near-peer OSCE.[179]

Telemedicine has long been appreciated as a mechanism to expand timely and cost-effective care, but few institutions had successfully incorporated telemedicine SP-based assessments prior to marked expansion in telemedicine care during the COVID-19 pandemic.[180,181] The need during the pandemic to rapidly convert OSCEs to virtual formats sped the adoption of telemedicine encounters within OSCEs, with the assessment of physical examination proving the greatest area of challenge, as learners were typically invited to describe the examinations they would ideally perform if they had been in person.[182–184] It is likely that with the return to in-person OSCEs, the incorporation of telemedicine encounters within SP assessments can find a more authentic application; for example, limiting the case platforms to those that would reasonably receive telemedicine care in real practice (e.g., the evaluation of common rashes or conjunctivitis as opposed to acute onset of chest pain that would require urgent in-person examination).

Expansion of Learner Groups

While initially developed for assessment of medical students, the advantages of SP-based assessments to evaluate clinical competence has led to a similar adoption by most healthcare disciplines, including podiatry, occupational therapy, dentistry, nursing, audiology, and pharmacy.[17,185–189] Several disciplines, such as podiatry, have taken a similar approach by implementing SP assessments as a standard practice in all training programs as well as in a certification examination.[17] As is the case in medical education, SP assessments have been used effectively to teach and assess skills relating to interpersonal communication, history, physical examination, and patient education, as well as to address specific competencies relevant for the individual healthcare field, such as dental students' ability to respond appropriately to medical emergencies in the dental office or midwives' ability to provide sensitive sexual health counseling.[190–193]

Interprofessional Collaboration

Traditionally, SP-based assessments have been used to evaluate the clinical skills of individual practitioners. However, patient care is ultimately provided by healthcare teams rather than individuals, and effective teamwork is increasingly seen as a key competency required to reduce healthcare errors and improve patient safety.[194] As a result, SPs are increasingly being employed for assessing teamwork skills,[195–197] necessitating the development of simulation scenarios that incorporate additional roles beyond a single provider and a single SP. For team-based assessments, SPs can assess the teamwork of learners brought together from different healthcare disciplines, or SPs may be trained to play the role of a healthcare team member. While the latter may be difficult to employ for higher-stakes assessments given the challenge of high-fidelity training for healthcare expertise, interprofessional OSCEs can serve a vital pedagogical role in developing and enhancing interprofessional skills, and in underlining their importance both for the initial training of healthcare workers and workplace-based continuing education.[198]

Multifaceted Simulation

The provision of healthcare services can be quite complex, involving numerous settings, multiple providers, and various technologies. Simulation modalities can be combined to create more authentic clinical experiences for complex scenarios. For example, one could simulate a tragic event with an electromechanical mannequin (e.g., patient death), then follow this with an SP-based simulation that requires the practitioner to break bad news to a relative. The use of multiple simulation modalities can allow for the assessment of skills that would be impossible to measure, at least with any degree of fidelity, with SP-based methods alone (see Chapter 13).

While SPs can be quite proficient in simulating symptoms, and even some examination findings (e.g., neurological examination abnormalities), they may not be able to simulate other signs as described. Many SP-based assessments include props and/or employ some form of moulage that can increase the fidelity of the simulation and allow the participant to better "suspend disbelief" attributable to the less than perfect modeling of certain patient conditions. There are several technological innovations that can expand the measurement domain and address concerns regarding the lack of physical findings in typical SP-based assessments. These include, among others, stethoscopes with programmed heart sounds and breast models (worn by an SP) that have palpable masses.

Technology can also be used to provide additional perspectives on the clinical encounter—for example, using virtual reality to simulate being truly immersed in the experience or technologies such as Google Glass to be able to experience the patient perspective as a part of formative feedback.[199] Combining simulation modalities and incorporating technologies that allow individuals to model patients with physical findings can help improve the content validity of SP-based assessments (see Chapter 13).

Scoring and Automation

Depending on what is being measured, the scoring of SP-based assessments has generally been accomplished with the use of checklists and/or rating scales. While these tools can yield valid and reliable measures of ability, they can be difficult to construct and expensive to use. As such, more automated scoring modalities would be helpful. Novel approaches applying machine learning to OSCE transcripts demonstrate the ability to score aspects of the interview content and even communication skills with potential to track student progress and inform learning goals.[200]

For SP-based assessments that utilize postencounter exercises (e.g., writing a patient note, completing an electronic record), automated scoring, as is done in other fields, is certainly possible.[201] Even if the technology for automated scoring is not perfect, it may be helpful for quality assurance procedures and could improve efficiency.

Over the past decade, systems to record simulation-based activities and store relevant data have become more user friendly and less expensive, enabling scoring activities to be done externally via video review and also including tools for tracking and comparing student and rater performance. Asynchronous external review adds efficiency and simplifies logistics for faculty and staff.

Conclusion

SP-based assessments require learners to "show" their clinical skills, corresponding to the third level of Miller's pyramid, in contrast to assessments of lower-level demonstration of knowledge. By focusing learners, educators, and institutions on the clinical encounter, SP assessments drive learning toward patient-centered skills within a safe educational environment. The ability of educators to control the simulated environment, unlike the clinical environment, allows for the development of a program of assessment that includes SPs, aligns with the assessment vision, applies a competency framework, and enables the collection of validity evidence to support high-stakes decisions. While there are challenges to the use of SP-based assessments, such as cost and logistical complexity, the expansion of SP assessments in the past decades speak to their many strengths as a tool for competency-based assessments. Despite recent changes in clinical licensure examinations, high-stakes OSCEs will likely remain a critical component in the assessment of health professions students.

Annotated Bibliography

1. Boursicot K, Roberts T. How to set up an OSCE. *Clin Teach.* 2005;2(1):16–20. doi:10.1111/j.1743-498X.2005.00053.x.
   This is a brief, user-friendly guide for developing an OSCE that includes many practical tips and diagrams. It includes a photo of multiple OSCE stations set up in what appears to be a museum with wood dividers between stations. Fortunately, many medical schools now have simulation centers where each station has its own dedicated exam room. Reference #92 below.
2. Cleland JA, Abe K, Rethans JJ. The use of simulated patients in medical education: AMEE Guide No 42. *Med Teach.* 2009 Jun;31(6):477–486. doi:10.1080/01421590903002821.
   This AMEE Guide is an overview of utilizing SPs in medical education. After a review of the evolution of SPs, it describes how to recruit, select, and train SPs. It also covers the many ways SPs are used from formative teaching sessions to high-stakes assessment. Reference #19 below.
3. Daniels VJ, Pugh D. Twelve tips for developing an OSCE that measures what you want. *Med Teach.* 2018 Dec;40(12):1208–1213. doi:10.1080/0142159X.2017.1390214.
   This Twelve Tips paper is a well-referenced and still easily comprehensible set of recommendations for developing an OSCE based on Kane's validity framework. The best practices described in this paper would be very valuable when developing a rigorous, high-stakes OSCE. Reference #38 below.
4. Khan KZ, Ramachandran S, Gaunt K, Pushkar P. The Objective Structured Clinical Examination (OSCE): AMEE Guide No. 81. Part I: an historical and theoretical perspective. *Med Teach.* 2013 Sep;35(9):e1437–e1446. doi:10.3109/0142159X.2013.818634.
   This is the first of a two-part AMEE Guide that provides an authoritative overview of OSCEs. Part I focuses on the theoretical underpinnings and educational principles of OSCEs. It also reviews the history of OSCEs and the evolution of OSCEs over time. Reference #22 below.
5. Khan KZ, Gaunt K, Ramachandran S, Pushkar P. The Objective Structured Clinical Examination (OSCE): AMEE Guide No. 81. Part II: organisation & administration. *Med Teach.* 2013 Sep;35(9): e1447–e1463. doi:10.3109/0142159X.2013.818635.
   This is Part II of the AMEE Guide on OSCEs. This part is a practical guide that covers the logistics of developing an OSCE. It includes blueprinting, case development, checklist development, scoring, rater training, administering the OSCE, and follow-up tasks. Reference #40 below.
6. Pugh D, Smee S. Medical Council of Canada: Guidelines for the Development of Objective Structured Clinical Examination (OSCE) Cases. Accessed September 25, 2022. https://mcc.ca/media/OSCE-Booklet-2014.pdf.
   This booklet from the Medical Council of Canada provides step-by-step instructions for creating a high-stakes OSCE. It contains many clear and specific examples including samples of checklists, rating scales, patient encounter probes for use after the SP encounter, and a basic case template. Reference #98 below.

7. Yudkowsky R. Performance tests. In: Yudkowsky R, Park YS, Downing SM, eds. *Assessment in Health Professions Education*. 2nd ed. Routledge; 2020:141–159.
This chapter is a rigorous overview of performance tests with a focus on SP-based assessments and OSCEs. The explanations are exceptionally clear and concise. Even educators with long experience in developing and running OSCEs will benefit from reading this chapter. Reference #33 below.

References

1. Ilgen JS, Ma IW, Hatala R, Cook DA. A systematic review of validity evidence for checklists versus global rating scales in simulation-based assessment. *Med Educ*. 2015 Feb;49(2):161–173. doi:10.1111/medu.12621.
2. Varkey P, Natt N, Lesnick T, Downing S, Yudkowsky R. Validity evidence for an OSCE to assess competency in systems-based practice and practice-based learning and improvement: a preliminary investigation. *Acad Med*. 2008 Aug;83(8):775–780. doi:10.1097/ACM.0b013e31817ec873.
3. AAMC Data SP/OSCE Required Final Examinations. AAMC. Accessed September 24, 2022. https://www.aamc.org/data-reports/curriculum-reports/interactive-data/sp/osce-required-final-examinations.
4. Reznick RK, Blackmore D, Dauphinée WD, Rothman AI, Smee S. Large-scale high-stakes testing with an OSCE: report from the Medical Council of Canada. *Acad Med J Assoc Am Med Coll*. 1996 Jan;71(1 Suppl):S19–S21. doi:10.1097/00001888-199601000-00031.
5. Whelan GP. Educational commission for foreign medical graduates: clinical skills assessment prototype. *Med Teach*. 1999;21(2):156–160. doi:10.1080/01421599979789.
6. Wallace J, Rao R, Haslam R. Simulated patients and objective structured clinical examinations: review of their use in medical education. *Adv Psychiatr Treat*. 2002;8(5):342–348. doi:10.1192/apt.8.5.342.
7. Swanson DB, Roberts TE. Trends in national licensing examinations in medicine. *Med Educ*. 2016 Jan;50(1):101–114. doi:10.1111/medu.12810.
8. Zimmermann P, Kadmon M. Standardized examinees: development of a new tool to evaluate factors influencing OSCE scores and to train examiners. *GMS J Med Educ*. 2020 Jun 15;37(4):Doc40. doi:10.3205/zma001333.
9. Dillon GF, Boulet JR, Hawkins RE, Swanson DB. Simulations in the United States Medical Licensing Examination (USMLE). *Qual Saf Health Care*. 2004 Oct;13(Suppl 1):i41–i45. doi:10.1136/qhc.13.suppl_1.i41 Suppl 1.
10. Hawkins RE, Swanson DB, Dillon GF, Clauser B. The introduction of clinical skills assessment into the United States Medical Licensing Examination (USMLE): a description of USMLE Step 2 Clinical Skills (CS). *J Med Licens Discip*. 2005;91:22–25. doi:10.30770/2572-1852-91.3.22.
11. Katsufrakis PJ, Chaudhry HJ. Evolution of clinical skills assessment in the USMLE: looking to the future after Step 2 CS discontinuation. *Acad Med*. 2021 Sep 1;96(9):1236–1238. doi:10.1097/ACM.0000000000004214.
12. Nevins AB, Boscardin CK, Kahn D, et al. A call to action from the California Consortium for the Assessment of Clinical Competence: making the case for regional collaboration. *Acad Med*. 2022 Sep 1;97(9):1289–1294. doi:10.1097/ACM.0000000000004663.
13. Barrows HS, Abrahamson S. The programmed patient: a technique for appraising student performance in clinical neurology. *Acad Med*. 1964 Aug;39(8):802–805. PMID: 14180699.
14. Barrows HS. An overview of the uses of standardized patients for teaching and evaluating clinical skills. *Acad Med*. 1993 Jun;68(6):443–451. doi:10.1097/00001888-199306000-00002 discussion 451–453.
15. Jacobson AN, Bratberg JP, Monk M, Ferrentino J. Retention of student pharmacists' knowledge and skills regarding overdose management with naloxone. *Subst Abuse*. 2018;39(2):193–198. doi:10.1080/08897077.2018.1439797.
16. Luke S, Petitt E, Tombrella J, McGoff E. Virtual evaluation of clinical competence in nurse practitioner students. *Med Sci Educ*. 2021 May 24;31(4):1267–1271. doi:10.1007/s40670-021-01312-z.
17. Errichetti A, Eckles R, Beto J, Gross GA, Lorion AM. The use of patient simulations to teach and assess clinical competencies in colleges of podiatric medicine: a survey of US podiatric medical schools. *J Am Podiatr Med Assoc*. 2022 Apr 27;112(2):20–077. doi:10.7547/20-077.
18. Han SY, Lee SH, Chae H. Developing a best practice framework for clinical competency education in the traditional East-Asian medicine curriculum. *BMC Med Educ*. 2022 May 10;22(1):352. doi:10.1186/s12909-022-03398-4.
19. Cleland JA, Abe K, Rethans JJ. The use of simulated patients in medical education: AMEE Guide No 42. *Med Teach*. 2009 Jun;31(6):477–486. doi:10.1080/01421590903002821.
20. ASPEducators.org. Accessed September 24, 2022. https://www.aspeducators.org/
21. Harden RM, Stevenson M, Downie WW, Wilson GM. Assessment of clinical competence using objective structured examination. *Br Med J*. 1975 Feb 22;1(5955):447–451. doi:10.1136/bmj.1.5955.447.
22. Khan KZ, Ramachandran S, Gaunt K, Pushkar P. The Objective Structured Clinical Examination (OSCE): AMEE Guide No. 81. Part I: an historical and theoretical perspective. *Med Teach*. 2013 Sep;35(9):e1437–e1446. doi:10.3109/0142159X.2013.818634.
23. Hauer KE, Teherani A, Kerr KM, O'Sullivan PS, Irby DM. Impact of the United States Medical Licensing Examination Step 2 Clinical Skills exam on medical school clinical skills assessment. *Acad Med*. 2006 Oct;81(10 Suppl):S13–S16. doi:10.1097/01.ACM.0000236531.32318.02.
24. Gilliland WR, La Rochelle J, Hawkins R, et al. Changes in clinical skills education resulting from the introduction of the USMLE step 2 clinical skills (CS) examination. *Med Teach*. 2008;30(3):325–327. doi:10.1080/01421590801953026.
25. Boulet JR, Smee SM, Dillon GF, Gimpel JR. The use of standardized patient assessments for certification and licensure decisions. *Simul Heal*. 2009 Spring;4(1):35–42. doi:10.1097/SIH.0b013e318182fc6c.
26. Holmboe ES. Faculty and the observation of trainees' clinical skills: problems and opportunities. *Acad Med*. 2004 Jan;79(1):16–22. doi:10.1097/00001888-200401000-00006.
27. Hauer KE, O'Sullivan PS, Fitzhenry K, Boscardin C. Translating theory into practice: implementing a program of assessment. *Acad Med*. 2018 Mar;93(3):444–450. doi:10.1097/ACM.0000000000001995.
28. Mookherjee S, Chang A, Boscardin CK, Hauer KE. How to develop a competency-based examination blueprint for longitudinal standardized patient clinical skills assessments. *Med Teach*. 2013 Nov;35(11):883–890. doi:10.3109/0142159X.2013.809408.

29. Chalabian J, Garman K, Wallace P, Dunnington G. Clinical breast evaluation skills of house officers and students. *Am Surg.* 1996 Oct;62(10):840–845. PMID: 8813167.
30. Colletti L, Gruppen L, Barclay M, Stern D. Teaching students to break bad news. *Am J Surg.* 2001 Jul;182(1):20–23. doi:10.1016/s0002-9610(01)00651-1.
31. Foley KL, George G, Crandall SJ, Walker KH, Marion GS, Spangler JG. Training and evaluating tobacco-specific standardized patient instructors. *Fam Med.* 2006 Jan;38(1):28–37. PMID: 16378256.
32. Nestel D, Clark S, Tabak D, et al. Defining responsibilities of simulated patients in medical education. *Simul Heal.* 2010 Jun;5(3):161–168. doi:10.1097/SIH.0b013e3181de1cb6.
33. Yudkowsky R. Performance tests. In: Yudkowsky R, Park YS, Downing SM, eds. *Assessment in Health Professions Education.* 2nd ed. Routledge; 2020:141–159.
34. Cook DA, Brydges R, Ginsburg S, Hatala R. A contemporary approach to validity arguments: a practical guide to Kane's framework. *Med Educ.* 2015 Jun;49(6):560–575. doi:10.1111/medu.12678.
35. Tavares W, Brydges R, Myre P, et al. Applying Kane's validity framework to a simulation based assessment of clinical competence. *Adv Health Sci Educ Theory Pract.* 2018 May;23(2):323–338. doi:10.1007/s10459-017-9800-3.
36. Epstein RM, Hundert EM. Defining and assessing professional competence. *JAMA.* 2002 Jan 9;287(2):226–235. doi:10.1001/jama.287.2.226.
37. Cooke M, Irby DM, Sullivan W, Ludmerer KM. American medical education 100 years after the flexner report. *N Engl J Med.* 2006 Sep 28;355(13):1339–1344. doi:10.1056/NEJMra055445.
38. Daniels VJ, Pugh D. Twelve tips for developing an OSCE that measures what you want. *Med Teach.* 2018 Dec;40(12):1208–1213. doi:10.1080/0142159X.2017.1390214.
39. Moreau KA. Exploring the connections between programmatic assessment and program evaluation within competency-based medical education programs. *Med Teach.* 2021 Mar;43(3):250–252. doi:10.1080/0142159X.2020.1841128.
40. Khan KZ, Gaunt K, Ramachandran S, Pushkar P. The Objective Structured Clinical Examination (OSCE): AMEE Guide No. 81. Part II: organisation & administration. *Med Teach.* 2013 Sep;35(9):e1447–e1463. doi:10.3109/0142159X.2013.818635.
41. Patricio MF, Juliao M, Fareleira F, Carneiro AV. Is the OSCE a feasible tool to assess competencies in undergraduate medical education? *Med Teach.* 2013 Jun;35(6):503–514. doi:10.3109/0142159X.2013.774330.
42. Morrison LJ, Barrows HS. Developing consortia for clinical practice examinations: the macy project. *Teach Learn Med.* 1994;6:23–27. doi:10.1080/10401339409539638.
43. Fernandez A, Wang F, Braveman M, Finkas LK, Hauer KE. Impact of student ethnicity and primary childhood language on communication skill assessment in a clinical performance examination. *J Gen Intern Med.* 2007 Aug;22(8):1155–1160. doi:10.1007/s11606-007-0250-0.
44. Berg K, Blatt B, Lopreiato J, et al. Standardized patient assessment of medical student empathy: ethnicity and gender effects in a multi-institutional study. *Acad Med.* 2015 Jan;90(1):105–111. doi:10.1097/ACM.0000000000000529.
45. Chalabian J, Dunnington G. Do our current assessments assure competency in clinical breast evaluation skills? *Am J Surg.* 1998 Jun;175(6):497–502. doi:10.1016/s0002-9610(98)00075-0.
46. Bell K, Boshuizen HP, Scherpbier A, Dornan T. When only the real thing will do: junior medical students' learning from real patients. *Med Educ.* 2009 Nov;43(11):1036–1043. doi:10.1111/j.1365-2923.2009.03508.x.
47. Rethans JJ, Sturmans F, Drop R, Vleuten C, Hobus P. Does competence of general practitioners predict their performance? Comparison between examination setting and actual practice. *BMJ.* 1991 Nov 30;303(6814):1377–1380. doi:10.1136/bmj.303.6814.1377.
48. Kopelow ML, Schnabl GK, Hassard TH. Assessing practicing physicians in two settings using standardized patients. *Acad Med.* 1992 Oct;67(10 Suppl):S19–S21. doi:10.1097/00001888-199210000-00026.
49. Dong T, Zahn C, Saguil A, et al. The associations between clerkship objective structured clinical examination (OSCE) grades and subsequent performance. *Teach Learn Med.* 2017 Jul-Sep;29(3):280–285. doi:10.1080/10401334.2017.1279057.
50. Pugh D, Bhanji F, Cole G, et al. Do OSCE progress test scores predict performance in a national high-stakes examination? *Med Educ.* 2016 Mar;50(3):351–358. doi:10.1111/medu.12942.
51. van der Vleuten CPM, Schuwirth LWT, Driessen EW, et al. A model for programmatic assessment fit for purpose. *Med Teach.* 2012;34(3):205–214. doi:10.3109/0142159X.2012.652239.
52. Schuwirth LWT, Van der Vleuten CPM. Programmatic assessment: from assessment of learning to assessment for learning. *Med Teach.* 2011;33(6):478–485. doi:10.3109/0142159X.2011.565828.
53. van der Vleuten CPM, Schuwirth LWT, Driessen EW, Govaerts MJB, Heeneman S. Twelve tips for programmatic assessment. *Med Teach.* 2015 Jul;37(7):641–646. doi:10.3109/0142159X.2014.973388.
54. Swan Sein A, Rashid H, Meka J, Amiel J, Pluta W. Twelve tips for embedding assessment for and as learning practices in a programmatic assessment system. *Med Teach.* 2021 Mar;43(3):300–306. doi:10.1080/0142159X.2020.1789081.
55. Torre D, Rice NE, Ryan A, et al. Ottawa 2020 consensus statements for programmatic assessment–2. Implementation and practice. *Med Teach.* 2021 Oct;43(10):1149–1160. doi:10.1080/0142159X.2021.1956681.
56. Ross S, Hauer KE, Wycliffe-Jones K, et al. Key considerations in planning and designing programmatic assessment in competency-based medical education. *Med Teach.* 2021 Jul;43(7):758–764. doi:10.1080/0142159X.2021.1925099.
57. Schuwirth L, van der Vleuten C, Durning SJ. What programmatic assessment in medical education can learn from healthcare. *Perspect Med Educ.* 2017 Aug;6(4):211–215. doi:10.1007/s40037-017-0345-1.
58. Iobst WF, Holmboe ES. Programmatic assessment: the secret sauce of effective CBME implementation. *J Grad Med Educ.* 2020 Aug;12(4):518–521. doi:10.4300/JGME-D-20-00702.1.
59. Edgar L, Roberts S, Holmboe E. Milestones 2.0: a step forward. *J Grad Med Educ.* 2018 Jun;10(3):367–369. doi:10.4300/JGME-D-18-00372.1.
60. Swing S. The ACGME outcome project: retrospective and prospective. *Med Teach.* 2007 Sep;29(7):648–654. doi:10.1080/01421590701392903.
61. CanMEDS Framework: The Royal College of Physicians and Surgeons of Canada. Accessed September 25, 2022. https://www.royalcollege.ca/rcsite/canmeds/canmeds-framework-e
62. General Medical Council: Outcomes for Graduates. Accessed September 25, 2022. https://www.gmc-uk.org/education/standards-guidance-and-curricula/standards-and-outcomes/outcomes-for-graduates/outcomes-for-graduates.

63. Hauff SR, Hopson LR, Losman E, et al. Programmatic assessment of level 1 milestones in incoming interns. *Acad Emerg Med.* 2014 Jun;21(6):694–698. doi:10.1111/acem.12393.
64. Beeson MS, Vozenilek JA. Specialty milestones and the next accreditation system: an opportunity for the simulation community. *Simul Healthc.* 2014 Jun;9(3):184–191. doi:10.1097/SIH.0000000000000006.
65. Peña A. The Dreyfus model of clinical problem-solving skills acquisition: a critical perspective. *Med Educ Online.* 2010;15. doi:10.3402/meo.v15i0.4846.
66. MD Competency Milestones | UCSF Medical Education. Accessed September 29, 2022. https://meded.ucsf.edu/md-program/current-students/curriculum/md-competency-milestones.
67. Lie D, Bereknyei S, Braddock CHI, Encinas J, Ahearn S, Boker JR. Assessing medical students' skills in working with interpreters during patient encounters: a validation study of the interpreter scale. *Acad Med.* 2009 May;84(5):643–650. doi:10.1097/ACM.0b013e31819faec8.
68. Brown RS, Graham CL, Richeson N, Wu J, McDermott S. Evaluation of medical student performance on objective structured clinical exams with standardized patients with and without disabilities. *Acad Med.* 2010 Nov;85(11):1766–1771. doi:10.1097/ACM.0b013e3181f849dc.
69. McEvoy M, Schlair S, Sidlo Z, Burton W, Milan F. Assessing third-year medical students' ability to address a patient's spiritual distress using an OSCE case. *Acad Med.* 2014 Jan;89(1):66–70. doi:10.1097/ACM.0000000000000061.
70. Bloom-Feshbach K, Casey D, Schulson L, Gliatto P, Giftos J, Karani R. Health literacy in transitions of care: an innovative objective structured clinical examination for fourth-year medical students in an internship preparation course. *J Gen Intern Med.* 2016 Feb;31(2):242–246. doi:10.1007/s11606-015-3513-1.
71. Jefferies A, Simmons B, Tabak D, et al. Using an objective structured clinical examination (OSCE) to assess multiple physician competencies in postgraduate training. *Med Teach.* 2007 Mar;29(2-3):183–191. doi:10.1080/01421590701302290.
72. Hingle ST, Robinson S, Colliver JA, Rosher RB, McCann-Stone N. Systems-based practice assessed with a performance-based examination simulated and scored by standardized participants in the health care system: feasibility and psychometric properties. *Teach Learn Med.* 2011 Apr;23(2):148–154. doi:10.1080/10401334.2011.561751.
73. Ginsburg LR, Tregunno D, Norton PG, et al. Development and testing of an objective structured clinical exam (OSCE) to assess socio-cultural dimensions of patient safety competency. *BMJ Qual Saf.* 2015 Mar;24(3):188–194. doi:10.1136/bmjqs-2014-003277.
74. Sukalich S, Elliott JO, Ruffner G. Teaching medical error disclosure to residents using patient-centered simulation training. *Acad Med.* 2014 Jan;89(1):136–143. doi:10.1097/ACM.0000000000000046.
75. Wagner DP, Hoppe RB, Lee CP. The patient safety OSCE for PGY-1 residents: a centralized response to the challenge of culture change. *Teach Learn Med.* 2009 Jan-Mar;21(1):8–14. doi:10.1080/10401330802573837.
76. Chen JG, Mistry KP, Wright MC, Turner DA. Postoperative handoff communication: a simulation-based training method. *Simul Healthc.* 2010 Aug;5(4):242–247. doi:10.1097/SIH.0b013e3181e3bd07.
77. McQueen-Shadfar L, Taekman J. Say what you mean to say: improving patient handoffs in the operating room and beyond. *Simul Healthc.* 2010 Aug;5(4):248–253. doi:10.1097/SIH.0b013e3181e3f234.
78. Bonnell S, Macauley K, Nolan S. Management and handoff of a deteriorating patient from primary to acute care settings: a nursing academic and acute care collaborative case scenario. *Simul Healthc.* 2013 Jun;8(3):180–182. doi:10.1097/SIH.0b013e3182859fc6.
79. Oza SK, Boscardin CK, Wamsley M, et al. Assessing 3rd year medical students' interprofessional collaborative practice behaviors during a standardized patient encounter: a multi-institutional, cross-sectional study. *Med Teach.* 2015;37(10):915–925. doi:10.3109/0142159X.2014.970628.
80. Siassakos D, Draycott T. Measuring the impact of simulation-based training on patient safety and quality of care: lessons from maternity. *Resuscitation.* 2011 Jun;82(6):782–783. doi:10.1016/j.resuscitation.2010.12.026.
81. Yuasa M, Nagoshi M, Oshiro-Wong C, Tin M, Wen A, Masaki K. Standardized patient and standardized interdisciplinary team meeting: validation of a new performance-based assessment tool. *J Am Geriatr Soc.* 2014 Jan;62(1):171–174. doi:10.1111/jgs.12604.
82. Odegard PS, Robins L, Murphy N, et al. Interprofessional initiatives at the University of Washington. *Am J Pharm Educ.* 2009 Jul 10;73(4):63. doi:10.5688/aj730463.
83. Curran V, Casimiro L, Banfield V, et al. Research for interprofessional competency-based evaluation (RICE). *J Interprof Care.* 2009 May;23(3):297–300. doi:10.1080/13561820802432398.
84. Norcini J, Boulet J. Status of standardized patient assessment: methodological issues in the use of standardized patients for assessment. *Teach Learn Med.* 2003 Fall;15(4):293–297. doi:10.1207/S15328015TLM1504_12.
85. Harrison CJ, Könings KD, Molyneux A, Schuwirth LWT, Wass V, van der Vleuten CPM. Web-based feedback after summative assessment: how do students engage? *Med Educ.* 2013 Jul;47(7):734–744. doi:10.1111/medu.12209.
86. Harrison CJ, Molyneux AJ, Blackwell S, Wass VJ. How we give personalised audio feedback after summative OSCEs. *Med Teach.* 2015 Apr;37(4):323–326. doi:10.3109/0142159X.2014.932901.
87. Newble DI, Swanson DB. Psychometric characteristics of the objective structured clinical examination. *Med Educ.* 1988 Jul;22(4):325–334. doi:10.1111/j.1365-2923.1988.tb00761.x.
88. Vargas AL, Boulet JR, Errichetti A, van Zanten M, López MJ, Reta AM. Developing performance-based medical school assessment programs in resource-limited environments. *Med Teach.* 2007 Mar;29(2-3):192–198. doi:10.1080/01421590701316514.
89. Baker TK. The end of Step 2 CS should be the beginning of a new approach to clinical skills assessment. *Acad Med.* 2021 Sep 1;96(9):1239–1241. doi:10.1097/ACM.0000000000004187.
90. Kogan JR, Hauer KE, Holmboe ES. The dissolution of the Step 2 Clinical Skills examination and the duty of medical educators to step up the effectiveness of clinical skills assessment. *Acad Med.* 2021 Sep 1;96(9):1242–1246. doi:10.1097/ACM.0000000000004216.
91. Yudkowsky R, Szauter K. Farewell to the Step 2 Clinical Skills Exam: new opportunities, obligations, and next steps. *Acad Med.* 2021 Sep 1;96(9):1250–1253. doi:10.1097/ACM.0000000000004209.
92. Boursicot K, Kemp S, Wilkinson T, et al. Performance assessment: consensus statement and recommendations from the 2020 Ottawa Conference. *Med Teach.* 2021 Jan;43(1):58–67. doi:10.1080/0142159X.2020.1830052.

93. Coderre S, Woloschuk W, McLaughlin K. Twelve tips for blueprinting. *Med Teach.* 2009 Apr;31(4):322–324. doi:10.1080/01421590802225770.
94. Boursicot K, Roberts T. How to set up an OSCE. *Clin Teach.* 2005;2(1):16–20. doi:10.1111/j.1743-498X.2005.00053.x.
95. Boulet J. Using National Medical Care Survey data to validate examination content on a performance-based clinical skills assessment for osteopathic physicians. *J Am Osteopath Assoc.* 2003 May;103(5):225–231. doi:10.7556/jaoa.2003.103.5.225.
96. Dieckmann P, Gaba D, Rall M. Deepening the theoretical foundations of patient simulation as social practice. *Simul Healthc.* 2007 Fall;2(3):183–193. doi:10.1097/SIH.0b013e3180f637f5.
97. Rudolph JW, Raemer DB, Simon R. Establishing a safe container for learning in simulation: the role of the presimulation briefing. *Simul Healthc.* 2014 Dec;9(6):339–349. doi:10.1097/SIH.0000000000000047.
98. Pugh D, Smee S. Medical Council of Canada: Guidelines for the development of Objective Structured Clinical Examination (OSCE) cases. Accessed September 25, 2022. https://mcc.ca/media/OSCE-Booklet-2014.pdf.
99. Lewis KL, Bohnert CA, Gammon WL, et al. The Association of Standardized Patient Educators (ASPE) Standards of Best Practice (SOBP). *Adv Simul.* 2017 Jun 27;2(1):10. doi:10.1186/s41077-017-0043-4.
100. van Merriënboer JJG, Sweller J. Cognitive load theory in health professional education: design principles and strategies. *Med Educ.* 2010 Jan;44(1):85–93. doi:10.1111/j.1365-2923.2009.03498.x.
101. MedEdPORTAL. Accessed September 25, 2022. https://www.mededportal.org/.
102. Case Development Template. Accessed January 31, 2023. https://www.aspeducators.org/aspe-case-development-template
103. Chambers KA, Boulet JR, Gary NE. The management of patient encounter time in a high-stakes assessment using standardized patients. *Med Educ.* 2000 Oct;34(10):813–817. doi:10.1046/j.1365-2923.2000.00752.x.
104. USMLE Step 2 Clinical Skills (CS) Content Description and General Information 2014. Accessed September 24, 2022. https://www.evms.edu/media/departments/medical_education/STEP2CS_info.pdf.
105. Pugh D, Halman S, Desjardins I, Humphrey-Murto S, Wood TJ. Done or almost done? Improving OSCE checklists to better capture performance in progress tests. *Teach Learn Med.* 2016 Oct-Dec;28(4):406–414. doi:10.1080/10401334.2016.1218337.
106. Gorter S, Rethans JJ, Scherpbier A, van der Heijde D, Houben H, van der Vleuten C. Developing case-specific checklists for standardized-patient-based assessments in internal medicine: a review of the literature. *Acad Med.* 2000 Nov;75(11):1130–1137. doi:10.1097/00001888-200011000-00022.
107. Nendaz MR, Gut AM, Perrier A, et al. Degree of concurrency among experts in data collection and diagnostic hypothesis generation during clinical encounters. *Med Educ.* 2004 Jan;38(1):25–31. doi:10.1111/j.1365-2923.2004.01738.x.
108. Hettinga AM, Denessen E, Postma CT. Checking the checklist: a content analysis of expert- and evidence-based case-specific checklist items. *Med Educ.* 2010 Sep;44(9):874–883. doi:10.1111/j.1365-2923.2010.03721.x.
109. Daniels VJ, Bordage G, Gierl MJ, Yudkowsky R. Effect of clinically discriminating, evidence-based checklist items on the reliability of scores from an Internal Medicine residency OSCE. *Adv Health Sci Educ.* 2014 Oct;19(4):497–506. doi:10.1007/s10459-013-9482-4.
110. Wilkinson TJ, Frampton CM, Thompson-Fawcett M, Egan T. Objectivity in objective structured clinical examinations: checklists are no substitute for examiner commitment. *Acad Med.* 2003 Feb;78(2):219–223. doi:10.1097/00001888-200302000-00021.
111. Young JQ, Van Merrienboer J, Durning S, ten Cate O. Cognitive load theory: implications for medical education: AMEE Guide No. 86. *Med Teach.* 2014 May;36(5):371–384. doi:10.3109/0142159x.2014.889290.
112. Boulet JR, van Zanten M, De Champlain A, Hawkins R, Peitzman SJ. Checklist content on a standardized patient assessment: an ex post facto review. *Adv Health Sci Educ Theory Pr.* 2008 Mar;13(1):59–69. doi:10.1007/s10459-006-9024-4.
113. Hodges B, Regehr G, McNaughton N, Tiberius R, Hanson M. OSCE checklists do not capture increasing levels of expertise. *Acad Med.* 1999;74:1129–1134. doi:10.1097/00001888-199910000-00017.
114. Croskerry P. A universal model of diagnostic reasoning. *Acad Med.* 2009 Aug;84(8):1022–1028. doi:10.1097/ACM.0b013e3181ace703.
115. Vu NV, Marcy MM, Colliver JA, Verhulst SJ, Travis TA, Barrows HS. Standardized (simulated) patients' accuracy in recording clinical performance check-list items. *Med Educ.* 1992 Mar;26(2):99–104. doi:10.1111/j.1365-2923.1992.tb00133.x.
116. McLaughlin K, Ainslie M, Coderre S, Wright B, Violato C. The effect of differential rater function over time (DRIFT) on objective structured clinical examination ratings. *Med Educ.* 2009 Oct;43(10):989–992. doi:10.1111/j.1365-2923.2009.03438.x.
117. Yudkowsky R, Downing S, Klamen D, Valaski M, Eulenberg B, Popa M. Assessing the head-to-toe physical examination skills of medical students. *Med Teach.* 2004 Aug;26(5):415–419. doi:10.1080/01421590410001696452.
118. Chan J, Humphrey-Murto S, Pugh DM, Su C, Wood T. The objective structured clinical examination: can physician-examiners participate from a distance? *Med Educ.* 2014 Apr;48(4):441–450. doi:10.1111/medu.12326.
119. Isaak R, Stiegler M, Hobbs G, et al. Comparing real-time versus delayed video assessments for evaluating ACGME sub-competency milestones in simulated patient care environments. *Cureus.* 2018 Mar 4;10(3):e2267. doi:10.7759/cureus.2267.
120. van Zanten M, Boulet JR, McKinley DW, DeChamplain A, Jobe AC. Assessing the communication and interpersonal skills of graduates of international medical schools as part of the United States Medical Licensing Exam (USMLE) Step 2 Clinical Skills (CS) Exam. *Acad Med.* 2007 Oct;82(10 Suppl):S65–S68. doi:10.1097/ACM.0b013e318141f40a.
121. Boulet JR, Ben-David MF, Ziv A, et al. Using standardized patients to assess the interpersonal skills of physicians. *Acad Med.* 1998 Oct;73(10 Suppl):S94–S96. doi:10.1097/00001888-199810000-00057.
122. Swanson DB, van der Vleuten CPM. Assessment of clinical skills with standardized patients: state of the art revisited. *Teach Learn Med.* 2013;25(Suppl 1):S17–S25. doi:10.1080/10401334.2013.842916.
123. Rothman AI, Blackmore D, Dauphinee WD, Reznick R. The use of global ratings in OSCE station scores. *Adv Health Sci Educ Theory Pr.* 1997 Jan;1(3):215–219. doi:10.1007/BF00162918.
124. Solomon DJ, Szauter K, Rosebraugh CJ, Callaway MR. Global ratings of student performance in a standardized patient ex-

amination: is the whole more than the sum of the parts? *Adv Health Sci Educ Theory Pr.* 2000;5(2):131–140. doi:10.1023/A:1009878124073.

125. Makoul G. The SEGUE Framework for teaching and assessing communication skills. *Patient Educ Couns.* 2001 Oct;45(1):23–34. doi:10.1016/S0738-3991(01)00136-7.
126. Stillman PL, Brown DR, Redfield DL, Sabers DL. Construct validation of the Arizona Clinical Interview Rating Scale. *Educ Psychol Meas.* 1977;37(4):1031–1038. doi:10.1177/001316447703700427.
127. van Thiel J, Kraan HF, Van Der Vleuten CP. Reliability and feasibility of measuring medical interviewing skills: the revised Maastricht History-Taking and Advice Checklist. *Med Educ.* 1991 May;25(3):224–229. doi:10.1111/j.1365-2923.1991.tb00055.x.
128. Novack DH, Dubé C, Goldstein MG. Teaching medical interviewing: a basic course on interviewing and the physician-patient relationship. *Arch Intern Med.* 1992;152(9):1814–1820. doi:10.1001/archinte.1992.00400210046008.
129. Frankel RM, Stein T. Getting the most out of the clinical encounter: the four habits model. *J Med Pract Manag.* 2001 Jan-Feb;16(4):184–191. doi:10.7812/TPP/99-020.
130. Makoul G. Essential elements of communication in medical encounters: the Kalamazoo consensus statement. *Acad Med.* 2001 Apr;76(4):390–393. doi:10.1097/00001888-200104000-00021.
131. Kurtz S, Silverman J, Benson J, Draper J. Marrying content and process in clinical method teaching: enhancing the Calgary-Cambridge guides. *Acad Med.* 2003 Aug;78(8):802–809. doi:10.1097/00001888-200308000-00011.
132. Makoul G, Krupat E, Chang CH. Measuring patient views of physician communication skills: development and testing of the Communication Assessment Tool. *Patient Educ Couns.* 2007 Aug;67(3):333–342. doi:10.1016/j.pec.2007.05.005.
133. van Zanten M, Boulet JR, McKinley D. Using standardized patients to assess the interpersonal skills of physicians: six years' experience with a high-stakes certification examination. *Health Commun.* 2007;22(3):195–205. doi:10.1080/10410230701626562.
134. Sandilands (Dallie) D, Gotzmann A, Roy M, Zumbo BD, De Champlain A. Weighting checklist items and station components on a large-scale OSCE: is it worth the effort? *Med Teach.* 2014 Jul;36(7):585–590. doi:10.3109/0142159X.2014.899687.
135. Association of SP Educators (ASPE) Center for SP Methodology. Accessed September 24, 2022. https://www.aspeducators.org/the-center-for-sp-methodology
136. Vu NV, Steward DE, Marcy M. An assessment of the consistency and accuracy of standardized patients' simulations. *Acad Med.* 1987;62(12):1000–1002. https://journals.lww.com/academicmedicine/Fulltext/1987/12000/An_assessment_of_the_consistency_and_accuracy_of.10.aspx.
137. Howley L. Focusing feedback on interpersonal skills: a workshop for standardized patients. *MedEdPORTAL.* 2007;3:339. doi:10.15766/mep_2374-8265.339.
138. Bokken L, Linssen T, Scherpbier A, Van Der Vleuten C, Rethans JJ. Feedback by simulated patients in undergraduate medical education: a systematic review of the literature. *Med Educ.* 2009 Mar;43(3):202–210. doi:10.1111/j.1365-2923.2008.03268.x.
139. Roy M, Wojcik J, Bartman I, Smee S. Augmenting physician examiner scoring in objective structured clinical examinations: including the standardized patient perspective. *Adv Health Sci Educ Theory Pract.* 2021 Mar;26(1):313–328. doi:10.1007/s10459-020-09987-6.
140. Swartz MH, Colliver JA, Robbs RS. The interaction of examinee's ethnicity and standardized patient's ethnicity: an extended analysis. *Acad Med.* 2001 Oct;76(10 Suppl):S96. doi:10.1097/00001888-200110001-00032.
141. Vora S, Dahlen B, Adler M, et al. Recommendations and guidelines for the use of simulation to address structural racism and implicit bias. *Simul Healthc.* 2021 Aug 1;16(4):275–284. doi:10.1097/SIH.0000000000000591.
142. Picketts L, Warren MD, Bohnert C. Diversity and inclusion in simulation: addressing ethical and psychological safety concerns when working with simulated participants. *BMJ Simul Technol Enhanc Learn.* 2021 May 6;7(6):590–599. doi:10.1136/bmjstel-2020-000853.
143. Preusche I, Schmidts M, Wagner-Menghin M. Twelve tips for designing and implementing a structured rater training in OSCEs. *Med Teach.* 2012;34(5):368–372. doi:10.3109/0142159X.2012.652705.
144. Moineau G, Power B, Pion AMJ, Wood TJ, Humphrey-Murto S. Comparison of student examiner to faculty examiner scoring and feedback in an OSCE. *Med Educ.* 2011 Feb;45(2):183–191. doi:10.1111/j.1365-2923.2010.03800.x.
145. Bergus GR, Woodhead JC, Kreiter CD. Trained lay observers can reliably assess medical students' communication skills. *Med Educ.* 2009 Jul;43(7):688–694. doi:10.1111/j.1365-2923.2009.03396.x.
146. Liew SC, Dutta S, Sidhu JK, et al. Assessors for communication skills: SPs or healthcare professionals? *Med Teach.* 2014 Jul;36(7):626–631. doi:10.3109/0142159X.2014.899689.
147. ten Cate O, Chen HC, Hoff RG, Peters H, Bok H, van der Schaaf M. Curriculum development for the workplace using Entrustable Professional Activities (EPAs): AMEE Guide No. 99. *Med Teach.* 2015;37(11):983–1002. doi:10.3109/0142159X.2015.1060308.
148. Talwalkar JS, Murtha TD, Prozora S, Fortin 6th AH, Morrison LJ, Ellman MS. Assessing advanced communication skills via objective structured clinical examination: a comparison of faculty versus self, peer, and standardized patient assessors. *Teach Learn Med.* 2020 Jun-Jul;32(3):294–307. doi:10.1080/10401334.2019.1704763.
149. Boulet JR, McKinley DW, Whelan GP, Hambleton RK. The effect of task exposure on repeat candidate scores in a high-stakes standardized patient assessment. *Teach Learn Med.* 2003 Fall;15(4):227–232. doi:10.1207/S15328015TLM1504_02.
150. Swygert KA, Balog KP, Jobe A. The impact of repeat information on examinee performance for a large-scale standardized-patient examination. *Acad Med.* 2010;85(9):1506–1510. https://journals.lww.com/academicmedicine/Fulltext/2010/09000/The_Impact_of_Repeat_Information_on_Examinee.25.aspx.
151. Gotzmann A, De Champlain A, Homayra F, et al. Cheating in OSCEs: the impact of simulated security breaches on OSCE performance. *Teach Learn Med.* 2017 Jan-Mar;29(1):52–58. doi:10.1080/10401334.2016.1202832.
152. Ghouri A, Boachie C, McDowall S, et al. Gaining an advantage by sitting an OSCE after your peers: a retrospective study. *Med Teach.* 2018 Nov;40(11):1136–1142. doi:10.1080/0142159X.2018.1458085.
153. Swanson DB, Clauser BE, Case SM. Clinical skills assessment with standardized patients in high-stakes tests: a framework for thinking about score precision, equating, and security. *Adv Health Sci Educ.* 1999;4(1):67–106. doi:10.1023/A:1009862220473.

154. Pell G, Fuller R, Homer M, Roberts T. How to measure the quality of the OSCE: A review of metrics – AMEE guide no. 49. *Med Teach.* 2010;32(10):802–811. doi:10.3109/0142159X.2010.507716.
155. Messick S. Validity. In: Linn RL, ed. *Educational Measurement.* 3rd ed. The American Council on Education/Macmillan series on higher education. American Council on Education; 1989:13–103.
156. Kane MT. Validating the interpretations and uses of test scores. *J Educ Meas.* 2013;50(1):1–73. doi:10.1111/jedm.12000.
157. Brannick MT, Erol-Korkmaz HT, Prewett M. A systematic review of the reliability of objective structured clinical examination scores. *Med Educ.* 2011 Dec;45(12):1181–1189. doi:10.1111/j.1365-2923.2011.04075.x.
158. van der Vleuten CPM, Norman GR, De Graaff E. Pitfalls in the pursuit of objectivity: issues of reliability. *Med Educ.* 1991 Mar;25(2):110–118. doi:10.1111/j.1365-2923.1991.tb00036.x.
159. van der Vleuten CPM. The assessment of professional competence: developments, research and practical implications. *Adv Health Sci Educ.* 1996 Jan;1(1):41–67. doi:10.1007/BF00596229.
160. Stillman P, Swanson D, Regan MB, et al. Assessment of clinical skills of residents utilizing standardized patients. *Ann Intern Med.* 1991 Mar 1;114(5):393–401. doi:10.7326/0003-4819-114-5-393.
161. Petrusa ER, Blackwell TA, Ainsworth MA. Reliability and validity of an objective structured clinical examination for assessing the clinical performance of residents. *Arch Intern Med.* 1990;150(3):573–577. doi:10.1001/archinte.1990.00390150069014.
162. van der Vleuten CPM, Swanson DB. Assessment of clinical skills with standardized patients: state of the art. *Teach Learn Med.* 1990;2(2):58–76. doi:10.1080/10401339009539432.
163. Whelan GP, McKinley DW, Boulet JR, Macrae J, Kamholz S. Validation of the doctor–patient communication component of the Educational Commission for Foreign Medical Graduates Clinical Skills Assessment. *Med Educ.* 2001 Aug;35(8):757–761. doi:10.1046/j.1365-2923.2001.00977.x.
164. Boulet JR, De Champlain AF, McKinley DW. Setting defensible performance standards on OSCEs and standardized patient examinations. *Med Teach.* 2003 May;25(3):245–249. doi:10.1080/0142159031000100274.
165. McKinley DW, Norcini JJ. How to set standards on performance-based examinations: AMEE Guide No. 85. *Med Teach.* 2014 Feb;36(2):97–110. doi:10.3109/0142159X.2013.853119.
166. Yousuf N, Violato C, Zuberi RW. Standard setting methods for pass/fail decisions on high-stakes objective structured clinical examinations: a validity study. *Teach Learn Med.* 2015;27(3):280–291. doi:10.1080/10401334.2015.1044749.
167. Smee SM, Blackmore DE. Setting standards for an objective structured clinical examination: the borderline group method gains ground on Angoff. *Med Educ.* 2001;35(11):1009–1010. doi:10.1111/j.1365-2923.2001.01047.x.
168. Williams RG. Have standardized patient examinations stood the test of time and experience? *Teach Learn Med.* 2004 Spring;16(2):215–222. doi:10.1207/s15328015tlm1602_16.
169. Tavakol M, Dennick R. Post-examination analysis of objective tests. *Med Teach.* 2011;33(6):447–458. doi:10.3109/0142159X.2011.564682.
170. Boulet JR, McKinley DW, Whelan GP, Hambleton RK. Quality assurance methods for performance-based assessments. *Adv Health Sci Educ.* 2003;8(1):27–47. doi:10.1023/A:1022639521218.
171. De Champlain AF, Margolis MJ, King A, Klass DJ. Standardized patients' accuracy in recording examinees' behaviors using checklists. *Acad Med.* 1997 Oct;72(10 Suppl 1):S85–S87. doi:10.1097/00001888-199710001-00029.
172. Tamblyn RM, Grad R, Gayton D, Petrella L, Reid T. McGill Drug Utilization Research Group. Impact of inaccuracies in standardized patient portrayal and reporting on physician performance during blinded clinic visits. *Teach Learn Med.* 1997;9(1):25–38. doi:10.1080/10401339709539809.
173. Bouter S, van Weel-Baumgarten E, Bolhuis S. Construction and validation of the Nijmegen Evaluation of the Simulated Patient (NESP): assessing simulated patients' ability to role-play and provide feedback to students. *Acad Med.* 2013 Feb;88(2):253–259. doi:10.1097/ACM.0b013e31827c0856.
174. Greene RE, Blasdel G, Cook TE, Gillespie C. How do OSCE cases activate learners about transgender health? *Acad Med.* 2020 Dec;95(12S):S156–S162. doi:10.1097/ACM.0000000000003704.
175. Vance SR, Buckelew SM, Dentoni-Lasofsky B, Ozer E, Deutsch MB, Meyers M. A pediatric transgender medicine curriculum for multidisciplinary trainees. *MedEdPORTAL J Teach Learn Resour.* 2020 Apr 3;16:10896. doi:10.15766/mep_2374-8265.10896.
176. John JT, Block L, Stein A, Vasile E, Barilla-LaBarca ML. Caring for patients with physical disabilities: assessment of an innovative spinal cord injury session that addresses an educational gap. *Am J Phys Med Rehabil.* 2019 Nov;98(11):1031–1035. doi:10.1097/PHM.0000000000001251.
177. Kelekar A, Rubino I, Kavanagh M, et al. Vaccine hesitancy counseling-an educational intervention to teach a critical skill to preclinical medical students. *Med Sci Educ.* 2022 Jan 21;32(1):141–147. doi:10.1007/s40670-021-01495-5.
178. Morato TMR, Mendes PHM, Ghosn DSNB, et al. Teaching medical students to choose wisely through simulation. *Eur J Pediatr.* 2022 Mar;181(3):1125–1131. doi:10.1007/s00431-021-04305-7.
179. Emin EI, Emin E, Bimpis A, et al. Teaching and assessment of medical students during complex multifactorial team-based tasks: the "Virtual on Call" case study. *Adv Med Educ Pract.* 2022 May 5;13:457–465. doi:10.2147/AMEP.S357514.
180. Shortridge A, Steinheider B, Ciro C, Randall K, Costner -Lark Amy, Loving G. Simulating interprofessional geriatric patient care using telehealth: a team-based learning activity. *MedEdPORTAL.* 2016 Jun 17;12:10415. doi:10.15766/mep_2374-8265.10415.
181. Sartori DJ, Olsen S, Weinshel E, Zabar SR. Preparing trainees for telemedicine: a virtual OSCE pilot. *Med Educ.* 2019 May;53(5):517–518. doi:10.1111/medu.13851.
182. Farrell SE, Junkin AR, Hayden EM. Assessing clinical skills via telehealth objective standardized clinical examination: feasibility, acceptability, comparability, and educational value. *Telemed E-Health.* 2022 Feb;28(2):248–257. doi:10.1089/tmj.2021.0094.
183. Kunutsor SK, Metcalf EP, Westacott R, Revell L, Blythe A. Are remote clinical assessments a feasible and acceptable method of assessment? A systematic review. *Med Teach.* 2022 Mar;44(3):300–308. doi:10.1080/0142159X.2021.1987403.
184. Lawrence K, Hanley K, Adams J, Sartori DJ, Greene R, Zabar S. Building telemedicine capacity for trainees during the novel coronavirus outbreak: a case study and lessons learned. *J Gen Intern Med.* 2020 Sep;35(9):2675–2679. doi:10.1007/s11606-020-05979-9.

185. Fu CP, Chi HY, Li MW, et al. Development of an objective structured clinical examination station for pediatric occupational therapy and an evaluation of its quality. *Am J Occup Ther*. 2022 Mar 1;76(2):7602205010. doi:10.5014/ajot.2022.043521.
186. Hofer SH, Schuebel F, Sader R, Landes C. Development and implementation of an objective structured clinical examination (OSCE) in CMF-surgery for dental students. *J Craniomaxillofac Surg*. 2013 Jul;41(5):412–416. doi:10.1016/j.jcms.2012.11.007.
187. Rushforth HE. Objective structured clinical examination (OSCE): review of literature and implications for nursing education. *Nurse Educ Today*. 2007 Jul;27(5):481–490. doi:10.1016/j.nedt.2006.08.009.
188. Nickbakht M, Amiri M, Latifi SM. Study of the reliability and validity of objective structured clinical examination (OSCE) in the assessment of clinical skills of audiology students. *Glob J Health Sci*. 2013 Jan 31;5(3):64–68. doi:10.5539/gjhs.v5n3p64.
189. Horton N, Payne KD, Jernigan M, et al. A standardized patient counseling rubric for a pharmaceutical care and communications course. *Am J Pharm Educ*. 2013 Sep 12;77(7):152. doi:10.5688/ajpe777152.
190. Broder HL, Janal M. Promoting interpersonal skills and cultural sensitivity among dental students. *J Dent Educ*. 2006 Apr;70(4):409–416. doi:10.1002/j.0022-0337.2006.70.4.tb04095.x.
191. Wilson L, Gallagher Gordon M, Cornelius F, et al. The standardized patient experience in undergraduate nursing education. *Stud Health Technol Inform*. 2006;122:830. doi:10.1016/j.ecns.2022.10.003.
192. Manton JW, Kennedy KS, Lipps JA, Pfeil SA, Cornelius BW. Medical Emergency Management in the Dental Office (MEMDO): a pilot study assessing a simulation-based training curriculum for dentists. *Anesth Prog*. 2021 Jun 1;68(2):76–84. doi:10.2344/anpr-67-04-04.
193. Khadivzadeh T, Ardaghi Sefat Seighalani M, Mirzaii K, Mazloum SR. The effect of interactive educational workshops with or without standardized patients on the clinical skills of midwifery students in providing sexual health counseling. *Simul Healthc*. 2020 Aug;15(4):234–242. doi:10.1097/SIH.0000000000000439.
194. Samuriwo R. Interprofessional collaboration—time for a new theory of action? *Front Med*. 2022 Mar 18;9:876715. doi:10.3389/fmed.2022.876715.
195. Siassakos D, Bristowe K, Hambly H, et al. Team communication with patient actors: findings from a multisite simulation study. *Simul Healthc*. 2011 Jun;6(3):143–149. doi:10.1097/SIH.0b013e31821687cf.
196. King S, Carbonaro M, Greidanus E, Ansell D, Foisy-Doll C, Magus S. Dynamic and routine interprofessional simulations: expanding the use of simulation to enhance interprofessional competencies. *J Allied Health*. 2014 Aug;43(3):169–175. PMID: 25194064.
197. González-Pascual JL, López-Martín I, Saiz-Navarro EM, Oliva-Fernández Ó, Acebedo-Esteban FJ, Rodríguez-García M. Using a station within an objective structured clinical examination to assess interprofessional competence performance among undergraduate nursing students. *Nurse Educ Pract*. 2021 Oct;56:103190. doi:10.1016/j.nepr.2021.103190.
198. Cyr PR, Schirmer JM, Hayes V, Martineau C, Keane M. Integrating interprofessional case scenarios, allied embedded actors, and teaching into formative observed structured clinical exams. *Fam Med*. 2020 Mar;52(3):209–212. doi:10.22454/FamMed.2020.760357.
199. Youm J, Wiechmann W. Formative feedback from the first-person perspective using Google Glass in a family medicine objective structured clinical examination station in the United States. *J Educ Eval Health Prof*. 2018 Mar 7;15:5. doi:10.3352/jeehp.2018.15.5.
200. Jani KH, Jones KA, Jones GW, Amiel J, Barron B, Elhadad N. Machine learning to extract communication and history-taking skills in OSCE transcripts. *Med Educ*. 2020 Dec;54(12):1159–1170. doi:10.1111/medu.14347.
201. Williamson DM, Xi X, Breyer FJ. A framework for evaluation and use of automated scoring. *Educ Meas Issues Pract*. 2012;31(1):2–13. doi:10.1111/j.1745-3992.2011.00223.x.

7

Assessing Clinical Reasoning *In Vitro* (Nonworkplace Assessment)

THILAN WIJESEKERA, MD, MHS, AND STEVEN J. DURNING, MD, PHD

CHAPTER OUTLINE

Background

Each year approximately 12 million Americans experience a diagnostic error in ambulatory care and 40,000 to 80,000 die from missed diagnoses in hospitals.[1,2] A majority of delayed, wrong, and missed diagnoses can lead to severe harm due to delayed, inappropriate, or missed treatment.[3] In its landmark report *Improving Diagnosis in Health* Care, the National Academy of Medicine (NAM) defined diagnostic error as the "failure to (a) establish an accurate and timely explanation of a patient's health care problem(s) or (b) communicate that explanation to the patient."[4] With cognitive errors estimated to be part of approximately 75% of diagnostic errors, clinical reasoning has become an increasingly deliberate part of medical education curricula.[5,6] In this chapter we discuss the nonworkplace assessment of clinical reasoning.

Definition and a Basic Model for Clinical Reasoning

Assessing clinical reasoning can be a challenge because there are several scientific traditions that have explored this construct, thus influencing ways of understanding and defining it.[7,8] For the purpose of this chapter, we will use an inclusive definition that can be summarized as the cognitive and physical process by which a healthcare professional consciously and subconsciously interacts with the patient and environment to collect and interpret patient data, weigh the benefits and risks of actions, and understand patient preferences to determine a working diagnostic and therapeutic management plan whose purpose is to improve a patient's well-being.[9] While there are many ways to delineate the clinical reasoning process, some of its commonly described components include data collection, problem representation, generating and prioritizing a differential diagnosis, and management (Fig. 7.1).[4,10,11] Recent work has also emphasized the importance of the situation (or context).[12] Though often framed as proceeding in this order, it is important to note that these cognitive steps are intertwined (e.g., hypothesis-driven data collection), cycle iteratively during a clinical encounter, are highly dependent on content, and occur within the specific context (e.g., an environment).[13]

Data collection is the process of acquiring the clinical information necessary to inform a diagnosis.[10] For the classroom-based assessments that will be described, data collection will generally include reading a case and identifying pertinent history, physical examination, laboratory, or imaging results. While learners will be prompted to ask for

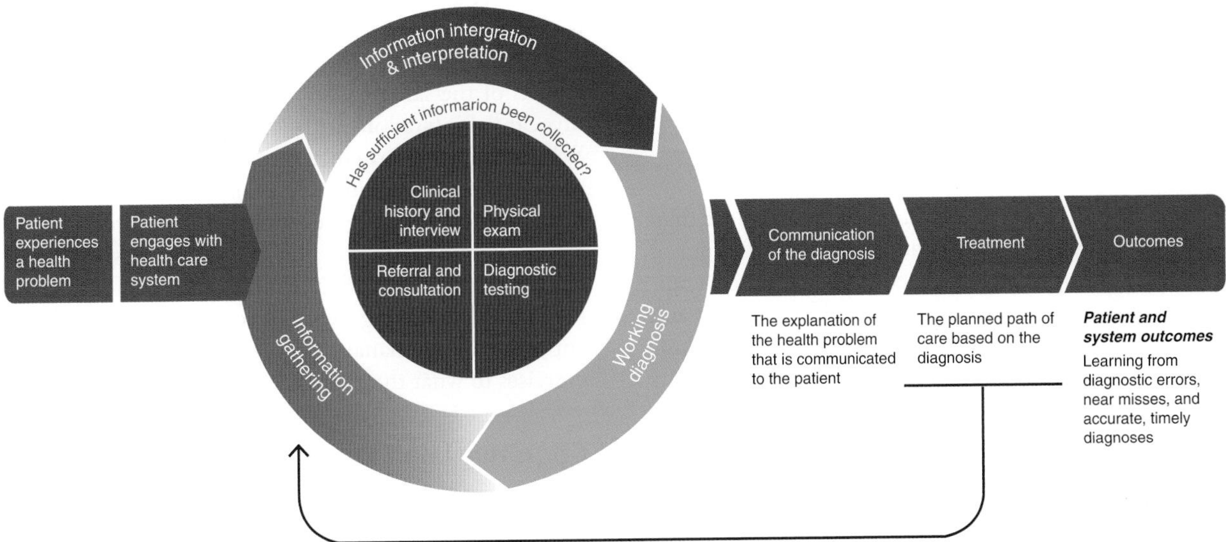

• **Fig. 7.1** The diagnostic process. From *Improving Diagnosis in Health Care*. National Academies of Sciences, Engineering, and Medicine; Institute of Medicine; Board on Health Care Services; et al., eds. National Academies Press; 2016.

pertinent data, it is important to note that most of a case's data are typically provided to learners in classroom assessments, unlike the clinical encounter where a provider has to acquire most information through their own history taking and physical examination on a patient. Problem representation describes how a clinician synthesizes relevant information from a case, which has often been synonymized with the one-line "assessment" of a presentation.[10] The problem representation generally transitions patient- or case-derived language into more abstract and medical terminology that is more consistent with how diseases are described in health professions education. Problem representations require an open-ended answer or verbal response format, making a problem representation more challenging to assess (exceptions include concept maps, modified essay questions, and essay questions).

Numerous terms are related to diagnosis, which can be described as a label for a pathological medical condition explained by underlying causes and pathophysiology.[14] During a real patient encounter or clinical case, the provider will develop a differential diagnosis of the possible diagnoses that could explain the patient's or case's presentation. Prioritizing a differential diagnosis begins with hypothesis generation, which is the process of iteratively identifying possible diagnoses, using that information to identify additional pertinent information, and further refining the differential diagnosis. Diagnostic justification occurs by identifying which diseases are most likely within a differential diagnosis and weighing how supporting and refuting information in a patient's case fits with that clinician's understanding of each diagnosis.[15] Eventually the provider will identify leading or working diagnoses that are of a high enough probability to engage in management.[16–18] During assessments of clinical reasoning, learners are most often asked for their leading diagnosis in a given clinical encounter, though more open-ended assessments allow them to share other diagnostic possibilities.

Management reasoning appears to be a different cognitive task than diagnostic reasoning, as the former is more of a prioritization task while the latter is more of a classification task.[19,20] Unlike diagnostic reasoning, management is fluid and depends more on the context (or specifics of the situation), has multiple solutions, and requires shared decision-making with the patient.[19] Though the cognitive process of management reasoning is still being understood, management can largely be described as prognostication, diagnostic testing, treatment, and prevention strategies around a patient's medical condition.[21–23] In clinical practice, upon identifying the condition, there appears to be an initial identification of possible interventions but only performing them when it crosses the provider's testing or treatment thresholds.[11,17,18] The testing and treatment thresholds are when a physician's probability of a given disease has crossed their threshold to pursue additional testing or to initiate treatment, respectively.[17] Given the complexity of management decisions, it can be challenging to assess this aspect of clinical reasoning, particularly in the classroom, which is likely why many if not most clinical reasoning assessments focus on diagnosis.

Pertinent Theories for Assessment of Clinical Reasoning

Our understanding of clinical reasoning has been shaped by many different fields, among them expertise, education, and cognitive psychology. While some theories overlap, among the most notable are deliberate practice theory, script theory, cognitive load theory, dual process theory, metacognition, and situativity theory. Each has aspects that can help educators not only develop or select the appropriate assessment method but also understand the factors that might affect learner performance.

Historical Perspective

The history of clinical reasoning education spans more than half a century, beginning with the problem-solving era of the 1960s.[24] During this period, educators believed clinical reasoning was a general skill that could be taught and applied to various educational or clinical scenarios regardless of a case's specific content or presentation. Scholars eventually trended away from this understanding of clinical reasoning after performance on certain types of assessment (e.g., patient management problems) was not consistent for an expert across different cases or for different experts across the same case.[25,26] These findings suggested that clinical reasoning performance was dependent on a specific case's content (i.e., content or case specificity) as well as the context around an individual activity (i.e., specifics of the situation or context specificity).[12,27,28]

Realizing the integral nature of medical knowledge to clinical reasoning, educators and researchers then focused on how information was acquired, synthesized, and organized. Accordingly, information processing theory suggested that the more organized medical knowledge was for a clinician, the more efficient and accurate their clinical reasoning would be.[29] Script theory advanced our understanding of knowledge organization by describing an individual's mental representations of a disease along parameters of epidemiology, pathophysiology, and clinical features (i.e., an illness script).[30] The contemporarily burgeoning cognitive load theory expanded on information processing by describing memory and highlighting the cognitive demands on a provider during the clinical reasoning process.[31–33]

Despite the previously mentioned implications of context specificity and the considerations of cognitive load, it was not until the 2000s that researchers emphasized the role of environment on clinical reasoning. Situated cognition explained that, in each encounter, factors including the patient, provider, healthcare team, and system interact in the diagnostic process.[12,34] These situativity theories moved the field away from the notion of the "cognitively isolated" clinician, instead framing expertise as a state that is impacted by the clinical situation.

Dual Process Theory

Dual process theory describes two modes of thinking: system 1 and system 2.[35] System 1 (fast or nonanalytical thinking) is reflexive and low effort, often incorporating pattern recognition and heuristics (i.e., cognitive shortcuts or rules of thumb).[36–38] For instance, a seasoned clinician might employ system 1 thinking to immediately diagnose a myocardial infarction in a patient with chest pain, diaphoresis, shortness of breath, and elevated cardiac enzymes. System 2 (slow or analytical thinking) is conscious and effortful and is usually employed in unfamiliar situations. As an example, a first-year student might need more time to consider the aspects of the same patient case before deciding between a myocardial infarction, acid reflux, or pulmonary embolism. While expert performance is often seen in the transition to more system 1 thinking, clinicians use both analytical and nonanalytical thinking depending on the situation. Learners should receive instruction on dual process theory while being assessed in ways that use both analytical (i.e., challenging clinical reasoning exercises requiring a more deliberate approach) and nonanalytical (i.e., familiar clinical reasoning exercises to what they have seen previously).[39–42]

Cognitive Load Theory

Cognitive load theory describes the limited nature of human memory and explains the cognitive demands of an individual during a complex task like clinical reasoning.[43] The cognitive load of clinical reasoning includes intrinsic load (i.e., mental resources directly related to clinical reasoning), germane load (i.e., mental resources for learning how to clinically reason in various patient scenarios), and extraneous load (i.e., mental resources not related to the clinical reasoning process).[44] For example, when a learner is diagnosing a patient with shortness of breath in the simulation center, the extraneous load would be represented by a suboptimally functioning electronic health record (EHR) and/or ambient noise; the intrinsic load would be the clinical reasoning process of understanding the patient information, synthesizing it, and coming up with the most likely diagnosis for a patient presenting with shortness of breath; and the germane load would be how the learner links the features of the current patient to diagnoses that can cause shortness of breath. Since an individual has only limited working, or short-term, memory, it can be challenging to overcome the various forms of cognitive load in each situation. Educators should be mindful of cognitive load in clinical reasoning assessment both in arranging test-taking conditions (e.g., time, distractions) and in item selection (e.g., straightforward versus challenging).[45]

One strategy for overcoming cognitive load is chunking, or organizing information into larger units that can be stored and accessed better through long-term memory.[33] Examples of chunking and schema (i.e., frameworks for organizing larger information) in clinical reasoning include semantic qualifiers, encapsulation, and illness scripts. Semantic qualifiers are abstract descriptors that can be used to understand a presentation more holistically (e.g., acute vs. chronic, unilateral vs. bilateral, mild vs. moderate vs. severe).[10] Encapsulation uses pathophysiology to describe a syndrome (e.g., sepsis).[46] An Illness script is a schema of an individual's "mental file" or understanding of a given condition including its epidemiology, pathophysiology, and clinical features of a disease (e.g., myocardial infarction [coronary artery disease, crushing chest pain, electrocardiogram abnormalities, and elevated cardiac enzymes]).[30,47] There has even been new literature supporting the notion of a management script to describe the options and process of diagnostic and therapeutic interventions.[11,23,48–50] Incorporating knowledge organization and script theory into clinical reasoning assessment can be achieved by compare-and-contrast assignments and exercises that require an understanding of both typical and atypical aspects of a given condition.[30,51]

Expertise

Expert performance in clinical reasoning requires not only deep knowledge and experience on a wide array of conditions but also the *application* of that knowledge and experience efficiently across many situations. Deliberate practice theory proposes that to develop expertise in any task, such as diagnosing and treating patients, a learner must perform its component parts in a time-intensive, purposeful, and supported fashion.[52,53] In clinical reasoning education, deliberate practice thus requires engaging in a sufficient number of (real or fictional) cases across a significant number of hours while reflecting before, during, and after a patient encounter, ideally with feedback from a coach.[54] Utilizing deliberate practice in the assessment of clinical reasoning might include both incorporating a wide range of cases and returning to similar types of cases for reinforcement. Reviewing performance individually, with peers and/or faculty, can further improve the educational yield from a given exercise.

Unfortunately, deliberate practice in many clinical reasoning educational settings can be limited by supervision and/or time (e.g., duration of clinical rotations for students) to fully experience the increasing complexity in patient care.[55] Given these growing challenges in developing clinical reasoning, the role of adaptive expertise has become increasingly valuable. Adaptive expertise encourages learners to use known solutions efficiently when applicable, but to also be capable of learning new information, create alternative strategies, and innovate problem-solving when appropriate.[56,57] This requires that learners have procedural fluency to draw on past experience (e.g., diagnosing congestive heart failure in a patient with shortness of breath after seeing a patient with it in clinic) in addition to a conceptual understanding to draw on in new situations where problem-solving is needed (e.g., using the pathophysiology of heart failure to diagnose it in a patient with leg swelling despite never seeing that condition previously) and incorporating evidence-based guidelines to inform their diagnostic and management practices (see Chapter 10 for additional discussion). Strategies for encouraging adaptive expertise in clinical reasoning assessment include guided discovery, contrasting cases, and productive failure (i.e., attempting to solve challenging problems ahead of explicit instruction).[55,58,59]

Situativity Theory

Given these theories' limitations with context specificity, the incorporation of a family of social cognitive theories known as situativity theory can help the educator.[12] Situativity theory includes embodied cognition, ecological psychology, situated cognition, and distributed cognition, and these theories can be valuable in providing the most accurate assessment of clinical reasoning.[60,61] Embodied cognition describes how a clinician's mind and body are connected to the environment, which can impact the perception of key data and subsequent action in clinical reasoning.[62] Situated cognition postulates that clinical reasoning is the result of bidirectional and context-specific interactions between participants and their environment, which can impact outcomes in diagnosis and management.[34] Distributed cognition explores how interactions between large numbers of individuals (e.g., patient, healthcare workers, consultants) and artifacts (e.g., EHR, laboratory equipment) allows information to be accessed and advanced across an entire healthcare system in medical decision-making.[63] Ecological psychology explains how providers are given affordances—opportunities (e.g., history, physical, laboratory, and imaging findings) to make a diagnosis—but do not always have the effectivities—knowledge or ability to identify affordances—to make a diagnosis.[64] Educators can incorporate these cognitive theories into clinical reasoning assessment by being mindful of the environment and how a learner interacts with it in making a diagnosis.

Principles of and Validity in Assessing Clinical Reasoning

Despite increasing consensus on the components of clinical reasoning, assessing it is still quite challenging for educators,[15,65] not only because clinical reasoning includes medical knowledge, problem-solving, and decision-making but also because thinking cannot be directly observed. Thus, for nonworkplace-based (in vitro) assessments, clinical reasoning needs to be inferred from the choices learners make with written or verbal questions related to clinical cases.[41]

When evaluating the validity evidence in any single form of clinical reasoning assessment, it can be helpful to consider the steps in Messick's framework for validity evidence, which include content, internal structure, response process, relationship to other variables, and consequences.[66] In content, a plan of how many questions for each pertinent topic on the assessment needs to be identified. Then the items need to be written in a way that measures problem-solving ability while avoiding items that yield false positives (answering despite insufficient ability) and false negatives (answering incorrectly despite sufficient ability). The scoring system needs to be considered carefully, including whether to assign differing weights to certain questions.[67,68] Internal structure considerations include the number of items, which need to be high enough for generalizability and to avoid construct underrepresentation. Additionally, the questions need to be difficult enough to discriminate between high and low performers. The response process—the way learners

Five-item multiple-choice question

1. An 8-year-old girl with migrating polyarthralgia, rash, and fever develops a holosystolic apical murmur, grade 4/6, with radiation to the axilla. Which of the following is the most likely diagnosis?
   a) Aortic stenosis
   b) Ebstein's anomaly
   c) Mitral regurgitation
   d) Mitral stenosis
   e) Ventricular septal defect

Two-item extended-matching question

a) Aortic regurgitation
b) Aortic stenosis
c) Atrial septal defect
d) Coarctation of the aorta
e) Ebstein's anomaly
f) Hypertrophic obstructive cardiomyopathy
g) Mitral regurgitation
h) Mitral stenosis
i) Patent ductus arteriosus
j) Pulmonary stenosis
k) Tetralogy of Fallot
l) Tricuspid regurgitation
m) Truncus arteriosus
n) Ventricular septal defect

For each patient with a murmur, select the most likely diagnosis.

1. An 8-year-old girl with migrating polyarthralgia, rash, and fever develops a holosystolic apical murmur, grade 4/6, with radiation to the axilla.
2. A 28-year-old woman at 7 months' gestation reports excessive fatigability and dyspnea. Blood pressure is 118/74 mmHg, pulse is 110/min and regular, and lungs are clear to auscultation. S1 is loud, there is a sharp sound after S2, and a low frequency diastolic murmur is heard at the apex, which increases in intensity before S1.

• **Fig. 7.2** Comparison between five-item multiple-choice and extended-matching questions. From Case (Academic Medicine, 2004).

provide answers—needs to be formulated (i.e., how questions are written) in a way to avoid errors that decrease performance and are not necessarily reflective of learner ability. The consequences or stakes of an assessment should also be reflective of the quality of data, with high-stakes assessments needing to collect high-quality information to adequately reflect a learner's clinical reasoning. Finally, any given assessment should be compared to other assessments (relationship to other variables) of clinical reasoning to best triangulate a learner's actual ability.[41]

Further complicating the assessment of clinical reasoning is that clinical reasoning is typically a nonlinear process and there may be multiple acceptable solutions to the correct answer. This means learners can get the correct diagnosis with flawed intermediate steps and can take appropriate steps to reveal an incorrect (albeit reasonable) answer.[15] To account for the different clinical reasoning paths to an answer, it is important that the assessment items are developed in a way that can lend toward a correct answer or that the gold standard has a range of answers to compensate for appropriate credit relative to the "correctness" of a given answer. In doing so, developing gold standards for clinical reasoning in nonworkplace-based assessments can potentially be resource intensive, including in terms of faculty time and expertise. For that reason, it can be helpful to have multiple forms of clinical reasoning assessment and be mindful of which components of the clinical reasoning process the assessment tests.[41]

Methods of Assessing Clinical Reasoning in the Classroom

In this section, we will describe several common types of nonworkplace-based assessments, including a general description, associated evidence, advantages, and disadvantages.

Multiple-Choice Questions

With a format that is familiar for educators to create and learners to take, multiple-choice questions (MCQs) have been the most common form of clinical assessment since the 1960s.[69,70] Despite concerns that they only test medical knowledge, MCQs have shown potential to evaluate higher-level clinical reasoning tasks too.[71] There are several formats to MCQs, including extended matching questions, which will also be described in this section.[72]

Overview

When developed to assess clinical reasoning, MCQs typically begin with some form of case vignette (Fig. 7.2). The case vignette includes patient information (e.g., medical history, physical examination), though the amount and type can vary depending on the goal of the question (e.g., diagnosis, management). Question types include single best alternative, combinations of alternatives, matching, and true/false, though the most common type is single best alternative.[15] Based on the vignette and associated question, learners then typically select from up to five potential answer choices. Extended-matching questions (EMQs) (Fig. 7.2) differ slightly in that there are more answer choices (i.e., at least eight), which are listed at the beginning of a question and can be enabled by free text in computerized formats.[73–75] Often based on a theme, a lead-in question (e.g., "For each of the following cases, choose the appropriate type of headache") then asks the learner to match a clinical vignette to the appropriate answer option. Both MCQs and EMQs are typically scored either full or no credit and with each item weighted equally. Though some items might be more difficult than others within the test and items might be different between tests, the entire form should be similar in difficulty overall across comparable sets of learners. While MCQs and EMQs can be taken in written or computerized format, they often can be scored electronically.[15]

Evidence

Writing MCQs and EMQs can be straightforward but requires steps to ensure content validity, including evidence-based material, consensus through experts, training for question writers, decisions about question difficulty (e.g., Angoff method), and evaluation of items postperformance.[76] Some studies have suggested that MCQs can be associated with problem-solving and clinical performance, in addition to medical knowledge.[71,77] A significant threat to validity is from cueing, given the limited number of options compared to an actual clinical presentation.[72,78,79] In regard to cueing, EMQs benefit from the additional number of choices available, though it is important that the choices are viable.[72] Curiously, EMQs have also shown previous correlation with diagnostic thinking inventory (DTI) and short-answer questions, while having inconsistent correlation to MCQs, particularly in regard to difficulty.[72,74] Reliability studies for both MCQs and EMQs have been favorable, likely because of the large number of items that can be included in the same examination.[15] Additionally, the ability to include many items in MCQ or EMQ examinations reduces the limitations around content (case) specificity when assessing clinical reasoning. For those reasons, MCQs have been and continue to be used in high-stakes examinations such as licensing examinations conducted by the National Board of Medical Examiners (NBME) and the Medical Council of Canada (MCC).

Advantages and Disadvantages

The biggest advantages of MCQs and EMQs are how straightforward they are to write and score, though EMQs can be more time intensive based on the number of answer choices.[41] They also can cover a wide range of content in a short period of time, increasing the feasibility of test administration and serving as a way to address content specificity. As previously mentioned, a noteworthy disadvantage of MCQs is cueing, which can artificially inflate performance by rewarding guessing.[79] Since MCQs and EMQs require learners to select from a list of provided answers, they cannot explain their clinical reasoning process. For these reasons, clinical reasoning experts have noted that MCQs and EMQs are particularly limited in their ability to assess hypothesis generation, problem presentation, and diagnostic justification, even if they can be helpful in evaluating a learner's leading diagnosis and management plans.[15]

Essay Questions

Essay questions have long been a staple of educational assessment with some examples of its use in evaluating clinical practice beginning in the mid-1900s, including modified essay questions (MEQs) (Fig. 7.3) in the 1970s.[80–83] While the basis of essay questions is an open response from the learner, there are other formats in addition to MEQs, including long-answer short-answer essay questions. However, open-response questions were thought to better allow learners to demonstrate higher-order clinical reasoning processes beyond medical knowledge recall.[84]

Part 1:
A 46-year-old woman presents to the emergency department with a 3-month history of early satiety and anorexia. Over the last 2 weeks, she has been vomiting most days and has been unable to eat or drink much over the last few days. Describe what other information you would seek from the history that would help you establish a diagnosis, and justify your answers.

Part 2 (revealed after answering Part 1):
From the history, you think the patient has gastric outlet obstruction. Describe the physical findings you would look for on an examination and why they might occur.

Part 3 (revealed after answering Part 2):
What diagnoses are highest on your differential diagnosis and why?

• **Fig. 7.3** Modified essay question example. Modified from Palmer EJ, Devitt PG. Assessment of higher order cognitive skills in undergraduate education: modified essay or multiple choice questions? Research paper. *BMC Med Educ*. 2007 Nov 28;7(1):1–7. doi:10.1186/1472-6920-7-49.

Overview

When used to assess clinical reasoning, long- and short-answer essay questions typically begin with some sort of clinical vignette. The goal of an item can vary from describing medical knowledge around a topic to comparing diagnoses in a differential to explaining management reasoning.[85] Based on the question stem, learners are expected to explain their clinical reasoning in a response with a word limit that can be short (i.e., fewer than three sentences) or long (i.e., up to five pages).[15] Given the length of possible responses, each essay question can take upward of 15 minutes, making it challenging to include more than 20 essay questions in a given examination. While essays can be completed by learners in a computer or handwritten format, the complexity of answers—even with a rubric—requires an educator to read and grade each answer. Scoring methods can be either global (i.e., based on the overall quality of the answer) or analytical (i.e., based on their inclusion of essential elements in their answer), which have shown some correlation.[85,86] Global grading schemes are performed by clinicians and do not require preparation. Analytical grading schemes can be performed comparably by clinicians and nonclinicians but require clear delineation and training around a previously determined rubric, which is determined by subject matter experts as is the passing score.[86]

MEQs also begin with a brief case vignette in which the learner is provided a clinical role but are then followed by a series of both open-response questions *and* MCQs. In a serial-structured format with both types of items nested into a case, the learner has to complete each item before further information is revealed and is unable to go back to change a previous answer.[83] There are typically three to six items per case, with an MEQ paper potentially including a wide range of cases depending on the scope of the paper, the word limit of the open-response items, and the overall time limit. Each item in an MEQ is graded as satisfactory (i.e., 1 point) or unsatisfactory (i.e., 0 points) based on a rubric and minimum level of competence determined by educators. For example, if a learner got the first two items of a case correct but the last time was incorrect, then they would get a total of 2 out of 3 points for the case (Fig. 7.3). The scores for each item are added up within cases and across the cases, with passing scores typically ranging from 40% to 70%.[83]

Evidence

Despite offering learners the ability to fully explain their clinical reasoning, essay questions generally have weak assessment characteristics. The open-ended nature of each answer can also make it challenging to create a consistent rubric, though this can be alleviated with a global rating scale.[86] Each answer's length and associated time requirement can lead to undersampling, which limits an essay test's ability to be representative of a content domain.[87] Though reliability can be achieved, it can sometimes require over 20 cases that can take more than 5 hours to complete.[86] Even when essay tests are well constructed, they do not necessarily correlate with supervisor ratings and can be impacted by the writing of the learner (e.g., language, grammar).[87,88] The open-response items in MEQs face similar threats to validity and reliability, with some studies also finding that they do not necessarily test higher-order clinical reasoning better than MCQs.[84,89] For these reasons MEQs, short-answer essay questions, and particularly long-answer essay questions are only used in formative assessment and not high-stakes examinations.

Advantages and Disadvantages

Unfortunately, highly reliable essay or MEQ tests are resource intensive to both develop and grade, limiting their overall feasibility. Despite being resource intensive, a significant advantage of essay questions over other forms of clinical reasoning assessment is the lack of cueing, which can arguably make essay questions a more reflective assessment of a learner's clinical reasoning. Because of the lack of cueing, experts do find both essays and MEQs strong in assessing most clinical reasoning components of diagnosis (e.g., differential, leading, and justification), and management with MEQs also gives flexibility to incorporate information gathering.[15]

Script Concordance Test

The script concordance test (SCT) was introduced in the late 1990s with a focus on evaluating how learners interpreted information during uncertain clinical situations that resembled actual medical practice.[90] Based on the illness script literature, SCTs were designed to highlight how medical knowledge is organized, accessed, and interpreted by a clinician.[91,92]

Overview

SCTs comprise a brief case vignette followed by a collection of items. Each question is formatted along the structure of "if you were considering this [e.g., possible diagnosis or treatment]", "and you learned [new clinical information]", "this [aspect of the case] becomes [question on change in likelihood]" (Fig. 7.4). For the second part of the item ("new clinical information"), additional history, physical examination, laboratory, or imaging findings are provided. The question in the third part of the item is based on a type of judgment, which can be a diagnosis, investigation,

(A. Diagnosis Example): A 58-year-old woman presents to the emergency department with a two-week history of intermittent vertigo. She feels well between episodes						
If you were thinking of:	And then you find:	The diagnosis becomes:				
Q1. Benign paroxysmal positional vertigo	Episodes of vertigo lasting 30 minutes	-2	-1	0	1	2
Q2. Transient ischemic attacks	History of hypertension	-2	-1	0	1	2
Q3. Meniere's syndrome	Recent surgical removal of a skin lesion	-2	-1	0	1	2
(B. Investigation Example): A 33-year-old woman with polycystic ovarian syndrome and previous pregnancy-associated hypertension has been referred for evaluation of postpartum headaches, visual disturbances, and paresthesia of the arms. Her blood pressure in your office is 180/100						
If you were thinking of:	And then you find:	The diagnosis becomes:				
Q4. Ordering magnetic resonance venography (MRV)	The patient's headaches worsen when she lies flat	-2	-1	0	1	2
Q5. Ordering a 24-hour urinary protein collection	The patient underwent a spontaneous vaginal delivery 4 weeks ago	-2	-1	0	1	2
Q6. Performing a lumbar puncture	The patient underwent caesarian section 1 week ago	-2	-1	0	1	2
(C. Treatment Example): You have been asked to see a hypertensive 74-year-old woman on hydrochlorothiazide and aspirin 80mg daily who experienced a 15-minute episode of slurred speech and clumsiness of the left hand. Carotid dopplers demonstrate 90% stenosis of the right internal carotid artery.						
If you were thinking of:	And then you find:	The diagnosis becomes:				
Q7. Sending her for a right carotid endarterectomy	70% stenosis of the left internal carotid artery	-2	-1	0	1	2
Q8. Initiating stain therapy	LDL 1.97 mmol/L (normal range 2.00-3.40 mmol/L	-2	-1	0	1	2
Q9. Replacing aspirin with clopidogrel 75mg daily	Patient has a history of peptic ulcer disease	-2	-1	0	1	2

• **Fig. 7.4** Script concordance test: (A) diagnosis, (B) investigation, and (C) treatment. Modified from Lubarsky S, Dory V, Duggan P, Gagnon R, Charlin B. Script concordance testing: from theory to practice: AMEE Guide No.75. *Med Teach*. 2013;35(3):184–193. doi:10.3109/0142159X.2013.760036.

or treatment that is framed in the form of a Likert scale. The Likert scale usually includes five choices from −2 to +2, but some have used three choices. The score has different meanings depending on the type of question: in a diagnosis question, −2 means ruled out and +2 means certain; in an investigation question, −2 means contraindicated whereas +2 means indicated; in a treatment question, −2 means unnecessary and +2 means necessary (Fig. 7.4).[91,93,94]

Grading is based on faculty who complete the same test, with the learner receiving full, partial, or no credit depending on how frequently faculty chose the answer the learner selected. For example, if 10 faculty took a test and on a particular item five of them chose the answer correlated to 0, three chose the answer correlated to +1, and two chose the answer correlated to −1, a learner would receive 1 point for selecting 0, 0.6 points for choosing +1, 0.4 points for choosing −1, and no points for choosing −2 or +2. Tests can be taken in written or computer format, with each test typically taking 60 to 90 minutes and including 20 to 30 items.[94] Passing scores vary but are anywhere from two to four standard deviations below the faculty score depending on how much of a novice the learner is.[94]

Evidence

The SCT has some strong evidence as a clinical reasoning assessment format, albeit with some notable caveats. It appears to have stronger face validity in that it mimics realistic clinical scenarios, moves beyond the retrieval of facts, and is grounded in actual clinician responses. SCTs weakly correlate with fact-based exams, suggesting a construct validity that may be closer to the clinical reasoning process.[15,95] To optimize reliability, SCTs should include around 25 cases with at least three items per case, each created with a level of ambiguity or incompleteness.[96,97] Development of the answer key is best when at least 10 panelists are involved, all of whom have expertise in the field and work in a similar setting to the learners', though some have used fewer panelists (e.g., five) with good results.[93,97,98] There have been some concerns about the scoring system, with some studies finding partial credit more reliable and others less reliable.[98,99] Additionally, it appears that anchors at the extremes of the scale often receive less credit than those in the middle.[100] Some have also called for a free-text box where the learner can explain their answer to better understand the grounding for their Likert rating. For those reasons, SCTs are less used today than previously in high-stakes medical examinations.

Advantages and Disadvantages

As previously described, one advantage of the SCT is that it can reflect the uncertainty in clinical practice more than other assessments. SCTs are also easy to administer and grade, though they do require clear explanations to learners given the unfamiliar answer format. They can be time intensive to develop, requiring multiple writers and a large group of panelists.[91] When evaluated on their clinical reasoning components, SCTs appear to best assess learners' ability to make a leading diagnosis or appropriately manage a patient but are weakest in their evaluation of data collection.[15]

Key Feature Examinations

Designed in the late 1980s and early 1990s, key feature examinations (KFEs) are a form of assessment targeted at a learner's clinical reasoning around the "key features" in a patient case.[101,102] These key features can be described as stages or decisions that could impact how a healthcare problem is resolved and where learners might be most likely to make errors.[103]

Overview

KFEs typically include 10 to 40 cases, usually with two to five items (i.e., questions) specific to a given case vignette.[104] Each case in a KFE begins with a patient's presentation, which is subsequently followed by questions around the important diagnostic and/or management decisions (Fig. 7.5) such as diagnoses being considered, relevant history information, or possible management options. Questions can be write-in (i.e., open response) or short menu (i.e., multiple options), with some cases including both types of question style. Short menu questions often include well over 10 possible options with at least several being incorrect to minimize cueing. Learners can choose multiple options, though only the key features are graded. Based on the number of key features identified, the learner receives zero, partial, or full credit. Each case within the exam and items within a case are weighted equally.[15] Selecting extra features outside the "key" features is not penalized unless it is one of the "poison responses" (e.g., a clinically unsafe intervention) for which the learner would lose all points for the case (Fig. 7.5). KFEs are written by a collection of medical educators. They can be taken in written or computer format and can similarly be scored by hand or electronically.[103]

Evidence

Compared to their predecessor, patient management problems, KFEs have demonstrated much better clinical reasoning assessment characteristics. The validation around a KFE requires a consensus process among the educators writing the exam that should be supported by the literature and appropriate piloting prior to administration, often through a blueprinting process.[103,105,106] Both educators and learners have generally endorsed face validity in the appropriateness of the items in previously studied KFEs. To ensure reliability, studies have reported that 30 to 40 cases (3 to 4 hours) might be necessary.[105] From among the types of questions, the write-in style tends to have a lower interrater reliability than the short menu questions. There appears to be some correlation to knowledge-based MCQs and clinical practice performance.[105,107] KFEs are currently used for high-stakes examinations in Canada and Australia.[108]

A 35-year-old mother of 3 presents to your office at 17.00 hours with complaints of severe, watery diarrhea. On questioning, she indicates that she has been ill for about 24 hours. She has had 15 watery bowel movements in the past 24 hours, has been nauseated, but not vomited. She works during the day as a cook in a long-term care facility but left work to come to your office. On her chart, your office nurse notes a resting blood pressure of 105/50 mmHg supine (a pulse of 110/minute), 90/40 standing, and an oral temperature of 36.8°. On physical examination, you find she has dry mucous membranes and active bowel sounds. A urinalysis (urine microscopy) was normal, with a specific gravity of 1.030.

1. What clinical problems would you focus on in your immediate management of this patient? List up to 3

2. How should you treat this patient at this time? Select up to 3

a) Antidiarrheal medication
b) Antiemetic medication
c) Intravenous 0.9% NaCl
d) Intravenous 2/3–1/3
e) Intravenous gentamicin
f) Intravenous metronidazole
g) Intravenous Ringer lactate
h) Nasogastric tube and suction
i) Nothing by mouth
j) Oral ampicillin
k) Oral chloramphenicol
l) Oral fluids
m) Rectal tube
n) Send home with close follow-up
o) Surgical consultation
p) Transfer to hospital

• **Fig. 7.5** Key feature examination question example. Modified from Farmer EA, Page G. A practical guide to assessing clinical decision-making skills using the key features approach. *Med Educ*. 2005 Dec;39(12):1188–1194. doi:10.1111/j.1365-2929.2005.02339.x.

Advantages and Disadvantages

As described, KFEs appear to assess clinical practice performance in addition to medical knowledge, a strength compared to other forms of clinical reasoning assessment. They also can be completed in a less burdensome amount of time, which suggests more feasibility in application. Unfortunately, they can be very resource intensive to develop, including the number of and time required from educators and the complicated grading system.[41] Experts in clinical reasoning rate KFEs favorably in their assessment of creating a differential and management plan but describe it as weaker in problem representation and diagnostic justification.[15] For those reasons, key features might be helpful to use as an adjunct form of clinical reasoning assessment in a health professions program.

Simulation

Part of educational practice since the 1980s, technology-enhanced simulation is an assessment tool that mimics clinical care in a way that requires learner interaction.[109]

Ranging from in-person to virtual experiences, simulation allows learners to practice deliberately in a realistic environment without harming a patient[110,111] (see Chapter 13 for additional discussion). Used to evaluate different types of procedural and clinical skills across fields (e.g., nursing, physician) and learners (e.g., student, fellow, practicing clinician), simulation has also shown potential in assessing clinical reasoning.[112,113]

Overview

There is significant variation among different technology-enhanced simulations depending on setting (i.e., in person or virtual) and platform (i.e., institution or program).[109] In-person simulations usually take place in some form of classroom designed to resemble clinical practice. While being observed, learner(s) interview and examine a high-fidelity mannequin with responses automated or provided by an educator. They are then asked to provide appropriate diagnostic and/or management interventions (and occasionally supporting information) during and/or after the clinical encounter. The educators then typically grade the learner's clinical reasoning performance globally or by different components—most notably including their data collection and its sequence—using a rubric or action log based on expert consensus. Learners can then potentially complete multiple stations in a similar format for different cases.[15]

Computer-based simulations can range from a clinical vignette with electronic media to virtual patients, which specifically require a learner to interact with the case for more information to unfold.[114-117] Computer-based simulation exams can be taken at scheduled times (e.g., during class hours) or at the learner's discretion depending on the educator's preferences. The automated scoring from virtual cases is based on a blueprint or answer key created by faculty experts. Most computer-based simulations include several cases, particularly as they are usually less time and resource intensive than in-person simulations.[114,115]

Evidence

Technology-enhanced simulation, particularly when conducted in person, can have high face validity for clinical reasoning as it can better account for situational factors that affect clinical reasoning in practice. Some studies have shown improvement in learner clinical reasoning through simulation, which can be best promoted by authentic case development at a difficulty that can discriminate between learners.[117,118] Reliability requires a well-designed scoring rubric and trained faculty graders, which can be limited in the in-person setting compared to the automated scoring from computer-based simulations.[119] While most technology-enhanced simulation is used formatively in evaluation, there are some notable high-stakes summative evaluations, including the United States Medical Licensing Examination (USMLE) Step 3 evaluation in the United States.[15]

Advantages and Disadvantages

The most significant advantage of technology-enhanced simulations is how comparable they are to real clinical experiences. This allows faculty to not only better evaluate a learner's clinical reasoning but also collect rich data from which to evaluate. Unfortunately, they can be very resource intensive, including time and cost, which can be important to ensure enough cases to accurately assess clinical reasoning.[15,41] Computer-based simulations potentially offer a balance of improved face validity from most clinical reasoning assessments (e.g., MCQs and SCTs) while requiring fewer resources.[114] Both in-person and computer-based simulations have also shown some versatility in adapting to the challenges of the COVID-19 pandemic.[120,121] When educators have evaluated technology-enhanced simulation, they noted they felt they were helpful in evaluating data collection, diagnostic justification, and management but were less useful for evaluating problem representation.[15]

Interesting Tools for Consideration

While no clinical reasoning test is perfect, utilizing each based on the resources and needs of the health professions program can allow educators to triangulate their learners' clinical reasoning effectively. Two promising and additional tools that might be worth considering despite limited evidence to date in their assessment include concept maps and clinical integrative puzzles.

Concept Maps

Concept maps were first developed in the 1980s as a graphical diagramming exercise for displaying and organizing knowledge.[122] Meant to foster deeper learning, concept maps were intended to enable learners to understand new concepts and connect them to previous knowledge on the topic.

Overview

When creating a concept map (Fig. 7.6), the learner is first presented a case (e.g., a 79-year-old with diabetes presenting with shortness of breath) or a topic (e.g., heart failure, pneumonia) prompt. From that case or topic, the learner identifies the most important concepts at the top of the map, which can be drawn on a sheet of paper or entered into a computer program.[123,124] Depending on the prompt and setting, each concept can vary in its clarity (e.g., concrete, abstract, general, specific) or category (e.g., epidemiological factor [age, comorbidities], pathophysiology [decreased cardiac contractility], clinical feature [dyspnea on exertion]). The learner then writes additional related and

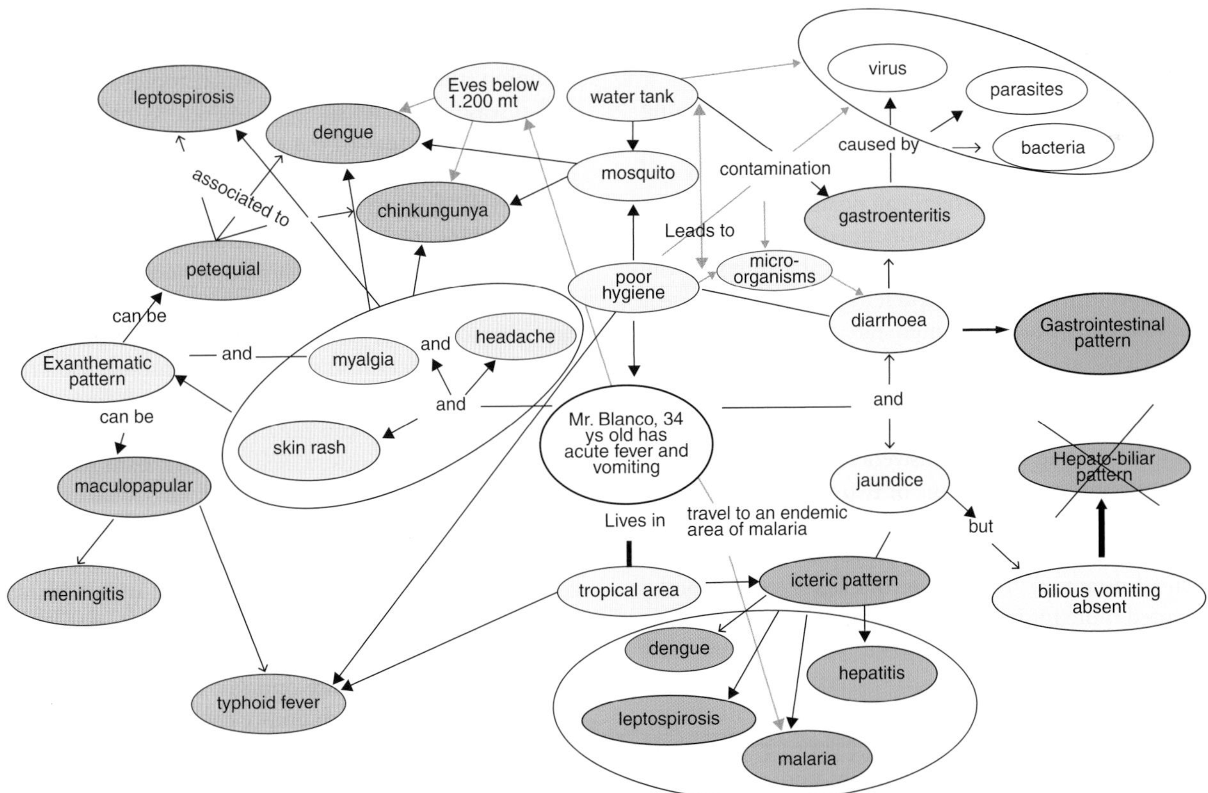

• **Fig. 7.6** Concept map. From Peñuela-Epalza M, De la Hoz K. Incorporation and evaluation of serial concept maps for vertical integration and clinical reasoning in case-based learning tutorials: perspectives of students beginning clinical medicine. *Med Teach*. 2019 Apr;41(4):433–440. doi:10.1080/0142159X.2018.1487046.

more specific concepts and connects them with an arrow (Fig. 7.6). Arrows are typically unidirectional and indicate some level of causality, which can be more explicitly written out on the concept map (i.e., [general concept] → leads to → [specific concept]). The learner then identifies cross-linkages that tie concepts from the left to the right sides of the map.[123] Concept maps can also be partially or nearly filled in when students start them, which can help faculty focus on a particular aspect of a learner's knowledge (e.g., a pathophysiologic mechanism). Some additional variations of concept maps include placement of concepts (e.g., core concepts in the middle), timing (e.g., prior to or during a session), number of learners collaborating on one concept map (e.g., problem-based learning), and use for teaching or assessment.[125,126]

When concept maps are used for assessment, they can be scored in different ways. Sometimes they might be graded broadly on content, presentation, and logic.[127] More specifically, learners can also be graded on depth of the information, connections between concepts, internal consistency, comparisons to instructor concept maps, and relationship to final examinations.[128] There have also been examples of serial concept maps, which are performed at different times during a course and graded on improvement.[129,130] It appears that scoring focused on the quality of the map and its concepts is more important than solely the *structure* of map, which is harder to standardize.[15,131] Most importantly, it is imperative that students and faculty understand the directions for completing and grading the concept map.

Evidence

Concept maps appear to have some promise in assessing clinical reasoning, albeit with certain limitations.[132] There can potentially be high content validity given the depth and connection of knowledge learners can demonstrate, particularly across the knowledge components of an illness script (i.e., epidemiology, pathophysiology, clinical features) or the synthesis aspects of a problem representation (if case based). The face validity appears to be moderate, with students having mixed views on concept map effectiveness, albeit perhaps limited by its possibly challenging construction.[133] They are also impacted by limitations in content and situation (context) sampling as the time intensiveness of creating a concept map prevents more than one or two to be completed in a single session. Reliability across graders for concept maps (interrater) and consistency of a single assessor grading concept maps (intrarater) has been favorable.[134,135] Ultimately, they are used more for low-stakes formative assessment than high-stakes summative assessment.[123]

Advantages and Disadvantages

The biggest advantage of concept maps appears to be their ability to display the depth, elaboration, and connections of a learner's knowledge on a particular subject or how they identify and synthesize the most salient features of a case. They can also be particularly helpful in assessment *for* learning with students showing improved performance after receiving feedback on prior concept maps.[136] The biggest disadvantage is the previously mentioned time intensiveness for students to create concept maps and, to a lesser extent, for educators to grade them. Other notable disadvantages include the emphasis on System 2 (slow, hypotheticodeductive) processing. Experts in clinical reasoning rate concept maps as moderate in assessing for problem representation and differential diagnosis, but as poor in information gathering and hypothesis generation, though that depends on the concept map's prompt.[15]

Clinical or Comprehensive Integrative Puzzles

The comprehensive integrative puzzle (CIP) was first developed in the 1990s as a form of clinical reasoning assessment that could integrate basic science and clinical knowledge by comparing different diagnoses.[137]

Overview

Each CIP is a "grid" that includes selected diagnoses on one axis (rows) and various disease characteristics on the other axis (columns) (Fig. 7.7).[137,138] The grid can be flexible depending on the goals and setting of the assessment (e.g., topic, timing, scoring, stage of learner). The content of a CIP is typically created by a team of educators with various backgrounds, potentially including clinicians, pathologists, pharmacologists, and radiologists. Topics for the CIP can be based on different specialties (e.g., internal medicine, pediatrics), systems (e.g., cardiovascular, pulmonary), or symptoms (e.g., chest pain, shortness of breath). After the topic is chosen, the creators decide which topics (e.g., diagnoses and disease characteristics) to include as response options (Fig. 7.2).[138] Similar to the content and organization of an illness script, the common categories of response options with a CIP focused on establishing the diagnosis include history taking, physical examination, laboratory tests, imaging studies, treatment, follow-up, and pathophysiology. After deciding on the diagnoses and the categories of disease characteristics, the educators create response options that are not only typical of a common presentation for that respective diagnosis but also distinguishing from the other diagnoses. Educators can potentially include additional distractor response options, which are not meant to be used, to increase the CIP's difficulty.[138]

The CIP can be taken in paper or computer format. Multiple CIPs can be completed in the same examination. To complete each CIP, learners are provided with a blank CIP table (e.g., 5 × 5, 5 × 6, 4 × 6, not including the diagnoses) and response option list of disease characteristics (Fig. 7.2). After reading the response options, learners are expected to record an answer for each empty cell in the CIP table. Each response can be used once, multiple times, or zero times depending on the course's preferences.[138] Of note, if each response option is used only once the test becomes easier because potential response options can be subsequently eliminated as the learner completes the CIP. Scoring a CIP similarly depends on the course's objectives and difficulty, but

Student's name ___________

Student's number ___________

Matching columns

Diagnosis	I: Medical history	II: Physical Examination	III: Chest X-ray and ECG	IV: Laboratory and other tests	V: Treatment and follow-up	VI: Pathology
Unstable angina	1(d)	2(c)	3(c)	4(c)	5(d)	6(c)
Myocardial infarction	11(a)	12(a)	13(a)	14(a)	15(c)	16(a)
Rheumatic mitral stenosis	21(b)	22(d)	23(b)	24(d)	25(b)	26(e)
Acute pericarditis	31(f)	32(e)	33(f)	34(f)	35(e)	36(f)
Infective endocarditis	41(e)	42(f)	43(e)	44(e)	45(f)	46(b)
Hypertrophic cardiomyopathy	51(c)	52(b)	53(d)	54(b)	55(a)	56(d)

Section I: History (Abbreviated)
(a) 55-year-old man arrived at the emergency room because of chest pressure, which began three hours beforehand while resting
(b) 28-year-old woman, in her third month of pregnancy, arrived at the emergency room because of severe shortness of breath (dyspnea)
(c) 25-year-old man complains of shortness of breath and dizziness on exertion
(d) 5-year-old man arrived at the emergency room because of 15 minutes of chest pain and sweating, which began without any prior exertion
(e) 32-year-old woman, with known congenital heart defect, was hospitalized with a three-week history of fever, malaise, night sweats, and increasing shortness of breath
(f) 40-year-old woman, suffering for the last three weeks from flulike symptoms, complains of continuous anterior chest pain during the last week

Section V: Treatment (Abbreviated)
(a) Treatment with beta-blockers improved the dyspnea
(b) Immediate catheterization and ballooning of the valve resulted in rapid improvement
(c) Infusion of 2,000 mL resulted in a rise in blood pressure
(d) Treatment with aspirin, heparin, and ACE inhibitors resulted in gradual improvement
(e) Pericardial tap yielded 750 mL of clear yellow fluid and improved symptoms
(f) Penicillin G was given intravenously every 12 hours for four weeks

NOTE: Sections II (Physical Exam), III (X-ray and EKG), IV (Other Diagnostic Tests), and VI (Pathology) not demonstrated

• **Fig. 7.7** Abbreviated comprehensive integrative puzzle. Modified from Ber R. The CIP (comprehensive integrative puzzle) assessment method. *Med Teach*. 2003 Mar;25(2):171–176. doi:10.1080/0142159031000092571.

generally students need to correctly match a predetermined number of cells horizontally and vertically. For instance, in a five-row (diagnosis) by five-column (disease characteristics) CIP, a passing score might be 40% (10 correct cells), 60% (15 correct cells), or 80% (20 correct cells).[138] There can also be a minimum passing number of correct cells for each row or column. CIP results are usually scored manually, and passing scores vary based on the writers' recommendations.

Evidence

There are limited studies evaluating the validity and reliability of the CIP, with the results being mixed in those available. There appears to be some face validity given the structural similarities to an illness script and the typical disease characteristics of the CIP table.[138,139] The content validity of each CIP depends on the expertise of the educators who write the CIP, which is why it can be helpful for the writers to review the CIP together after the responses are initially created.[138] One study showed increasing performance with increasing experience across medical students, residents, and attendings, which seemed to avoid the "intermediate" effect of some clinical reasoning assessment forms.[140] Each CIP's representativeness of a learner's clinical reasoning for that topic depends on how they use their basic science and clinical knowledge to differentiate between the diagnoses. To optimize the response process, students should receive clear instructions about the testing format, which can vary according to different types of content, timing, and scoring parameters, as described earlier. CIP results are usually scored manually and passing scores vary based on the writers' recommendations. Of the few studies that evaluated the CIPs, their reliability has been found to be moderate, with one study demonstrating high Cronbach's alphas[140] and another study finding moderate variation in odd–even reliability for each individual CIP item.[139] Limited, if any, correlation has been seen between CIPs and academic performance in medical students.[139]

Advantages and Disadvantages

CIPs have several advantages. Structurally they offer the benefit of testing both basic science and clinical knowledge while pushing learners to discriminate between those aspects for each diagnosis. They also have high feasibility, typically taking less time to write than many forms of clinical reasoning assessment. Similarly, when learners have been timed taking CIPs they have been able to complete them in a manageable amount of time (e.g., 10–15 minutes).[140] The biggest disadvantage of CIPs is the limited number of studies on their psychometric properties. Structurally some might have concerns that all the data are provided, unlike in real-life clinical reasoning where a learner has to identify the diagnoses, salient features of the presentation, and their own relevant medical knowledge to diagnose and manage a patient. For those considerations, experts have rated the CIP strongest for assessing a learner's ability to identify a leading diagnosis but poorest for assessing a learner's information gathering, hypothesis generation, and diagnostic justification.[15] CIPs might thus be recommended to be incorporated into more formative assessments when there is not sufficient time to develop a more rigorous assessment and/or interest in the assessment is in evaluating the steps prior to the diagnosis (intermediate steps).

Conclusion

Despite being such an important skill to all healthcare providers, clinical reasoning remains challenging to assess in the classroom setting (in vitro). Each type of in vitro clinical reasoning assessment has strengths and weakness in both evidence and resource intensiveness. Educators would be best served utilizing multiple types of assessment over their learners' training in both formative and summative fashion to best triangulate weaknesses and build educational plans accordingly. Moving forward, it would be unsurprising for institutions to perform more types of technology-based assessment that can provide higher-volume and higher-quality data, particularly targeted at components in the clinical reasoning process. Grounding future assessments in clinical reasoning components as well as relevant theory can offer potential for new types of clinical reasoning assessment in the future.

References

1. Leape L, Berwick D, Bates D. Counting deaths due to medical errors–reply. *JAMA*. 2002;288(19):2405.
2. Singh H, Meyer AN, Thomas EJ. The frequency of diagnostic errors in outpatient care: estimations from three large observational studies involving US adult populations. *BMJ Qual Saf.* 2014 Sep;23(9):727–731. doi:10.1136/bmjqs-2013-002627.
3. Singh H, Giardina TD, Meyer AND, Forjuoh SN, Reis MD, Thomas EJ. Types and origins of diagnostic errors in primary care settings. *JAMA Intern Med.* 2013 Mar 25;173(6):418–425. doi:10.1001/jamainternmed.2013.2777.
4. *Improving Diagnosis in Health Care.* National Academies of Sciences, Engineering, and Medicine; Institute of Medicine; Board on Health Care Services; et al., eds. National Academies Press; 2016.
5. Graber ML, Franklin N, Gordon R. Diagnostic error in internal medicine. *Arch Intern Med.* 2005 Jul 11;165(13):1493–1499. doi:10.1001/archinte.165.13.1493.
6. Rencic J, Trowbridge Jr RL, Fagan M, Szauter K, Durning S. Clinical reasoning education at us medical schools: results from a national survey of internal medicine clerkship directors. *J Gen Intern Med.* 2017 Nov;32(11):1242–1246. doi:10.1007/s11606-017-4159-y.
7. Young M, Thomas A, Lubarsky S, et al. Drawing boundaries: the difficulty in defining clinical reasoning. *Acad Med.* 2018 Jul;93(7):990–995. doi:10.1097/ACM.0000000000002142.
8. Young M, Thomas A, Gordon D, et al. The terminology of clinical reasoning in health professions education: implications and considerations. *Med Teach.* 2019 Nov;41(11):1277–1284. doi:10.1080/0142159X.2019.1635686.
9. Wimmers PF, Mentkowski M. *Assessing Competence in Professional Performance Across Disciplines and Professions.* Springer; 2016.
10. Bowen JL. Educational strategies to promote clinical diagnostic reasoning. *N Engl J Med.* 2006 Nov 23;355(21):2217–2225. doi:10.1056/NEJMra054782.
11. Parsons AS, Wijesekera TP, Rencic JJ. The management script: a practical tool for teaching management reasoning. *Acad Med.* 2020 Aug;95(8):1179–1185. doi:10.1097/ACM.0000000000003465.
12. Durning SJ, Artino AR. Situativity theory: a perspective on how participants and the environment can interact: AMEE Guide no. 52. *Med Teach.* 2011;33(3):188–199. doi:10.3109/0142159X.2011.550965.
13. Rencic J, Schuwirth LWT, Gruppen LD, Durning SJ. Clinical reasoning performance assessment: using situated cognition theory as a conceptual framework. *Diagnosis (Berl).* 2020 Aug 27;7(3):241–249. doi:10.1515/dx-2019-0051.
14. Croskerry P, Cosby K, Graber ML, Singh H. *Diagnosis: Interpreting the Shadows.* CRC Press; 2017.
15. Daniel M, Rencic J, Durning SJ, et al. Clinical reasoning assessment methods: a scoping review and practical guidance. *Acad Med.* 2019 Jun;94(6):902–912. doi:10.1097/ACM.0000000000002618.
16. Stojan JN, Daniel M, Hartley S, Gruppen L. Dealing with uncertainty in clinical reasoning: a threshold model and the roles of experience and task framing. *Med Educ.* 2022 Feb;56(2):195–201. doi:10.1111/medu.14673.
17. Pauker SG, Kassirer JP. The threshold approach to clinical decision making. *N Engl J Med.* 1980 May 15;302(20):1109–1117. doi:10.1056/NEJM198005153022003.
18. Stojan JN, Daniel M, Morgan HK, Whitman L, Gruppen LD. A randomized cohort study of diagnostic and therapeutic thresholds in medical student clinical reasoning. *Acad Med.* 2017;92(11S Association of American Medical Colleges Learn Serve Lead: Proceedings of the 56th Annual Research in Medical Education Sessions):S43–S47. doi:10.1097/ACM.0000000000001909.
19. Cook DA, Sherbino J, Durning SJ. Management reasoning: beyond the diagnosis. *JAMA.* 2018 Jun 12;319(22):2267–2268. doi:10.1001/jama.2018.4385.
20. Cook DA, Durning SJ, Sherbino J, Gruppen LD. Management reasoning: implications for health professions educators and a research agenda. *Acad Med.* 2019 Sep;94(9):1310–1316. doi:10.1097/ACM.0000000000002768.
21. Goldszmidt M, Minda JP, Bordage G. Developing a unified list of physicians' reasoning tasks during clinical encounters. *Acad Med.* 2013 Mar;88(3):390–394. doi:10.1097/ACM.0b013e31827fc58d.
22. Cook DA, Blachman MJ, Price DW, et al. Educational technologies for physician continuous professional development: a national survey. *Acad Med.* 2018 Jan;93(1):104–112. doi:10.1097/ACM.0000000000001817.
23. Cook DA, Stephenson CR, Gruppen LD, Durning SJ. Management reasoning scripts: qualitative exploration using simulated physician-patient encounters. *Perspect Med Educ.* 2022 Aug;11(4):196–206. doi:10.1007/s40037-022-00714-y.
24. Norman G. Research in clinical reasoning: past history and current trends. *Med Educ.* 2005 Apr;39(4):418–427. doi:10.1111/j.1365-2929.2005.02127.x.
25. McCarthy WH, Gonnella JS. The simulated patient management problem: a technique for evaluating and teaching clinical competence. *Br J Med Educ.* 1967 Dec;1(5):348–352. doi:10.1111/j.1365-2923.1967.tb01730.x.
26. Newble D, Hoare J, Baxter A. Patient management problems Issues of validity. *Med Educ.* 1982 May;16(3):137–142. doi:10.1111/j.1365-2923.1982.tb01073.x.
27. Eva KW, Neville AJ, Norman GR. Exploring the etiology of content specificity: factors influencing analogic transfer and problem solving. *Acad Med.* 1998 Oct;73(10 Suppl):S1–S5. doi:10.1097/00001888-199810000-00028.
28. Durning SJ, Artino AR, Boulet JR, Dorrance K, van der Vleuten C, Schuwirth L. The impact of selected contextual factors on experts' clinical reasoning performance (does context impact clinical reasoning performance in experts?). *Adv Health Sci Educ Theory Pract.* 2012 Mar;17(1):65–79. doi:10.1007/s10459-011-9294-3.
29. Bordage G. Elaborated knowledge: a key to successful diagnostic thinking. *Acad Med.* 1994 Nov;69(11):883–885. doi:10.1097/00001888-199411000-00004.
30. Custers EJ. Thirty years of illness scripts: theoretical origins and practical applications. *Med Teach.* 2015 Mar;37(5):457–462. doi:10.3109/0142159X.2014.956052.

31. Sweller J. Cognitive load theory, learning difficulty, and instructional design. *Learn Instruct.* 1994;4(4):295–312. doi:10.1016/0959-4752(94)90003-5.
32. Paas F, Van Gog T, Sweller J. Cognitive load theory: new conceptualizations, specifications, and integrated research perspectives. *Educ Psychol Rev.* 2010;22(2):115–121. doi:10.1007/s10648-010-9133-8.
33. Young JQ, Van Merrienboer J, Durning S, ten Cate O. Cognitive load theory: implications for medical education: AMEE Guide No. 86. *Med Teach.* 2014 May;36(5):371–384. doi:10.3109/0142159X.2014.889290.
34. Daniel M, Durning SJ, Wilson E, Abdoler E, Torre D. Situated cognition: clinical reasoning and error are context dependent. *Diagnosis (Berl).* 2020 Aug 27;7(3):341–342. doi:10.1515/dx-2020-0011.
35. Kahneman D. *Thinking, Fast and Slow.* Macmillan; 2011.
36. Croskerry P. A universal model of diagnostic reasoning. *Acad Med.* 2009 Aug;84(8):1022–1028. doi:10.1097/ACM.0b013e3181ace703.
37. Croskerry P. Clinical cognition and diagnostic error: applications of a dual process model of reasoning. *Adv Health Sci Educ Theory Pract.* 2009 Sep;14(Suppl 1):27–35. doi:10.1007/s10459-009-9182-2.
38. Pelaccia T, Tardif J, Triby E, Charlin B. An analysis of clinical reasoning through a recent and comprehensive approach: the dual-process theory. *Med Educ Online.* 2011 Mar 14;16. doi:10.3402/meo.v16i0.5890.
39. Mamede S, et al. Conscious thought beats deliberation without attention in diagnostic decision-making: at least when you are an expert. *Psychol Res.* 2010;74(6):586–592. doi:10.1007/s00426-010-0281-8.
40. Mamede S, Hautz WE, Berendonk C, et al. Think twice: effects on diagnostic accuracy of returning to the case to reflect upon the initial diagnosis. *Acad Med.* 2020 Aug;95(8):1223–1229. doi:10.1097/ACM.0000000000003153.
41. Trowbridge RL, Rencic JJ, Durning SJ. *Teaching Clinical Reasoning.* American College of Physicians; 2015.
42. Croskerry P, Petrie DA, Reilly JB, Tait G. Deciding about fast and slow decisions. *Acad Med.* 2014 Feb;89(2):197–200. doi:10.1097/ACM.0000000000000121.
43. Van Merrienboer JJ, Sweller J. Cognitive load theory and complex learning: recent developments and future directions. *Educ Psych Rev.* 2005;17(2):147–177. doi:10.1007/s10648-005-3951-0.
44. Van Merrienboer J, Sweller J. Cognitive load theory in health professional education: design principles and strategies. *Med Educ.* 2010 Jan;44(1):85–93. doi:10.1111/j.1365-2923.2009.03498.x.
45. Szulewski A, Howes D, van Merriënboer JJG, Sweller J. From theory to practice: the application of cognitive load theory to the practice of medicine. *Acad Med.* 2021 Jan 1;96(1):24–30. doi:10.1097/ACM.0000000000003524.
46. Bordage G, Lemieux M. Semantic structures and diagnostic thinking of experts and novices. *Acad Med.* 1991 Sep;66(9 Suppl):S70–S72. doi:10.1097/00001888-199109000-00045.
47. Custers EJ, Regehr G, Norman GR. Mental representations of medical diagnostic knowledge: a review. *Acad Med.* 1996 Oct;71(10 Suppl):S55–S61. doi:10.1097/00001888-199610000-00044.
48. Schmidt HG, Rikers RM. How expertise develops in medicine: knowledge encapsulation and illness script formation. *Med Educ.* 2007 Dec;41(12):1133–1139. doi:10.1111/j.1365-2923.2007.02915.x.
49. Abdoler EA, O'Brien BC, Schwartz BS. Following the script: an exploratory study of the therapeutic reasoning underlying physicians' choice of antimicrobial therapy. *Acad Med.* 2020 Aug;95(8):1238–1247.doi:10.1097/ACM.0000000000003498.
50. Cook DA, Stephenson CR, Gruppen LD, Durning SJ. Management reasoning: empirical determination of key features and a conceptual model. *Acad Med.* 2023 Jan 1;98(1):80–87. doi:10.1097/ACM.0000000000004810.
51. Mamede S, van Gog T, Sampaio AM, de Faria RM, Maria JP, Schmidt HG. How can students' diagnostic competence benefit most from practice with clinical cases? The effects of structured reflection on future diagnosis of the same and novel diseases. *Acad Med.* 2014 Jan;89(1):121–127. doi:10.1097/ACM.0000000000000076.
52. Ericsson KA. Deliberate practice and the acquisition and maintenance of expert performance in medicine and related domains. *Acad Med.* 2004 Oct;79(10 Suppl):S70–S81. doi:10.1097/00001888-200410001-00022.
53. Ericsson KA. Deliberate practice and acquisition of expert performance: a general overview. *Acad Emerg Med.* 2008 Nov;15(11):988–994. doi:10.1111/j.1553-2712.2008.00227.x.
54. Rencic J. Twelve tips for teaching expertise in clinical reasoning. *Med Teach.* 2011;33(11):887–892. doi:10.3109/0142159X.2011.558142.
55. Mylopoulos M. Preparing future adaptive experts: why it matters and how it can be done. *Med Sci Educ.* 2020 Sep 30;30(Suppl 1):11–12. doi:10.1007/s40670-020-01089-7.
56. Mylopoulos M, Kulasegaram K, Woods NN. Developing the experts we need: fostering adaptive expertise through education. *J Eval Clin Pract.* 2018 Jun;24(3):674–677. doi:10.1111/jep.12905.
57. Mylopoulos M, Woods NN. When I say … adaptive expertise. *Med Educ.* 2017 Jul;51(7):685–686. doi:10.1111/medu.13247.
58. Mylopoulos M, Steenhof N, Kaushal A, Woods NN. Twelve tips for designing curricula that support the development of adaptive expertise. *Med Teach.* 2018 Aug;40(8):850–854. doi:10.1080/0142159X.2018.1484082.
59. Steenhof N, Woods NN, Van Gerven PWM, Mylopoulos M. Productive failure as an instructional approach to promote future learning. *Adv Health Sci Educ Theory Pract.* 2019 Oct;24(4):739–749. doi:10.1007/s10459-019-09895-4.
60. Holmboe ES, Durning SJ. Understanding the social in diagnosis and error: a family of theories known as situativity to better inform diagnosis and error. *Diagnosis (Berl).* 2020 Aug 27;7(3):161–164. doi:10.1515/dx-2020-0080.
61. Merkebu J, Battistone M, McMains K, et al. Situativity: a family of social cognitive theories for understanding clinical reasoning and diagnostic error. *Diagnosis (Berl).* 2020 Aug 27;7(3):169–176. doi:10.1515/dx-2019-0100.
62. Daniel M, Wilson E, Torre D, Durning SJ, Lang V. Embodied cognition: knowing in the head is not enough. *Diagnosis (Berl).* 2020 Aug 27;7(3):337–338. doi:10.1515/dx-2020-0004.
63. Wilson E, Seifert C, Durning SJ, Torre D, Daniel M. Distributed cognition: interactions between individuals and artifacts. *Diagnosis (Berl).* 2020 Aug 27;7(3):343–344. doi:10.1515/dx-2020-0012.
64. Daniel M, Torre D, Durning SJ, Wilson E, Rencic JJ. Ecological psychology: diagnosing and treating patients in complex environments. *Diagnosis (Berl).* 2020 Aug 27;7(3):339–340. doi:10.1515/dx-2020-0008.
65. Olson AP, Graber ML. Improving diagnosis through education. *Acad Med.* 2020 Aug;95(8):1162. doi:10.1097/ACM.0000000000003172.
66. Downing SM. Validity: on meaningful interpretation of assessment data. *Med Educ.* 2003 Sep;37(9):830–837. doi:10.1046/j.1365-2923.2003.01594.x.

67. Schuwirth LW, Van der Vleuten SP. Programmatic assessment: from assessment of learning to assessment for learning. *Med Teach.* 2011;33(6):478–485. doi:10.3109/0142159X.2011.565828.
68. Van der Vleuten CP, Norman GR, De Graaff E. Pitfalls in the pursuit of objectivity: issues of reliability. *Med Educ.* 1991 Mar;25(2):110–118. doi:10.1111/j.1365-2923.1991.tb00036.x.
69. Joorabchi B, Chawhan AR. Multiple choice questions. The debate goes on. *Br J Med Educ.* 1975 Dec;9(4):275–280. doi:10.1111/j.1365-2923.1975.tb01938.x.
70. Norcini JJ, Swanson DB, Grosso LJ, Shea JA, Webster GD. A comparison of knowledge, synthesis, and clinical judgment. Multiple-choice questions in the assessment of physician competence. *Eval Health Prof.* 1984 Dec;7(4):485–499. doi:10.1177/016327878400700409.
71. Coderre SP, Harasym P, Mandin H, Fick G. The impact of two multiple-choice question formats on the problem-solving strategies used by novices and experts. *BMC Med Educ.* 2004 Nov 5;4:23. doi:10.1186/1472-6920-4-23.
72. Case SM, Swanson DB, Ripkey DR. Comparison of items in five-option and extended-matching formats for assessment of diagnostic skills. *Acad Med.* 1994 Oct;69(10 Suppl):S1–S3. doi:10.1097/00001888-199410000-00023.
73. Beullens J, Struyf E, Van Damme B. Do extended matching multiple-choice questions measure clinical reasoning? *Med Educ.* 2005 Apr;39(4):410–417. doi:10.1111/j.1365-2929.2005.02089.x.
74. Beullens J, Struyf E, Van Damme B. Diagnostic ability in relation to clinical seminars and extended-matching questions examinations. *Med Educ.* 2006 Dec;40(12):1173–1179. doi:10.1111/j.1365-2929.2006.02627.x.
75. Brailovsky CA, Bordage G, Allen T, Dumont H. Writing vs coding diagnostic impressions in an examination: short-answer vs long-menu responses. *Res Med Educ.* 1988;27:201–206.
76. Jozefowicz RF, Koeppen BM, Case S, Galbraith R, Swanson D, Glew RH. The quality of in-house medical school examinations. *Acad Med.* 2002 Feb;77(2):156–161. doi:10.1097/00001888-200202000-00016.
77. Norcini JJ, Boulet JR, Opalek A, Dauphinee WD. The relationship between licensing examination performance and the outcomes of care by international medical school graduates. *Acad Med.* 2014 Aug;89(8):1157–1162. doi:10.1097/ACM.0000000000000310.
78. Heemskerk L, Norman G, Chou S, Mintz M, Mandin H, McLaughlin K. The effect of question format and task difficulty on reasoning strategies and diagnostic performance in internal medicine residents. *Adv Health Sci Educ Theory Pract.* 2008 Nov;13(4):453–462. doi:10.1007/s10459-006-9057-8.
79. Schuwirth LW, van der Vleuten CP, Donkers HH. A closer look at cueing effects in multiple-choice questions. *Med Educ.* 1996 Jan;30(1):44–49. doi:10.1111/j.1365-2923.1996.tb00716.x.
80. Starch D, Elliott EC. Reliability of the grading of high-school work in English. *School Rev.* 1912;20(7):442–457. doi:10.1086/435971.
81. Starch D, Elliott EC. Reliability of grading work in mathematics. *School Rev.* 1913;21(4):254–259. doi:10.1086/436086.
82. Abrahamson S. A study of the objectivity of the essay examination. *Acad Med.* 1964 Jan;39(1):65–68.
83. Feletti GI. Reliability and validity studies on modified essay questions. *J Med Educ.* 1980 Nov;55(11):933–941. doi:10.1097/00001888-198011000-00006.
84. Palmer EJ, Devitt PG. Assessment of higher order cognitive skills in undergraduate education: modified essay or multiple choice questions? Research paper. *BMC Med Educ.* 2007 Nov 28;7(1):1–7. doi:10.1186/1472-6920-7-49.
85. Oermann M. Developing and scoring essay tests. *Nurse Educ.* 1999 Mar-Apr;24(2):29–32. doi:10.1097/00006223-199903000-00010.
86. Norcini JJ, Diserens D, Day SC, et al. The scoring and reproducibility of an essay test of clinical judgment. *Acad Med.* 1990 Sep;65(9 Suppl):S41–S42. doi:10.1097/00001888-199009000-00035.
87. Day SC, Norcini JJ, Diserens D, et al. The validity of an essay test of clinical judgment. *Acad Med.* 1990 Sep;65(9 Suppl):S39–S40. doi:10.1097/00001888-199009000-00034.
88. de Graaff E, Post G, Drop M. Validation of a new measure of clinical problem-solving. *Med Educ.* 1987 May;21(3):213–218. doi:10.1111/j.1365-2923.1987.tb00693.x.
89. Reinert A, Berlin A, Swan-Sein A, Nowygrod R, Fingeret A. Validity and reliability of a novel written examination to assess knowledge and clinical decision making skills of medical students on the surgery clerkship. *Am J Surg.* 2014 Feb;207(2):236–242. doi:10.1016/j.amjsurg.2013.08.024.
90. Charlin B, Brailovsky C, Leduc C, Blouin D. The Diagnosis Script questionnaire: a new tool to assess a specific dimension of clinical competence. *Adv Health Sci Educ Theory Pract.* 1998;3(1):51–58. doi:10.1023/A:1009741430850.
91. Lubarsky S, Dory V, Duggan P, Gagnon R, Charlin B. Script concordance testing: from theory to practice: AMEE Guide No.75. *Med Teach.* 2013;35(3):184–193. doi:10.3109/0142159X.2013.760036.
92. Lubarsky S, Dory V, Audétat M-C, Custers E, Charlin B. Using script theory to cultivate illness script formation and clinical reasoning in health professions education. *Can Med Educ J.* 2015 Dec 11;6(2):e61–e70.
93. Kelly W, Durning S, Denton G. Comparing a script concordance examination to a multiple-choice examination on a core internal medicine clerkship. *Teach Learn Med.* 2012;24(3):187–193. doi:10.1080/10401334.2012.692239.
94. Dory V, Gagnon R, Vanpee D, Charlin B. How to construct and implement script concordance tests: insights from a systematic review. *Med Educ.* 2012 Jun;46(6):552–563. doi:10.1111/j.1365-2923.2011.04211.x.
95. Collard A, Gelaes S, Vanbelle S, et al. Reasoning versus knowledge retention and ascertainment throughout a problem-based learning curriculum. *Med Educ.* 2009 Sep;43(9):854–865. doi:10.1111/j.1365-2923.2009.03410.x.
96. Fournier JP, Demeester A, Charlin B. Script concordance tests: guidelines for construction. *BMC Med Inform Decis Mak.* 2008 May 6;8:18. doi:10.1186/1472-6947-8-18.
97. Gagnon R, Charlin B, Coletti M, Sauvé E, van der Vleuten C. Assessment in the context of uncertainty: how many members are needed on the panel of reference of a script concordance test? *Med Educ.* 2005 Mar;39(3):284–291. doi:10.1111/j.1365-2929.2005.02092.x.
98. Charlin B, Gagnon R, Pelletier J, et al. Assessment of clinical reasoning in the context of uncertainty: the effect of variability within the reference panel. *Med Educ.* 2006 Sep;40(9):848–854. doi:10.1111/j.1365-2929.2006.02541.x.
99. Charlin B, Desaulniers M, Gagnon R, Blouin D, van der Vleuten C. Comparison of an aggregate scoring method with a consensus scoring method in a measure of clinical reasoning capacity. *Teach Learn Med.* 2002 Summer;14(3):150–156. doi:10.1207/S15328015TLM1403_3.
100. Lineberry M, Kreiter CD, Bordage G. Threats to validity in the use and interpretation of script concordance test scores. *Med Educ.* 2013 Dec;47(12):1175–1183. doi:10.1111/medu.12283.

101. Page G, Bordage G. The Medical Council of Canada's key features project: a more valid written examination of clinical decision-making skills. *Acad Med.* 1995 Feb;70(2):104–110. doi:10.1097/00001888-199502000-00012.
102. Page G, Bordage G, Allen T. Developing key-feature problems and examinations to assess clinical decision-making skills. *Acad Med.* 1995 Mar;70(3):194–201. doi:10.1097/00001888-199503000-00009.
103. Farmer EA, Page G. A practical guide to assessing clinical decision-making skills using the key features approach. *Med Educ.* 2005 Dec;39(12):1188–1194. doi:10.1111/j.1365-2929.2005.02339.x.
104. Hrynchak P, Takahashi SG, Nayer M. Key-feature questions for assessment of clinical reasoning: a literature review. *Med Educ.* 2014 Sep;48(9):870–883. doi:10.1111/medu.12509.
105. Fischer MR, Kopp V, Holzer M, Ruderich F, Jünger J. A modified electronic key feature examination for undergraduate medical students: validation threats and opportunities. *Med Teach.* 2005 Aug;27(5):450–455. doi:10.1080/01421590500078471.
106. Bordage G, Brailovsky C, Carretier H, Page G. Content validation of key features on a national examination of clinical decision-making skills. *Acad Med.* 1995 Apr;70(4):276–281. doi:10.1097/00001888-199504000-00010.
107. Tamblyn R, Abrahamowicz M, Dauphinee D, et al. Influence of physicians' management and communication ability on patients' persistence with antihypertensive medication. *Arch Intern Med.* 2010 Jun 28;170(12):1064–1072. doi:10.1001/archinternmed.2010.167.
108. Farmer EA, Hinchy J. Assessing general practice clinical decision making skills: the key features approach. *Aust Fam Physician.* 2005 Dec;34(12):1059–1061.
109. Ilgen JS, Sherbino J, Cook DA. Technology-enhanced simulation in emergency medicine: a systematic review and meta-analysis. *Acad Emerg Med.* 2013 Feb;20(2):117–127. doi:10.1111/acem.12076.
110. Ziv A, Wolpe PR, Small SD, Glick S. Simulation-based medical education: an ethical imperative. *Acad Med.* 2003 Aug;78(8):783–788. doi:10.1097/00001888-200308000-00006.
111. Abdulnour RE, Parsons AS, Muller D, Drazen J, Rubin EJ, Rencic J. Deliberate practice at the virtual bedside to improve clinical reasoning. *N Engl J Med.* 2022 May 19;386(20):1946–1947. doi:10.1056/NEJMe2204540.
112. Cook DA, Hatala R, Brydges R, et al. Technology-enhanced simulation for health professions education: a systematic review and meta-analysis. *JAMA.* 2011 Sep 7;306(9):978–988. doi:10.1001/jama.2011.1234.
113. Jensen R. Clinical reasoning during simulation: comparison of student and faculty ratings. *Nurse Educ Pract.* 2013 Jan;13(1):23–28. doi:10.1016/j.nepr.2012.07.001.
114. Cook DA, Triola MM. Virtual patients: a critical literature review and proposed next steps. *Med Educ.* 2009 Apr;43(4):303–311. doi:10.1111/j.1365-2923.2008.03286.x.
115. Waechter J, Allen J, Lee CH, Zwaan L. Development and pilot testing of a data-rich clinical reasoning training and assessment tool. *Acad Med.* 2022 Oct 1;97(10):1484–1488. doi:10.1097/ACM.0000000000004758.
116. Watari T, Tokuda Y, Owada M, Onigata K. The utility of virtual patient simulations for clinical reasoning education. *Int J Environ Res Public Health.* 2020 Jul 24;17(15):5325. doi:10.3390/ijerph17155325.
117. Plackett R, Kassianos AP, Timmis J, Sheringham J, Schartau P, Kambouri M. Using virtual patients to explore the clinical reasoning skills of medical students: mixed methods study. *J Med Internet Res.* 2021 Jun 4;23(6):e24723. doi:10.2196/24723.
118. Mutter MK, Martindale JR, Shah N, Gusic ME, Wolf SJ. Case-based teaching: does the addition of high-fidelity simulation make a difference in medical students' clinical reasoning skills? *Med Sci Educ.* 2020 Jan 10;30(1):307–313. doi:10.1007/s40670-019-00904-0.
119. Cook DA, Brydges R, Zendejas B, Hamstra SJ, Hatala R. Technology-enhanced simulation to assess health professionals: a systematic review of validity evidence, research methods, and reporting quality. *Acad Med.* 2013 Jun;88(6):872–883. doi:10.1097/ACM.0b013e31828ffdcf.
120. Ray JM, Wong AH, Yang TJ, et al. Virtual telesimulation for medical students during the COVID-19 pandemic. *Acad Med.* 2021 Oct 1;96(10):1431–1435. doi:10.1097/ACM.0000000000004129.
121. Hege I, Sudacka M, Kononowicz AA, et al. Adaptation of an international virtual patient collection to the COVID-19 pandemic. *GMS J Med Educ.* 2020 Nov 3;37(7):Doc92. doi:10.3205/zma001385.
122. Novak JD, Gowin DB. *Learning How to Learn.* Cambridge University Press; 1984.
123. Daley BJ, Torre DM. Concept maps in medical education: an analytical literature review. *Med Educ.* 2010 May;44(5):440–448. doi:10.1111/j.1365-2923.2010.03628.x.
124. Ertmer PA, Nour AY. Teaching basic medical sciences at a distance: strategies for effective teaching and learning in internet-based courses. *J Vet Med Educ.* 2007 Summer;34(3):316–324. doi:10.3138/jvme.34.3.316.
125. Hsu LL. Developing concept maps from problem-based learning scenario discussions. *J Adv Nurs.* 2004 Dec;48(5):510–518. doi:10.1111/j.1365-2648.2004.03233.x.
126. Williams M. Concept mapping—a strategy for assessment. *Nurs Stand.* 2004 Nov;19(9):33–38. doi:10.7748/ns2004.11.19.9.33.c3754.
127. Moni RW, Moni KB. Student perceptions and use of an assessment rubric for a group concept map in physiology. *Adv Physiol Educ.* 2008 Mar;32(1):47–54. doi:10.1152/advan.00030.2007.
128. McGaghie WC, McCrimmon DR, Mitchell G, Thompson JA, Ravitch MM. Quantitative concept mapping in pulmonary physiology: comparison of student and faculty knowledge structures. *Adv Physiol Educ.* 2000 Jun;23(1):72–81. doi:10.1152/advances.2000.23.1.S72.
129. Peñuela-Epalza M, De la Hoz K. Incorporation and evaluation of serial concept maps for vertical integration and clinical reasoning in case-based learning tutorials: perspectives of students beginning clinical medicine. *Med Teach.* 2019 Apr;41(4):433–440. doi:10.1080/0142159X.2018.1487046.
130. González HL, Palencia AP, Umaña LA, Galindo L, Villafrade M LA. Mediated learning experience and concept maps: a pedagogical tool for achieving meaningful learning in medical physiology students. *Adv Physiol Educ.* 2008 Dec;32(4):312–316. doi:10.1152/advan.00021.2007.
131. Srinivasan M, McElvany M, Shay JM, Shavelson RJ, West DC. Measuring knowledge structure: reliability of concept mapping assessment in medical education. *Acad Med.* 2008 Dec;83(12):1196–1203. doi:10.1097/ACM.0b013e31818c6e84.
132. Pierce C, Corral J, Aagaard E, Harnke B, Irby DM, Stickrath C. A BEME realist synthesis review of the effectiveness of teaching strategies used in the clinical setting on the development of clinical skills among health professionals: BEME Guide No. 61.

Med Teach. 2020 Jun;42(6):604–615. doi:10.1080/0142159X.2019.1708294.

133. Edmondson KM, Smith DF. Concept mapping to facilitate veterinary students' understanding of fluid and electrolyte disorders. *Teach Learn Med.* 1998;10(1):21–33.
134. Pottier P, Hardouin J-B, Hodges BD, et al. Exploring how students think: a new method combining think-aloud and concept mapping protocols. *Med Educ.* 2010 Sep;44(9):926–935. doi:10.1111/j.1365-2923.2010.03748.x.
135. Vink S, van Tartwijk J, Verloop N, Gosselink M, Driessen E, Bolk J. The articulation of integration of clinical and basic sciences in concept maps: differences between experienced and resident groups. *Adv Health Sci Educ Theory Pract.* 2016 Aug;21(3):643–657. doi:10.1007/s10459-015-9657-2.
136. Morse D, Jutras F. Implementing concept-based learning in a large undergraduate classroom. *CBE Life Sci Educ.* 2008 Summer;7(2):243–253. doi:10.1187/cbe.07-09-0071.
137. Ber R. Design of an integrative course and assessment method: the CIP (comprehensive integrative puzzle). *Advances in Medical Education*. Springer; 1997:84–86.
138. Ber R. The CIP (comprehensive integrative puzzle) assessment method. *Med Teach.* 2003 Mar;25(2):171–176. doi:10.1080/0142159031000092571.
139. Capaldi VF, Durning SJ, Pangaro LN, Ber R. The clinical integrative puzzle for teaching and assessing clinical reasoning: preliminary feasibility, reliability, and validity evidence. *Mil Med.* 2015 Apr;180(4 Suppl):54–60. doi:10.7205/MILMED-D-14-00564.
140. Groothoff JW, Frenkel J, Tytgat GAM, Vreede WB, Bosman DK, ten Cate OT. Growth of analytical thinking skills over time as measured with the MATCH test. *Med Educ.* 2008 Oct;42(10):1037–1043. doi:10.1111/j.1365-2923.2008.03152.x.

8

Assessing Clinical Reasoning in the Workplace

JAMES G. BOYLE, MBCHB, MD, MSC, FRCP, ERIC S. HOLMBOE, MD, AND STEVEN J. DURNING, MD, PHD

CHAPTER OUTLINE

Introduction

Chapter 7 discussed cognitive assessment in more standardized and controlled situations, highlighting the different methods and techniques—including multiple-choice, essay, concept mapping, script concordance testing, and key feature approaches—one can use to explore constructs such as clinical reasoning in written formats. Additional chapters in this book have addressed other standardized performance formats, such as objective structured clinical examinations (OSCEs), for assessing topics like clinical reasoning.

In this chapter we discuss assessment of clinical reasoning (i.e., a construct of assessment) from an in vivo or workplace perspective and build upon discussions from prior chapters and germane findings from the literature (Appendix 8.1). While clinical reasoning will be used as the construct of focus for this chapter, aspects of this discussion may also apply to other important assessment constructs germane to the workplace the reader might have in mind, such as professionalism and teamwork. We will begin with a background, followed by a theoretical framework and then a description of selected emerging methods for workplace assessment at both the individual learner and program levels that could be used in the local context. We will end with notable challenges and opportunities with these emerging methods.

Background

We have witnessed dramatic changes in both clinical practice and medical education over the past several decades and even since the first edition of this book. These changes have been fueled in part by advances in science and technology as well as evolution in how we approach the assessment of our learners and programs to include competencies, milestones, Entrustable Professional Activities EPAs), electronic health records (EHRs), and point-of-care resources, to just name a few (see Chapter 1).

Despite profound advances in technological capability, the human process of clinical reasoning leading to accurate diagnosis and management remains essential to high-quality and safe patient care in the clinical environment. For example, studies over the past 30 years have demonstrated the centrality of the medical interview in making a correct diagnosis.[1,2] Furthermore, results on high-stakes, written examinations often only explain a small fraction of the wide variation currently seen in clinical practice. Diagnostic errors remain a serious and vexing problem for patients and the healthcare system despite decades of rigorous high-stakes examinations.[3] The recent National Academy of Medicine (NAM) report, "Improving Diagnosis in Medicine," highlighted diagnostic error as a pernicious and persistent patient safety problem. The report noted that almost every patient can expect to experience at least one diagnostic error in their lifetime.[4] Makary and Daniel, in a review of studies focused on medical error, concluded that medical error may be the third leading cause of death in the United States, with diagnostic error a substantial source of medical errors.[5] Regardless of where errors actually rank as a cause of death, almost everyone agrees that too many patients are harmed by diagnostic errors. While we have made great strides with in vitro assessment practices as outlined in Chapter 7, these recent data on diagnostic error suggest use of standardized assessments of clinical reasoning is necessary but not sufficient to ensure effective assessment of clinical reasoning.

Flaws in clinical reasoning continue to be a primary contributor to diagnostic errors. Patients consult healthcare professionals with the expectation of receiving an accurate diagnosis and sound clinical management, in an affordable and timely fashion, and without experiencing harm. Practitioners, scholars, funders, and regulatory bodies alike are concerned with these outcomes. Since the publication of the "To Err is Human" report of the Institute of Medicine in 1999, the incidence rate of harm of approximately 25 per 100 hospital patient admissions did not change over a 10-year period.[6,7] Although miscommunication and poor communication are important sources of medical error[8] (as is prescribing error), Graber states in his recent review that "a wide variety of research studies suggest that breakdowns in the diagnostic process result in a staggering toll of harm and patient deaths."[9] The authors of another recent review of 25 years of US malpractice claims note that ". . . diagnostic errors appear to be the most common, most costly and most dangerous of medical mistakes."[10]

We believe that all these findings when coupled with emerging theoretical lenses can shed light onto why in vitro assessments may not sufficiently capture performance in actual practice. These emerging theories can serve as guiding forces behind the development of better workplace or workplace-based assessments (WBAs). We refer to WBAs as "in vivo" assessments occurring in authentic clinical environments, to include assessing the domain of clinical reasoning. Clinical reasoning entails the steps leading up to and including arriving at a diagnosis (diagnostic reasoning) and management (management reasoning). The concept of management reasoning is relatively new in clinical reasoning literature and has been defined as "the cognitive processes by which clinicians integrate clinical information (history, physical exam findings, and test results), preferences, medical knowledge, and contextual (situational) factors to make decisions about the management of an individual patient, including decisions about treatment, further testing, follow-up visits, and allocation of limited resources."[11] Clinical reasoning emphasizes the process (steps up to) and output (diagnostic or management "answer") and thus contrasts with related fields such as decision-making and errors that tend to place more focus on outcome (physician's behavior). These are different but related fields and we recommend that the reader consider the NAM report[4] and the Graber review[9] for a more in-depth discussion of distinctions.

In this chapter we focus on assessing diagnostic clinical reasoning in the workplace. We do so for a number of reasons. Applying a diagnostic "label" is often less value based and nuanced than patient-specific management decisions that need to take into account a patient's circumstances and preferences and requires shared decision-making. Typically, successful management requires the application of an accurate diagnostic label. Just like diagnosis, there is the possibility of getting the right answer for the wrong reason. For example, the patient gets better despite an incorrect diagnosis and/or management plan. In contrast to diagnosis, there can be multiple correct answers in management, and in the assessment of management reasoning careful blueprinting will be required for new domains of performance. While not the focus of this chapter, it is still important to understand the domains of management reasoning that will be impacted by the diagnostic reasoning process. The 12 domains of management reasoning identified thus far through empirical work include:[12]

- Contrasting and selection among multiple solutions
- Prioritization of patient, clinician, and system preferences and constraints
- Communication and shared decision-making
- Ongoing monitoring and adjustment of the management plan
- Dynamic interplay among people, systems, and competing priorities
- Illness-specific knowledge
- Process knowledge
- Management scripts
- Clinician roles as patient, teacher, and salesperson
- Clinician–patient relationship
- Prognostication
- Organization of the clinical encounter (sequencing and time management)

Chapter 10 explores how quality indicators can be used to assess the output of management reasoning. While our understanding of diagnostic reasoning has advanced, there are still challenges to be addressed, and this is even more so with management reasoning.

A Theoretical Framework

To effectively use existing WBA approaches and instruments, a basic understanding of theory is essential and can serve as the lens to see why workplace performance may vary from using in vitro methods that were described in Chapter 6 and Chapter 7. In this section we begin with a brief discussion of theory to assist the teacher with assessing the construct of clinical reasoning in the workplace. In a sense, theory provides the framework to enable the teacher to provide some order to the many moving parts of the authentic clinical environment and can provide confidence to the teacher, learner, program, and accreditor that the domain under inspection (in this case clinical reasoning) is being assessed with rigor within our complex and at times chaotic workplaces.

Perhaps the most commonly cited theory in clinical reasoning is dual process theory. Dual process theory argues

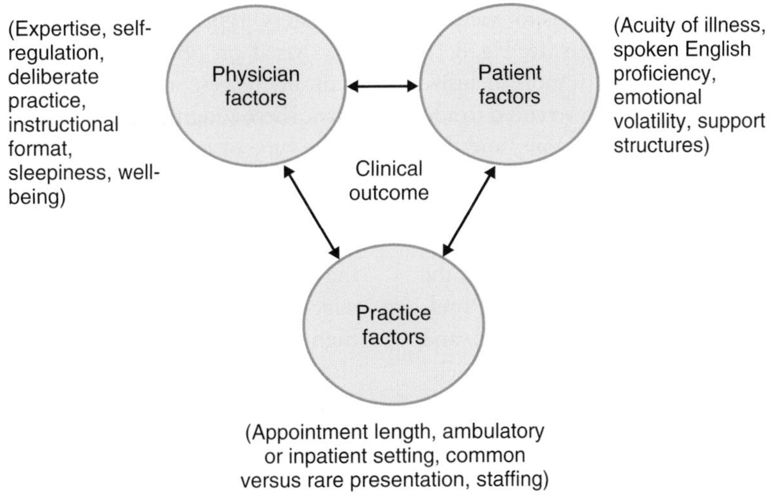

• **Fig. 8.1** Workplace-based assessment of clinical reasoning: a situated cognition approach.

that we use two processes to reason: system 1 or fast thinking, which is described as low effort and rapid; and system 2 or slow thinking, which is high effort. Fast thinking is also known as nonanalytic reasoning and slow thinking is referred to as analytic reasoning.[13] Related to dual process theory is script theory. Scripts are believed to represent organized knowledge (e.g., chunks of memory). A diagnostic script contains all the symptoms and findings generally comprising a diagnosis, the range of each symptom and finding for a given diagnosis, and the most likely or "default" presentation of each symptom and finding. Management scripts are believed to be distinct from diagnostic scripts and represent organized knowledge of the courses of action that clinicians take to manage a patient's health problems. Components of management scripts may include laboratory and imaging studies, procedures, input from specialists, medications, and monitoring.[14] Finally, cognitive load theory refers to our limited cognitive architecture whereby we can only hold or process so many (typically 4+/−2) pieces of information at a given time. Indeed, these theories converge on the notion that we constantly chunk or group information together (constantly create patterns) leading to scripts (enabling fast thinking) as well as freeing up our working memory (cognitive load). To learn more about these theories and others that relate to clinical reasoning, we refer the reader to Trowbridge et al.,[15] Eva,[16] Bowen,[17] and Young et al.[18]

We have chosen an inclusive framework for optimally assessing clinical reasoning in the workplace that also encompasses the aforementioned theories. We have done so in part given emerging findings in clinical reasoning research to include the phenomenon of context specificity. Context specificity refers to the recurrent finding that a physician can see two patients with the same chief complaint, the same (or nearly identical) symptoms and findings (physical exam, laboratory, etc.) and the same underlying diagnosis, and yet the physician attaches two *different* diagnostic labels. In other words, something beyond the essential content (i.e., *content* specificity) of the presentation needed to establish the diagnosis is driving the processes and outputs of the physician's reasoning; these other "things" are often referred to as contextual factors by some (see Fig. 8.1 for examples of contextual factors). We therefore believe that our view of assessing clinical reasoning in the workplace should be inclusive of the content as well as the environment (system) and interactions between participants that play a role in underpinning context specificity. We believe this can be useful as we move from the standardized assessment setting to what happens in complex and often ill-structured clinical practice settings (i.e., context specificity).

The theoretical framework we will briefly describe to assist in the assessment of clinical reasoning in the workplace is situated cognition.[19,20] There is limited extant literature on inclusive theoretical frameworks for assessing clinical reasoning in the workplace, and situated cognition represents one of several potential inclusive theoretical frameworks that can be used for assessing clinical reasoning in clinical settings. Situated cognition argues that thinking (cognition) emerges from individual(s) acting in concert with their environment. It shifts the emphasis from the physician to the physician interacting with the patient in the context of a specific setting or encounter. Viewed through this lens, the component parts of reasoning and how these parts can and sometimes do interact become apparent. This can help with defining where and when reasoning goes awry and better understanding when it goes well, which also offers a means to help physicians and trainees in the messy and, at times, complex nature of clinical practice.

In the clinical encounter, the participants (in Fig. 8.1, the physician and patient) interact with each other and the environment or setting; in vivo assessment of clinical reasoning is situation specific, and this model provides a means of "dissecting" the component parts, which can lead to a better understanding of context specificity. The figure represents just a sample of contextual factors one might include. Additional circles can be added based on the clinical setting and may include the patient's family, trainees, nurses, or other interprofessional team members. Like assessing each individual competency, we would put forth the notion that you should assess the factors displayed with multiple methods over time. This theoretical framework provides an expanded lens for viewing frameworks that have been articulated by others (see Fig. 8.1).

For example, this framework expands on (is more inclusive than) the notion of context in the model by Bowen need to add the figure - Bowen 8.2A - not sure where if has gone? and that of Gruppen and Frohna;[17,21] Fig. 8.2B; situated cognition (our approach) would argue that clinical reasoning is more emergent and interactive in the workplace than what is shown in Fig. 8.2A and B. Through the lens of situated cognition, the assessment of clinical reasoning is seen as dynamic and multifactorial, and recent work has described dyadic, triadic, and quadratic interactions between six different performance elements or contextual factors: clinician or assessee, patient, rater, assessment method, task, and environment;[22] Fig. 8.2B.

Now that we have provided a lens for viewing the assessment of clinical reasoning in the workplace, we will describe several methods for doing so. As these methods are emerging, several have limited reliability and validity data to date. We have grouped these methods into example categories.

Expert Assessments

Expert assessments are sometimes called global summaries. They typically occur at the end of a learning experience and are overall or quasisummative assessments performed by raters, typically faculty. Longitudinal evaluations, usually based on observations over a defined period of time, typically represent a collective and gestalt assessment of faculty. These judgments have traditionally been expressed on some type of rating scale, such as a 5-point Likert scale, or more commonly today, an entrustment scale. There are data that suggest that global ratings have value, particularly for complex constructs where devising a checklist can be vexing and situation specific. Global ratings of medical knowledge by programs variably correlate with performance on high-stakes examinations[23–25] (see Chapter 6). Limitations also have been noted in the use of these scales for assessing clinical reasoning, the most significant being poor interrater reliability ranging from 0.25 to 0.37.[26,27] Several factors help explain these poor correlations. First, the faculty's own clinical skills as well as the lack of standardization of the clinical content and context have been shown to affect faculty ratings and judgments. Kogan et al. demonstrated that faculty clinical skills positively correlated with their rating stringency.[28] Faculty come with their own strengths, weaknesses and idiosyncrasies that can affect their judgment of clinical reasoning[29] (see Chapter 4).

Second, faculty often fail to appropriately recognize the important role and impact of contextual factors on the clinical reasoning process, which is a reason why we believe a theoretical frame such as situated cognition could improve workplace assessments of clinical reasoning. Take, for example, a learner who is struggling with their clinical reasoning. While we often conclude that the learner has insufficient knowledge or experience, the above diagram Fig. 8.1 points out many factors that may come into play, including the environment or practice, as well as factors unique to the physician (e.g., burnout or sleepiness) and the patient (e.g., acuity of illness or emotional volatility over the visit). One can also quickly surmise how these factors in combination can lead to clinical reasoning going awry, such as a tired resident who is late to the start of the appointment interacting with a nervous patient with an EHR that is not optimally supportive.

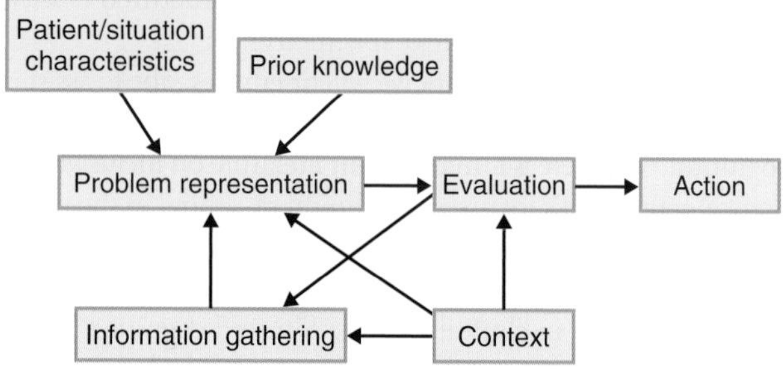

• **Fig. 8.2a** Gruppen and Frohna model of clinical reasoning. From Gruppen LD, Frohna AZ. Clinical reasoning. In: Norman GR, Van Der Vleuten CP, Newble DI, eds. *International Handbook of Research in Medical Education. Part 1.* Kluwer Academic; 2002:205–230.

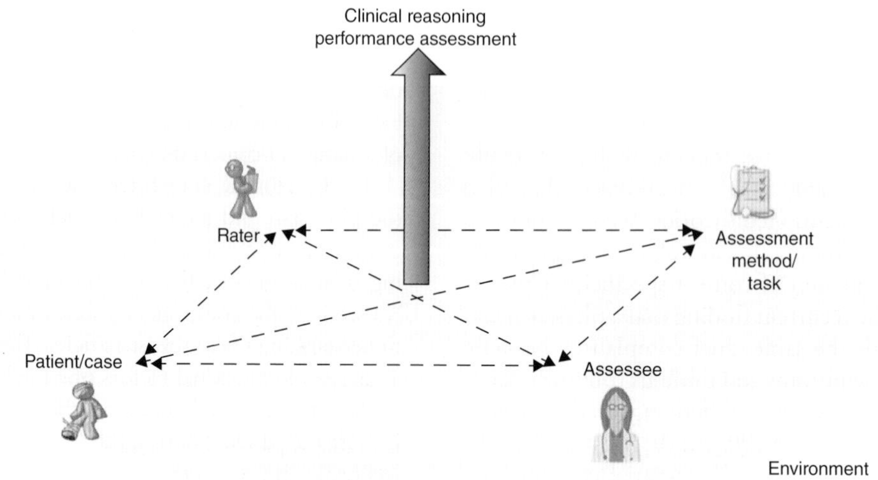

• **Fig. 8.2b** Try clinical reasoning performance assessment emerges from the interactions of contextual factors, including the assessee, the patient, the assessment method, and the task.

In fact, a recent study found heath information technology vulnerabilities that contributed to errors.[30] Such factors may be missed unless explicitly labeled, and these factors are not easily distillable to a linear psychometric approach. Indeed, such factors can represent much of the "noise" that standardized assessments seek to eliminate. We believe an important advantage with using situated cognition is providing a means of diagnosing when a clinical reasoning situation goes poorly or well. What are the component parts? What may have led to success (or lack therein)? What might the teacher suggest for the future?

Third, in our review of several global-type scales and instruments used to capture ratings of clinical reasoning, the use of any educational theories such as those highlighted earlier were notably absent. As we will discuss further shortly, the mini clinical evaluation exercise (mini-CEX), a common and extensively studied tool for direct observation, contains a clinical judgment category using a 9-point scale (1–3 = unsatisfactory; 4–6 = satisfactory; 7–9 = superior) with little definition of what the scale descriptors mean or the theory(ies) informing the assessment of clinical judgment (see Chapter 4).

Finally, faculty are assessing clinical reasoning in a very different context than that of standardized tests. Faculty most often assess clinical reasoning through a complex combination of precepting (e.g., as when a resident presents a patient to a faculty member on inpatient rounds or in an ambulatory clinic), semiformal presentations (e.g., morning report about patients admitted the night before, case rounds, etc.), and various forms of questioning during patient care activities.

The challenge is that most faculty often do not use systematic approaches to assessing clinical reasoning during these activities. The result is an idiosyncratic mix that the faculty member translates into an overall rating at the end of a curricular experience. While data are quite limited, we provide structured approaches in the following sections that may help faculty attain a better judgment of a learner's clinical reasoning. These approaches can inform assessment of clinical reasoning and can serve as important "input" into an overall rating.

SNAPPS

Of all the teaching frameworks, SNAPPS is one of the most studied. Box 8.1 outlines the SNAPPS steps. SNAPPS is designed to help the learner more systematically present a patient's clinical situation while concomitantly facilitating a faculty member's ability to assess the learner's clinical reasoning.[31–33]

SNAPPS has been mostly studied with medical students and much less so with residents, so it is not known how SNAPPS might work with higher-level learners such as residents and fellows. However, several studies have demonstrated that the use of SNAPPS can improve the learner's ability to describe their clinical reasoning process. It is not known how the use of SNAPPS affects overall faculty judgment of clinical reasoning other than that faculty find the technique helpful and feasible to use. SNAPPS has also been combined with the PICO (Patient-Intervention-Comparator-Outcome) approach to evidence-based medicine (see Chapter 9) to enhance the generation of a well-formulated clinical question.

• BOX 8.1 The SNAPPS Model to Facilitate Assessment of Clinical Reasoning

S: Summarize history and findings.
N: Narrow the differential.
A: Analyze the differential.
P: Probe preceptor about uncertainties.
P: Plan management.
S: Select case related issues for self-study.

One-Minute Preceptor and Written Notes

Other, less studied frameworks from an assessment perspective include the 1-minute preceptor and written notes (Box 8.2)[34] One study gathered validity evidence and demonstrated high feasibility and reliability for the use of a structured postencounter form (PEF) to assess clinical reasoning in students after an objective structured clinical examination (OSCE).[35] This work inspired the development of a postencounter rating tool (PERT) for students during clinical practice encounters.[36] Another study gathered initial validity and reliability evidence for a patient note scoring rubric that provides detailed and specific criteria to help standardize and facilitate scoring of raters of medical students in the United States Medical Licensing Examination (USLME) three-step clinical examination.[37] Finally, one study also investigated use of the interpretive summary, differential diagnosis, explanation of reasoning, and alternatives (IDEA) framework to judge the quality of student admission notes. Using a 15-item instrument, the investigators found moderate reliability and a positive correlation with final clerkship grades.[38–40]

ART and REACT

The Assessment of Reasoning Tool (ART) was recently developed by an expert opinion subcommittee within the Society to Improve Diagnosis in Medicine (SIDM).[41] The goal of the tool was to facilitate the formative assessment of clinical reasoning during oral presentations using behaviorally anchored rating scales (BARS) for five domains of diagnostic reasoning: hypothesis-directed information gathering, problem representation, prioritized differential diagnosis, high-value testing, and metacognition (see Appendix 8.2). The tool can provide a structure for the feedback conversation with learners and is supported by faculty development tools. A description of the development of the tool and small pilot evaluation of learners has provided validity evidence for content and response processes. A reconstructed version (ART-R) is a 15-item instrument that has

• BOX 8.2 Examples of Assessment of Clinical Reasoning Frameworks

One-Minute Preceptor

- Get a commitment.
- Probe for supporting evidence
- Teach a general rule.
- Reinforce what was done right.
- Correct mistakes.

IDEA

- I – interpretive summary
- D – Differential diagnosis
- E – Explanation of reasoning for selecting the most likely diagnosis
- A – Alternative diagnoses with an explanation of reasoning

Post-Encounter Form

Summary statement (1 point; in one sentence, summarize the most important history and physical exam features in this patient's presentation)

Problem list (3 points; one point for each reasonable problem listed)

1.
2.
3.

Differential diagnosis (3 points; list diagnoses that would explain all the problems you have listed)

1.
2.
3.

MOST likely diagnosis (1 point)

1.

Supporting data for MOST likely diagnosis (2 points)

Provide four key history and/or PE facts to support the MOST likely diagnosis (1 point for each fact provided)

1.
2.
3.
4.

Patient Note Scoring Rubric

Documentation of findings in history and physical examination (30 points)

1 Key history and physical examination findings are missing or incorrect
2 Most key positive findings present but poorly documented or disorganized or missing pertinent negatives
3 Most key positive findings well documented and organized, may miss a few pertinent negatives
4 All key information present, concise and well organized with little irrelevant information

DDX

Justification of differential diagnosis (60 points)

1. Unreasonable differential diagnosis
2. Appropriate differential diagnosis weakly supported, or several incorrect links between findings and diagnosis
3. Appropriate differential diagnosis well supported, may have a few missing or incorrect attributions that would not impact diagnosis
4. Excellent differential diagnosis well supported, links to diagnoses are correct and complete

Workup Plan for immediate diagnostic workup (10 points)

1. Diagnostic workup places patient in unnecessary risk or danger
2. Ineffective plan for diagnostic workup, essential tests missed, irrelevant tests included
3. Reasonable plan for diagnostic workup, may have some unnecessary tests
4. Plan for diagnostic workup is effective and efficient, includes all essential tests, and few or no unnecessary testsEach score category is worth 25% of the maximum points for its dimension. Points for scores by dimension: Documentation, 1 = 7, 2 = 15, 3 = 23, 4 = 30; DDX, 1 = 15, 2 = 30, 3 = 45, 4 = 60; and Workup, 1 = 2, 2 = 5, 3 = 8, 4 = 10

undergone additional psychometric validation of the internal structure and the relationship to other variables[42] (see Appendix 8.3). A similar tool called REACT (Rapid Evaluation Assessment of Clinical Reasoning Tool) includes the additional domains of management reasoning and communication. REACT was recently reported to have reliability and content validity for the formative assessment of students in simulated urgent clinical situations.[43]

More research is needed to determine whether use of these structured frameworks leads to more reliable and valid determinations of clinical reasoning ability. Providing faculty a structure on which to probe clinical reasoning in the workplace would be a reasonable and logical place to start.

We did find another unique expert-based assessment tool with some validity evidence used in nursing that merits mention. The Lasater Clinical Judgment Rubric (LCJR)[44,45] is a promising developmental framework for assessing clinical judgment that corresponds to clinical reasoning and has some validity and reliability data,[44–46] although it needs to be tested in larger and more diverse groups to confirm these preliminary findings. This tool includes the assessment of information seeking, deviations from expectations, prioritizing data, making sense of data, and communicating findings, which are elements of clinical reasoning. The rubric describes performance in four categories: beginning, developing, accomplished, and exemplary. More information is provided in Appendix 8.3.

Direct Observation

Direct observation has long been a mainstay method for the assessment of clinical skills. As noted earlier, multiple observations can inform a global or expert summary judgment. Other assessment tools exist to capture judgments related to one-on-one patient care encounters. Although many tools exist, the mini-CEX is perhaps the most used form[47] (see Chapter 4). The original mini-CEX contains the rating domain of Clinical Judgment. Assessing clinical judgment through observation commonly incorporates an assessment of data-gathering skills such as medical interviewing and physical examination, which is lacking in the other tools described. The advantage of direct observation, when combined with an assessment of data-gathering skills, allows faculty to assess integration of all the steps up to and including establishing the diagnosis (diagnostic reasoning). For example, if the learner gathers data poorly, it substantially lowers the probability they can create an accurate differential diagnosis. The same principles described with SNAPPS, the 1-minute preceptor, and IDEA frameworks can also be applied to point-of-encounter assessments such as the mini-CEX.

While the mini-CEX and other observation tools have been shown to possess reasonable reliability and validity evidence for judging clinical skills, much less is known about their psychometric properties regarding assessment of clinical reasoning.[36] One study gathered feasibility, validity, and reliability evidence for an 11-item observation rating tool (ORT).[48] The ORT was developed from qualitative data where 11 main indicators of clinical reasoning ability were abstracted from medical students' observable acts during history taking. Direct observation can also be combined with other assessments of clinical reasoning; for example, combining the ORT with a multiple-choice questions (MCQ) examination on the content area being observed. Regardless of the direct observation tool, combining observation with effective use of questions or other adjuncts can provide meaningful feedback to learners.

Chart-Stimulated Recall

Chart-stimulated recall (CSR) can be considered a structured "oral examination" that uses the medical record of an actual patient encounter to retrospectively review the clinical reasoning process of healthcare professionals.[49] We recently referred to CSR as a form of "game tape review" for healthcare providers.[50] Typically, the medical record of a clinical encounter, chosen by the health professional, trainee, or assessor, is first reviewed by the assessor against a structured template that produces a series of questions designed to probe the "why" behind the health professional's actions and decisions.[50–53] The assessor uses these questions in a one-on-one session with the health professional, eliciting and documenting the health professional's rationale and reasoning for the choices reflected in the medical record plus any additional pertinent information not documented. The challenge with such assessments, in addition to time requirements and training the assessors, is obtaining an adequate sampling of patient encounters and associated contexts. Sufficient sampling when using situated practice-based assessments is essential for high-stakes assessment but is less critical when used to support assessment for learning (or formative assessment).

CSR and a variant known as case-based discussion (CBD) are currently used in several contexts. CSR was originally developed for use in the American Board of Emergency Medicine (ABEM) certification in the early 1980s. While CSR was found to possess favorable psychometric properties, it was ultimately abandoned due to cost and the logistical difficulties (e.g., scheduling, recruiting sufficient faculty to perform the CSR) in operating a CSR-based high-stakes examination.[54] The main issues were the number of examiners needed and the growing number of physicians entering emergency medicine. Currently, CSR is a component of the Physician Assessment Review (PAR) program in Canada (most notably the province of Alberta) with validity evidence, and CBD has been studied as part of the United Kingdom's Foundation Programme.[55–58] Both techniques, used mostly for lower-stakes, formative assessments, have been found to be reliable and perceived as useful by examiners and examinees alike. CSR has also been recently compared with chart audit among a group of family medicine physicians in Quebec. Agreement between CSR and chart audit in a limited sample for diagnostic accuracy was 81% but CSR predictably provided more useful information on clinical reasoning.[58] Reddy and colleagues also provided useful cautions in using CSR, especially around the validity issues of construct underrepresentation (e.g., insufficient sampling, inconsistent case difficulty) and construct irrelevant variance (examiner bias and cognitive errors).[59] In our view, CSR and CBD are probably underutilized assessment methods to probe clinical reasoning in the clinical workplace. Useful templates exist to guide questioning, and CSR can be particularly useful in identifying deficiencies in struggling learners.

CSR may also be particularly useful in this era of electronic medical records (EMRs). EMRs can undermine the ability of assessing clinical reasoning for several reasons (see Chapter 10). First, many EMRs use a template function to standardize data entry that often does not effectively reflect the nuances of the learners' reasoning. Second, EMRs allow for cut-and-paste of previous notes, which further distorts the accurate representation of the patient's current clinical state and condition. Therefore CSR enables faculty to probe around information gaps in the EMR that can affect clinical reasoning ability.

One good example of this comes from a study that examined the reasons and causes for patients returning to a clinical care setting (clinic, emergency department, or hospitalization) unexpectedly within 14 days of an index visit to a clinic. In that study more than 25% of the patients returned as a result of diagnostic error.[60] These types of events lend themselves very well to combining CSR with root cause analysis (RCA; see Chapter 10) to explore why the error occurred, from the clinical reasoning contribution (CSR) to how the environment and system may have also contributed to the diagnostic error (RCA).

Think Aloud

Think Aloud is a research method whereby participants are asked to voice the unfiltered thoughts they have (or had) while performing a discrete task. Think Aloud has potential as a teaching and assessment approach for clinical reasoning as it can make explicit all the steps in clinical reasoning up to and including diagnosis and management. Think Aloud is a straightforward method where you (1) need a task with a clear beginning and end; (2) need to train the person doing the Think Aloud;[3] (3) need to tell the individual to think aloud (a useful prompt is to ask clinicians to pretend they don't have a frontal lobe); and (4) say "Think aloud" if the individual doesn't. A useful warmup that readers might find helpful is: "Describe the last time you had a meal at a restaurant. Describe all the steps involved in getting and consuming the meal until you left the establishment." Think Aloud can be used during a task or immediately after a task. An example would be: "Say your thought processes out loud as you review this patient's EHR. Don't try to explain or plan what you say, just act as if you were speaking to yourself. If you are silent for a long time, I'll ask you to think aloud." This approach when used individually or in a small group can uncover common errors that can lead to targeted remediation for learners. Also, faculty modeling the uncertainty and vulnerability of the narration of their cognition with Think Aloud may enhance learners' ability to think aloud and in turn facilitate their formative assessment and feedback. Further research is required to collect the psychometric properties of this approach.[61–64]

Work-Based Related Assessments

This section provides examples of clinical reasoning assessment methods that are not truly centered on the care of actual patients (in vitro assessments) but can be potentially adapted and used by programs in their local environment as adjunctive methods to those described earlier. These methods can be particularly helpful in determining where a learner might be developmentally along a continuum in a competency-based world and provide information to help tailor a faculty member's approach to assessing clinical reasoning in the clinical setting.

OSCE and High-Fidelity Simulations

The objective structured clinical examination (OSCE) is probably the most common format in which standardized patients (SPs) are employed to assess clinical skills. SPs are live actors trained to portray a range of clinical scenarios. OSCEs are usually delivered as a series of stations where the learner is given 15 to 20 minutes to perform a focused medical history, physical examination, and review of pertinent radiologic or laboratory data with or without discussion or counseling with the SP.[65] Chapter 5 covers standardized patients and OSCEs in greater detail. For example, both formative and summative formats may include an assessment of clinical reasoning that incorporates a "patient note" where the OSCE taker provides a differential diagnosis. Similar techniques are also used in lower-stakes OSCEs, including brief oral exams by faculty, interpretation of additional clinical material, and presentation of treatment plans to either the SP or faculty (Chapter 5).

High-fidelity simulation is also increasingly incorporating clinical reasoning into the assessment process. High-fidelity simulations often do not involve an SP, but instead employ sophisticated mannequins, virtual reality, and other computer-based simulations. Like OSCEs, clinical reasoning through multiple approaches can be incorporated into the simulation[66] (see Chapter 6). Recently, the American Board of Anesthesiology (ABA) added a simulation to its Maintenance of Certification program, designed to help practicing anesthesiologists practice difficult and less common clinical scenarios in a controlled environment.[67] Virtual patients and virtual reality are also enabling the creation of avatars that can be programmed to act like real patients and move along various pathways depending on the learner's clinical decisions.[68,69] What is less well known is whether this type of assessment effectively transfers to actual clinical practice. Regardless, simulation holds significant promise as an assessment method.

Emerging Strategies in Clinical Reasoning Assessment

A number of emerging means of assessing clinical reasoning are appearing in the literature. Here we will briefly describe three such techniques, recognizing that there are many others and that these methods have limited validity evidence thus far. The first two represent an important advancement with our assessment tools in that they explicitly incorporate educational theory. The latter shows promise by allowing for a more direct introspection of the reasoning process. Programs considering using one or more of these strategies should carefully weigh the pros and cons of adding this approach to their overall program of assessment.

Concept Mapping

Concept mapping is a technique for visually representing a learner's thinking or knowledge organization.[70] In a concept map, the learner connects several ideas (concepts) with specific phrases (linking words) to demonstrate how they put their ideas together (Fig. 8.3A and B). Concept maps can be unstructured (draw a concept map on the topic of anemia), partially structured (draw a concept map on the topic of anemia that includes hemoglobin, peripheral blood smear, microcytic, and bone marrow biopsy), or completely structured (whereby the learner fills in specific concepts or linking words, somewhat like a partially completed crossword puzzle). A number of recent publications on concept mapping have appeared in the medical education literature.[71,72] The reader is also encouraged to review Chapter 7 for more on concept maps.

Script Concordance Test

The script concordance test (SCT) is designed to assess clinical reasoning that incorporates, to the extent possible, practice-like conditions. The SCT is designed to produce a bounded range of responses based on information provided sequentially to the examinee, in effect trying to simulate what might happen in an actual clinical encounter. The hypothesis is that SCT more effectively captures the uncertainty commonly encountered in real clinical practice.

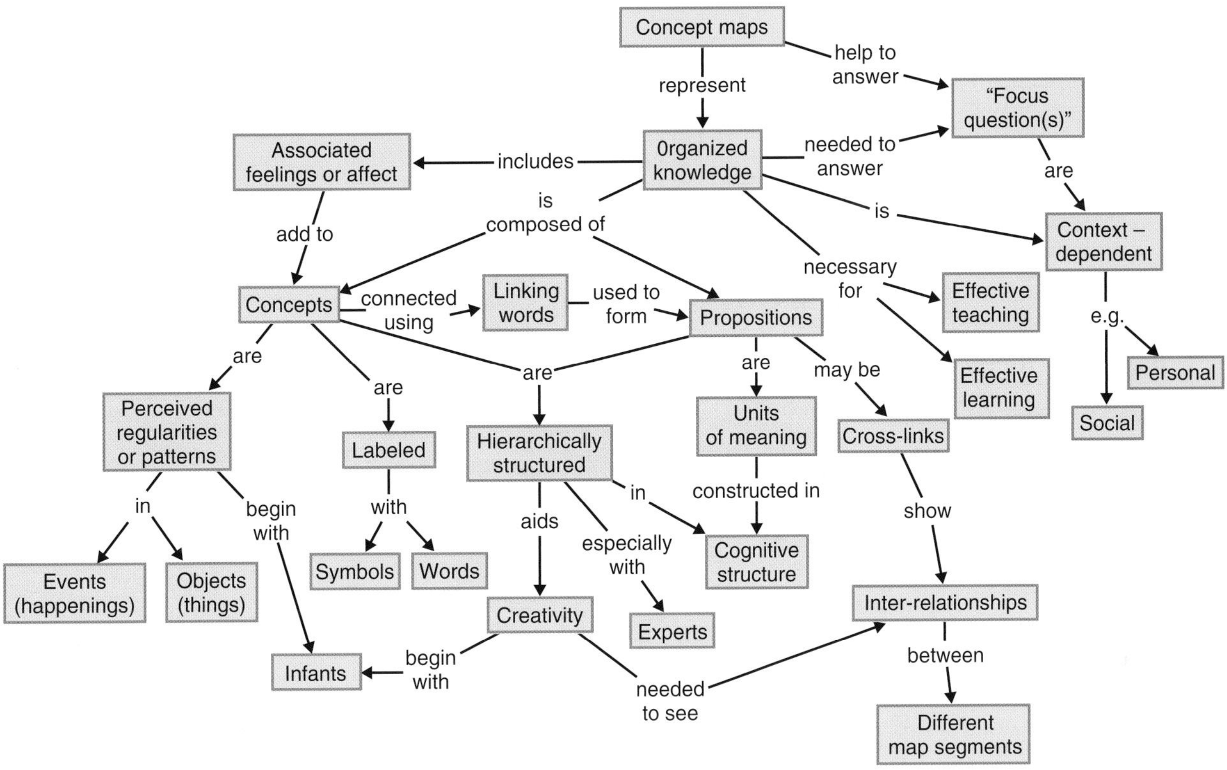

• **Fig. 8.3a** Concept map.

In an SCT, the learner is presented with a brief clinical scenario followed by questions that allow for learner to list (or choose) several diagnostic or treatment options and estimate their impact on the likelihood of different diagnoses. Dory and colleagues provide the following example in their review:[73]

A 25-year-old man presents to your general practice surgery. He has a severe retrosternal chest pain that began the previous night. There is nothing of note in his medical history. He does not smoke. His father, aged 60 years, and his mother, aged 55 years, are both in good health. The possible response options are:

If you were thinking of:	And the patient reports or you find upon clinical examination:	This hypothesis becomes:
Pericarditis	Normal chest auscultation	−2 − 1 0 + 1 + 2
Pneumothorax	Decreased breath sounds in the left chest area with hyperresonant chest percussion	−2 − 1 0 + 1 + 2
Panic attack	Yellow deposits around the eyelids	−2 − 1 0 + 1 + 2

Key: −2 = ruled out or almost ruled out; −1 = less likely; 0 = neither more nor less likely; +1 = more likely; +2 = certain or almost certain

Uncertainty can be built into the case to create a series of answers with a range of reasonable possibilities. SCT can also incorporate confidence ratings regarding the diagnosis, somewhat mimicking the probabilistic nature of clinical reasoning in real-world settings. The learner's answers are compared to the choices of an expert panel that systematically generates a range of acceptable answers.

Lubarsky and colleagues have published a useful AMEE Guide on SCT as well as a review of the current evidence for SCT.[74,75] They concluded that some validity evidence exists for using SCT to assess clinical reasoning under the conditions of uncertainty and ambiguity, specifically the sequential interpretation of clinical information and data.[75] When using SCT, traditional psychometric methods may not be fully up to the task for analyzing more complex assessment methodologies that may not be linear. We recommend exercising caution before prematurely deploying new methods for routine use in assessing clinical reasoning.[76,77] Chapter 7 covers SCT in more detail.

Self-Regulated Learning

Self-regulated learning (SRL) is defined as a set of processes learners use to moderate their own learning and performance. The processes are typically divided into several elements in each of three phases: forethought (before), performance (during), and reflection (after).[78–81] These elements interact, and from this model, learning and performance are believed to emerge. More recently,

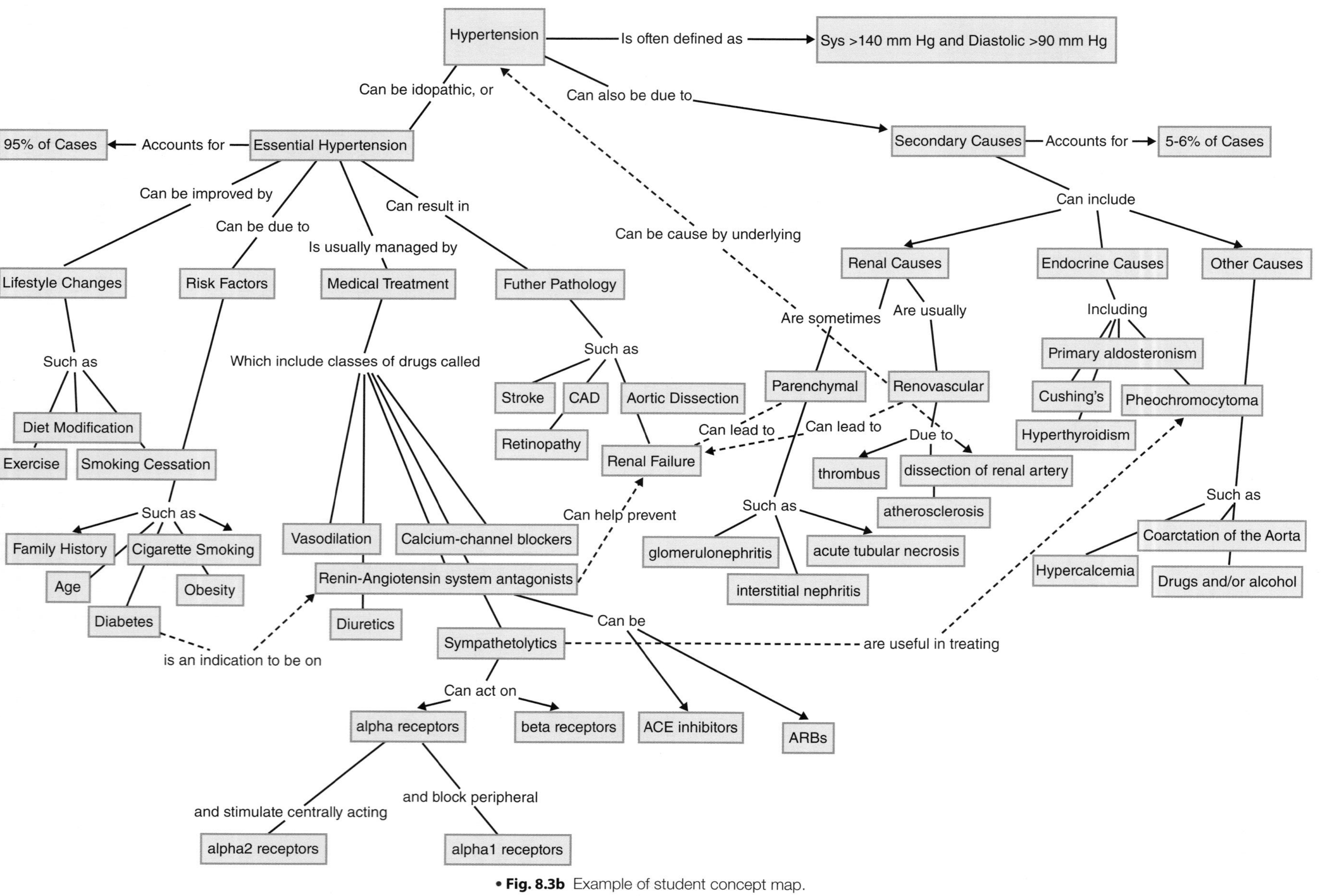

• **Fig. 8.3b** Example of student concept map.

medical education researchers have turned to theories of SRL—in particular, SRL microanalytic assessment techniques—to help understand and explain why and how some trainees succeed while others do not.[82] In the SRL microanalytic technique the learner is asked specific questions about their preparation (before), performance (during), and reflection (after) on completing a task with a beginning and an end (e.g., reaching the most likely diagnosis for a consultation in clinic). Examples of selected phase-specific SRL microanalytic questions in each phase might include:

Forethought (before)—Goal setting: "Do you have a goal in mind as you prepare to consult with this patient?

Strategic planning: "What do you think you need to do to perform well during this patient consultation?"

Self-efficacy: "How confident are you that you can reach the most likely diagnosis for this patient on your first try?"

Performance (during)—Metacognitive monitoring: "As you have been going through this process of reaching the most likely diagnosis, what has been the primary thing you have been thinking about or focusing on?"

Self-reflection (after)—Self-evaluation: "Why do you think you were unable to arrive at the most likely diagnosis during this consultation?"

Neuroanatomical Correlation

A promising area of research is increasing our understanding of clinical reasoning assessment through more direct means such as functional MRI.[83] Functional MRI is particularly promising as it permits the inspection of neuroanatomical changes that occur during cognition (in this case the assessment of clinical reasoning in the workplace). Returning to dual process theory, recent work suggests that functional MRI may show particular promise for nonanalytical reasoning that is not believed to be completely subject to introspection.

Team-Based Diagnosis

Diagnosis has almost exclusively been viewed as the domain of the physician and as a "solo act." While this continues to occur in some settings for some patients, most notably ambulatory care in the form of a medical visit, this is not as true for settings such as the hospital, rehabilitation facilities, and other forms of institutionally based care such as ambulatory surgical centers. Many residents, for example, can recall an incident in the ICU, ward, or emergency department when an astute observation by a nurse, physician assistant, or nurse practitioner led to the correct diagnosis or a revision in a diagnosis. A second theoretical framework, distributed cognition, has potential as a lens with which to better understand individual clinicians' clinical reasoning within teams or a team-based diagnosis.[84–86] Distributed cognition is a member of the same family of theories as situated cognition and widens the lens further to argue that there is a way to see (and therefore assess) cognition (in this case, clinical reasoning) in an interprofessional team working in a dynamic system like the clinical environment. The theory goes further to posit that clinical reasoning is (1) distributed across the members of a diagnostic team and artifacts such as personal computers that host the EHR; (2) coordinated by interactions between individual members of the team and with artifacts; and (3) propagated as multiple information structures such as gestures verbal utterances and the EHR, where the products of past events can transform the outcome of future related events (e.g., during handoffs). Distributed cognition also asserts that the clinical reasoning of a team is different from the individual members and may be explained as the pattern of interactions (e.g., team communication) and resultant social organization. For example, team-based diagnosis clinical reasoning is likely to be influenced by how individual members of a team share knowledge and information from multiple perspectives depending on their horizon of observation (or what is visible to different members of the team), leading to overlapping or idiosyncratic situational awareness. One example would be the assessment of team clinical reasoning during the rapid adaption to telediagnosis during the COVID-19 pandemic.[87]

Theory-informed work through this lens could lead to the development of assessments with reliability and validity evidence of an individual clinician working within a team as well as team-based clinical reasoning performance within a specific system. Examples could be a resident working within a rounding team and multiple interdisciplinary clinicians working collectively on a tumor board. Examples of existing assessments for teams include direct observation and feedback from multiple faculty and ratings with narrative reports such as 360-degree feedback tools. Through a distributed cognition lens, we could extend our understanding of rater cognition for teams (see Lockyer MSF chapter). The horizons of observation of each assessor may explain differences in individual assessment rater cognition. Through a distributed cognition lens, we could also inform how we define the competencies and EPAs of team clinical reasoning. Another avenue for research in the area of assessment of clinical reasoning would be to increase the number of simulated roles over time within sequential OSCE stations (e.g., two simulated clinicians in a handover followed by a linked encounter with a simulated patient and relative).

At this juncture, however, we simply do not have any well-studied methods or tools to assess and capture the nature of team-based diagnosis. In the meantime, we would encourage faculty to be attentive to the phenomenon and use oral techniques such as the 1-minute preceptor and Think Aloud to probe for group understanding and to use frameworks for written notes such as IDEA to judge the cumulative quality of the written notes by the multiple learners involved in caring for the patient.

Audio and Video Review of Diagnostic Reasoning

In this age of smartphones, mini cameras, iPads, and the like, video (or audio) review of the clinical encounter would seem to hold substantial promise in assessing the steps up to and including establishing the diagnosis. Video is routinely used for SPs as a debriefing tool and increasingly in the clinical program (e.g., residents asking patients for consent to videotape the patient encounter for feedback on history, physical exam, and counseling skills).

Previous studies have shown that presentations by learners to faculty preceptors often do not accurately reflect what happened in the exam room between the resident and patient.[88] In several cases, the discordances had substantial implications for the patient's care. Although little work has been done in this area, audiotaping the patient encounter and learner–preceptor sign-out and then comparing and contrasting the learner presentation with the information collected in the exam room could be very helpful in examining how the data that were collected—especially the history and physical exam if captured on video—affected clinical reasoning and the learner's decisions. Many of the techniques discussed earlier (e.g., stimulated recall) could be combined to probe clinical reasoning.

Conclusion

Assessment in the workplace can be challenging. We believe an understanding of theory is important as it can serve as a lens when standardization in the "messy" clinical environment is not feasible and has been magnified during the COVID-19 pandemic.[89] Faculty also need some basic understanding of key theories in clinical reasoning to guide their assessment and judgment. This chapter provided an inclusive theoretical model that can help us better understand context specificity so that one can optimize workplace assessment of clinical reasoning—both for diagnosis and management. We suggested that distributed cognition may be a fruitful additional lens for exploring how we could assess team-based clinical reasoning. We described several educational frameworks and assessments to help the reader. Despite the advances in high-stakes standardized testing, we still see many challenges and opportunities for assessing clinical reasoning; we do not believe standardized written tests provide a complete assessment of clinical reasoning. Therefore, despite the lack of robust evidence for workplace assessment of clinical reasoning, it is critical to conduct this in clinical settings. We hope this chapter demonstrates that there has been considerable progress in the assessment of clinical reasoning in the workplace but that much work remains to be done.[90]

Annotated Bibliography

1. National Academy of Medicine. *Improving Diagnosis in Medicine*: National Academy Press; 2015.
This report calls out diagnostic error as an important national patient safety issue. The figures presented in the report are staggering with regard to the yearly impact and harm on patients. The report calls for better methods of assessment. The executive summary and Chapter 1 should be read by all educators and shared with learners.
2. Rencic J, Durning S, Holmboe E, Gruppen LD. Assessing competence in professional performance across disciplines and professions. In: Wimmers PF, Mentkowski M, eds. *Innovation and Change in Professional Education Editors*: Springer International Publishing; 2016:209–224.
This book chapter provides a comprehensive overview of the different methods for assessing competence in a variety of professions and is specifically focused on clinical reasoning. This is a very useful chapter for educators wanting to take a deeper dive into clinical reasoning assessment.
3. Holmboe ES, Durning SJ. Assessing clinical reasoning: moving from in vitro to in vivo. *Diagnosis (Berl)*. 2014 Jan 1;1(1):111–117. doi:10.1515/dx-2013-0029.
This overview article may be helpful to frontline faculty to help them improve their approach to assessing clinical reasoning in the workplace. In the inaugural edition of the journal Diagnosis, readers will find other useful articles detailing the scope of the problem and challenges moving forward.
4. Schuwirth L, Durning SJ, King SM. Assessment of clinical reasoning: three evolutions of thought. *Diagnosis (Berl)*. 2020 Aug 27;7(3):191–196. doi:10.1515/dx-2019-0096.
This article explores how we might achieve a shift in the assessment of clinical reasoning as a linear predictable process with instruments that predominately collect quantitative measurements to a complex, dynamic process that could be complemented to include qualitative narratives.
5. Gordon D, Rencic JJ, Lang VJ, Thomas A, Young M, Durning SJ. Advancing the assessment of clinical reasoning across the health professions: definitional and methodological recommendations. *Perspect Med Educ*. 2022 Mar;11(2):108–114. doi:10.1007/s40037-022-00701-3.
A useful review outlining the fractured literature on clinical reasoning assessment with inconsistencies due to (1) a wide array of clinical reasoning–like terms that were rarely defined or informed by a conceptual framework, (2) limited details of assessment methodology, and (3) inconsistent reporting of the steps taken to establish validity evidence for clinical reasoning assessments. Recommendations to better support the development, description, study, and reporting of clinical reasoning assessments are provided.
6. Schipper S, Ross S. Structured teaching and assessment. A new chart stimulated recall worksheet for family medicine residents. *Can Fam Physician*. 2010 Sep;56:958–959.
This article describes CSR in the context of family medicine and provides a useful sample worksheet that can be accessed at www.practicaldoc.ca/wp-content/uploads/2012/10/chart.pdf. Another example for radiation oncology based on the Schipper article can be accessed at https://www.acgme.org/globalassets/430_ChartStimulatedRecall.pdf.
7. Daniel M, Rencic J, Durning SJ, et al. Clinical reasoning assessment methods: a scoping review and practical guidance. *Acad Med*. 2019 Jun;94(6):902–912. doi:10.1097/ACM.0000000000002618.
This scoping review provides helpful information on other tools that did not meet an evidence threshold to be included in this chapter but may be of interest to the reader. In addition, the review provides a very helpful table on the strengths and weaknesses of each tool and what aspect of the clinical reasoning process the tool best addresses. Appendix 8.1 provides the synopsis table of the various assessment methods.
8. Daniel M, Daniel M, Durning SJ, Wilson E, Abdoler E, Torre D. Situated cognition: clinical reasoning and error are context dependent.

Diagnosis (Berl). 2020 Aug 27;7(3):341–342. doi:10.1515/dx-2020-0011. *Appendix 8.4 provides two useful diagrams illustrating how both situated and distributed cognition can work in the healthcare workplace.*

9. Wilson E, Seifert C, Durning SJ, Torre D, Daniel M. Distributed cognition: interactions between individuals and artifacts. *Diagnosis (Berl)*. 2020 Aug 27;7(3):343–344. doi:10.1515/dx-2020-0012. *Appendix 8.4 provides two useful diagrams illustrating how both situated and distributed cognition can work in the healthcare workplace.*

References

1. Hampton JR, Harrison MJG, Mitchell JRA, Prichard JS, Seymour C. Relative contributions of history-taking, physical examination, and laboratory investigation to diagnosis and management of medical outpatients. *BMJ*. 1975 May 31;2(5969):486–489. doi:10.1136/bmj.2.5969.486.
2. Peterson MC, Holbrook JH, Hales DV, Smith NL, Staker LV. Contributions of the history, physical examination, and laboratory investigation in making medical diagnoses. *West J Med*. 1992 Feb;156(2):163–165.
3. Holmboe ES, Weng W, Arnold G, et al. The Comprehensive Care Project: measuring physician performance in ambulatory practice. *Health Serv Res*. 2010 Dec;45(6 Pt 2):1912–1933. doi:10.1111/j.1475-6773.2010.01160.x.
4. National Academy of Medicine. *Improving Diagnosis in Medicine*. National Academy Press; 2016.
5. Makary M, Daniel M. Medical error – the third leading cause of death in the US. *BMJ*. 2016 May 3;353:i2139. doi:10.1136/bmj.i2139.
6. Institute of Medicine. *To Err is Human*. National Academy Press; 1999.
7. Landrigan CP, Parry GJ, Bones CB, Hackbarth AD, Goldmann DA, Sharek PJ. Temporal trends in rates of patient harm resulting from medical care. *N Engl J Med*. 2010 Nov 25;363(22):2124–2134. doi:10.1056/NEJMsa1004404.
8. Starmer AJ, Spector ND, Srivastava R, et al. Changes in medical errors after implementation of a handoff program. *N Engl J Med*. 2014 Nov 6;371(19):1803–1812. doi:10.1056/NEJMsa1405556.
9. Graber ML. The incidence of diagnostic error in medicine. *BMJ Qual Saf*. 2013 Oct;22(Suppl 2):ii21–ii27. doi:10.1136/bmjqs-2012-001615.
10. Saber Tehrani AS, Lee H, Mathews SC, et al. 25-year summary of US malpractice claims for diagnostic errors 1986-2010: an analysis from the National Practitioner Data Bank. *BMJ Qual Saf*. 2013 Aug;22(8):672–680. doi:10.1136/bmjqs-2012-001550.
11. Cook DA, Sherbino J, Durning SJ. Management reasoning: beyond the diagnosis. *JAMA*. 2018 Jun 12;319(22):2267–2268. doi:10.1001/jama.2018.4385.
12. Cook DA, Stephenson CR, Gruppen LD, Durning SJ. Management reasoning: empirical determination of key features and a conceptual model. *Acad Med*. 2023 Jan 1;98(1):80–87. doi:10.1097/ACM.0000000000004810.
13. Kahneman D. *Thinking, Fast and Slow*. Farrar, Strauss and Giroux; 2011:19–97.
14. Cook DA, Stephenson CR, Gruppen LD, Durning SJ. Management reasoning scripts: qualitative exploration using simulated physician-patient encounters. *Perspect Med Educ*. 2022 Aug;11(4):196–206. doi:10.1007/s40037-022-00714-y.
15. Trowbridge RL, Rencic JJ, Durning SJ. *Teaching Clinical Reasoning*. ACP Press; 2015.
16. Eva KW. What every teacher needs to know about clinical reasoning. *Med Educ*. 2005 Jan;39(1):98–106. doi:10.1111/j.1365-2929.2004.01972.x.
17. Bowen JL. Educational strategies to promote clinical diagnostic reasoning. *N Engl J Med*. 2006 Nov 23;355(21):2217–2225. doi:10.1056/NEJMra054782.
18. Young JQ, Van Merrienboer J, Durning S, ten Cate O. Cognitive load theory: implications for medical education: AMEE Guide No. 86. *Med Teach*. 2014 May;36(5):371–384. doi:10.3109/0142159X.2014.889290.
19. Bredo E. Reconstructing educational psychology: situated cognition and Deweyian pragmatism. *Educ Psychol*. 1994;29(1):23–35.
20. Durning SJ, Lubarsky S, Torre D, Dory V, Holmboe E. Considering "nonlinearity" across the continuum in medical education assessment: supporting theory, practice, and future research directions. *J Cont Educ Health Prof*. 2015 Summer;35(3):232–243. doi:10.1002/chp.21298.
21. Gruppen LD, Frohna AZ. Clinical reasoning. In: Norman GR, Van Der Vleuten CP, Newble DI, eds. *International Handbook of Research in Medical Education. Part 1*. Kluwer Academic; 2002:205–230.
22. Rencic J, Schuwirth LWT, Gruppen LD, Durning SJ. Clinical reasoning performance assessment: using situated cognition theory as a conceptual framework. *Diagnosis (Berl)*. 2020 Aug 27;7(3):241–249. doi:10.1515/dx-2019-0051.
23. Tamblyn R, Abrahamowicz M, Dauphinee WD, et al. Association between licensure examination scores and practice in primary care. *JAMA*. 2002 Dec 18;288(23):3019–3026. doi:10.1001/jama.288.23.3019.
24. Norcini JJ, Lipner RS, Kimball HR. Certifying examination performance and patient outcomes following acute myocardial infarction. *Med Educ*. 2002 Sep;36(9):853–859. doi:10.1046/j.1365-2923.2002.01293.x.
25. Holmboe ES, Wang Y, Meehan TP, et al. Association between maintenance of certification examination scores and quality of care for Medicare beneficiaries. *Arch Intern Med*. 2008 Jul 14;168(13):1396–1403. doi:10.1001/archinte.168.13.1396.
26. Hawkins RE, Sumption KF, Gaglione M, Holmboe ES. The in-training examination in internal medicine: resident perceptions and correlation between resident scores and faculty predictions of resident performance. *Am J Med*. 1999 Feb;106(2):206–210. doi:10.1016/s0002-9343(98)00392-1.
27. Striener DL. Global rating scales. In: Neufeld VR, Norman GR, eds. *Assessing Clinical Competence*. Springer; 1985.
28. Kogan JR, Hess BJ, Conforti LN, Holmboe ES. What drives faculty ratings of residents' clinical skills? The impact of faculty's own clinical skills. *Acad Med*. 2010 Oct;85(10 Suppl):S25–S28. doi:10.1097/ACM.0b013e3181ed1aa3.
29. Gingerich A, Kogan J, Yeates P, Govaerts M, Holmboe E. Seeing the 'black box' differently: assessor cognition from three research perspectives. *Med Educ*. 2014 Nov;48(11):1055–1068. doi:10.1111/medu.12546.
30. Graber ML, Siegal D, Riah H, Johnston D, Kenyon K. Electronic health record-related events in medical malpractice claims. *J Patient Saf*. 2015 Nov 6 [Epub ahead of print].
31. Wolpaw TM, Wolpaw DR, Papp KK. SNAPPS: a leaner-centered model for outpatient education. *Acad Med*. 2003 Sep;78(9):89398. doi:10.1097/00001888-200309000-00010.
32. Wolpaw T, Papp KK, Bordage G. Using SNAPPS to facilitate expression of clinical reasoning and uncertainties: a randomized comparison group trial. *Acad Med*. 2009 Apr;84(4):517–524. doi:10.1097/ACM.0b013e31819a8cbf.

33. Nixon J, Wolpaw T, Schwartz A, Duffy B, Menk J, Bordage G. SNAPPS-Plus: an educational prescription to facilitate formulating and answering clinical questions. *Acad Med.* 2014 Aug;89(8):1174–1179.doi:10.1097/ACM.0000000000000362.
34. Neher JO, Stevens NG. The one-minute preceptor: shaping the teaching conversation. *Fam Med.* 2003 Jun;35(6):391–393 PMID: 12817861.
35. Durning SJ, Artino A, Boulet J, et al. The feasibility, reliability, and validity of a post-encounter form for evaluating clinical reasoning. *Med Teach.* 2012;34(1):30–37. doi:10.3109/0142159X.2011.590557.
36. Haring CM, Klaarwater CCR, Bouwmans GA, et al. Validity, reliability and feasibility of a new observation rating tool and a post encounter rating tool for the assessment of clinical reasoning skills of medical students during their internal medicine clerkship: a pilot study. *BMC Med Educ.* 2020 Jun 19;20(1):198. doi:10.1186/s12909-020-02110-8.
37. Park YS, Lineberry M, Hyderi A, Bordage G, Riddle J, Yudkowsky R. Validity evidence for a patient note scoring rubric based on the new patient note format of the United States Medical Licensing Examination. *Acad Med.* 2013 Oct;88(10):1552–1557. doi:10.1097/ACM.0b013e3182a34b1e.
38. Baker E, Riddle J. IDEA in evolution: an attempt to use RIME to more accurately assess medical student write-ups. *JGIM.* 2005; 20(Suppl 1):157.
39. Baker E, Ledford C, Liston B. Teaching, evaluating and remediating clinical reasoning. *Acad Int Med Insight.* 2010;8:12–17.
40. Baker EA, Ledford CH, Fogg L, Way DP, Park YS. The IDEA assessment tool: assessing the reporting, diagnostic reasoning, and decision-making skills demonstrated in medical students' hospital admission notes. *Teach Learn Med.* 2015;27(2):163–173. doi: 10.1080/10401334.2015.1011654.
41. Thammasitboon S, Rencic JJ, Trowbridge RL, Olson APJ, Sur M, Dhaliwal G. The Assessment of Reasoning Tool (ART): structuring the conversation between teachers and learners. *Diagnosis (Berl).* 2018 Nov 27;5(4):197–203. doi:10.1515/dx-2018-0052.
42. Thammasitboon S, Sur M, Rencic JJ, et al. Psychometric validation of the reconstructed version of the assessment of reasoning tool. *Med Teach.* 2021 Feb;43(2):168–173. doi:10.1080/0142159X.2020.1830960.
43. Peterson BD, Magee CD, Martindale JR, et al. REACT: Rapid Evaluation Assessment of Clinical Reasoning Tool. *J Gen Intern Med.* 2022 Jul;37(9):2224–2229. doi:10.1007/s11606-022-07513-5.
44. Lasater K. Clinical judgment development: using simulation to create an assessment rubric. *J Nurs Educ.* 2007 Nov;46(11):269–276. doi:10.3928/01484834-20071101-04.
45. Lasater K. Clinical judgment: the last frontier for evaluation. *Nurss Educ Pract.* 2011 Mar;11(2):86–92. doi:10.1016/j.nepr.2010.11.013.
46. Adamson KA, Gubrud P, Sideras S, Lasater K. Assessing the reliability, validity, and the use the Lasater clinical judgment rubric: three approaches. *J Nurs Educ.* 2012 Feb;51(2):66–73. doi:10.3928/01484834-20111130-03.
47. Kogan JR, Holmboe ES, Hauer KR. Tools for direct observation and assessment of clinical skills of medical trainees: a systematic review. *JAMA.* 2009 Sep 23;302(12):1316–1326. doi:10.1001/jama.2009.1365.
48. Haring CM, Cools BM, van Gurp PJM, van der Meer JWM, Postma CT. Observable phenomena that reveal medical students' clinical reasoning ability during expert assessment of their history taking: a qualitative study. *BMC Med Educ.* 2017 Aug 29;17(1):147. doi:10.1186/s12909-017-0983-3.
49. Norcini JJ, McKinley DW. Assessment methods in medical education. *Teach Teach Educ.* 2007;23:239–250.
50. Holmboe ES, Durning SJ. Assessing clinical reasoning: moving from in vitro to in vivo. *Diagnosis (Berl).* 2014 Jan 1;1(1):111–117. doi:10.1515/dx-2013-0029.
51. Hall W, Violato C, Lewkonia R, et al. Assessment of physician performance in Alberta: the physician achievement review. *Can Med Assoc J.* 1999 Jul 13;161(1):52–57.
52. Jennett P, Affleck L. Chart audit and chart stimulated recall as methods of needs assessment in continuing professional health education. *J Cont Educ Health Prof.* 1998;18:163–171. doi:10.1002/chp.1340180306.
53. Schipper S, Ross S. Structured teaching and assessment: a new chart-stimulated recall worksheet for family medicine residents. *Can Fam Physician.* 2010 Sep;56(9):958–959.
54. Munger BS, Krome RL, Maatsch JC, Podgorny G. The certification examination in emergency medicine: an update. *Ann Emerg Med.* 1982 Feb;11(2):91–96. doi:10.1016/s0196-0644(82)80304-1.
55. Davies H, Archer J, Southgate L, Norcini J. Initial evaluation of the first year of the Foundation Assessment Program. *Med Educ.* 2009 Jan;43(1):74–81. doi:10.1111/j.1365-2923.2008.03249.x.
56. Norcini J, Burch V. Workplace-based assessment as an educational tool: AMEE Guide No. 31. *Med Teach.* 2007 Nov;29(9):855–871. doi:10.1080/01421590701775453.
57. Cunnington JP, Hanna E, Turnbull J, Kaigas TB, Norman GR. Defensible assessment of the competency of the practicing physician. *Acad Med.* 1997 Jan;72(1):9–12.
58. Goulet F, Gagnon R, Gingras ME. Influence of remedial professional development for poorly performing physicians. *J Cont Educ Health Prof.* 2007 Winter;27(1):42–48. doi:10.1002/chp.93.
59. Reddy ST, Endo J, Gupta S, Tekian A, Park YS. A case for caution: chart-stimulated recall. *J Grad Med Educ.* 2015 Dec;7(4):531–535. doi:10.4300/JGME-D-15-00011.1.
60. Singh H, Giardina TD, Meyer AN, Forjuoh SN, Reis MD, Thomas EJ. Types and origins of diagnostic errors in primary care settings. *J Am Med Assoc Intern Med.* 2013 Mar 25;173(6):418–425. doi:10.1001/jamainternmed.2013.2777.
61. Pinnock R, Young L, Spence F, Henning M, Hazell W. Can Think Aloud be used to teach and assess clinical reasoning in graduate medical education? *J Grad Med Educ.* 2015 Sep;7(3):334–337. doi:10.4300/JGME-D-14-00601.1.
62. Audétat MC, Dory V, Nendaz M, et al. What is so difficult about managing clinical reasoning difficulties? *Med Educ.* 2012 Feb;46(2):216–227. doi:10.1111/j.1365-2923.2011.04151.x.
63. Jagannath AD, Dreicer JJ, Penner JC, Dhaliwal G. The cognitive apprenticeship: advancing reasoning education by thinking aloud. *Diagnosis (Berl).* 2022 Dec 1;10(1):9–12. doi:10.1515/dx-2022-0043.
64. Johnson WR, Artino Jr AR, Durning SJ. Using the think aloud protocol in health professions education: an interview method for exploring thought processes: AMEE Guide No. 151. *Med Teach.* 2022 Dec 19:1–12. doi:10.1080/0142159X.2022.2155123.
65. Cleland JA, Abe K, Rethans JJ. The use of simulated patients in medical education: AMEE Guide No 42. *Med Teach.* 2009 Jun;31(6):477–486. doi:10.1080/01421590903002821.
66. Walsh CM, Sherlock ME, Ling SC, Carnahan H. Virtual reality simulation training for health professions trainees in gastrointestinal endoscopy. *Cochrane Database Syst Rev.* 2012 Jun 13;6:CD008237. doi:10.1002/14651858.CD008237.pub2.

67. American Board of Anesthesia. MOCA 2.0 Part 4: Improvement in Medical Practice. Accessed May 14, 2016. https://www.theaba.org/maintain-certification/moca-eligibility/.
68. Satter KM, Butler AC. Finding the value of immersive, virtual environments using competitive usability analysis. *J Comput Inf Sci Eng.* 2012 Jun;12(2):024504. doi:10.1115/1.4005722.
69. Courteille O, Bergin R, Stockeld D, Ponzer S, Fors U. The use of a virtual patient case in an OSCE-based exam—a pilot study. *Med Teach.* 2008;30(3):e66–e76. doi:10.1080/01421590801910216.
70. Pinto AJ, Zeitz HJ. Concept mapping: a strategy for promoting meaningful learning in medical education. *Med Teach.* 2009 Jul;19(2):114–121. doi:10.3109/01421599709019363.
71. Daley B, Torre D. Concept maps in medical education: an analytical literature review. *Med Educ.* 2010 May;44(5):440–448. doi:10.1111/j.1365-2923.2010.03628.x.
72. Torre D, Daley B. Using concept maps in medical education. In: Walsh K, ed. *Oxford Textbook of Medical Education.* Oxford University Press; 2003.
73. Dory V, Gagnon R, Vanpeez D, Charlin B. How to construct and implement script concordance tests: insights from a systematic review. *Med Educ.* 2012 Jun;46(6):552–563. doi:10.1111/j.1365-2923.2011.04211.x.
74. Lubarsky S, Dory V, Duggan P, Gagnon R, Charlin B. Script concordance testing: from theory to practice: AMEE Guide no. 75. *Med Teach.* 2013;35(3):184–193. doi:10.3109/0142159X.2013.760036.
75. Lubarsky S, Durning S, Charlin B. AM last page. The script concordance test: a tool for assessing clinical data interpretation under conditions of uncertainty. *Acad Med.* 2014 Jul;89(7):1089. doi:10.1097/ACM.0000000000000315.
76. Lineberry M, Kreiter CD, Bordage G. Threats to validity in the use and interpretation of script concordance test scores. *Med Educ.* 2013 Dec;47(12):1175–1183. doi:10.1111/medu.12283.
77. Lineberry M, Kreiter CD, Bordage G. Script concordance tests: strong inferences about examinees require stronger evidence. *Med Educ.* 2014 Apr;48(4):452–453. doi:10.1111/medu.12417.
78. Brydges R, Butler D. A reflective analysis of medical education research on self-regulation in learning and practice. *Med Educ.* 2012 Jan;46(1):71–79. doi:10.1111/j.1365-2923.2011.04100.x.
79. Cleary TJ, Durning SJ, Hemmer PA, Gruppen LD, Artino AR. Self-regulated learning in medical education. In: Walsh K, ed. *Oxford Textbook of Medical Education.* Oxford University Press; 2013:465–477.
80. Durning SJ, Cleary TJ, Sandars J, Hemmer PA, Kokotala P, Artino AR. Viewing strugglers through a different lens: how a self-regulated learning perspective can help medical educators with assessment and remediation. *Acad Med.* 2011 Apr;86(4):488–495. doi:10.1097/ACM.0b013e31820dc384.
81. Zimmerman B, Schunk D, eds. *Handbook of Self-Regulation of Learning and Performance.* Routledge; 2011.
82. Cleary TJ, Durning SJ, Artino Jr AR. Microanalytic assessment of self-regulated learning during clinical reasoning tasks: recent developments and next steps. *Acad Med.* 2016 Nov;91(11):1516–1521. doi:10.1097/ACM.0000000000001228.
83. Durning SJ, Costanzo M, Artino Jr AR, et al. Using functional magnetic imaging to improve how we understand, teach, and assess clinical reasoning. *J Contin Educ Health Prof.* 2014 Winter;34(1):76–82. doi:10.1002/chp.21215.
84. Hutchins E. *Cognition in the Wild.* MIT Press; 1996.
85. Boyle JG, Walters MR, Jamieson S, Durning SJ. Sharing the bandwidth in cognitively overloaded teams and systems: mechanistic insights from a walk on the wild side of clinical reasoning. *Teach Learn Med.* 2022 Apr-May;34(2):215–222. doi:10.1080/10401334.2021.1924723.
86. Olson A, Rencic J, Cosby K, et al. Competencies for improving diagnosis: an interprofessional framework for education and training in health care. *Diagnosis (Berl).* 2019 Nov 26;6(4):335–341. doi:10.1515/dx-2018-0107.
87. Boyle JG, Walters MR, Jamieson S, Durning SJ. Distributed cognition: a framework for conceptualizing telediagnosis in teams. *Diagnosis (Berl).* 2021 Sep 16;9(1):143–145. doi:10.1515/dx-2021-0111.
88. Gennis VM, Gennis MA. Supervision in the outpatient clinic: effects on teaching and patient care. *J Gen Intern Med.* 1993 Jul;8(7):378–380. doi:10.1007/BF02600077.
89. Boyle JG, Walters MR, Jamieson S, Durning SJ. Clinical reasoning in the wild: premature closure during the COVID-19 pandemic. *Diagnosis (Berl).* 2020 Aug 27;7(3):177–179. doi:10.1515/dx-2020-0061.
90. Daniel M, Rencic J, Durning SJ, et al. Clinical reasoning assessment methods: a scoping review and practical guidance. *Acad Med.* 2019 Jun;94(6):902–912. doi:10.1097/ACM.0000000000002618.

9

Workplace-Based Assessment of Procedural Skills

STANLEY J. HAMSTRA, PHD

CHAPTER OUTLINE

Introduction

The purpose of this chapter is to help program directors and core faculty in medical education, especially graduate medical education (GME) programs, by providing practical guidance for using and selecting assessment instruments for procedural skills in surgical and related disciplines. To guide the discussion, the chapter will highlight two major developments in medical education in recent years: (1) a reconceptualization of the idea of validity in assessment, and (2) a new approach to creating assessment tools that incorporate entrustability. Both of these recent developments should help faculty and program directors manage the sometimes daunting task of producing rigorous and defensible assessment data of our trainees in the busy clinical setting. The chapter will focus on the assessment of residents (i.e., learners in their postgraduate training years) but the principles are equally applicable to the assessment of medical students and physicians in practice.

Introduction to Assessment Tools for Procedural Skills

One of the original and most influential tools for assessing procedural skills in surgery has been the objective structured assessment of technical skill (OSATS),[1,2] which has been widely adapted for use in a variety of specialties and different contexts[3–8] and has been reviewed extensively elsewhere.[9–12] Since these early developments in the 1980s and 1990s, medical education has become dominated by competency-based medical education (CBME), and that has led to national mandates for specific forms of assessment across all specialties (see Chapter 1).[13–15] CBME has compelled program directors to select, use, and/or adapt assessment tools for their programs to meet the expectations of certification and accrediting bodies. Fortunately, several recent developments have made this task easier, and they are the focus of this chapter.

Validity Lies in the Process of Assessment, Not in the Instrument Itself

The single most important development in the assessment literature over the past 20 years has been the recognition that there is no such thing as a validated assessment tool.[16–18] Validity does not rest in the assessment instrument itself, but depends on the process of assessment and how the scores are used. While the structure and layout of assessment tools remain critical, it is now well recognized that the raters themselves, and the context in which the raters observe and make judgments, are also critical to obtaining valid assessment data. This simple idea alone should help program directors and faculty in creating the best environment for valid and reliable assessment. Raters should not be so concerned about choosing a "validated" instrument, but rather selecting and adapting existing tools and assessment processes to take advantage of the unique nature of their local context.* This attitude alone will help improve the validity of assessment data so that the ratings are considered defensible and can stand up to any challenges that might arise in making decisions about learners and their future. In addition to high-stakes summative decisions about resident progression, graduation, and need for remediation, these principles also apply to formative feedback to help individual learners improve.

In this new framework, validity includes not only (1) the content and language of the assessment tool but also (2) the behaviors and characteristics of the raters and (3) how well the ratings predict future performance in the clinical setting. This *unitary framework of validity* for assessment instruments is reviewed in Chapter 2 of this volume by Clauser et al. and has been endorsed as the new standard for educational and psychological testing by national measurement organizations since 1999.[18] Cook and Beckman[21] provide an excellent introduction and summary of the unitary validity framework as applied to medical education.

While the number of published assessment tools for procedural skills has increased dramatically since the early 2000s,[22] few of those tools were developed with the unitary validity framework in mind, and these standards have been slow to gain traction in the literature on procedural skills assessment,[23,24] leaving surgical educators with little guidance as to best practices for implementation. Fortunately, an excellent review of assessment tools for technical skills is available (Ghaderi et al.),[25] which reviews many assessment instruments useful for a standardized national curriculum in surgery in terms of the unitary validity framework. Ghaderi and colleagues were able to classify a total of 23 assessment instruments for the 35 curriculum modules for technical skills that were recently adopted by the American College of Surgeons (ACS) and the Association of Program Directors in Surgery (APDS).[26,27] Their analysis showed that relatively few of the studies describing the development of these tools or their use in the field provided adequate evidence for validity, but were able to isolate a short list of three tools that were designed according to these standards. Updates to Ghaderi and colleagues' review can be found in gynecologic surgery[28] and laparoscopic surgery.[29,30] Other research has reviewed the Accreditation Council for Graduate Medical Education (ACGME) Milestones according to this validity framework.[31]

Simplifying the Assessment Tools Using Construct-Aligned Scales

Another important and emerging development is the concept of construct-aligned scales, which involves developing assessment tools with much more natural language (such as "I had to provide some guidance") than was typically seen in the past. Many of our older tools were peppered with "psychometric jargon" and required faculty to make a difficult translation onto scales with nonspecific anchors (e.g., from "unsatisfactory" to "superior"; see Chapter 4). Crossley and colleagues[32] developed a new approach to help reduce the burden on raters and on the need for faculty development sessions for core faculty with no particular interest in psychometrics. The idea is that a rater using these scales can quickly and easily adapt to the new requirements for assessment by using rating scales with more natural language. An example is the Ottawa Surgical Competency Operating Room Evaluation (O-SCORE), which is highlighted in Fig. 9.1.[33] The goal of using this framework to design tools is to assist raters by using natural language and leveraging the expertise and priorities of the rater, rather than to focus too much on traditional assessment language and psychometric jargon that is prevalent in so many of the assessment tools developed in the past. In fact, the O-SCORE was developed by conducting interviews in the surgical lounge with surgeons following a day in the OR to get a sense of the natural language they would normally use to describe residents they had just worked with. Using a rater's natural way of speaking about a trainee allows for instrument design that is easier to use without the need for extensive rater training about the scale, while maintaining expected standards for validity.[34] Another way to describe this is the use of a "shared mental model" between the instrument's designers and the raters who will actually use it (see Chapter 1).

Construct-aligned scales that make use of a shared mental model in the design phase help address the "usability" problem of assessment tools often faced by raters (see also response process validity[21]). To put it another way, if raters cannot reach consensus or don't agree with adverbs such as *frequently*, *occasionally*, or *consistently* (see e.g., the wording on the original OSATS),[2] or don't normally use such jargon in the same way as the person who designed the tool, it literally reduces the statistical evidence for validity obtained from those tools. For example, in Fig. 9.1 the behavioral anchor language for the O-SCORE is more natural and objective, with phrases such as "I had to talk them through" or "I had to prompt them from time to time," and reflects the way surgeons naturally talk to one another about their residents following a case. This is consistent with related research in the field, where researchers have found that valid assessments depend more on the raters than on the instruments themselves.[35] Thus, rather than asking raters to make assessments using scales with abstract psychometric language, construct-aligned scales provide raters with behavioral anchors that are framed in the day-to-day ordinary language the raters would typically use in a busy clinical setting. Additional research has found that errors arising in the use of assessment tools are often due to raters' disagreement on translating implicit categorical judgments into the interval judgments traditionally required by abstract psychometric scales (i.e., "on a scale of 1–5"), thus highlighting the advantage of this approach.[36,37]

*A review of how to select and adapt existing assessment tools for a new assessment environment can be found in published resources by Hamstra.[19,20]

Evaluation of Resident Readiness for Independent Surgical Performance

Trainee:	Level: 1 2 3 4 5	Staff:
Procedure:		Date:

Relative complexity of this procedure to average of same procedure Low Medium High

The purpose of this scale is to evaluate the trainee's ability to perform this procedure safely and independently. With that in mind please use the scale below to evaluate each item, irrespective of the resident's level of training in regards to this case.

Scale
1 – "I had to do the case" – *i.e. Requires complete hands-on guidance, did not do, or not given the opportunity to do*
2 – "I had to talk them through the case" – *i.e. Able to perform tasks but requires constant direction*
3 – "I had to prompt them from time to time" – *i.e. Demonstrates some independence but requires intermittent direction*
4 – "I needed to be in the room just in case" – *i.e. Independence but unaware of risks and still requires supervision for safe practice*
5 – "I did not need to be there" – *i.e. Complete independence, understands risks and performs safely, practice ready*

1. Overall Level of Supervision required for optimal outcome of this procedure?	1	2	3	4	5
2. Preoperative Plan Gathers/assesses required information to reach diagnosis and determine correct procedure required	1	2	3	4	5
3. Case Preparation Patient correctly prepared and positioned, understands approach and required instruments, prepared to deal with probable complications	1	2	3	4	5
4. Knowledge of Specific Procedural Steps Understands steps of procedure, potential risks, and means to avoid/overcome them	1	2	3	4	5
5. Technical Performance Efficiently performs steps, avoiding pitfalls	1	2	3	4	5
6. Technical Skills (shows how) Soft tissue and instrument handling	1	2	3	4	5
7. Visuospatial Skills 3D spatial orientation and able to position instruments/hardware where intended	1	2	3	4	5
8. Postoperative Plan Appropriate complete postoperative plan	1	2	3	4	5
9. Efficiency and Flow Obvious planned course of procedure with economy of movement and flow	1	2	3	4	5
10. Communication Professional and effective communication/utilization of staff	1	2	3	4	5

11. Resident understands his or her limitations when performing this procedure	Y	N
12. Resident is able to safely perform this procedure independently (circle)	Y	N

13. Give at least 1 specific aspect of procedure done well

14. Give at least 1 specific suggestion for improvement

This evaluation has been reviewed with the trainee	Y	N

• **Fig. 9.1** The Ottawa Surgical Competency Operating Room scale. Reproduced with permission from Gofton W, Dudek N, Wood T, Balaa F, Hamstra SJ. The Ottawa Surgical Competency Operating Room Evaluation (O-SCORE): a tool to assess surgical competence. *Acad Med*. 2012 Oct;87(10):1401-1440. doi:10.1097/ACM.0b013e3182677805.

Embedding Entrustment Language Into the Rating Process

Besides the increased ease of use by raters, a benefit of construct-aligned scales is that they are often written in a language that enables entrustment decisions, thus allowing for bestowing (or withholding) clinically relevant responsibilities.[38] For example, the O-SCORE uses the rating "I did not need to be there" and the original Zwisch scale[39,40] uses "Dumb Help" and "No Help" to describe attending behaviors during observation. A modestly revised Zwisch scale is now part of the System for Improving and Measuring Procedural Learning (SIMPL) app (see Fig. 9.2A to C).[†] Since these examples were developed, many assessment tools make use of such language using simply worded entrustment descriptors tied to numerical rating options;[41] a good summary of how to do this can be found in Rekman et al.[42]

One of the benefits of construct-aligned scales written in the language of entrustability is that raters find increased meaning in their assessment decisions: rather than requiring an attending physician to translate their professional judgment of competence into typical terms or phrases such as *inconsistently*, *regularly*, or *the vast majority of time*, raters can acknowledge the categorical judgment they implicitly make while working with the resident; that is, to entrust or not to entrust with patients.[43] In this way, the rater is effectively making a series of high-stakes microdecisions about the trainee while observing and guiding their performance.[42] In the end, this cumulative evidence is more valid

[†]More can be learned about SIMPL at https://reports.simpl.org/.

Zwisch Stage of Supervision	Attending Behaviors	Resident Behaviors Commensurate with This Level of Supervision
Show and Tell	Does majority of key portions as the surgeon Narrates the case (i.e., thinks out loud) Demonstrates key concepts, anatomy, and skills	Opens and closes First assists and observes
Cues to advancement		When first assisting, begins to actively assist (i.e., anticipates surgeons' needs)
Smart Help	Shifts between surgeon and first assist roles When first assisting, leads the resident in surgeon role (active assist) Optimizes the field/exposure Demonstrates the plane or structure Coaches for specific technical skills Coaches regarding the next steps Continues to Idenity anatomical landmarks for the resident	The above, plus: Shifts between surgeon and first assist roles Knows all the component technical skills Demonstrates an increasing ability to perform different key parts of the operation with attending assistance
Cues to advancement		Can execute the majority steps of procedure with active assistance
Dumb Help	Assists and follows the lead of the resident (passive assist) Coaching regarding polishing and refinement of skills Follows the resident's lead throughout the operation	The above, plus: Can "set up" and accomplish the next step for the entire case with increasing efficiency Recognizes critical transition point issues
Cues to advancement		Can transition between all steps with passive assist from faculty
No Help	Largely provides no unsolicited advice Assisted by a junior resident or an attending acting like a junior resident Monitors progress and patient safety*	The above plus: Can work with inexperienced first assistant Can safely complete a case without faculty Can recover most errors Recognizes when to seek help/advice

* Implicit in all of those stages is the responsibility that the attending has to enure optimol patient safety and outcomes. To that end, they may at any time correct behaviors that may load to errors or, if on error has already occurrod, to "take over" and correct the error.

• Fig. 9.2a Original Zwisch scale. Reproduced with permission from DaRosa DA, Zwischenberger JB, Meyerson SL, et al. A theory-based model for teaching and assessing residents in the operating room. *J Surg Educ*. 2013 Jan-Feb;70(1):24-30. doi:10.1016/j.jsurg.2012.07.007.

Zwisch scale	Faculty and resident behavior
Show and tell	• Resident observes and assists • Faculty narrates the operation, demonstrating key anatomy and steps
Active help	• Resident actively assists and performs noncritical steps of the operation • Faculty guides resident through the operation, optimizes exposure, and coaches skills
Passive help	• Resident controls flow of the case, anticipates next steps and critical steps with minimal assistance • Faculty actively assists resident, coaches/refines surgical skills
Supervision only	• Resident performs operation with minimal faculty assistance or with junior resident • Faculty supervises, monitoring progress and safety

• Fig. 9.2b Revised Zwisch scale. Copyright © 2018 by the American College of Surgeons. Used with permission.

and hence more defensible when making decisions about resident progression or the need for specific remediation. In addition, by reverse-engineering the raters' existing categorical schemas into common language behavioral descriptors, construct-aligned scales using entrustability language can increase assessment reliability.[34,44] A final note here should be made about Entrustable Professional Activities (EPAs).[45] While this approach to assessment has become very popular lately, it should be noted that many of the principles that underlie EPAs can be incorporated into more familiar assessment tools by using entrustment language, as in the earlier examples with the O-SCORE and Zwisch scales. In other words, it is not necessary to completely transform one's assessment system into a series of EPAs, but simply to ensure that better entrustability language is incorporated into the rating scales faculty currently use to make their judgments about performance. A good overview of EPAs can be found in Chapter 1.

Procedural Competence Is Multidimensional

There is no question that competence in performing invasive procedures involves psychomotor skills. However, there has been considerable research that clearly

Topic addressed	Question	Answer choices
Resident intraoperative autonomy: Zwisch scale	How much guidance did you provide for the majority of the critical portion of this procedure?	• Show and tell • Active help • Passive help • Supervision only
Resident intraoperative performance	What was this resident's performance for the majority of the critical portion of this procedure?	• Unprepared/critical deficiency • Inexperienced with procedure • Intermediate performance • Practice-ready performance • Exceptional performance
Case complexity	How complex was the case relative to similar procedures?	• Easiest 1/2 • Average • Hardest 1/3

• **Fig. 9.2c** SIMPL assessment questions and scales. Copyright © 2018 by the American College of Surgeons. Used with permission.

demonstrates the importance of other dimensions of competence that are critical in achieving a high level of performance. So-called technical ability depends on a number of interdependent dimensions of ability, including both cognitive and psychomotor. Successful performance of technical skills also requires (1) a deep knowledge of functional anatomy, (2) facility in preprocedure planning, (3) intra-perative decision-making, (4) procedural flow, and (5) interprofessional communication skills involving a diverse team.[46–50] Nevertheless, most of the assessment tools available in surgery emphasize the psychomotor aspects of technical performance or related aspects of manual skill. Like any other complex skill, surgical skill is highly dependent on the specific context of performance and is acquired through hours of deliberate practice involving a combination of cognitive, psychomotor, communication, and management skills. In this sense, the process of acquiring expertise in surgery appears to be consistent with previous research on expertise in other domains of human activity.[51,52]

When considering the use of an assessment tool, it is critically important to reflect on whether the items in the assessment tool directly target the "construct of interest" that one is attempting to sample from the trainee's performance. The term *construct* is widely used in some of the social and behavioral sciences, such as psychology. Thoughtful consideration of the construct of interest by content experts is critical when designing an assessment instrument or selecting an existing tool for use in your local context. Not all tools are readily adaptable to local needs. The construct of interest is essentially the target of your "biopsy" of underlying ability in your learner; that is, just like a biopsy we must always remember that assessment often yields an imperfect sample of what you are trying to measure.

To be useful in the educational context, the construct of interest should represent a performance domain for which there is important and meaningful variance among individuals based on experience or training. Without observed variance among trainees on multiple dimensions of competence, decisions about progression would be impossible (as would the ability to provide useful feedback to trainees); indeed, the entire process of education would be of questionable value. It may be necessary to acquire or develop assessment tools for each of these dimensions of performance (see Appendix 9.1 for a more complete discussion of the importance of variance in assessment).

Useful Tools for Assessing Procedural Skills

For program directors, the production of well-documented, reliable, and valid assessments of procedural skills for each resident has become a critical component of expected best practice, especially with the rise of CBME. The expectations for clinical competency committees (CCCs) can be found in the standards set by the ACGME in the United States,[53] as well as frameworks adopted in other jurisdictions (e.g., the CanMEDS roles in Canada, the Scottish Doctor, and the GMC guidelines in the United Kingdom; see Chapter 1). Luckily, there are many articles in specialty journals designed to help program directors understand the principles and practices of procedural skills assessment in a variety of specialties, including anesthesia,[54] surgery,[55–57] and emergency medicine.[58] In addition, the

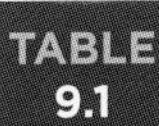

TABLE 9.1 Summary of Technical Skills Toolbox

Purpose of the Review:

- To create a technical skills assessment toolbox to support the ACS/APDS surgical skills curriculum
- To provide a critical summary of these tools, using the unitary validity framework endorsed by the American Educational Research Association (AERA), American Psychological Association (APA), and National Council on Measurement in Education (NCME)

Major Findings:

- Only a handful of tools meet the criteria outlined in the unitary validity framework for validity evidence to support high-stakes decisions.

Conclusion:

- Need further research to correct flaws in most of the existing assessment tools

Takeaway Message:

- Program directors should select tools that are easy to use and for which there are well-established sources of validity evidence.

The Top Three Tools Identified in This Review Are:

1. OPRS (Operative Performance Rating Scale)[a]
   a. Purpose: To provide detailed information that goes beyond end-of-rotation evaluations, which are subject to forgetting and selective recall
   b. Designed to measure and interpret individual operative performance, as supplementary information for the resident's operative case log
   c. Designed to assess all levels of trainee in a general surgery program
   d. Need to balance between obtaining a stable estimate across several performances and limiting the time interval to where performance does not change due to continued learning
   e. Has been used to assess central venous access, arterial line placement, surgical biopsy, laparoscopic ventral hernia repair, sentinel node biopsy and axillary lymph node dissection, open inguinal/femoral hernia repair, laparoscopic inguinal hernia, laparoscopic/open cholecystectomy, thyroidectomy, and parathyroidectomy
   f. Shows good evidence for validity for most procedures
2. MCSAT (Mayo Clinical Skills Assessment Test)[b]
   a. Designed for the assessment of cognitive and motor skills
   b. Focused on colonoscopy performance of surgical fellows, primarily for routine screening exams
   c. Provides typical learning curve data for fellows through first 400 procedures
   d. Provides very detailed evidence for validity, including construction and design of instrument
3. O-SCORE (Ottawa Surgical Competency Operating Room Evaluation)[33]
   a. Designed to measure individual operative performance, as supplementary information for simple case logs in providing timely formative feedback and for making high-stakes decisions for resident progression
   b. Designed for all level of resident trainees
   c. Designed for any surgical procedure, beyond technical skill to include overall surgical competence
   d. Good validity evidence, especially regarding design of instrument based on explicit input from focus group of surgeons
   e. Makes use of construct-aligned scales to avoid tendency to rate highly
   f. Relies on expert knowledge more than psychometric language in behavioral anchors

From Ghaderi I, Manji F, Park YS, et al. Technical skills assessment toolbox: a review using the unitary framework of validity. *Ann Surg*. 2015 Feb;261(2):251-262. doi:10.1097/SLA.0000000000000520.

[a]Williams RG, Verhulst S, Colliver JA, Sanfey H, Chen X, Dunnington GL. A template for reliable assessment of resident operative performance: assessment intervals, numbers of cases and raters. *Surgery*. 2012 Oct;152(4):517-527. doi:10.1016/j.surg.2012.07.004.

[b]Sedlack RE. The Mayo Colonoscopy Skills Assessment Tool: validation of a unique instrument to assess colonoscopy skills in trainees. *Gastrointest Endosc*. 2010 Dec;72(6):1125-1133. doi:10.1016/j.gie.2010.09.001.

literature specific to simulation-based assessment has been reviewed extensively by Cook and colleagues[22] and is covered in Chapter 13.

Methods to assess procedural competence range from informal assessments, such as procedure logs or unstructured observational assessments, to highly structured performance-based examinations. A good starting point for selecting or comparing assessment tools for procedural skills can be found in an excellent review by Ghaderi and colleagues[25] (see Table 9.1). Whichever method is used, one should consider the purpose of the assessment and examine the evidence for the validity of the scores obtained from that method. For those interested in pursuing these ideas in more detail, numerous guides and reviews on assessment in medical education are available.[17–19,59,60]

Practical Issues in the Design and Selection of Assessment Instruments

Among the practical issues that need to be addressed are (1) feasibility issues, including who exactly will rate the learner's performance and in what context; (2) faculty development (i.e., even with construct-aligned scales and embedded natural entrustment language, there is still a need to orient faculty to arrive at a shared mental model for effective use of the assessment tool); (3) details on the type of validity data to collect in each context and by different groups of raters; and (4) reporting issues, such as where the assessment data will be stored, and to whom, when, and how the data will be reported. Although some of these questions appear to be logistical in nature, all are critically important for making valid (i.e., accurate and defensible) decisions. The risk of providing invalid ratings of performance to competency committees and program directors is highlighted by recent challenges to decisions about trainees' advancement and remediation that are being brought forward for appeal by learners across the continuum.[61,62] By understanding and following the validity principles described in this chapter and elsewhere in this book, the program director can help insulate themselves from these challenges and build an assessment toolbox that meets defensible standards for reliability and validity.

When deciding to select, develop, or revise an assessment instrument for a particular construct of interest, it is important that content experts (e.g., your local faculty colleagues) and stakeholders are provided adequate opportunity to discuss the definition and the boundaries of the construct at length and that some consensus be achieved before adoption of the instrument.[63] If content experts or stakeholder groups do not share a common definition of the construct of interest, this will likely cause uncertainty and open the door to criticism and challenges of results from the instrument, which could then paradoxically lead to lower-quality assessment data.[37] Again, this is a good example of the effectiveness of using a shared mental model among raters. Finally, this is a good place to emphasize the point made earlier: valid assessment is more about the process than the tool itself.

As a program director, it is in your best interest to maintain buy-in and enthusiasm for teaching and assessment among your local faculty, as lack of acceptance for an instrument you select now could damage your ability to engage your core faculty in the future (see Chapter 1). For example, in a laparoscopic surgery environment, one aspect of the construct "visuospatial ability" could be defined as the ability to identify surgical planes effectively to allow for efficient dissection and access to the target tissue. Note that in this example, it would be useful to engage content experts to discuss what exactly is meant by the terms *surgical planes* and *visuospatial* according to some behavioral criteria. If your expert panel does not agree on what is meant by one or both terms, it may prove difficult to generate reliable ratings among your faculty raters. In an ideal assessment instrument, all the variance in test results will be construct-relevant variance. In other words, the test will only measure qualities related to the construct of interest and filter out unwanted sources of influence in ratings of performance, such as disagreement among raters, irrelevant contextual factors, or confusing language in the rating scales.

Future Trends in Assessment of Procedural Skills

Embedding Comprehensive Assessment in Training

One of the biggest challenges in making comprehensive assessments of competence in a busy clinical setting is the lack of standard, easy-to-use platforms for gathering information that can be embedded easily into daily workflow. Fortunately, several recent efforts have shown promise in addressing this problem. A recent guide for the use of smartphones in making workplace-based assessments (WBAs) provides an overview of mobile technologies to support entrustment decisions.[64] The ABS has partnered with leading-edge researchers to implement an easy-to-use smartphone app into all its training programs using an EPA format that will tie in directly to the ACGME Milestones.[65,66] This app will allow for a simple and user-friendly approach to collecting comprehensive assessment data using the Zwisch scale (discussed earlier) combined with a modified Dreyfus performance rating scale.[9]

Linking Resident Performance to Patient Outcomes

Surgeons have long sought to link performance in the OR to patient outcomes. Although this type of research is very difficult to do, there has been some incremental success. In a landmark study in general surgery, Birkmeyer and colleagues demonstrated a direct link between individual surgeon technical skill and complication rates by those very same surgeons.[67] A larger and more comprehensive analysis by Asch and colleagues demonstrated a linkage between site of training and obstetrician complication rates.[68] It is clear we need research that combines both approaches to understand whether a specialist's *individual* skills acquired during training can be linked to subsequent performance and outcomes following graduation. While the latter study focused on an indirect linkage between training program exposure and ultimate performance, the former demonstrated a proximal linkage between technical skills and performance that needs to be followed up with a cohort of learners.

With the new mandate for CBME and all its focus on assessment, it should be possible to collect detailed and comprehensive data on resident performance during training and link that with performance and patient outcomes following training. Each specialty collects patient outcomes data in unique ways, and often lacks the kind of specificity required to link back to detailed measures of competence during training. Fortunately for surgery, given the discrete nature of assessment, patient treatment, and outcomes, this specialty may be one of the first to demonstrate such a linkage. In a recent study looking at complication rates in vascular surgery, Smith et al. have shown that ACGME Milestone ratings collected during training can predict complication rates in endovascular aortic aneurysm repair using a detailed patient outcomes database.[69] In another study linking ACGME Milestones in general surgery and Medicare data, Kendrick et al. found no correlation but made several suggestions for how to modify their approach.[70] In principle, this is a promising approach, as both studies follow on from the earlier work on seeking outcomes that relate back to assessments of performance during training, which has been identified as a necessary line of research and will no doubt be an area of considerable research activity for the foreseeable future.[31,71,72]

Overcoming the Burden of Assessment Using Video and Machine Learning

One side effect of CBME is the additional burden of assessment. There have been calls for reducing this burden not only on the trainees but also on faculty raters.[73,74] Certainly in the surgical education literature, surgeons have long called for automated approaches to assessment to reduce the time pressure on their already busy days. Video-based review has been an acknowledged option for several decades and the literature shows that it can be feasible and effective, under the right circumstances.[75,76] Researchers are now studying whether preexisting embedded audio and video recording platforms developed to enhance patient safety, such as the OR Black Box, could be used for assessment purposes, not only of teamwork and efficiency but also for rating technical skill utilizing a panel of dedicated and trained raters.[77]

These video-based platforms are also now being explored to study the feasibility and validity of artificial intelligence (AI) and machine learning (ML) approaches to assessment.[78,79] While this area of research is still in its infancy, there is already a systematic review available on AI and ML approaches to automated assessment of procedural skills.[80] So far, only direct sensor-based kinematic data and video-based data using surgical instrument and hand motion have been studied, thus somewhat limiting the generalizability and validity of this approach.[81] Video-based data require substantial preprocessing to identify target structures in the video feed, and kinematic data are currently not feasible for open or even laparoscopic surgery given that position/motion sensors need to be mounted on or embedded on the surgical instruments.

Another interesting option for removing some of the burden from assessment is crowdsourcing. This involves submitting videos of performance for review by nonexperts. With enough ratings, it appears that a reasonable average of performance can be identified. In this sense, it is similar to AI and ML in that it is a data-driven approach, it does not require the direct judgment of an expert, and patterns emerge from the large volume of data that is fed into the system. Questions about the validity of these approaches remain, however; thus further research is required before they are applied to make high-stakes decisions.[82]

Given that surgery is one of the few disciplines that results in a tangible "product" (e.g., a functioning hip or repaired laceration), crowdsourcing lends itself to automated assessment of the final product of any surgical intervention. Frischknecht et al.[83] developed a proof of concept for this that could then be supplemented by expert review, used for self-directed learning, or indeed, submitted for crowdsourcing. It would be interesting to see if crowdsourced judgments correlated with judgments from expert raters or automated results from ML methods.

A relevant question to ask regarding all of these automated approaches is whether they should be restricted to in vitro simulation settings or could be used in vivo in the OR with live patients. Although questions of assessment in a simulation setting are addressed in Chapter 13, it is worth mentioning here that the assessment of procedural skills in a workplace context can result in very different ratings than assessment in vitro. Attempts to bridge this gap include both theoretical[84] and practical solutions.[85,87]

Conclusion

Assessment of procedural competence can be resource intensive. One way to justify the allocation of resources to the assessment process is to gather evidence to support the validity of the decisions made on the basis of them (i.e., in support of the current move toward CBME and increased public accountability). This requires knowledge of the peer-reviewed literature and resources to help sift through the myriad choices according to the most recent standards for quality, feasibility, and validity. This chapter provides access to these resources and standards and as such should be a useful guide for program directors.

Takeaway Messages

- Make liberal use of content experts in choosing your assessment instrument. It is important that the definition and the boundaries of the construct be discussed at length and that some degree of consensus be achieved before moving on.
- Put some effort into pilot-testing any instrument you choose. You will learn a lot about the construct of interest and the particular competencies you are trying to assess from doing this.
- Keep an eye on reliability, validity, and feasibility as you develop and work with your assessment instrument. Collect data for continuous quality improvement to support your validity argument.

Other Resources

Many medical schools now have medical education research units, typically with an expert in assessment (i.e., a psychometrician). Table 9.2 provides a checklist for developing a good assessment instrument. This checklist can also be adapted to evaluate the quality of existing assessment tools.

TABLE 9.2 Seven-Step Checklist for Developing a Good Assessment Instrument

1. Determine the purpose of your assessment.
   - Will the instrument be used for formative or summative (standard setting/criteria) assessment or research?
   - Do you want to assess knowledge, skills, or attitudes (e.g., performance, teamwork, anxiety)?
2. Identify the main construct of interest and stakeholders to help establish content validity.
3. Review the construct with content experts using a consensus method such as focus groups.
   - Obtain a representative sample from different institutions and disciplines.
   - Work towards thematic saturation and address political issues.
   - Set preliminary standards: What does perfect/borderline performance look like?
4. Develop and write the items, drawing on related existing tests if applicable.
5. If necessary, train the raters (and assess interrater reliability).
6. Pilot test the instrument (with a representative sample) for validity.
   - Check the feasibility of the instrument (length, clarity, cost).
   - If necessary, go back to step 4 (modify the items) and then pilot-test again.
7. Implement the modified test and measure its reliability and validity with a larger sample.
   - Assess construct validity.

Note: We can never achieve perfect validity, so consider this to be an ongoing process whereby you are constantly checking performance statistics for reliability and validity.

Modified from Hamstra SJ. The focus on competencies and individual learner assessment as emerging themes in medical education research. *Acad Emerg Med.* 2012;19(12):1336-1343. doi:10.1111/acem.12021.

For those interested in further studying the issues presented in this chapter, Appendix 9.2 includes an annotated bibliography of relevant literature.

References

1. Winckel CP, Reznick RK, Cohen R, Taylor B. Reliability and construct-validity of a structured technical skills assessment form. *Am J Surg.* 1994 Apr;167:423–427. doi:10.1016/0002-9610(94)90128-7.
2. Martin JA, Regehr G, Reznick R, et al. Objective structured assessment of technical skill (OSATS) for surgical residents. *Br J Surg.* 1997 Feb;84(2):273–278. doi:10.1046/j.1365-2168.1997.02502.x.
3. Vassiliou MC, Feldman LS, Andrew CG, et al. A global assessment tool for evaluation of intraoperative laparoscopic skills. *Am J Surg.* 2005 Jul;190(1):107–113. doi:10.1016/j.amjsurg.2005.04.004.
4. Mackay S, Datta V, Chang A, Shah J, Kneebone R, Darzi A. Multiple Objective Measures of Skill (MOMS): a new approach to the assessment of technical ability in surgical trainees. *Ann Surg.* 2003 Aug;238(2):291–300. doi:10.1097/01.sla.0000080829.29028.c4.
5. Cremers SL, Lora AN, Ferrufino-Ponce ZK. Global Rating Assessment of Skills in Intraocular Surgery (GRASIS). *Ophthalmology.* 2005 Oct;112(10):1655–1660. doi:10.1016/j.ophtha.2005.05.010.
6. Doyle JD, Webber EM, Sidhu RS. A universal global rating scale for the evaluation of technical skills in the operating room. *Am J Surg.* 2007 May;193(5):551–555. doi:10.1016/j.amjsurg.2007.02.003.
7. Goff BA, Lentz GM, Lee D, Houmard B, Mandel LS. Development of an objective structured assessment of technical skills for obstetric and gynecology residents. *Obstet Gynecol.* 2000 Jul;96(1):146–150. doi:10.1016/s0029-7844(00)00829-2.
8. Leong JJ, Leff DR, Das A, et al. Validation of orthopaedic bench models for trauma surgery. *J Bone Joint Surg Br.* 2008 Jul;90(7):958–965. doi:10.1302/0301-620X.90B7.20230.
9. Williams RG, Sanfey H, Chen XP, Dunnington GL. A controlled study to determine measurement conditions necessary for a reliable and valid operative performance assessment: a controlled prospective observational study. *Ann Surg.* 2012 Jul;256(1):177–187. doi:10.1097/SLA.0b013e31825b6de4.
10. Hamstra SJ. Workplace-based assessment of procedural skills. In: Holmboe ES, Durning SJ, Hawkins RE, eds. *Practical Guide to the Evaluation of Clinical Competence.* 2nd ed. Elsevier Health Sciences; 2018:155–164.
11. Hatala R, Cook DA, Brydges R, Hawkins R. Constructing a validity argument for the objective structured assessment of technical skills (OSATS): a systematic review of validity evidence. *Adv Health Sci Educ Theory Pract.* 2015 Dec;20(5):1149–1175. doi:10.1007/s10459-015-9593-1. Erratum in: *Adv Health Sci Educ Theory Pract.* 2015 Dec;20(5):1177-118. PMID: 25702196.
12. Hatala R, Cook DA, Brydges R, Hawkins R. Erratum to: constructing a validity argument for the objective structured assessment of technical skills (OSATS): a systematic review of validity evidence. *Adv Health Sci Educ Theory Pract.* 2015 Dec;20(5):1177–1218. doi:10.1007/s10459-015-9636-7. Erratum for: *Adv Health Sci Educ Theory Pract.* 2015 Dec;20(5):1149–1175. PMID: 26374730.
13. Frank J, ed. *The CanMEDS 2005 Physician Competency Framework: Better Standards. Better Physicians. Better Care.* The Royal College of Physicians and Surgeons of Canada; 2005.
14. Nasca TJ, Philibert I, Brigham T, Flynn TC. The next GME accreditation system: rationale and benefits. *N Engl J Med.* 2012 Mar 15;366(11):1051–1056. doi:10.1056/NEJMsr1200117.
15. Swing SR. The ACGME outcome project: retrospective and prospective. *Med Teach.* 2007 Sep;29(7):648–654. doi:10.1080/01421590701392903.
16. Downing SM. Validity: on meaningful interpretation of assessment data. *Med Educ.* 2003 Sep;37(9):830–837. doi:10.1046/j.1365-2923.2003.01594.x.
17. Messick S. Validation of inferences from persons' responses and performances as scientific inquiry into score meaning. *Am Psychol.* 1995;50:741–749.
18. American Educational Research Association, American Psychological Association, National Council on Measurement in Education. *Standards for Educational and Psychological Testing.* American Educational Research Association; 1999.
19. Hamstra SJ. Designing and selecting assessment instruments for competency-based medical education. In: Bandiera G, Dath D, eds. *The Royal College Program Directors Handbook: A Practical Guide for Leading an Exceptional Program.* Royal College of Physicians and Surgeons of Canada; 2014.
20. Hamstra SJ. The focus on competencies and individual learner assessment as emerging themes in medical education research. *Acad Emerg Med.* 2012 Dec;19(12):1336–1343. doi:10.1111/acem.12021.

21. Cook DA, Beckman TJ. Current concepts in validity and reliability for psychometric instruments: theory and application. *Am J Med.* 2006 Feb;119(2):166.e7–e16. doi:10.1016/j.amjmed.2005.10.036.
22. Cook DA, Brydges R, Zendejas B, Hamstra SJ, Hatala R. Technology-enhanced simulation to assess health professionals: a systematic review of validity evidence, research methods, and reporting quality. *Acad Med.* 2013 Jun;88(6):872–883. doi:10.1097/ACM.0b013e31828ffdcf.
23. Korndorffer Jr JR, Kasten SJ, Downing SM. A call for the utilization of consensus standards in the surgical education literature. *Am J Surg.* 2010 Jan;199(1):99–104. doi:10.1016/j.amjsurg.2009.08.018.
24. Cook DA, Zendejas B, Hamstra SJ, Hatala R, Brydges R. What counts as validity evidence? Examples and prevalence in a systematic review of simulation-based assessment. *Adv Health Sci Ed Theory Pract.* 2014 May;19(2):233–250. doi:10.1007/s10459-013-9458-4.
25. Ghaderi I, Manji F, Park YS, et al. Technical skills assessment toolbox: a review using the unitary framework of validity. *Ann Surg.* 2015 Feb;261(2):251–262. doi:10.1097/SLA.0000000000000520.
26. Scott DJ, Dunnington GL. The new ACS/APDS Skills Curriculum: moving the learning curve out of the operating room. *J Gastrointest Surg.* 2008 Feb;12(2):213–221. doi:10.1007/s11605-007-0357-y.
27. ACS Division of Education. ACS/APDS Surgical Skills Curriculum for Residents. Accessed May 21, 2023. https://www.facs.org/for-medical-professionals/education/programs/acsapds-surgery-resident-skills-curriculum/.
28. Hennings LI, Sørensen JL, Hybscmann J, Strandbygaard J. Tools for measuring technical skills during gynaecologic surgery: a scoping review. *BMC Med Educ.* 2021 Jul 26;21(1):402. doi:10.1186/s12909-021-02790-w.
29. Bilgic E, Endo S, Lebedeva E, et al. A scoping review of assessment tools for laparoscopic suturing. *Surg Endosc.* 2018 Jul;32(7):3009–3023. doi:10.1007/s00464-018-6199-8.
30. Watanabe Y, Bilgic E, Lebedeva E, et al. A systematic review of performance assessment tools for laparoscopic cholecystectomy. *Surg Endosc.* 2016 Mar;30(3):832–844. doi:10.1007/s00464-015-4285-8.
31. Hamstra SJ, Yamazaki K. A validity framework for effective analysis and interpretation of milestones data. *J Grad Med Educ.* 2021 Apr;13(2 Suppl):75–80. doi:10.4300/JGME-D-20-01039.1.
32. Crossley J, Johnson G, Booth J, Wade W. Good questions, good answers: construct alignment improves the performance of workplace-based assessment scales. *Med Educ.* 2011 Jun;45(6):560–569. doi:10.1111/j.1365-2923.2010.03913.x.
33. Gofton WT, Dudek NL, Wood TJ, Balaa F, Hamstra SJ. The Ottawa Surgical Competency Operating Room Evaluation (O-SCORE): a tool to assess surgical competence. *Acad Med.* 2012 Oct;87(10):1401–1407. doi:10.1097/ACM.0b013e3182677805.
34. Crossley J, Jolly B. Making sense of work-based assessment: ask the right questions, in the right way, about the right things, of the right people. *Med Educ.* 2012 Jan;46(1):28–37. doi:10.1111/j.1365-2923.2011.04166.x.
35. van der Vleuten C, Verhoeven B. In-training assessment developments in postgraduate education in Europe. *ANZ J Surg.* 2013 Jun;83(6):454–459. doi:10.1111/ans.12190.
36. MacRae CN, Bodenhausen GV. Social cognition: thinking categorically about others. *Ann Rev Psychol.* 2000;51:93–120. doi:10.1146/annurev.psych.51.1.93.
37. Apramian T, Cristancho S, Sener A, Lingard L. How do thresholds of principle and preference influence surgeon assessments of learner performance? *Ann Surg.* 2018 Aug;268(2):385–390. doi:10.1097/SLA.0000000000002284.
38. ten Cate O, Scheele F. Competency-based postgraduate training: can we bridge the gap between theory and clinical practice? *Acad Med.* 2007 Jun;82(6):542–547. doi:10.1097/ACM.0b013e31805559c7.
39. DaRosa DA, Zwischenberger JB, Meyerson SL, et al. A theory-based model for teaching and assessing residents in the operating room. *J Surg Educ.* 2013 Jan-Feb;70(1):24–30. doi:10.1016/j.jsurg.2012.07.007.
40. George BC, Teitelbaum EN, Meyerson SL, et al. Reliability, validity, and feasibility of the Zwisch scale for the assessment of intraoperative performance. *J Surg Educ.* 2014 Nov-Dec;71(6):e90–e96. doi:10.1016/j.jsurg.2014.06.018.
41. Rekman J, Hamstra SJ, Dudek N, Seabrook C, Gofton W. A new instrument for assessing resident competence in surgical clinic: the Ottawa Clinic Assessment Tool (OCAT). *J Surg Educ.* 2016 Jul-Aug;73(4):153–160. doi:10.1016/j.jsurg.2016.02.003.
42. Rekman J, Gofton W, Dudek N, Gofton T, Hamstra SJ. Entrustability scales: outlining their usefulness for competency-based clinical assessment. *Acad Med.* 2016 Feb;91(2):186–190. doi:10.1097/ACM.0000000000001045.
43. Yeates P, O'Neill P, Mann K, Eva K. Seeing the same thing differently: mechanisms that contribute to assessor differences in directly-observed performance assessments. *Adv Health Sci Educ Theory Pract.* 2013 Aug;18(3):325–341. doi:10.1007/s10459-012-9372-1.
44. Beard JD, Marriott J, Purdie H, Crossley J. Assessing the surgical skills of trainees in the operating theatre: a prospective observational study of the methodology. *Health Technol Assess.* 2011 Jan;15(1):i–xxi, 1–162. doi:10.3310/hta15010.
45. ten Cate O. Entrustability of professional activities and competency-based training. *Med Educ.* 2005 Dec;39(12):1176–1177. doi:10.1111/j.1365-2929.2005.02341.x.
46. Anastakis DJ, Hamstra SJ, Matsumoto ED. Visual-spatial abilities in surgical training. *Am J Surg.* 2000 Jun;179(6):469–471. doi:10.1016/s0002-9610(00)00397-4.
47. Wanzel KR, Hamstra SJ, Caminiti MF, Anastakis DJ, Grober ED, Reznick RK. Visual-spatial ability correlates with efficiency of hand motion and successful surgical performance. *Surgery.* 2003 Nov;134(5):750–757. doi:10.1016/s0039-6060(03)00248-4.
48. Sidhu RS, Tompa D, Jang RW, et al. Interpretation of three-dimensional structure from two-dimensional endovascular images: implications for educators in vascular surgery. *J Vasc Surg.* 2004 Jun;39(6):1305–1311. doi:10.1016/j.jvs.2004.02.024.
49. Moulton CA, Regehr G, Lingard L, Merritt C, MacRae H. Operating from the other side of the table: control dynamics and the surgeon educator. *J Am Coll Surg.* 2010 Jan;210(1):79–86. doi:10.1016/j.jamcollsurg.2009.09.043.
50. Moulton CA, Regehr G, Mylopoulos M, MacRae HM. Slowing down when you should: a new model of expert judgment. *Acad Med.* 2007 Oct;82(10 Suppl):S109–S116. doi:10.1097/ACM.0b013e3181405a76.
51. Ericsson KA. Deliberate practice and the acquisition and maintenance of expert performance in medicine and related domains. *Acad Med.* 2004 Oct;79(10 Suppl):S70–S81. doi:10.1097/00001888-200410001-00022.
52. Norman GR, Grierson L, Sherbino J, Hamstra SJ, Schmidt H, Mamede S. Expertise in medicine and surgery. In: Ericsson KA,

Hoffman RR, Kozbelt A, Williams AM, eds. *The Cambridge Handbook on Expertise and Expert Performance.* 2nd ed. Cambridge University Press; 2018.

53. Andolsek K, Padmore J, Hauer KE, Ekpenyong A, Edgar L, Holmboe E. *Clinical Competency Committees: A Guidebook for Programs.* Accreditation Council for Graduate Medical Education; 2020. Accessed May 22, 2023. https://www.acgme.org/milestones/resources/.
54. Boulet JR, Murray D. Review article: assessment in anesthesiology education. *Can J Anaesth.* 2012 Feb;59(2):182–192. doi:10.1007/s12630-011-9637-9.
55. Hamstra SJ, Dubrowski A. Effective training and assessment of surgical skills, and the correlates of performance. *Surg Innov.* 2005 Mar;12(1):71–77. doi:10.1177/155335060501200110.
56. Sidhu RS, Grober ED, Musselman LJ, Reznick RK. Assessing competency in surgery: where to begin? *Surgery.* 2004 Jan;135(1):6–20. doi:10.1016/s0039-6060(03)00154-5.
57. Fried GM, Feldman LS. Objective assessment of technical performance. *World J Surg.* 2008 Feb;32(2):156–160. doi:10.1007/s00268-007-9143-y.
58. Farrell SE. Evaluation of student performance: clinical and professional performance. *Acad Emerg Med.* 2005 Apr;12(4):302e6–e10. doi:10.1197/j.aem.2004.05.037.
59. Wass V, Van der Vleuten C, Shatzer J, Jones R. Assessment of clinical competence. *Lancet.* 2001 Mar 24;357(9260):945–949. doi:10.1016/S0140-6736(00)04221-5.
60. Epstein RM, Hundert EM. Defining and assessing professional competence. *JAMA.* 2002 Jan 9;287(2):226–235. doi:10.1001/jama.287.2.226.
61. Packer CD, Duca NS, Dhaliwal G, et al. Grade appeals in the internal medicine clerkship: a national survey and recommendations for improvement. *Am J Med.* 2021 Jun;134(6):817–822.e7. doi:10.1016/j.amjmed.2021.02.002.
62. Thomas LA, Milburn N, Kay A, Hatch E. Factors associated with grade appeals: a survey of psychiatry clerkship directors. *Acad Psychiatry.* 2018 Jun;42(3):354–356. doi:10.1007/s40596-017-0764-7.
63. Edgar L, Jones Jr MD, Harsy B, Passiment M, Hauer KE. Better decision-making: shared mental models and the clinical competency committee. *J Grad Med Educ.* 2021 Apr;13(2 Suppl):51–58. doi:10.4300/JGME-D-20-00850.1.
64. Marty AP, Linsenmeyer M, George B, Young JQ, Breckwoldt J, ten Cate O. Mobile technologies to support workplace-based assessment for entrustment decisions: guidelines for programs and educators: AMEE Guide No. 154. *Med Teach.* 2023 Jan 27:1–11. doi:10.1080/0142159X.2023.2168527.
65. American Board of Surgery. ABS Selects the Society for Improving Medical Professional Learning to Provide EPA Technology Solution. 2022. Accessed February 14, 2023. https://www.absurgery.org/default.jsp?news_epatech0922.
66. George BC, Bohnen JD, Williams RG, et al. Readiness of US general surgery residents for independent practice. *Ann Surg.* 2017 Oct;266(4):582–594. doi:10.1097/SLA.0000000000002414. Erratum in: *Ann Surg.* 2018 Mar;267(3):e63. PMID: 28742711.
67. Birkmeyer JD, Finks JF, O'Reilly A, et al. Surgical skill and complication rates after bariatric surgery. *N Engl J Med.* 2013 Oct 10;369(15):1434–1442. doi:10.1056/NEJMsa1300625.
68. Asch DA, Nicholson S, Srinivas S, Herrin J, Epstein AJ. Evaluating obstetrical residency programs using patient outcomes. *JAMA.* 2009 Sep 23;302(12):1277–1283. doi:10.1001/jama.2009.1356.
69. Smith BK, Yamazaki K, Tekian A, et al. ACGME Milestone ratings during training predict surgeons' early outcomes. *JAMA Surgery.* 2023 Submitted May 23.
70. Kendrick DE, Thelen AE, Chen X, et al. Association of surgical resident competency ratings with patient outcomes. *Acad Med.* 2023 Jul 1;98(7):813–820. doi:10.1097/ACM.0000000000005157.
71. Phillips Jr RL, George BC, Holmboe ES, Bazemore AW, Westfall JM, Bitton A. Measuring graduate medical education outcomes to honor the social contract. *Acad Med.* 2022 May 1;97(5):643–648. doi:10.1097/ACM.0000000000004592.
72. Smith BK, Hamstra SJ, Yamazaki K. Expert consensus on the conceptual alignment of Accreditation Council for Graduate Medical Education competencies with patient outcomes after common vascular surgical procedures. *J Vasc Surg.* 2022 Nov;76(5):1388–1397. doi:10.1016/j.jvs.2022.06.091.
73. Ott MC, Pack R, Cristancho S, Chin M, Van Koughnett JA, Ott M. "The most crushing thing": understanding resident assessment burden in a competency-based curriculum. *J Grad Med Educ.* 2022 Oct;14(5):583–592. doi:10.4300/JGME-D-22-00050.1.
74. Ames SE, Ponce BA, Marsh JL, Hamstra SJ. Orthopaedic surgery residency milestones: initial formulation and future directions. *J Am Acad Orthop Surg.* 2020 Jan 1;28(1):e1–e8. doi:10.5435/JAAOS-D-18-00786.
75. Dath D, Regehr G, Birch D, et al. Toward reliable operative assessment: the reliability and feasibility of videotaped assessment of laparoscopic technical skills. *Surg Endosc.* 2004 Dec;18(12):1800–1804. doi:10.1007/s00464-003-8157-2.
76. Tousignant MR, Liu X, Ershad Langroodi M, Jarc AM. Identification of main influencers of surgical efficiency and variability using task-level objective metrics: a five-year robotic sleeve gastrectomy case series. *Front Surg.* 2022 May 2;9:756522. doi:10.3389/fsurg.2022.756522.
77. Fecso AB, Kuzulugil SS, Babaoglu C, Bener AB, Grantcharov TP. Relationship between intraoperative non-technical performance and technical events in bariatric surgery. *Br J Surg.* 2018 Jul;105(8):1044–1050. doi:10.1002/bjs.10811.
78. Khalid S, Goldenberg MG, Grantcharov TP, Taati B, Rudzicz F. Evaluation of deep learning models for identifying surgical actions and measuring performance. *JAMA Netw Open.* 2020 Mar 2;3(3):e201664. doi:10.1001/jamanetworkopen.2020.1664.
79. Kasa K, Burns D, Goldenberg MG, Selim O, Whyne C, Hardisty M. Multi-modal deep learning for assessing surgeon technical skill. *Sensors (Basel).* 2022 Sep 27;22(19):7328. doi:10.3390/s22197328.
80. Yanik E, Intes X, Kruger U, et al. Deep neural networks for the assessment of surgical skills: a systematic review. *J Def Model Simul Appl Methodol Technol.* 2021;19:159–171. doi:10.1177/15485129211034.
81. Loftus TJ, Vlaar APJ, Hung AJ, et al. Executive summary of the artificial intelligence in surgery series. *Surgery.* 2022 May;171(5):1435–1439. doi:10.1016/j.surg.2021.10.047.
82. Olsen RG, Genét MF, Konge L, Bjerrum F. Crowdsourced assessment of surgical skills: a systematic review. *Am J Surg.* 2022 Nov;224(5):1229–1237. doi:10.1016/j.amjsurg.2022.07.008.
83. Frischknecht AC, Kasten SJ, Hamstra SJ, et al. The objective assessment of experts' and novices' suturing skills using an image analysis program. *Acad Med.* 2013 Feb;88(2):260–264. doi:10.1097/ACM.0b013e31827c3411.
84. Hamstra SJ, Brydges R, Hatala R, Zendejas B, Cook DA. Reconsidering fidelity in simulation-based training. *Acad Med.* 2014 Mar;89(3):387–392. doi:10.1097/ACM.0000000000000130.
85. Kneebone R, Kidd J, Nestel D, Asvall S, Paraskeva P, Darzi A. An innovative model for teaching and learning clinical procedures. *Med Educ.* 2002 Jul;36(7):628–634. doi:10.1046/j.1365-2923.2002.01261.x.

86. Kneebone R, Nestel D, Yadollahi F, et al. Assessing procedural skills in context: exploring the feasibility of an integrated procedural performance instrument (IPPI). *Med Educ.* 2006 Nov;40(11):1105–1114. doi:10.1111/j.1365-2929. 2006. 02612.x.
87. Nagy E, Luta GMM, Huhn D, et al. Teaching patient-centred communication skills during clinical procedural skill training—a preliminary pre-post study comparing international and local medical students. *BMC Med Educ.* 2021 Sep 3;21(1):469. doi:10.1186/s12909-021-02901-7.
88. Williams RG, Verhulst S, Colliver JA, Sanfey H, Chen X, Dunnington GL. A template for reliable assessment of resident operative performance: assessment intervals, numbers of cases and raters. *Surgery.* 2012 Oct;152(4):517–527. doi:10.1016/j.surg.2012.07.004.
89. Sedlack RE. The Mayo Colonoscopy Skills Assessment Tool: validation of a unique instrument to assess colonoscopy skills in trainees. *Gastrointest Endosc.* 2010 Dec;72(6):1125–1133. doi:10.1016/j.gie.2010.09.001.
90. Case SM, Swanson DB. *Constructing Written Test Questions for the Basic And Clinical Sciences.* 3rd ed. National Board of Medical Examiners; 2002.
91. Streiner DL. Global rating scales. In: Neufeld VR, Norman GR, eds. *Assessing Clinical Competence.* Springer; 1985:119–141.
92. Maxim BR, Dielman TE. Dimensionality, internal consistency and interrater reliability of clinical performance ratings. *Med Educ.* 1987 Mar;21(2):130–137. doi:10.1111/j.1365-2923.1987.tb00679.x.
93. Dauphinee WD. Assessing clinical performance: where do we stand and what might we expect? *JAMA.* 1995 Sep 6;274(9):741–743. doi:10.1001/jama.274.9.741.

10

Evaluating Evidence-Based Practice

LOAI ALBARQOUNI, MD, MSC, PHD, AND DRAGAN ILIC, PHD

CHAPTER OUTLINE

Introduction

Evidence-based practice (EBP) has emerged as a paradigm of clinical practice to improve healthcare quality by shifting emphasis from unsystematic clinical experience and pathophysiologic rationale to critical examination of scientific evidence from empirical patient-relevant clinical research.[1–3] EBP provides a framework for "the integration of the best research evidence with patients' values and clinical expertise and circumstances in clinical decision making."[4] In a consensus statement, the authors preferred the term *evidence-based practice* over *evidence-based medicine* to "reflect wider adoption of these concepts among other healthcare disciplines and the benefits of entire healthcare teams and organizations adopting a shared evidence-based approach."[5]

This ideal, however, remains far from realization. Clinicians leave the majority of their clinical questions unanswered,[6–8] often consult nonevidence-based sources for information, witness their up-to-date medical knowledge and practice performance deteriorate over the years following their training,[9,10] and often fail to use research evidence to inform clinical decisions.[11–13] Traditional didactic-based continuing medical education (CME) remains of limited utility as a remedy.[14–18]

In response, health professional organizations and accreditation councils have called for increased integration of EBP training in the curricula of undergraduate, postgraduate, and continuing healthcare education and require all health professionals to be competent in EBP for accreditation and licensing purposes.[19,20] For instance, the Accreditation Council for Graduate Medical Education (ACGME) recognized EBP in its "outcomes project,"[20] which shifted the currency of accreditation from structure and process to educational outcomes corresponding to six competencies. EBP is represented most prominently in the Patient Care and Practice-based Learning and Improvement general competencies. Similarly, the Institute of Medicine (now the National Academy of Medicine; NAM) included "employ evidence-based practice" and "utilize informatics"[21] among five essential competencies for all health professions; the American Association of Colleges and Universities (AAC&U) included "form clinical questions and retrieve evidence to advance patient care"[22] among 13 Entrustable Professional Activities (EPAs)[23] for entering residency; and in the Canadian Medical Education Directives for Specialists (CanMEDS) 2015 framework, EBP found representation in the scholar and medical expert roles (see Chapter 1).[24]

Steps in Practicing EBP

Evidence-based clinicians often follow a number of main steps to deliver evidence-based healthcare, alliteratively phrased as the five A's. Let's take a clinical example, which we will return to throughout the chapter:

> *A 70-year-old man visits his physician for a periodic health examination. His only new complaint is a 3-month history of a mild intermittent nonproductive cough. His medical history includes benign prostatic hypertrophy, osteoarthritis, and isolated systolic hypertension. In the past he smoked about one pack of cigarettes per day but stopped at age 60. He has received all of the routinely recommended preventive healthcare procedures, including*

a normal colonoscopy, a Pneumovax, and yearly influenza vaccines. Near the end of the visit, he tells you that his bocce partner was recently hospitalized emergently for a ruptured abdominal aortic aneurysm (AAA). He asks, "Can you check me for that, doc?"

First, clinicians must recognize emerging information needs. An important step is the recognition of personal knowledge gaps and uncertainties. Unaware of recent evidence to address the patient's question, the clinician in the previous example encounters a personal knowledge gap. A systematic review has found that on average, clinicians encountered 0.57 questions per patient seen,[25] yet they only pursued 51% of questions and successfully found answers for 78% of those pursued questions. In the end, only about one-third of questions encountered were successfully pursued and answered. Main barriers include clinicians' lack of time and doubt that a useful answer exists.[25]

The clinician must then *ask* the clinical question in an answerable structured format. Clinical questions can be classified as background (general) or foreground (specific, patient based)[26] and associated with particular clinical tasks, such as therapy, diagnosis, or prognosis.[27] Furthermore, foreground questions can be constructed in the Patient-Intervention-Comparator-Outcome (PICO) format, explicitly identifying characteristics of the patient, intervention, comparison, and outcome. Clinicians then must *acquire* the best available evidence that is pertinent to the clinical question and critically *appraise* the evidence for its validity, clinical relevance, and applicability. Clinicians must then *apply* the evidence to their decision-making for an individual patient. In this, clinicians use principles of shared decision-making to integrate patients' values, preferences, and circumstances in the decision-making process.[28] Finally, the clinician *assesses* their performance in the entire EBP process.

For the clinical scenario presented earlier, we might ask: "In a 70-year-old patient with a history of hypertension and smoking, will screening for AAA with abdominal ultrasound result in a decreased risk of death from AAA rupture?" Asking such questions may help in selecting information resources, choosing search terms, knowing when to stop searching, applying the evidence in decision-making, and communicating with other providers.[29,30]

Modes of Practicing EBP

There are three modes of incorporating evidence into practice depending on the nature of the encountered condition, time constraints, level of EBP expertise, and personal preference. For frequently encountered conditions with little or no time constraints, we may operate in the "doing" mode, following all five steps of EBP including seeking and critically appraising original clinical research reports.

For less common conditions or for more rushed clinical situations, we might eliminate the critical appraisal step and operate in the "user" mode, conserving our time by restricting our search to rigorously preappraised evidence. Editors of these evidence-based secondary information resources search, select, appraise, and summarize evidence from original research in the form of syntheses (systematic reviews) and synopses of studies and systematic reviews, adhering to accepted explicit methodological criteria.[31,32] Finally, in the "replicator" mode we trust and directly follow the recommendations of respected EBP consultants or champions (abandoning at least the search for evidence and its detailed appraisal).

Doctors may practice in any of these modes at various times, but their activity will probably fall predominantly into one category. In a survey of UK general practitioners, 72% reported practicing at least part of their time in the user mode, using evidence-based summaries generated by others.[33] On the other hand, fewer claimed to understand the appraising tools of number needed to treat (35%) and confidence intervals (20%). Finally, only 5% believed that learning the skills of evidence-based medicine (all five steps) was the most appropriate method for "moving from opinion-based medicine to evidence-based medicine."[33] Therefore with the increased availability of trustworthy resources of preappraised evidence, clinicians can practice EBP without being fully competent in detailed critical appraisal of original clinical research reports.[34,35]

Competency-Based EBP Education

CBME is an outcomes-based framework for design, implementation, assessment, and evaluation of clinical training programs (see Chapter 1).[36,37] Core competencies have been defined as the essential minimal set of a combination of attributes, such as applied knowledge, skills, and attitudes, that enable clinicians to perform a set of tasks to an appropriate standard efficiently and effectively.[38]

A consensus-based, contemporary set of 86 core competencies in EBP has been identified through a systematic, multistage, modified Delphi study that should inform the curriculum development of entry-level EBP teaching and learning programs for clinicians. Table 10.1 provides the 86 core competencies grouped into the main EBP step mentioned before (the five A's: *ask*; *acquire*; *appraise* and interpret; *apply*; and *assess*). Assessment instruments and strategies should be aligned with the core competencies and leaning objectives. Fig. 10.1 depicts how these

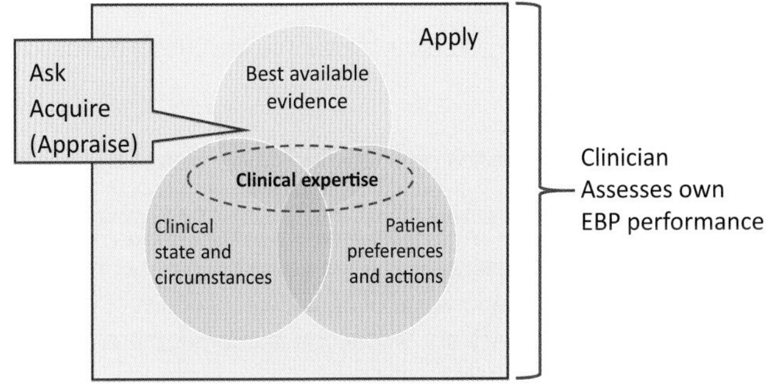

• **Fig. 10.1** Evidence-based practice at the bedside.

TABLE 10.1 Core Competencies for Evidence-Based Practice Grouped Into the Main EBP Domains

EBP core competencies	
0. Introductory	
0.1 Understand evidence-based practice (EBP) defined as the integration of the best research evidence with clinical expertise and patients' unique values and circumstances.	E
0.2 Recognize the rationale for EBP.	M
This competency includes the need to recognize:	
• The daily clinical need for valid information to inform decision-making, and the inadequacy of traditional sources for this information.	*M*
• The disparity between diagnostic skills and clinical judgment, which increase with experience, and up-to-date knowledge and clinical performance, which decline with age and experience.	*M*
• Lack of time to find and assimilate evidence as a clinician.	*M*
• The gaps between evidence and practice can lead to suboptimal practice and quality of care.	*M*
• The potential discordance between a pathophysiological and empirical approach to thinking about whether something is effective.	*M*
0.3 For each type of clinical question, identify the preferred order of study designs, including the pros and cons of the major study designs.	E
This competency includes:	
• Classify the major study designs for each type of clinical question.	*E*
0.4 Practice the 5 steps of EBP: Ask, Acquire, Appraise and Interpret, Apply, and Evaluate.	P
0.5 Understand the distinction between using research to inform clinical decision-making versus conducting research.	M
1. Ask	
1.1 Explain the difference between the types of questions that cannot typically be answered by research (background questions) and those that can (foreground questions).	E
1.2 Identify different types of clinical questions, such as questions about treatment, diagnosis, prognosis, and etiology.	P
1.3 Convert clinical questions into structured, answerable clinical questions using PICO.	P
This competency includes:	
• Recognize the importance of and strategies for identifying and prioritizing uncertainties or knowledge gaps in practice.	*M*
• Understand the rationale for using structured clinical questions.	*E*
• Identify the elements of PICO questions and use variations of it when appropriate (e.g., PICOT, PO, PECO – Exposure) to structure answerable clinical questions.	*P*
2. Acquire	
2.1 Outline the different major categories of sources of research information, including biomedical research databases or databases of filtered or preappraised evidence or resources.	E
This competency includes:	
• Outline the advantages of using filtered or preappraised evidence sources and recognize relevant resources.	*E*
• Indicate the differences between the hierarchy of evidence, level of processing of evidence, and types of EBM resources.	*E*
2.2 Construct and carry out an appropriate search strategy for clinical questions.	P
This competency includes:	
• Know where to look first to address a clinical question. [P]	*P*
• When necessary, construct a search strategy that reflects the purpose of the search. [P]	*P*
• Apply a general search strategy including the use of search terms, and the role of Boolean operators, truncation, and search filters for more efficient searches. [E]	*E*
2.3 State the differences in broad topics covered by the major research databases.	M
2.4 Outline strategies to obtain the full text of articles and other evidence resources.	E
3. Appraise and Interpret	
3.1 Identify key competencies relevant to the critical evaluation of the integrity, reliability, and applicability of health-related research.	E
This competency includes	
• Understand the difference between random error and systematic error (bias).	*E*
• Identify the major categories of bias and the impact of these biases on the results.	*E*
• Interpret commonly used measures of uncertainty, in particular, confidence intervals.	*P*
• Recognize that association does not imply causation and explain why.	*E*
• Recognize the importance of considering conflict of interest/funding sources.	*M*
• Recognize the uses and limitations of subgroup analysis and how to interpret its results.	*M*

TABLE 10.1 Core Competencies for Evidence-Based Practice Grouped Into the Main EBP Domains—Cont'd

Competency	
3.2 Interpret different types of measures of association and effect, including key graphical presentations.	P
This competency includes	
• Identify the basic types of data such as categorical and continuous.	*E*
• Recognize the meaning of some basic frequency measures.	*M*
• Identify the difference between "statistical significance" and "importance", and between a lack of evidence of an effect and "evidence of no effect."	*E*
3.3 Critically appraise and interpret a systematic review.	P
This competency includes	
• Recognize the difference between systematic reviews, metaanalyses, and nonsystematic reviews.	*M*
• Identify and critically appraise key elements of a systematic review.	*P*
• Interpret presentations of the pooling of studies such as a forest plot and summary of findings table.	*P*
3.4 Critically appraise and interpret a treatment study.	P
This competency includes	
• Identify and appraise key features of a controlled trial.	*P*
• Interpret the results including measures of effect.	*P*
• Identify the limitations of observational studies as treatment studies and recognize the basics of adjustment methods and its limitations.	*E*
3.5 Critically appraise and interpret a diagnostic accuracy study.	P
This competency includes	
• Identify and appraise key features of a diagnostic accuracy study.	*P*
• Interpret the results including interpret measures to evaluate diagnostic accuracy.	*P*
• Recognize the purpose and use of clinical prediction rules.	*M*
3.6 Distinguish evidence-based from opinion-based clinical practice guidelines.	P
3.7 Identify the key features of, and be able to interpret, a prognostic study.	E
This competency includes	
• Identify and appraise key features of a prognostic study.	*E*
• Interpret the results including measures of effect (e.g., Kaplan Meier "survival" curves) and uncertainty.	*E*
• Recognize the purpose and use of clinical prediction rules.	*M*
3.8 Explain the use of a harm/etiologies study for (rare) adverse effects of interventions.	E
This competency includes	
• Indicate that common treatment harms can usually be observed in controlled trials, but some rare or late harms will only be seen in observational studies.	*E*
3.9 Explain the purpose and processes of a qualitative study.	E
This competency includes	
• Recognize how qualitative research can inform the decision-making process.	*M*
4. Apply	
4.1 Engage patients in the decision-making process, using shared decision-making, including explaining the evidence and integrating their preferences.	P
This competency includes:	
• Recognize the nature of the patient's dilemma, hopes, expectations, fears, and values and preferences.	*M*
• Understand and practice shared decision-making.	*P*
• Recognize how decision support tools such as patient decision aids can assist in shared decision-making.	*M*
4.2 Outline different strategies to manage uncertainty in clinical decision-making in practice.	E
This competency includes:	
• Recognize professional, ethical, and legal components/dimensions of clinical decision-making, and the role of clinical reasoning.	*M*
4.3 Explain the importance of baseline risk of individual patients when estimating individual expected benefit.	E
This competency includes:	
• Recognize different types of outcome measures (surrogate vs. composite endpoints measures).	*M*
4.4 Interpret the grading of the certainty in evidence and the strength of recommendations in healthcare.	E
5. Evaluate	
5.1 Recognize potential individual-level barriers to knowledge translation and strategies to overcome these.	M
This competency includes:	
• Recognize the process of reflective clinical practice.	*M*
5.2 Recognize the role of a personal clinical audit in facilitating evidence-based practice.	M

E, Explained; *EBP*, evidence-based practice; *M*, mentioned; *P*, practiced with exercises; *PECO*, Population-Exposure-Comparator-Outcome; *PICO*, Population-Intervention-Comparator-Outcome; *PICOT*, Population-Intervention-Comparator-Outcome-Time; *PO*, population, outcome.

essential EBP competencies across the EBP main steps are used in the context of clinical care at the bedside where EBP intersects with coproduction and patient centeredness to provide the highest quality of care possible (see Chapter 1),

In this chapter we review the psychometric properties of instruments and strategies to evaluate these core competencies and steps of EBP and offer recommendations for current educational practice and future research. In addition, we provide a list of resources in Appendix 10.1.

Alternatively, in the previous example the clinician may already be aware that the Unites States Preventive Services Task Force (USPSTF), based on a systematic review and metaanalysis of screening trials, now recommends a one-time screening abdominal ultrasound for men 65 years of age or older with a history of smoking.[39] In a retrospective investigation of clinical practice via a record audit, clinicians might discover that only 60% of elderly male patients with a smoking history have been screened for AAA. This evidence–practice gap would trigger a quality improvement initiative, which might include examining clinician, patient, and microsystem barriers to screening; a practice intervention such as a reminder system or audit and feedback; and an evaluation of its effect on screening rates. This aspect of practice-based learning and improvement is covered in Chapter 11.

General Issues of Evaluation in Medical Education

For the purposes of this chapter, we will use the classification developed by the Joint Committee on the Standards for Educational and Psychological Testing of the American Educational Research Association (AERA), American Psychological Association (APA), and National Council on Measurement in Education (NCME)[40,41] and Downing's recent methodological treatises[42–47] (Table 10.2) in analyzing and recommending instruments to evaluate EBP core competencies.

TABLE 10.2 Classification and Terminology for Types of Validity Evidence

Sources of Validity Evidence	Description	Analysis[a]
Based on test content	Analysis of the relationship between the instrument's content and the construct it is intended to measure. Content refers to the themes, wording, and format of the items, tasks, or questions on a test, as well as the procedures for administration and scoring.	Often determined by external review by experts (*content validity*)
Based on response processes	Data collected on the "processes" that examinees use in completing or that observers use in rating the instrument	
Based on internal structure	The degree to which the relationships among the test items and test components conform to the construct on which the proposed test core interpretations are based	Detection, among the items, of a unified latent construct or, if specified in advance, discreet subthemes, often determined with factor analysis (*dimensionality*) Relationship between items within either the entire instrument or a prespecified section of the instrument, often measured with Cronbach's alpha (*internal consistency*)
Based on relationship to other variables	Analysis of the relationship of test scores to external variables (criteria) hypothesized to measure or represent the same constructs. Two designs may be distinguished. A *predictive* study indicates how accurately test data can predict criterion scores obtained in the future. A *concurrent* study obtains predictor and criterion information at the same time.	Correlation with scores on another test with established psychometric properties (*criterion validity*) Comparison of scores between groups assumed to have different levels of expertise (*discriminative validity*) Comparison of pre versus post scores with respect to an educational intervention (*responsive validity*)

Note: Descriptive labels in italics in Analysis column represent terms in common use but are not taken from this source.

[a]Classification proposed by Joint Committee on Standards for Educational and Psychological Testing of the American Educational Research Association; the American Psychological Association; and the National Council on Measurement in Education. *Standards for Educational and Psychological Testing*. American Educational Research Association; 1999.

The use of construct validity to describe a particular type of validity evidence has been criticized.[42] Rather, all validity is construct validity, as it represents evidence that the instrument is accurately approximating an intangible psychologic "construct" that cannot be measured directly (see Chapter 2). This is certainly true for knowledge, skills, and attitudes. Behaviors, on the other hand, can be directly observed. However, because resource and time constraints often make such observations impractical, investigators resort to surrogate measures. In this case, evidence for validity should demonstrate that the surrogate measures approximate the actual behaviors.

There is no single hierarchy for preferred types of validity evidence. Rather, appropriate analyses should be dictated by the intended evaluation uses of the instrument. For example, responsive validity (see Table 10.2) may be more critical for an instrument to evaluate the programmatic effectiveness of an EBP curriculum, whereas instruments with established discriminative validity may be more appropriate to assess individual learners. Table 10.2 also crosswalks the specific types of validity used in this chapter with the Messick validity framework (see Chapter 2). Higher-stakes evaluations, such as certification or promotion, require more robust validity (multiple types of evidence from strong scientific studies) than formative evaluation used for corrective feedback.

EBP Evaluation Domains

The Classification Rubric for EBP Assessment Tools in Education (CREATE) framework (Table 10.3 outlines a framework for classifying EBP evaluation domains and

TABLE 10.3 EBP Evaluation Domains[a]

Psychometric Domain		Description (Based on EBP Practice "Mode")		
		Doer	User	Replicator
Knowledge and skills				
EBP step	Ask	Identifying emerging information needs		
		Discriminating between "background" and "foreground" questions		
		Recognizing the "clinical task" associated with the clinical question		
		Phrasing foreground questions in PICO format		
	Acquire	General computer/internet skills[157]		
		Recognizing and choosing between different "EBP modes"[68]		
		Searching databases of original research (e.g., Medline)	Appraising secondary databases of evidence-based summaries	Knowing EBP performance of consultants
			Searching secondary databases of evidence-based summaries (e.g., Cochrane Library)	
	Appraise	Primarily appraising study design and conduct	Understanding and appreciating a critical appraisal done by others	
	Apply	Individualizing measures of effect†		
		Considering patient's particular clinical state and circumstances		
		Considering patient's preferences		
	Assess	Assessing one's performance of EBP		
Attitudes		Attitudes toward EBP		
		Self-directed learning "readiness"		
Behaviors		Performing EBP steps in practice		
		Performing evidence-based clinical maneuvers in practice		
		Affecting desirable good patient outcomes		
Global ratings		Global rating of EBP competence		

EBP, Evidence-based practice; *PICO*, Patient-Intervention-Comparison-Outcome.

[a]See text for more detailed descriptions.

[b]From McGowan JJ, Berner ES. Proposed curricular objectives to teach physicians competence in using the world wide web. *Acad Med*. 2004 Mar;79(3):236-240. doi:10.1097/00001888-200403000-00007.

[c]Straus SE, Green ML, Bell DS, et al. Evaluating the teaching of evidence based medicine: conceptual framework. *BMJ*. 2004 Oct 30;329(7473):1029-1032. doi:10.1136/bmj.329.7473.1029.

[d]For example, recasting number needed to treat based on patient's baseline risk or determining posttest probability of disease using patient's pretest probability and likelihood ratio of diagnostic test.

outcome measures that considers the assessment category (e.g., patient outcomes, behavior, skills, knowledge, self-efficacy, attitudes, and reaction to the educational experience), type of assessment (e.g., patient-oriented outcomes, activity monitoring, performance assessment, cognitive testing, and self-report/opinion), and steps of EBP (i.e., ask, acquire, appraise, apply, assess).[4]

An evidence-based practitioner ("doing" mode) must have the knowledge and skills to perform all five steps of EBP. For clinicians practicing the "using" mode, detailed knowledge and skills in the critical *appraisal* of original research reports is not essential. In any of the modes, the clinician must be able to interpret and *apply* the evidence to the decision-making for an individual patient.

Attitude domains include points of view about the appropriateness, effectiveness, feasibility, practice preferences, advantages, untoward consequences, and perceived barriers to EBP. In addition, as a strategy for lifelong learning, EBP requires readiness or inclination for self-directed learning, a related construct borrowed from educational psychology.

We can consider EBP behaviors at two levels. First, we can ask, "Does a trainee perform the five EBP steps in their actual practice?" Alternatively, we can look further downstream and examine their clinical practice directly, asking, "Does a trainee perform evidence-based clinical maneuvers in their practice?" And finally, we can examine patient outcomes as a desired result of EBP.

EBP Evaluation Instruments

A 2006 systematic review covering all health professions education summarized the development, formats, learner levels, EBP domains, feasibility, and psychometric properties of 104 unique EBP evaluation instruments.[49] Despite the apparent abundance of EBP evaluation instruments, only a few were of high quality (11 out of 104 instruments; based on the type, extent, methods, and results of psychometric testing and the suitability for different evaluation purposes). More recently, a 2020 systematic review of validated instruments used to evaluate EBP in medical education identified 12 unique instruments (6 were of high quality).[50]

Although the identified instruments most commonly evaluated skills in critically appraising evidence (EBP Step 3), several new instruments have emerged to evaluate the *ask*, *acquire*, and *apply* steps. Within the *acquire* step, however, most of the instruments assess Medline searching ("doing" mode) and do not evaluate the appraisal, selection, and searching of resources containing preappraised summaries ("using" mode). Similarly, most of the *apply* instruments are limited to consideration of research evidence in decision-making, neglecting consideration of the particular clinical circumstances and patient preferences (e.g., shared decision-making skills).

EBP attitude, knowledge, and skills are the domains most frequently evaluated in the EBP evaluation instruments. Regarding EBP behaviors, the systematic review identified several new objective approaches to document the performance of EBP steps in practice and a few instruments that assess the performance of evidence-based clinical maneuvers. However, instruments rarely measure patient-related outcomes.

Evaluating EBP Knowledge and Skills

Instruments With Multiple Types of Evidence for Validity, Including Discriminative Validity

Table 10.4 summarizes the specific domains, format, and psychometric properties of the instruments supported by established interrater reliability (if applicable), objective (nonself-reported) outcome measures, and multiple (three or more) types of established validity evidence, including at least discriminative validity. Given their ability to distinguish between different levels of expertise, these instruments should be suitable to evaluate the EBP competence of individual trainees. Furthermore, the robust psychometric properties in general should support their use in formative or summative evaluations. However, local institutions will need to establish passing standards, using accepted procedures,[47,51,52] before these instruments can be used for high-stakes evaluations, like academic promotion or certification.

Among the instruments in Table 10.4, the Fresno Test[53] and two other instruments[54,55] represent the only ones that assess all four EBP steps. In taking the Fresno Test, trainees perform authentic EBP tasks, exposing their underlying thinking process through short-answer, essay, and calculation responses. However, this same feature requires more time and expertise to grade this instrument. Versions adapted for psychiatry residents,[56] occupational therapists,[57,58] physical therapists,[59] and entry-level allied health profession students[60] demonstrated acceptable psychometric properties. A Spanish translation of the Fresno Test has also been published.[61] The Fresno Test and grading template are available on the internet (see Appendix 10.1).

The multiple-choice format of the Berlin Test restricts assessment to EBP applied knowledge but also makes it easier to implement.[62] A Dutch translation of the Berlin Test demonstrated multiple types of validity evidence with the exception of a lower internal consistency (i.e., reliability).[63] The other instruments in Table 10.4 evaluate a narrower range of EBP steps as indicated. For all of these instruments, educators can engage in various standards-setting procedures[51,52] to determine passing scores for their own purposes.

Instruments With "Strong Evidence" for Responsive Validity

In addition to five of the instruments in Table 10.4,[62,64–67] seven additional instruments fulfill criteria for "strong evidence" of responsive validity (Table 10.5). These instruments are supported by (1) established interrater reliability (if applicable), (2) a randomized controlled trial or pre/postcontrolled trial design, and (3) an objective (nonself-reported) outcome measure. Generally, these instruments have less robust psychometric properties than those in Table 10.4, which enjoy support from multiple types of validity evidence. However, given their ability to detect knowledge and skill changes after an educational intervention, these instruments should be suitable to determine the

TABLE 10.4 EBP Knowledge and Skill Instruments With Multiple Types of Validity Evidence, Including Discriminative Validity

Instrument	Knowledge and Skill Domains	Description	Experience	Interrater Reliability[b]	Validity
Berlin Questionnaire[a] [62,63,158,159]	Knowledge about interpreting evidence (*appraise*) Skills to relate a clinical problem to a clinical question (*ask*) Best design to answer a question (*appraise*) Use quantitative information from research to solve specific patient problems (*apply*)	2 separate sets of 15 MCQs built around "typical" clinical scenarios	43 "experts," 20 third-year students, 203 participants in EBM course in development study 49 internal medicine residents in controlled trial of EBM curriculum 53 junior faculty and residents in various specialties 140 general practice trainees and 7 tutors in EBP course	N/A	Content Internal consistency Discriminative Responsive
Taylor Questionnaire[a] [67,77,97]	Knowledge of critical appraisal (*appraise*) Knowledge of Medline searching (*acquire*)	Sets of 6 MCQs with 3 potential answers, each requiring a true, false, or don't know response. Best score on each set = 18	152 "healthcare professionals" in development study[64] Modified and "revalidated" instrument on 55 delegates at international EBP conferences 175 students in RCT of self-directed versus workshop-based EBP curricula 145 general practitioners, hospital physicians, allied health professionals, and healthcare managers in RCT of critical appraisal training	N/A	Content Internal consistency Discriminative Responsive
Fresno Test[a] [53,56,57,59–61]	Formulate a focused question (*ask*) Identify appropriate research design for answering the question (*appraise*) Show knowledge of electronic database searching, including secondary sources (*acquire*) Identify issues important for the relevance and validity of an article (*appraise*) Discuss the magnitude and importance of research findings (*apply*)	Short-answer free-text questions and calculations relating to 2 pediatric clinical scenarios. Scored by using a standardized grading rubric	53 "experts" and 43 family practice residents and faculty in development study Modifications 56 psychiatry residents in uncontrolled trial of EBM curriculum and 5 EBP "experts/teachers" 114 occupational therapists in pre/post uncontrolled trial of 2-day EBP workshop combined with outreach support 108 participants (31 EBP-novice physical therapy students, 50 EBP-trained students, and 27 EBP-expert faculty) in cross-sectional study More significant modification testing only the *ask*, *acquire*, and *apply* steps and replacing essay question with short answer and multiple choice. 100 entry-level allied health professions students	Yes	Content Internal consistency Discriminative Responsive
MacRae[a] [66,160]	Critical appraisal skills (*appraise*)	55 short-answer questions and 7-point methodological ratings related to 3 articles	44 surgery residents in development study 55 surgeons in RCT of internet-based EBP curriculum	Yes	Internal consistency Discriminative Responsive
Weberschock[161]	EBP knowledge and skills (specific skills not specified)	5 sets of 20 MCQs (5 "easy," 10 "average," and 5 "difficult") linked to clinical scenarios and pertaining to data from published research articles	132 third-year medical students and 11 students with advanced training in "EBM working group" in development and pre/post uncontrolled study of peer teaching EBP curriculum	N/A	Internal consistency Discriminative Responsive Criterion
Bennett[64]	Critical appraisal skills (*appraise*)	Set of case-based problems that require a diagnostic or treatment decision matched with an article advocating the test or treatment. Students have to "take a stand" and "defend" it in writing. Graded on preset criteria	79 medical students on various clerkships in pre/post controlled trial	Yes	Content Discriminative Responsive

Continued

Instrument	Knowledge and Skill Domains	Description	Experience	Interrater Reliability[b]	Validity
Haynes[a] [65,98,99]	Medline searching skills (*acquire*)	Search output scored by comparison to searches (for same clinical questions) by an expert end-user physician and a librarian. "Relative recall" calculated as number of relevant citations from a given search divided by number of relevant citations from the 3 searches (subject, expert physician, and librarian). "Precision" calculated as the number of relevant citations retrieved in a search divided by the total citations retrieved in that search. Article "relevance" rated reliably on a 7-point scale	158 clinicians (novice end users), 13 "expert searcher" clinicians (expert end users), and 3 librarians 308 physicians and physicians in training in RCT of one-to-one precepting and searching feedback	Yes	Content Discriminative Responsive
Hendricson[162]	EBP knowledge EBP attitudes EBP confidence Self-reported evidence accessing methods (*acquire*)	MCQs for EBP knowledge Likert or other 5-point scales for other domains	472 dental students 54 dental residents 58 dental faculty	N/A	Content Internal consistency Discrimination Responsive
Ilic[54]	EBP knowledge and skills (*ask, acquire, appraise, apply*) EBP attitudes	15 yes/no questions related to a clinical scenario, search strategy, and article abstract	342 medical trainees representing novice, intermediate, and advanced EBM trainees	N/A	Content Internal consistency Discrimination
Chernick[55]	EBP knowledge and skills (*ask, acquire, appraise, apply*) EBP comfort level Self-reported EBP practice	Free-text responses based on clinical scenarios	56 pediatrics residents	Yes	Content Internal consistency Discrimination
Utrecht questionnaire [163]	Knowledge questions	Two sets of questionnaires consisting of 25 questions. Questions focused on "ask," "appraise," and "apply," with 6 open-ended questions and 19 MCQs	173 participants consisting of: –144 first-year GP trainees –39 third-year GP trainees –11 hospital trainees –14 GP supervisors –4 experts	N/A	Content Internal consistency Discriminative Responsive
Johnston KAB questionnaire[164]	Knowledge, attitudes, and skills	43-item questionnaire with domains across knowledge, attitude, practice, actual use of EBP, and anticipated use of EBP	–239 second- and third-year medical students –158 fifth-year medical students	N/A	Content Internal consistency Responsive
BACES[165]	Knowledge and skills	30 MCQs across study designs, critical appraisal and interpretation of results	–147 postgraduate medical trainees	N/A	Content Discriminative

Note: Superscript numbers in parentheses indicate references from this chapter's References section where the reader can get more information about the topic being discussed.
[a]Instruments evaluated in more than one study. Results from all the studies were used to determine the number of trainees, reliability, and validity.
[b]Interrater reliability testing was deemed "not applicable" for instruments, such as multiple-choice tests, that required no rater judgment to score (see Box 10.1).
EBM, Evidence-based medicine; *EBP*, evidence-based practice; *MCQ,* multiple-choice question; *RCT,* randomized controlled trial.
Modified from Shaneyfelt T, Baum KD, Bell D, et al. Instruments for evaluating education in evidence-based practice: a systematic review. *JAMA*. 2006 Sep 6;296(9):1116–1127. doi: 10.1001/jama.296.9.1116; and from Kumaravel B, Hearn JH, Jahangiri L, et al. A systematic review and taxonomy of tools for evaluating evidence-based medicine teaching in medical education. *Syst Rev*. 2020 Apr 24;9(1):91. doi: 10.1186/s13643-020-01311-y.

TABLE 10.5 EBP Knowledge and Skill Instruments Supported by "Strong Evidence" of Responsive Validity[a,b]

Instrument	Knowledge and Skill Domains	Description	Study Settings/Participants	Interrater Reliability[c]	Validity
Landry[d] [71]	Research design and critical appraisal knowledge (*appraise*)	10-item test	146 medical students in controlled trial of two 90-minute seminars	N/A	Content Responsive
	Skills in applying medical literature to clinical decision-making (*apply*)	Blinded review of patient "write-ups" looking for literature citations		No	
Green[70]	Skills in critical appraisal (*appraise*) Skills in applying evidence to individual patient decision-making (*apply*)	9-question test (requiring free-text response) relating to a case presentation and a redacted journal article	34 residents in controlled trial of a 7-session EBP curriculum	Yes	Content Responsive
Linzer[d] [72]	Epidemiology and biostatistics knowledge	Multiple-choice test (knowledge). 15 questions chosen so that perfect score would allow access to 81% of medical literature (1983)[163]	44 medical residents in RCT of journal club curriculum	N/A	Content Responsive
	Skills in critical appraisal (*appraise*)	Free-text critical appraisal of text article. Scoring based on "gold standard" criteria developed by consensus of faculty		Yes	Content Discriminative
Stevermer[128]	EBP behavior (performance of EBP steps in practice)	Test of awareness and recall of recently published articles reporting "important findings about common primary care problems" (selected by faculty physicians)	59 family practice residents in RCT of EBP "academic detailing"	N/A	Responsive
Smith[69]	Skills in formulating clinical questions (*ask*) Skills in Medline searching (*acquire*) Skills in critical appraisal (*appraise*) Skills in applying evidence to individual patient decision-making (*apply*) Knowledge of quantitative aspects of diagnosis and treatment studies	Test including sets of questions (format not specified) relating to 5 clinical cases	55 medical residents in pre/post controlled crossover trial of 7-week EBP curriculum, which included interactive sessions and computer lab training	Yes	Responsive[e]
Villanueva[74]	Skills in formulating clinical questions (*ask*)	Librarians identified elements of the Patient-Intervention-Comparison-Outcome (PICO) format in clinical question requests.[147] One point awarded for each of 4 elements included	39 healthcare professional participants in a library "evidence search and critical appraisal service" in an RCT of providing instructions and clinical question examples	Yes	Responsive
Ross[73]	EBP knowledge (specific steps not specified)	50-item "open book" multiple-choice test	48 family practice residents in controlled trial of 10-session EBP workshop (control residents in different program)	N/A	Content Responsive
	EBP behavior (enacting EBP steps in practice)	Analysis of audiotapes of resident–faculty interactions, looking for phrases related to literature searching, clinical epidemiology, or critical appraisal		No	Content Responsive

Note: Superscript numbers in parentheses indicate references from this chapter's References section where the reader can get more information about the topic being discussed.

[a]To qualify for "strong evidence," instruments must demonstrate interrater reliability (if applicable) and responsive validity must be established by studies with a randomized controlled trial or pre/post controlled trial design and an objective (nonself-reported) outcome measure.

[b]Four instruments from Table 10.4 also showed "strong evidence" of responsive validity.[62,64,66,67]

[c]Reliability testing was deemed "not applicable" for instruments, such as multiple-choice tests, that required no rater judgment to score (see Box 10.1).

[d]Met "strong evidence" criteria for the EBP knowledge portion of overall instrument, not for the EBP skill portion.

[e]Gains in skills persisted after 6 months, indicating both concurrent and predictive (responsive) validity.

EBP, Evidence-based practice; *RCT,* randomized controlled trial.

Modified from Shaneyfelt T, Baum KD, Bell D, et al. Instruments for evaluating education in evidence-based practice: a systematic review. *JAMA*. 2006 Sep 6;296(9):1116–1127. doi: 10.1001/jama.296.9.1116; and from Kumaravel B, Hearn JH, Jahangiri L. et al. A systematic review and taxonomy of tools for evaluating evidence-based medicine teaching in medical education. *Syst Rev*. 2020 Apr 24;9(1):91. doi: 10.1186/s13643-020-01311-y.

programmatic-level impact of EBP curricula. For this type of evaluation, the Society of General Internal Medicine (SGIM) EBP Task Force recommends tailoring evaluation strategies to the learners (including their level and particular needs), the intervention (including the curriculum objectives, intensity, delivery method, and targeted EBP steps), and the outcomes (including knowledge, skills, attitudes, behaviors, or patient-level outcomes).[68]

Among the instruments in Table 10.5, only Smith's EBP examination[69] measures all four EBP steps. Residents articulated clinical questions, conducted Medline searches, performed calculations, and answered free-text questions about critical appraisal and application of the evidence. In this study, gains in skills persisted on retesting at 6 months, indicating both concurrent and predictive responsive validity. The instrument described by Green and Ellis[70] required free-text responses about the appraisal of a redacted journal article and application of the results to a patient. The three multiple-choice tests[71–73] detected improvements in trainees' EBP knowledge. However, in two of the studies, this gain did not translate into improvements in critical appraisal skills as measured with a test article[72] or the incorporation of literature into admission notes.[71] Finally, in the study by Villanueva and colleagues,[74] librarians identified elements of the PICO format[26] in clinical question requests, awarding 1 point for each of the four elements included. This instrument detected improvements in a randomized controlled trial (RCT) of providing instructions and clinical question examples as part of an "evidence search and critical appraisal service."

Additional EBP Knowledge and Skill Instruments

The following instruments, in spite of their more limited psychometric testing, are worthy of mention because of either an innovative evaluation strategy or assessment of EBP steps other than *appraise*. (As we noted earlier, many older EBP evaluation instruments measured critical appraisal knowledge and skills, to the exclusion of the other EBP steps.)

EBP Evaluation Objective Structured Clinical Examinations

Objective structured clinical examinations (OSCEs) measure knowledge and skills as applied in a realistic clinical setting (the "shows how" level in Miller's classification[75]). Investigators have reported EBP OSCEs using standardized patients,[76–79] computer stations,[80–82] and written cases.[83,84] Tudiver and colleagues extended traditional OSCE stations with EBP tasks related to the cases.[78] Second-year residents, who had some EBP training, scored slightly better than first-year residents (6.95 vs. 5.65 out of 10) on a global rating item. In Berner and colleagues' study, students at a medical school with a "mature informatics curriculum" scored significantly higher, on 4 of the 11 tasks, than students (with higher MCAT and United States Medical Licensing Examination [USMLE] II scores) at another school that offered "no formal instruction."[80] A 2021 study explored the use of OSCEs in a spiral learning approach for an EBM curriculum within a medical program.[85] Students completed OSCEs across the 4 years of training, with each year focusing on a combination of EBM domains from *asking*, *acquiring*, *appraising*, and *applying*. Individual item total correlation (ITC) and internal consistency were demonstrated to be acceptable. Similarly, a 2020 RCT examining EBM education in a cohort of physician assistant students highlighted the value of utilizing OSCEs with the application domain of EBM.[86]

Critically Appraised Topic

A critically appraised topic (CAT) is a critical summary of the best available evidence on a focused clinical question. Kersten and colleagues sought to evaluate EBP knowledge and skills while reviewing their written CATs and subsequent presentations.[87] Interestingly, they developed a scoring rubric with anchors based on the Dreyfus and Dreyfus model of skill development. Psychometric testing, however, was limited to internal consistency and interrater reliability.

Evaluating Ask: Articulating Clinical Questions

In addition to the one instrument in Table 10.5,[74] three additional investigators developed approaches to evaluate formulation of clinical questions, using 4-point,[88] 2-point,[89] and 8-point[90] scales corresponding to inclusion of PICO elements. The later PICO conformity scale gives 2 points (yes, clearly stated), 1 point (somewhat), or 0 points (no) for each element. When applying this scale to students' educational prescriptions,[91] higher scores were associated with the presence of an answer and the quality of an answer.[90]

Evaluating Acquire: Searching for Evidence

In several studies, librarians rated trainees' Medline search strategies according to predetermined criteria, usually developed by consensus.[92–97] Search strategy criteria often include the efficient use of Boolean operators, Medical Subject Headings (MeSH), "explode" functions, and methodological (or publication-type) filters. Three studies demonstrated evidence of responsive validity,[93–95,97] one provided evidence of criterion validity,[94] and one demonstrated the interrater reliability[95] of these Medline search strategy ratings. As described in Haynes and colleagues' studies[65,98,99] in Table 10.4, we can reliably assess searching skills by looking beyond the intermediate outcome of the search strategy to the captured articles.

It is notable that nearly all the evaluation approaches for the *acquire* step exclusively assess Medline searching skills. Of the four instruments that assess consulting secondary preappraised evidence-based medical information resources, only the Fresno Test[53] (see Table 10.4) assesses skills, and the others[33,88,100] only include a few survey questions about "awareness of" or "preference for" these resources.

Evaluating Apply: Applying Evidence to Decision-Making

Evaluating this EBP step remains largely unexplored in most EBP evaluation instruments. Some of the general EBP instruments include one or two questions relating to applying evidence to an individual patient, but none comprehensively assesses skills in "individualizing" evidence and integrating it with the patient's particular clinical context, preferences, and potential actions. Some promising approaches to this type of evaluation include having standardized patients rate students' explanations of therapeutic decisions after reviewing research evidence,[76,77] scoring of residents' free-text justification of applying results of a study to a "paper case,"[70] and documenting decision-making before and after access to a research abstract[83,84] or Medline searching.[101]

Evaluating EBP Attitudes and Learning Climate

Although many EBP instruments include a few questions about attitudes, few explore this domain in depth.[33,102–110] McAlister and colleagues' survey assessed EBP attitudes, perceived barriers to EBP, preferred sources of information, and self-reported confidence in EBP skills.[102] The study reported correlations between some scales within the instrument, such as self-reported use of EBM and preference for primary research articles, as evidence for validity. In the attitude section of McColl and colleagues' survey, respondents reported their attitudes toward EBP, awareness of medical information resources, ability to access information databases, understanding of EBP terms, perceived barriers to EBP, and views on how to "move from opinion-based to evidence-based medicine."[33] In a subsequent RCT, EBP academic detailing did not influence general practitioners' attitudes (but did improve their scores on the multiple-choice knowledge section) as measured with this instrument.[111]

Young and Ward's survey addressed views of EBP, understanding of technical terms in EBP, barriers to EBP, preferred strategies to support EBP, and familiarity with information databases.[104] In Baum's uncontrolled study, residents' attitudes improved after an EBP workshop.[103] Additional instruments measure EBP beliefs and implementation;[105] EBP confidence;[108,109] self-reported EBP attitudes, knowledge, and practice in nurses;[110] and attitudes and utilization[106] and knowledge, skills, and beliefs[107] among complementary and alternative medicine practitioners. In addition to these quantitative surveys, investigators have employed qualitative techniques to analyze the responses of focus groups and structured interviews.[112–119]

The learning environment exerts a profound influence on learning in any educational setting. Many contextual barriers may undermine trainees' learning and practice of EBM. These include lack of personal time, lack of support and mentoring, lack of trained EBM faculty teachers, limited access to EBM resources, and difficulty with statistical concepts.[118,120] There are also barriers unique to residents positioned as trainees, including institutional culture and team dynamics.[118,121] Lack of attention to these factors may undermine EBM education initiatives.

Educators can defer to Mi's survey to characterize their local EBM learning environment. This 36-item instrument, with a Likert scale response format, showed excellent internal consistency (Cronbach's alpha = 0.86).[122] Scores were higher for residents with prior EBM training in medical school and in residency and discriminated among six residency programs. Factor analysis revealed seven factors: situational clues, learner role, utility and accountability, learning culture, resource availability, learning support, and social support.

• BOX 10.1 Strategies for Evaluating Physician EBP Behaviors and Patient Outcomes

Performing EBP Steps in Practice

- Retrospective self-reports of performing EBP steps
- Frequency of EBP terminology in analysis of recorded teaching interactions
- Recall and knowledge of recent articles important to particular practice and specialty
- Electronic capture of searching behavior, including number of "log-ons," searching volume, abstracts or articles viewed, and time spent searching
- EBP learning portfolios
- Direct observation and debriefing

Performing Evidence-Based Clinical Maneuvers in Practice and/or Affecting Desirable Patient Outcomes

- Record audit for primary diagnosis and therapy and determination of level of supporting evidence
- Record audit for quality performance indicators or patient outcomes
- Clinical vignettes

Note: See text for explanations.
EBP, Evidence-based practice.

Evaluating EBP Behaviors (Performance)

EBP behavior remains the most challenging domain for evaluators. Nonetheless, we must ensure that trainees implement their EBP skills in actual practice.[123] The range of evaluation strategies is summarized in Box 10.1.

Evaluating the Performance of EBP Steps in Practice

Regarding EBP steps, we can simply ask a trainee if they, for example, consistently search for the evidence to answer their clinical questions. However, retrospective self-reports of EBP behaviors remain extremely biased, because physicians tend to underestimate their information needs and overestimate their pursuit of them.[48] At the opposite extreme of rigor, we can shadow a trainee in the course of their patient encounters, document their emerging clinical questions, and follow up later to see if they have acquired, appraised, and applied the evidence. The question collection might involve passive "anthropologic" observation[124] or active debriefing.[48,125] Although this direct observation yields more valid data, it is generally not feasible outside of the research setting. Thus educators have looked for intermediate approaches to evaluating EBP performance.

In three studies, investigators analyzed audiotapes of resident–faculty interactions, looking for phrases related to EBP steps.[73,126,127] Family practice residents' "EBP utterances" increased from 0.21 per hour to 2.9 per hour after an educational intervention.[73] In another study, researchers rated interactions using a qualitative analytic template consisting of three criteria: (1) presence of clinical questions, (2) presence of an evidence-based process, and (3) resident ability to articulate a clinical question.[127] However, this outcome represents a poor surrogate for EBP performance. Taking a different approach, investigators questioned residents about their awareness and knowledge of findings in recent journal articles deemed relevant to primary care practice.[128] In this pre/post RCT, residents exposed to "academic detailing" recalled more articles and correctly answered more questions about them.

Educators can also electronically capture trainees' searching behaviors, including number of "log-ons," searching volume, abstracts or articles viewed, and time spent searching.[99,129] In an RCT, Cabell and colleagues demonstrated that these measures were responsive to an intervention including a 1-hour didactic session, the use of well-built clinical question cards, and practical sessions in clinical question building.[129] In the RCT by Haynes and colleagues, physicians receiving additional help from a personal clinical preceptor and feedback from a librarian did not search more often than controls receiving a 2-hour training session alone.[99] Although this approach is quite feasible, the crude measure of searching "volume" fails to capture the pursuit and application of information in response to particular clinical questions.

Another approach is to have trainees catalogue their EBP learning activities in "learning portfolios," which represent "a purposeful collection of student work that exhibits the student's efforts, progress, or achievement in (a) given area(s)" (see Chapter 15).[130] EBP portfolios might include "educational prescriptions," which faculty "dispense" when a moment of uncertainty arises in the course of patient care.[91,131–134] A typical educational prescription describes the clinical problem, states the question, specifies who is responsible for answering it, and reminds the trainee and faculty of a follow-up time. Some variations have the trainee articulate foreground questions in the PICO format, document the information resources searched, grade the level of evidence, or summarize what they learned. (See Appendix 10.2 for examples.) In Feldstein and colleagues' system,[132] residents electronically document their educational prescriptions and faculty grade them on the four EBP steps. The educational prescription can easily be translated to mobile device applications.

EBP learning portfolios can be maintained in sophisticated internet-based databases.[135–138] Educators implemented a Computerized Obstetrics and Gynecology Automated Learning Analysis (KOALA) at several residency programs.[136] This portfolio allowed residents to record their clinical encounters, directly link to information resources, and document "critical learning incidents." During a 4-month pilot period at four programs, 41 residents recorded 7049 patient encounters and 1460 critical learning incidents. Residents at one of the programs, which had a prior 1-year experience with KOALA, demonstrated higher "self-directed learning readiness."[139] In another program, internal medicine residents entered their clinical questions, accompanied by Medline reference links and article summaries, into a similar internet-based compendium.[135] The EBP exercises produced "useful information" for 82% and altered patient management for 39% of 625 clinical questions over 10 months. A study evaluated an internet-based point of care (POC) learning portfolio as an alternative to open-book multiple-choice exams for the American Board of Internal Medicine (ABIM) Maintenance of Certification (MOC) program. The study found t POC portfolio more relevant to their practice, helped them expand their information resources, and resulted in a significant number of planned practice changes, leading to its adoption as an elective option in MOC by the ABIM.[140]

Evaluating the Performance of Evidence-Based Clinical Maneuvers and Affecting Patient Outcomes

Sackett and colleagues devised a reliable method for determining the primary therapeutic intervention chosen by a practitioner and classifying the quality of evidence supporting it.[141] In this scheme, interventions are (1) supported by individual or systematic reviews of RCTs, (2) supported by "convincing nonexperimental evidence," or (3) lacking substantial evidence. This method has been employed in descriptive studies in inpatient medicine,[141,142] general outpatient practice,[143] emergency ophthalmology,[144] dermatology,[145] anesthesiology,[146] general surgery,[147] pediatric surgery,[148] and inpatient psychiatry settings.[149] Straus and colleagues' pre/post study of a multifaceted EBP educational intervention provides initial evidence of the "responsive" validity of this evaluation strategy.[150] Patients admitted after the intervention were more likely to receive therapies proven to be beneficial in RCTs (62% vs. 49%; $P = .016$). And of these trial-proven therapies, those offered after the EBM intervention were more likely to be based on high-quality RCTs (95% vs. 87%; $P = .023$).

Lucas and colleagues' study showed that this method of classifying the quality of supporting evidence may not be sensitive to clinicians' selections among evidence-based therapies.[151] On an inpatient medical service, 86% of inpatients of 33 providers received "evidence-based treatments" (Level 1 or 2 of the Ellis classification) at baseline. After performing a standardized literature search related to the primary diagnosis, the practitioners altered their treatment for 23 (18%) of the patients. However, the proportion of patients classified as receiving "evidence-based treatments" did not significantly change (86–87%). The Ellis "protocol" appears most suited to evaluate changes in EBP performance after an educational intervention or simply just over time. To use it to document some absolute threshold of performance, one would have to know, for every trainee's set of patients, the "denominator" of evidence-based therapeutic options, making it impractical on a programmatic scale.

We can also document the provision of evidence-based care by auditing records for adherence to evidence-based guidelines or quality indicators. Hardly a new development, this type of audit is commonly performed as part of internal quality initiatives or by third-party payers or regulatory agencies. Langham and colleagues used a quality audit to evaluate the impact of an EBP curriculum, documenting, in an RCT, improvements in practicing physicians' documentation, clinical interventions, and patient outcomes relating to cardiovascular risk factors.[152] Epling and colleagues showed improvements in residents' performance of recommended diabetes mellitus care measures after they participated in a curriculum that involved the development of a practice guideline.[153] Clinical vignettes may represent a more feasible, yet valid, alternative for measuring the quality of clinical practice.[154]

Finally, patient-level outcomes remain the most elusive to evaluators, remaining subject to myriad influences apart from physician performance. Nonetheless, investigators have documented changes in patient outcomes, albeit intermediate outcomes such as blood pressure, glycemic control, and serum lipids, following EBP educational interventions.[152,153,155]

Which Level of EBP Behaviors Should We Measure?

One could argue that trainees' enactment of EBP steps, however measured, represents an intermediate behavioral outcome. That is, we assume that physicians who consistently perform EBP steps will provide more evidence-based care, which, in turn, will lead to more EBP actions and better patient outcomes. But our clinical experience reminds us that intermediate outcomes may fail to guarantee the ultimate outcomes of interest. Should educators, then, "cast their line" beyond EBP steps to measures of EBP performance and, if possible, clinical outcomes in patients?

We believe we should document *both* types of EBP behavior outcomes. Although practice performance measures represent the ultimate outcome, they remain, by virtue of their "downstream" vantage, blunt instruments. A physician's performance, for instance, in screening their elderly male patients for abdominal aortic aneurysm represents the end result of myriad inputs, some of which remain beyond their control. Would a record audit "detect" that the patient did not adhere with their recommendation to undergo screening because of denied insurance coverage? Or perhaps the physician did *not* recommend screening but their decision reflected a careful consideration of the patient's particular clinical circumstances and preferences,[116] rather than a failure to consider the new guidelines supported by a systematic review of the evidence. Perhaps, for example, a chest radiograph revealed a pulmonary nodule, and the physician deferred screening until lung cancer was excluded. And finally, we should ensure trainees' inclination to consistently perform EBP steps in practice in anticipation that they will direct this behavior to the unforeseeable (and thus unauditable) clinical problems they will encounter in the future.

Conclusion

1. Educators should design EBP evaluation informed by granular understanding of the steps and core concepts of EBP[35] and available validated high-quality instruments.[50]
2. Educators should select instruments and strategies that are dictated by the purpose of evaluation, learners' level and needs, EBP domain of interest, feasibility (including cost), format, and compatibility with programmatic and institutional contextual variables.
3. Evaluating EBP knowledge and skills
   a. For evaluation of the competence of individual trainees, educators may utilize the instruments in Table 10.4, which discriminate between different levels of expertise. Their robust psychometric properties support their use in both formative and summative evaluations. Of these, the Fresno Test stands out because it assesses all four EBP steps; allows learners to authentically work through realistic cases with short-answer, essay, and calculation questions; and draws validity evidence from a spectrum of learners, languages, institutions, and health professions. Educators can engage in various standard-setting procedures[51,52] to determine "passing" scores for their own purposes.
   b. Educators can also take advantage of the efficiencies of integrating EBP evaluation into the course of clinical care and teaching. Although I am unaware of any published experience, educators could assess EBP skills as part of a mini clinical evaluation exercise (mini-CEX). These observations, described in Chapter 5, assess brief snapshots of real clinical encounters, show measurement characteristics similar to those of other performance assessments, permit evaluation based on a broader set of clinical settings and patient problems, and achieve sufficient reliability with multiple testing.[156] For example, a clinic preceptor, supervising the patient encounter described in the introduction, could prompt and then rate the resident's clinical question formulation, information gathering, or integration of the evidence for AAA screening into an informed decision-making discussion. Such items could be incorporated into customized mini-CEX forms. In addition, when the EBP "moment" cannot occur in real time, faculty can "dispense" and later rate educational prescriptions[132] (Appendix 10.2). This approach should be restricted to formative evaluation until more validity evidence accumulates.
   c. To determine the programmatic-level impact of specific curricula, educators may turn to instruments with strong evidence of responsive validity, including five of the instruments in Table 10.3[62,64–67] and

the seven instruments in Table 10.5.[69–73,128] Educators should choose instruments with outcome measures aligned with their curricula's learning objectives. Use of EBM-OSCEs provides an opportunity to evaluate learner performance in a "high-stakes" examination environment simulating realistic clinical situations.

4. EBP attitudes. Assessing attitudes may uncover hidden but potentially remediable barriers to trainees' EBP skill development and performance. In addition to surveys (or sections of surveys),[33,102–104] educators may use focus groups or structured interviews to determine trainees' attitudes and experiences.[112–119] Educators may also characterize their program's EBP learning environment.[122]
5. EBP behaviors
   a. Although EBP behaviors remain the most challenging domain, evaluators nonetheless must ensure that trainees implement their EBP skills in actual practice. The range of strategies to evaluate EBP behaviors appears in Box 10.1. A portfolio of educational prescriptions represents the most promising technology to document the performance of EBP steps in practice (see Appendix 10.2 for examples). With a simple system in place to dispense and collect the forms, the trainees can do most of the data entry. Internet-based systems may make tracking of information seeking and applying behavior more feasible. In addition unlike many other approaches, the prescription serves as an education intervention as well, particularly if the trainee reflects upon the "EBP moment" and reviews it with a faculty member. Program directors (or regulatory bodies) might consider *requiring* documentation of a minimum number of "EBP episodes," in much the same way they currently do for technical procedures.
   b. To document evidence-based practice performance, educators can borrow the quality data often already collected by healthcare organizations or teams with institutional officials to leverage resources for nascent efforts.

Acknowledgment

We are indebted to Dr. Michael Green, the author of this chapter for editions 1 and 2, for providing his original work for the revision and updating of this chapter.

Annotated Bibliography

A selected annotated bibliography is available online at www.expertconsult.com.

Articles

1. Shaneyfelt T, Baum KD, Bell D, et al. Instruments for evaluating education in evidence-based practice: a systematic review. *JAMA.* 2006 Sep 6;296(9):1116–1127. doi:10.1001/jama.296.9.1116.
   While now a bit dated, this systematic review still provides some useful guidance. The authors systematically reviewed 104 EBP evaluation instruments. Among EBP skills, acquiring evidence and appraising evidence were most commonly evaluated, but newer instruments evaluated asking answerable questions and applying evidence to individual patients. At least one type of validity evidence was demonstrated for 53% of instruments, but three or more types of validity evidence were established for only 10%. The authors identified instruments with the strongest validity evidence for evaluating the competence of individual trainees (including high-stakes assessment), determining the effectiveness of EBP curricula, and assessing EBP behaviors with objective outcome measures. We updated this systematic review for this chapter to include instruments developed after the publication. Reference #49 in printed list.
2. Kumaravel B, Hearn JH, Jahangiri L, Pollard R, Stocker CJ, Nunan D. A systematic review and taxonomy of tools for evaluating evidence-based medicine teaching in medical education. *Syst Rev.* 2020 Apr 24;9(1):91. doi:10.1186/s13643-020-01311-y.
   In this more recent systematic review of 77 studies, the authors developed a taxonomy of tools used for evaluating evidence-based medicine (EBM) teaching in medical education, based on three dimensions: the level of assessment (individual, program, or institutional), the type of tool (knowledge, skills, attitudes, or behavior), and the method of evaluation (self-assessment, peer assessment, or faculty assessment). The review found that a variety of tools have been used to evaluate EBM teaching, but most focus on assessing knowledge rather than skills, attitudes, or behavior. The authors recommend the use of a combination of tools to comprehensively evaluate EBM teaching in medical education. Reference #50 in printed list.
3. Straus SE, Green ML, Bell DS, et al. Evaluating the teaching of evidence based medicine: conceptual framework. *BMJ.* 2004 Oct 30;329(7473):1029–1032. doi:10.1136/bmj.329.7473.1029.
   The authors propose a framework for evaluating methods of teaching EBM, considering the learner, intervention, and outcome. Reference #68 in printed list.
4. Tilson J, Kaplan S, Harris J, et al. Sicily statement on classification and development of evidence-based practice learning assessment tools. *BMC Med Educ.* 2011 Oct 5;11(1):78. doi:10.1186/1472-6920-11-78.
   The authors identify key principles for designing EBP learning assessment tools, recommend a common taxonomy for new and existing tools, and present the Classification Rubric for EBP Assessment Tools in Education (CREATE). Examples place existing EBP assessments into the CREATE framework to demonstrate how a common taxonomy might facilitate purposeful development and use of EBP learning assessment tools. Reference #48 in printed list.
5. Albarqouni L, Hoffmann T, Straus S, et al. Core competencies in evidence-based practice for health professionals: consensus statement based on a systematic review and Delphi survey. *JAMA Netw Open.* 2018 Jun 1;1(2):e180281. doi:10.1001/jamanetworkopen.2018.0281.
   In this systematic, multistage, modified Delphi survey study, the authors identified a consensus set of 68 core competencies in EBP that should be covered in EBP teaching and learning programs, grouped into the main EBP domains. Reference #35 in printed list.

Helpful Textbooks

6. Fletcher GS. *Clinical Epidemiology: The Essentials.* 6th ed. Lippincott Connect; 2020.
7. Guyatt G, Rennie D, Meade MO et al, eds. *User's Guides to the Medical Literature: Essentials of Evidence-Based Clinical Practice,*

Third Edition (Uses Guides to Medical Literature). 3rd ed. McGraw Hill; 2015.
8. Straus SE, Glasziou P, Richardson WS, et al. *Evidence-Based Medicine: How to Practice and Teach EBM*. 5th ed. Elsevier; 2018.
9. Hoffmann T, Bennett S, Del Mar C. *Evidence-Based Practice Across the Health Professions*. 3rd ed. Elsevier; 2017.

References

1. Institute of Medicine. *Crossing the Quality Chasm: A New Health System for the 21st Century*. National Academies Press; 2001.
2. IOM (Institute of Medicine). Evidence-Based Medicine and the Changing Nature of Healthcare: 2007 IOM Annual Meeting Summary. 2008. *The National Academies Collection: Reports funded by National Institutes of Health*.
3. Montori VM, Guyatt GH. Progress in evidence-based medicine. *JAMA*. 2008 Oct 15;300(15):1814–1816. doi:10.1001/jama.300.15.1814.
4. Haynes RB, Devereaux PJ, Guyatt GH. Clinical expertise in the era of evidence-based medicine and patient choice. *ACP J Club*. 2002 Mar-Apr;136(2):A11–A14.
5. Dawes M, Summerskill W, Glasziou P, et al. Sicily statement on evidence-based practice. *BMC Med Educ*. 2005 Jan 5;5(1):1. doi:10.1186/1472-6920-5-1.
6. Del Fiol G, Workman TE, Gorman PN. Clinical questions raised by clinicians at the point of care: a systematic review. *JAMA Intern Med*. 2014 May;174(5):710–718. doi:10.1001/jamainternmed.2014.368.
7. Covell DG, Uman GC, Manning PR. Information needs in office practice: are they being met? *Ann Intern Med*. 1985 Oct;103(4):596–599. doi:10.7326/0003-4819-103-4-596.
8. Brassil E, Gunn B, Shenoy AM, Blanchard R. Unanswered clinical questions: a survey of specialists and primary care providers. *J Med Libr Assoc*. 2017 Jan;105(1):4–11. doi:10.5195/jmla.2017.101.
9. Choudhry NK, Fletcher RH, Soumerai SB. Systematic review: the relationship between clinical experience and quality of health care. *Ann Intern Med*. 2005 Feb 15;142(4):260. doi:10.7326/0003-4819-142-4-200502150-00008.
10. Ajmi SC, Aase K. Physicians' clinical experience and its association with healthcare quality: a systematised review. *BMJ Open Qual*. 2021 Nov;10(4):e001545. doi:10.1136/bmjoq-2021-001545.
11. McGlynn EA, Asch SM, Adams J, et al. The quality of health care delivered to adults in the United States. *N Engl J Med*. 2003 Jun 26;348(26):2635–2645. doi:10.1056/nejmsa022615.
12. Hayward RA, Asch SM, Hogan MM, Hofer TP, Kerr EA. Sins of omission: getting too little medical care may be the greatest threat to patient safety. *J Gen Intern Med*. 2005 Aug;20(8):686–691. doi:10.1111/j.1525-1497.2005.0152.x.
13. Clancy CM, Cronin K. Evidence-based decision making: global evidence, local decisions. *Health Aff (Millwood)*. 2005 Jan-Feb;24(1):151–162. doi:10.1377/hlthaff.24.1.151.
14. Davis D, O'Brien MA, Freemantle N, Wolf FM, Mazmanian P, Taylor-Vaisey A. Impact of formal continuing medical education: do conferences, workshops, rounds, and other traditional continuing education activities change physician behavior or health care outcomes? *JAMA*. 1999 Sep 1;282(9):867–874. doi:10.1001/jama.282.9.867.
15. Davis DA. Changing physician performance. A systematic review of the effect of continuing medical education strategies. *JAMA*. 1995 Sep 6;274(9):700–705. doi:10.1001/jama.274.9.700.
16. Buchanan H, Siegfried N, Jelsma J, Lombard C. Comparison of an interactive with a didactic educational intervention for improving the evidence-based practice knowledge of occupational therapists in the public health sector in South Africa: a randomised controlled trial. *Trials*. 2014 Jun 10;15:216. doi:10.1186/1745-6215-15-216.
17. Ilic D, Maloney S. Methods of teaching medical trainees evidence-based medicine: a systematic review. *Med Educ*. 2014 Feb;48(2):124–135. doi:10.1111/medu.12288.
18. Albarqouni L, Hoffmann T, Glasziou P. Evidence-based practice educational intervention studies: a systematic review of what is taught and how it is measured. *BMC Med Educ*. 2018 Aug 1; 18(1):177. doi:10.1186/s12909-018-1284-1.
19. General Medical Council. Education and Training. Accessed February 2023. www.gmc-uk.org/education/index.asp.
20. Accreditation Council of Graduate Medical Education. Program and Institutional Guidelines. Accessed February 2023. www.acgme.org/tabid/83/.
21. Institute of Medicine (US) Committee on the Health Professions Education Summit. Health professions education: a bridge to quality. In: Greiner AC, Knebel E, eds. *The Core Competencies Needed for Health Care Professionals*. National Academies Press; 2003.
22. Amiel JM, Andriole DA, Biskobing DM, et al. Revisiting the core Entrustable Professional Activities for entering residency. *Acad Med*. 2021 Jul 1;96(7s):S14–S21. doi:10.1097/acm.0000000000004088.
23. Chen HC, van den Broek WES, ten Cate O. The case for use of entrustable professional activities in undergraduate medical education. *Acad Med*. 2015 Apr;90(4):431–436. doi:10.1097/acm.0000000000000586.
24. Frank JR, Danoff D. The CanMEDS initiative: implementing an outcomes-based framework of physician competencies. *Med Teach*. 2007 Sep;29(7):642–647. doi:10.1080/01421590701746983.
25. Del Fiol G, Workman TE, Gorman PN. Clinical questions raised by clinicians at the point of care. *JAMA Int Med*. 2014 May 1;174(5):710. doi:10.1001/jamainternmed.2014.368.
26. Richardson WS, Murphy AL. Ask, and ye shall retrieve. *Evidence Based Medicine*. 1998 Aug;3(4):100–101. doi:10.1136/ebm.1998.3.100.
27. Straus SE, McAlister FA. Evidence-based medicine: a commentary on common criticisms. *CMAJ*. 2000 Oct 3;163(7):837–841.
28. Hoffmann TC, Montori VM, Del Mar C. The connection between evidence-based medicine and shared decision making. *JAMA*. 2014 Oct 1;312(13):1295–1296. doi:10.1001/jama.2014.10186.
29. Bergus GR. Does the structure of clinical questions affect the outcome of curbside consultations with specialty colleagues? *Arch Fam Med*. 2000 Jun 1;9(6):541–547. doi:10.1001/archfami.9.6.541.
30. McKibbon KA, Walker-Dilks CJ, Haynes RB. Finding the evidence in hematology. In: Crowther MA, Ginsberg J, Schünemann H, Meyer RM, Lottenberg R, eds. *Evidence-Based Hematology*. Wiley-Blackwell; 2009:23–31.
31. Dicenso A, Bayley L, Haynes RB. Accessing pre-appraised evidence: fine-tuning the 5S model into a 6S model. *Evid Based Nurs*. 2009 Oct;12(4):99–101. doi:10.1136/ebn.12.4.99-b.
32. Guyatt GH, Meade MO, Jaeschke RZ, Cook DJ, Haynes RB. Practitioners of evidence based care. Not all clinicians need to appraise evidence from scratch but all need some skills. *BMJ*. 2000 Apr 8;320(7240):954–955. doi:10.1136/bmj.320.7240.954.
33. McColl A, Smith H, White P, Field J. General practitioner's perceptions of the route to evidence based medicine: a questionnaire

survey. *BMJ.* 1998 Jan 31;316(7128):361–365. doi:10.1136/bmj.316.7128.361.
34. Tikkinen KAO, Guyatt GH. Understanding of research results, evidence summaries and their applicability-not critical appraisal-are core skills of medical curriculum. *BMJ Evid Based Med.* 2021 Oct;26(5):231–233. doi:10.1136/bmjebm-2020-111542.
35. Albarqouni L, Hoffmann T, Straus S, et al. Core competencies in evidence-based practice for health professionals: consensus statement based on a systematic review and Delphi survey. *JAMA Netw Open.* 2018 Jun 1;1(2):e180281. doi:10.1001/jamanetworkopen.2018.0281.
36. Holmboe ES. The transformational path ahead: competency-based medical education in family medicine. *Fam Med.* 2021 Jul 7;53(7):583–589. doi:10.22454/FamMed.2021.296914.
37. Frenk J, Chen L, Bhutta ZA, et al. Health professionals for a new century: transforming education to strengthen health systems in an interdependent world. *Lancet.* 2010 Dec 4;376(9756):1923–1958. doi:10.1016/S0140-6736(10)61854-5.
38. Moynihan S, Paakkari L, Valimaa R, Jourdan D, Mannix-McNamara P. Teacher competencies in health education: results of a Delphi study. *PloS One.* 2015 Dec 2;10(12):e0143703. doi:10.1371/journal.pone.0143703.
39. Owens DK, Davidson KW, Krist AH, et al. Screening for abdominal aortic aneurysm: US Preventive Services Task Force recommendation statement. *JAMA.* 2019 Dec 10;322(22):2211–2218. doi:10.1001/jama.2019.18928.
40. Association AER, Association AP. *Standards for Educational and Psychological Testing* Education NCoMi, Educational JCoSf, Testing P: American Educational Research Association; 2014.
41. Cook DA, Thompson WG, Thomas KG, Thomas MR, Pankratz VS. Impact of self-assessment questions and learning styles in web-based learning: a randomized, controlled, crossover trial. *Acad Med.* 2006 Mar;81(3):231–238. doi:10.1097/00001888-200603000-00005.
42. Downing SM. Validity: on the meaningful interpretation of assessment data. *Med Educ.* 2003 Sep;37(9):830–837. doi:10.1046/j.1365-2923.2003.01594.x.
43. Downing SM. Reliability: on the reproducibility of assessment data. *Med Educ.* 2004 Sep;38(9):1006–1012. doi:10.1111/j.1365-2929.2004.01932.x.
44. Downing SM. Threats to the validity of clinical teaching assessments: what about rater error? *Med Educ.* 2005 Apr;39(4):353–355. doi:10.1111/j.1365-2929.2005.02138.x.
45. Downing SM. Face validity of assessments: faith-based interpretations or evidence-based science? *Med Educ.* 2006 Jan;40(1):7–8. doi:10.1111/j.1365-2929.2005.02361.x.
46. Downing SM, Haladyna TM. Validity threats: overcoming interference with proposed interpretations of assessment data. *Med Educ.* 2004 Mar;38(3):327–333. doi:10.1046/j.1365-2923.2004.01777.x.
47. Downing SM, Tekian A, Yudkowsky R. Research methodology: procedures for establishing defensible absolute passing scores on performance examinations in health professions education. *Teach Learn Med.* 2006 Jan;18(1):50–57. doi:10.1207/s15328015tlm1801_11.
48. Tilson JK, Kaplan SL, Harris JL, et al. Sicily statement on classification and development of evidence-based practice learning assessment tools. *BMC Med Educ.* 2011 Oct 5;11:78. doi:10.1186/1472-6920-11-78.
49. Shaneyfelt T, Baum KD, Bell D, et al. Instruments for evaluating education in evidence-based practice: a systematic review. *JAMA.* 2006 Sep 6;296(9):1116–1127. doi:10.1001/jama.296.9.1116.
50. Kumaravel B, Hearn JH, Jahangiri L, Pollard R, Stocker CJ, Nunan D. A systematic review and taxonomy of tools for evaluating evidence-based medicine teaching in medical education. *Syst Rev.* 2020 Apr 24;9(1):91. doi:10.1186/s13643-020-01311-y.
51. Ben-David MF. AMEE Guide No. 18: Standard setting in student assessment. *Med Teach.* 2000 Jan;22(2):120–130. doi:10.1080/01421590078526.
52. McKinley DW, Norcini JJ. How to set standards on performance-based examinations: AMEE Guide No. 85. *Med Teach.* 2013 Nov 20;36(2):97–110. doi:10.3109/0142159x.2013.853119.
53. Ramos KD, Schafer S, Tracz SM. Validation of the Fresno Test of competence in evidence based medicine. *BMJ.* 2003 Feb 8;326(7384):319–321. doi:10.1136/bmj.326.7384.319.
54. Ilic D, Nordin RB, Glasziou P, Tilson JK, Villanueva E. Development and validation of the ACE tool: assessing medical trainees' competency in evidence based medicine. *BMC Med Educ.* 2014 Jun 9;14:114. doi:10.1186/1472-6920-14-114.
55. Chernick L, Pusic M, Liu H, Vazquez H, Kwok M. A pediatrics-based instrument for assessing resident education in evidence-based practice. *Acad Pediatr.* 2010 Jul-Aug;10(4):260–265. doi:10.1016/j.acap.2010.03.009.
56. Rothberg B, Feinstein RE, Guiton G. Validation of the Colorado psychiatry evidence-based medicine test. *J Grad Med Educ.* 2013 Sep;5(3):412–416. doi:10.4300/JGME-D-12-00193.1.
57. McCluskey A, Bishop B. The adapted Fresno Test of competence in evidence-based practice. *J Contin Educ Health Prof.* 2009 Spring;29(2):119–126. doi:10.1002/chp.20021.
58. McCluskey A, Lovarini M. Providing education on evidence-based practice improved knowledge but did not change behaviour: a before and after study. *BMC Med Educ.* 2005 Dec 19;5:40. doi:10.1186/1472-6920-5-40.
59. Tilson JK. Validation of the modified Fresno test: assessing physical therapists' evidence based practice knowledge and skills. *BMC Med Educ.* 2010 May 25;10:38. doi:10.1186/1472-6920-10-38.
60. Lewis LK, Williams MT, Olds TS. Development and psychometric testing of an instrument to evaluate cognitive skills of evidence based practice in student health professionals. *BMC Med Educ.* 2011 Oct 3;11:77. doi:10.1186/1472-6920-11-77.
61. Argimon-Pallàs JM, Flores-Mateo G, Jiménez-Villa J, Pujol-Ribera E. Psychometric properties of a test in evidence based practice: the Spanish version of the Fresno test. *BMC Med Educ.* 2010 Jun 16;10:45. doi:10.1186/1472-6920-10-45.
62. Fritsche L, Greenhalgh T, Falck-Ytter Y, Neumayer HH, Kunz R. Do short courses in evidence based medicine improve knowledge and skills? Validation of Berlin questionnaire and before and after study of courses in evidence based medicine. *BMJ.* 2002 Dec 7;325(7376):1338–1341. doi:10.1136/bmj.325.7376.1338.
63. Zwolsman SE, Wieringa-de Waard M, Hooft L, van Dijk N. Measuring evidence-based medicine knowledge and skills. The Dutch Berlin Questionnaire: translation and validation. *J Clin Epidemiol.* 2011 Aug;64(8):928–930. doi:10.1016/j.jclinepi.2011.02.005.
64. Bennett KJ. A controlled trial of teaching critical appraisal of the clinical literature to medical students. *JAMA.* 1987 May 8;257(18):2451–2454. doi:10.1001/jama.257.18.2451.
65. Haynes RB. Online access to Medline in clinical settings. *Ann Intern Med.* 1990 Jan 1;112(1):78. doi:10.7326/0003-4819-112-1-78.
66. MacRae HM, Regehr G, Brenneman F, McKenzie M, McLeod RS. Assessment of critical appraisal skills. *Am J Surg.* 2004 Jan;187(1):120–123. doi:10.1016/j.amjsurg.2002.12.006.

67. Taylor R, Reeves B, Mears R, et al. Development and validation of a questionnaire to evaluate the effectiveness of evidence-based practice teaching. *Med Educ*. 2001 Jun;35(6):544–547. doi:10.1046/j.1365-2923.2001.00916.x.
68. Straus SE, Green ML, Bell DS, et al. Evaluating the teaching of evidence based medicine: conceptual framework. *BMJ*. 2004 Oct 30;329(7473):1029–1032. doi:10.1136/bmj.329.7473.1029.
69. Smith CA, Ganschow PS, Reilly BM, et al. Teaching residents evidence-based medicine skills: a controlled trial of effectiveness and assessment of durability. *J Gen Intern Med*. 2000 Oct;15(10):710–715. doi:10.1046/j.1525-1497.2000.91026.x.
70. Green ML, Ellis PJ. Impact of an evidence-based medicine curriculum based on adult learning theory. *J Gen Intern Med*. 1997 Dec;12(12):742–750. doi:10.1046/j.1525-1497.1997.07159.x.
71. Landry FJ, Pangaro L, Kroenke K, Lucey C, Herbers J. A controlled trial of a seminar to improve medical student attitudes toward, knowledge about, and use of the medical literature. *J Gen Intern Med*. 1994 Aug;9(8):436–439. doi:10.1007/bf02599058.
72. Linzer M. Impact of a medical journal club on house-staff reading habits, knowledge, and critical appraisal skills. *JAMA*. 1988 Nov 4;260(17):2537. doi:10.1001/jama.1988.03410170085039.
73. Ross R, Verdieck A. Introducing an evidence-based medicine curriculum into a family practice residency—is it effective? *Acad Med*. 2003 Apr;78(4):412–417. doi:10.1097/00001888-200304000-00019.
74. Villanueva EV, Burrows EA, Fennessy PA, Rajendran M, Anderson JN. Improving question formulation for use in evidence appraisal in a tertiary care setting: a randomised controlled trial [ISRCTN66375463]. *BMC Med Inform Decis Mak*. 2001;1:4. doi:10.1186/1472-6947-1-4.
75. Miller GE. The assessment of clinical skills/competence/performance. *Acad Med*. 1990 Sep;65(9):S63–S67. doi:10.1097/00001888-199009000-00045.
76. Davidson RA, Duerson M, Romrell L, Pauly R, Watson RT. Evaluating evidence-based medicine skills during a performance-based examination. *Acad Med*. 2004 Mar;79(3):272–275. doi:10.1097/00001888-200403000-00016.
77. Bradley P, Humphris G. Assessing the ability of medical students to apply evidence in practice: the potential of the OSCE. *Med Educ*. 1999 Nov;33(11):815–817. doi:10.1046/j.1365-2923.1999.00466.x.
78. Tudiver F, Rose D, Banks B, Pfortmiller D. Reliability and validity testing of an evidence-based medicine OSCE station. *Fam Med*. 2009 Feb;41(2):89–91.
79. Asemota E, Winkel A, Vieira D, Gillespie C. A novel means of assessing evidence-based medicine skills. *Med Educ*. 2013 Apr 10;47(5):527. doi:10.1111/medu.12160.
80. Berner ES, McGowan JJ, Hardin JM, Spooner SA, Raszka WV, Berkow RL. A Model for Assessing Information Retrieval and Application Skills of Medical Students. *Academic Medicine*. 2002/06 2002;77(6):547–551. doi:10.1097/00001888-200206000-00014.
81. Frohna JG, Gruppen LD, Fliegel JE, Mangrulkar RS. Development of an evaluation of medical student competence in evidence-based medicine using a computer-based OSCE station. *Teach Learn Med*. 2006 Jun;18(3):267–272. doi:10.1207/s15328015tlm1803_13.
82. Fliegel JE, Frohna JG, Mangrulkar RS. A computer-based OSCE station to measure competence in evidence-based medicine skills in medical students. *Acad Med*. 2002 Nov;77(11):1157–1158. doi:10.1097/00001888-200211000-00022.
83. Schwartz A, Hupert J. Medical students' application of published evidence: randomised trial. *BMJ*. 2003 Mar 8;326(7388):536–538. doi:10.1136/bmj.326.7388.536.
84. Schwartz A, Hupert J. A decision making approach to assessing critical appraisal skills. *Med Teach*. 2005 Jan;27(1):76–80. doi:10.1080/01421590400016415.
85. Kumaravel B, Stewart C, Ilic D. Development and evaluation of a spiral model of assessing EBM competency using OSCEs in undergraduate medical education. *BMC Med Educ*. 2021 Apr 10;21(1):204. doi:10.1186/s12909-021-02650-7.
86. Stack MA, DeLellis NO, Boeve W, Satonik RC. Effects of teaching evidence-based medicine on physician assistant students' critical appraisal, self-efficacy, and clinical application: a randomized controlled trial. *J Physician Assist Educ*. 2020 Sep;31(3):159–165. doi:10.1097/jpa.0000000000000313.
87. Kersten HB, Frohna JG, Giudice EL. Validation of an Evidence-Based Medicine Critically Appraised Topic Presentation Evaluation Tool (EBM C-PET). *J Grad Med Educ*. 2013 Jun;5(2):252–256. doi:10.4300/JGME-D-12-00049.1.
88. Cheng GYT. Educational workshop improved information-seeking skills, knowledge, attitudes and the search outcome of hospital clinicians: a randomised controlled trial. *Health Info Libr J*. 2003 Jun 20;20(Suppl 1):22–33. doi:10.1046/j.1365-2532.20.s1.5.x.
89. Bergus GR, Emerson M. Family medicine residents do not ask better-formulated clinical questions as they advance in their training. *Fam Med*. 2005 Jul-Aug;37(7):486–490.
90. Nixon J, Wolpaw T, Schwartz A, Duffy B, Menk J, SNAPPS-Plus Bordage G. *Acad Med*. 2014 Aug;89(8):1174–1179. doi:10.1097/acm.0000000000000362.
91. Rucker L, Morrison E. The "EBM Rx". *Acad Med*. 2000 May;75(5):527–528. doi:10.1097/00001888-200005000-00050.
92. Burrows SC, Tylman V. Evaluating medical student searches of MEDLINE for evidence-based information: process and application of results. *Bull Med Libr Assoc*. 1999 Oct;87(4):471–476.
93. Gruppen LD, Rana GK, Arndt TS. A controlled comparison study of the efficacy of training medical students in evidence-based medicine literature searching skills. *Acad Med*. 2005 Oct;80(10):940–944. doi:10.1097/00001888-200510000-00014.
94. Toedter LJ, Thompson LL, Rohatgi C. Training surgeons to do evidence-based surgery: a collaborative approach1,2. *J Am Coll Surg*. 2004 Aug;199(2):293–299. doi:10.1016/j.jamcollsurg.2004.04.006.
95. Rana GK, Bradley DR, Hamstra SJ, et al. A validated search assessment tool: assessing practice-based learning and improvement in a residency program. *J Med Libr Assoc*. 2011 Jan;99(1):77–81. doi:10.3163/1536-5050.99.1.013.
96. Vogel EW, Block KR, Wallingford KT. Finding the evidence: teaching medical residents to search Medline. *J Med Libr Assoc*. 2002 Jul;90(3):327–330.
97. Bradley DR, Rana GK, Martin PW, Schumacher RE. Real-time, evidence-based medicine instruction: a randomized controlled trial in a neonatal intensive care unit. *J Med Libr Assoc*. 2002 Apr;90(2):194–201.
98. McKibbon KA, Haynes RB, Walker Dilks CJ, et al. How good are clinical Medline searches? A comparative study of clinical end-user and librarian searches. *Comput Biomed Res*. 1990 Dec;23(6):583–593. doi:10.1016/0010-4809(90)90042-b.
99. Haynes RB, Johnston ME, McKibbon KA, Walker CJ, Willan AR. A program to enhance clinical use of Medline. A randomized controlled trial. *Online J Curr Clin Trials*. 1993 May 11: Doc No 56 [4005 words; 39 paragraphs].

100. Forsetlund L, Bradley P, Forsen L, Nordheim L, Jamtvedt G, Bjørndal A. Randomised controlled trial of a theoretically grounded tailored intervention to diffuse evidence-based public health practice [ISRCTN23257060]. *BMC Med Educ.* 2003 Mar 13;3(2). doi:10.1186/1472-6920-3-2.
101. Reiter HI, Neville AJ, Norman G. Medline for medical students? Searching for the right answer. *Adv Health Sci Educ Theory Pract.* 2000;5(3):221–232. doi:10.1023/a:1009877514060.
102. McAlister FA, Graham I, Karr GW, Laupacis A. Evidence-based medicine and the practicing clinician. *J Gen Intern Med.* 1999 Apr;14(4):236–242. doi:10.1046/j.1525-1497.1999.00323.x.
103. Baum KD. The impact of an evidence-based medicine workshop on residents' attitudes towards and self-reported ability in evidence-based practice. *Med Educ Online.* 2003 Dec;8(1):4329. doi:10.3402/meo.v8i.4329.
104. Young JM, Ward JE. Evidence-based medicine in general practice: beliefs and barriers among Australian GPs. *J Eval Clin Pract.* 2001 May;7(2):201–210. doi:10.1046/j.1365-2753.2001.00294.x.
105. Melnyk BM, Fineout-Overholt E, Mays MZ. The evidence-based practice beliefs and implementation scales: psychometric properties of two new instruments. *Worldviews Evid Based Nurs.* 2008 Dec;5(4):208–216. doi:10.1111/j.1741-6787.2008.00126.x.
106. Leach MJ, Gillham D. Evaluation of the evidence-based practice attitude and utilization survey for complementary and alternative medicine practitioners. *J Eval Clin Pract.* 2008 Oct;14(5):792–798. doi:10.1111/j.1365-2753.2008.01046.x.
107. Hadley J, Hassan I, Khan KS. Knowledge and beliefs concerning evidence-based practice amongst complementary and alternative medicine health care practitioners and allied health care professionals: a questionnaire survey. *BMC Complement Altern Med.* 2008 Jul 23;8:45. doi:10.1186/1472-6882-8-45.
108. Salbach NM, Jaglal SB. Creation and validation of the evidence-based practice confidence scale for health care professionals. *J Eval Clin Pract.* 2010 Jul 13;17(4):794–800. doi:10.1111/j.1365-2753.2010.01478.x.
109. Salbach NM, Jaglal SB, Williams JI. Reliability and validity of the Evidence-Based Practice Confidence (EPIC) scale. *J Contin Educ Health Prof.* 2013 Winter;33(1):33–40. doi:10.1002/chp.21164.
110. Upton D, Upton P. Development of an evidence-based practice questionnaire for nurses. *J Adv Nurs.* 2006 Feb;53(4):454–458. doi:10.1111/j.1365-2648.2006.03739.x.
111. Markey P, Schattner P. Promoting evidence-based medicine in general practice—the impact of academic detailing. *Fam Pract.* 2001 Aug 1;18(4):364–366. doi:10.1093/fampra/18.4.364.
112. Freeman AC, Sweeney K. Why general practitioners do not implement evidence: qualitative study. *BMJ.* 2001 Nov 10;323(7321):1100–1102. doi:10.1136/bmj.323.7321.1100.
113. Montori VM, Tabini CC, Ebbert JO. A qualitative assessment of 1st-year internal medicine residents' perceptions of evidence-based clinical decision making. *Teach Learn Med.* 2002 Apr;14(2):114–118. doi:10.1207/s15328015tlm1402_08.
114. Tracy CS, Dantas GC, Upshur REG. Evidence-based medicine in primary care: qualitative study of family physicians. *BMC Fam Pract.* 2003 May 9;4:6. doi:10.1186/1471-2296-4-6.
115. Putnam W, Burge F, Tatemichi S, Twohig P. Asthma in primary care: making guidelines work. *Can Respir J.* 2001 Mar-Apr;8(Suppl A):29A–34A. doi:10.1155/2001/805379.
116. Oswald N, Bateman H. Treating individuals according to evidence: why do primary care practitioners do what they do? *J Eval Clin Pract.* 2000 May;6(2):139–148. doi:10.1046/j.1365-2753.2000.00243.x.
117. Lam WWT, Fielding R, Johnston JM, Tin KYK, Leung GM. Identifying barriers to the adoption of evidence-based medicine practice in clinical clerks: a longitudinal focus group study. *Med Educ.* 2004 Sep;38(9):987–997. doi:10.1111/j.1365-2929.2004.01909.x.
118. Green ML, Ruff TR. Why do residents fail to answer their clinical questions? A qualitative study of barriers to practicing evidence-based medicine. *Acad Med.* 2005 Feb;80(2):176–182. doi:10.1097/00001888-200502000-00016.
119. Bhandari M, Montori V, Devereaux PJ, Dosanjh S, Sprague S, Guyatt GH. Challenges to the practice of evidence-based medicine during residents' surgical training: a qualitative study using grounded theory. *Acad Med.* 2003 Nov;78(11):1183–1190. doi:10.1097/00001888-200311000-00022.
120. van Dijk N, Hooft L, Wieringa-de Waard M. What are the barriers to residents' practicing evidence-based medicine? A systematic review. *Acad Med.* 2010 Jul;85(7):1163–1170. doi:10.1097/acm.0b013e3181d4152f.
121. Sahu JK. Evidence based practice of pediatrics—right time to start. *Indian J Pediatr.* 2007 Jan;74(1):66. doi:10.1007/s12098-007-0030-1.
122. Mi M. Evidence based medicine teaching in undergraduate medical education: a literature review. *Evid Based Libr Inf Pract.* 2012 Sep 12;7(3):98. doi:10.18438/b88p6d.
123. Whitcomb ME. Research in medical education. *Acad Med.* 2002 Nov;77(11):1067–1068. doi:10.1097/00001888-200211000-00001.
124. Osheroff JA. Physicians' information needs: analysis of questions posed during clinical teaching. *Ann Intern Med.* 1991 Apr 1; 114(7):576. doi:10.7326/0003-4819-114-7-576.
125. Green ML, Ciampi MA, Ellis PJ. Residents' medical information needs in clinic: are they being met? *Am J Med.* 2000 Aug;109(3):218–223. doi:10.1016/s0002-9343(00)00458-7.
126. Flynn C, Helwig A. Evaluating an evidence-based medicine curriculum. *Acad Med.* 1997 May;72(5):454–455. doi:10.1097/00001888-199705000-00096.
127. Tilburt JC, Mangrulkar RS, Goold SD, Siddiqui NY, Carrese JA. Do we practice what we preach? A qualitative assessment of resident-preceptor interactions for adherence to evidence-based practice. *J Eval Clin Pract.* 2008 Oct;14(5):780–784. doi:10.1111/j.1365-2753.2008.00966.x.
128. Stevermer JJ, Chambliss ML, Hoekzema GS. Distilling the literature. *Acad Med.* 1999 Jan;74(1):70–72. doi:10.1097/00001888-199901001-00021.
129. Cabell CH, Schardt C, Sanders L, Corey GR, Keitz SA. Resident utilization of information technology. *J Gen Intern Med.* 2001 Dec;16(12):838–844. doi:10.1046/j.1525-1497.2001.10239.x.
130. Reckase MD. Portfolio assessment: a theoretical esthnate of score reliability. *Educ Meas.* 2005 Oct 25;14(1):12–14. doi:10.1111/j.1745-3992.1995.tb00846.x.
131. Khunti K. Teaching evidence-based medicine using educational prescriptions in general practice. *Med Teach.* 1998 Jan;20(4):380–381. doi:10.1080/01421599880841.
132. Feldstein DA, Mead S, Manwell LB. Feasibility of an evidence-based medicine educational prescription. *Med Educ.*

2009 Nov;43(11):1105–1106. doi:10.1111/j.1365-2923.2009.03492.x.

133. Philbrick AM, Hager KD, Lounsbery JL, et al. Educational prescriptions to document evidence-based medicine questions in ambulatory care advanced pharmacy practice experiences. *Am J Pharm Educ*. 2019 Oct;83(8):7299. doi:10.5688/ajpe7299.
134. Umscheid CA, Maenner MJ, Mull N, et al. Using educational prescriptions to teach medical students evidence-based medicine. *Med Teach*. 2016 Nov;38(11):1112–1117. doi:10.3109/0142159x.2016.1170775.
135. Crowley SD, Owens TA, Schardt CM, et al. A web-based compendium of clinical questions and medical evidence to educate internal medicine residents. *Acad Med*. 2003 Mar;78(3):270–274. doi:10.1097/00001888-200303000-00007.
136. Fung MFK, Walker M, Fung KFK, et al. An internet-based learning portfolio in resident education: the KOALA multicentre programme. *Med Educ*. 2000 Jun;34(6):474–479. doi:10.1046/j.1365-2923.2000.00571.x.
137. Campbell C, Parboosingh J, Gondocz T, Babitskaya G, Pham B. A study of the factors that influence physicians' commitments to change their practices using learning diaries. *Acad Med*. 1999 Oct;74(10):S34–S36. doi:10.1097/00001888-199910000-00033.
138. Campbell C, Parboosingh JT, Fox RD, Gondocz TS. Diary use for physicians to record self-directed continuing medical education. *J Contin Educ Health Prof*. 1995;15(4):209–216. doi:10.1002/chp.4750150404.
139. Guglielmino LM. *Development of the Self-Directed Learning Readiness Scale*. University of Georgia; 1977.
140. Green ML, Reddy SG, Holmboe E. Teaching and evaluating point of care learning with an Internet-based clinical-question portfolio. *J Contin Educ Health Prof*. 2009 Fall;29(4):209–219. doi:10.1002/chp.20039.
141. Sackett D, Ellis J, Mulligan I, Rowe J. Inpatient general medicine is evidence based. *Lancet*. 1995 Aug 12;346(8972):407–410.
142. Michaud G, McGowan JL, van der Jagt R, Wells G, Tugwell P. Are therapeutic decisions supported by evidence from health care research? *Arch Int Med*. 1998 Aug;158(15):1665. doi:10.1001/archinte.158.15.1665.
143. Gill P, Dowell AC, Neal RD, Smith N, Heywood P, Wilson AE. Evidence based general practice: a retrospective study of interventions in one training practice. *BMJ*. 1996 Mar 30;312(7034):819–821. doi:10.1136/bmj.312.7034.819.
144. Lai T, Wong V, Leung G. Is ophthalmology evidence based? A clinical audit of the emergency unit of a regional eye hospital. *Br J Ophthalmol*. 2003 Apr;87(4):385–390. doi:10.1136/bjo.87.4.385.
145. Jemec GBE, Thorsteinsdottir DMSH, Wulf HC. Evidence-based dermatologic out-patient treatment. *Int J Dermatol*. 1998 Nov;37(11):850–854. doi:10.1046/j.1365-4362.1998.00470.x.
146. Myles PS, Bain DL, Johnson F, McMahon R. Is anaesthesia evidence-based? A survey of anaesthetic practice. *Br J Anaesth*. 1999 Apr;82(4):591–595. doi:10.1093/bja/82.4.591.
147. Kingston MBSTR. Treatment of surgical patients is evidence-based. *Eur J Surg*. 2001 May;167(5):324–330. doi:10.1080/110241501750215168.
148. Kenny SE, Shankar KR, Rintala R, Lamont GL, Lloyd DA. Evidence-based surgery: interventions in a regional paediatric surgical unit. *Arch Dis Child*. 1997 Jan;76(1):50–53. doi:10.1136/adc.76.1.50.
149. Geddes JR, Game D, Jenkins NE, Peterson LA, Pottinger GR, Sackett DL. What proportion of primary psychiatric interventions are based on evidence from randomised controlled trials? *Qual Health Care*. 1996 Dec;5(4):215–217. doi:10.1136/qshc.5.4.215.
150. Straus SE, Ball C, Balcombe N, Sheldon J, McAlister FA. Teaching evidence-based medicine skills can change practice in a community hospital. *J Gen Intern Med*. 2005 Apr;20(4):340–343. doi:10.1111/j.1525-1497.2005.04045.x.
151. Lucas BP, Evans AT, Reilly BM, et al. The impact of evidence on physicians' inpatient treatment decisions. *J Gen Intern Med*. 2004 May;19(5 Pt 1):402–409. doi:10.1111/j.1525-1497.2004.30306.x.
152. Langham J, Tucker H, Sloan D, Pettifer J, Thom S, Hemingway H. Secondary prevention of cardiovascular disease: a randomised trial of training in information management, evidence-based medicine, both or neither: the PIER trial. *Br J Gen Pract*. 2002 Oct;52(483):818–824.
153. Epling JW, Heidelbaugh JJ, Woolever D, et al. Examining an evidence-based medicine culture in residency education. *Fam Med*. 2018 Nov;50(10):751–755. doi:10.22454/fammed.2018.576501.
154. Peabody JW, Luck J, Glassman P, et al. Measuring the quality of physician practice by using clinical vignettes: a prospective validation study. *Ann Int Med*. 2004 Nov 16;141(10):771. doi:10.7326/0003-4819-141-10-200411160-00008.
155. Holmboe ES, Prince L, Green M. Teaching and improving quality of care in a primary care internal medicine residency clinic. *Acad Med*. 2005 Jun;80(6):571–577. doi:10.1097/00001888-200506000-00012.
156. Norcini JJ, Blank LL, Duffy FD, Fortna GS. The mini-CEX: a method for assessing clinical skills. *Ann Int Med*. 2003 Mar 18;138(6):476. doi:10.7326/0003-4819-138-6-200303180-00012.
157. McGowan JJ, Berner ES. Proposed curricular objectives to teach physicians competence in using the world wide web. *Acad Med*. 2004 Mar;79(3):236–240. doi:10.1097/00001888-200403000-00007.
158. Wyer PC, Naqvi Z, Dayan PS, Celentano JJ, Eskin B, Graham MJ. Do workshops in evidence-based practice equip participants to identify and answer questions requiring consideration of clinical research? A diagnostic skill assessment. *Adv Health Sci Educ Theory Pract*. 2008 Oct;14(4):515–533. doi:10.1007/s10459-008-9135-1.
159. Akl EA, Izuchukwu IS, El-Dika S, Fritsche L, Kunz R, Schünemann HJ. Integrating an evidence-based medicine rotation into an internal medicine residency program. *Acad Med*. 2004 Sep;79(9):897–904. doi:10.1097/00001888-200409000-00018.
160. MacRae HM, Regehr G, McKenzie M, et al. Teaching practicing surgeons critical appraisal skills with an internet-based journal club: a randomized, controlled trial. *Surgery*. 2004 Sep;136(3):641–646. doi:10.1016/j.surg.2004.02.003.
161. Weberschock TB, Ginn TC, Reinhold J, et al. Change in knowledge and skills of year 3 undergraduates in evidence-based medicine seminars. *Med Educ*. 2005 July;39(7):665–671. doi:10.1111/j.1365-2929.2005.02191.x.
162. Hendricson WD, Rugh JD, Hatch JP, Stark DL, Deahl T, Wallmann ER. Validation of an instrument to assess evidence-based practice knowledge, attitudes, access, and confidence in the dental environment. *J Dent Educ*. 2011 Feb;75(2):131–144. doi:10.1002/j.0022-0337.2011.75.2.tb05031.x.

163. Kortekaas MF, Bartelink ME, Zuithoff NP, van der Heijden GJ, de Wit NJ, Hoes AW. Does integrated training in evidence-based medicine (EBM) in the general practice (GP) specialty training improve EBM behaviour in daily clinical practice? A cluster randomised controlled trial. *BMJ Open*. 2016 Sep 13;6(9):e010537. doi:10.1136/bmjopen-2015-010537.
164. Johnston JM, Leung GM, Fielding R, Tin KY, Ho LM. The development and validation of a knowledge, attitude and behaviour questionnaire to assess undergraduate evidence-based practice teaching and learning. *Med Educ*. 2003 Nov;37(11):992–1000. doi:10.1046/j.1365-2923.2003.01678.x.
165. Barlow PB, Skolits G, Heidel RE, Metheny W, Smith TL. Development of the Biostatistics and Clinical Epidemiology Skills (BACES) assessment for medical residents. *Postgrad Med J*. 2015 Aug;91(1078):423–430. doi:10.1136/postgradmedj-2014-133197.
166. Mi M, Moseley JL, Green ML. An instrument to characterize the environment for residents' evidence-based medicine learning and practice. *Fam Med*. 2012;44(2):98–104.

11

Clinical Performance Measures and Practice Review

ERIC S. HOLMBOE, MD, AND DANIEL J. SCHUMACHER, MD, PHD, MED

CHAPTER OUTLINE

Introduction

Assessing quality of care through review of clinical practice, historically referred to as a medical record or practice "audit," has grown substantially as an essential and important assessment method. In many countries and health systems quality and patient safety measures (aka indicators) have become the norm for practicing physicians. These measures are used for multiple purposes including quality improvement, patient safety, and public reporting. It follows that learners in undergraduate and graduate medical education programs must be introduced to, participate in, and perform reviews of their clinical practice using specific measures to guide their own professional development and prepare them for unsupervised practice.

However, to fully understand the importance and utility of clinical practice review, we need to start with an overview of quality improvement and patient safety (QIPS) science. The Institute of Medicine (now the National Academy of Medicine [NAM] in two seminal reports, *To Err is Human* and *Crossing the Quality Chasm*, highlighted the significant gaps in safety and quality over 20 years ago.[1,2] Unfortunately, progress in improving quality and safety continues to been painfully slow globally.[3–7] Furthermore, the COVID-19 pandemic that claimed millions of lives also further exposed substantial gaps and inequities in health and healthcare. Medical education must be part of the solution to address these persistent and pernicious gaps.[8,9]

Addressing these issues must begin in training for several reasons. First, it is well documented that the context of training—in other words, the quality and safety of care occurring within a training site—will "imprint" on trainees and impact care provided for *decades* following training.[10–13] Second, it is also well documented that graduates leave training with fundamental gaps in their abilities to provide the care that patients need.[14,15] Finally, evidence suggests that trainees play an important role in optimal and safe care delivery while in training.[16] This should not be surprising as trainees, especially in (post) graduate medical education (PGME and GME), provide substantial care during this training phase.

Beyond improving care provision during and following training, additional considerations underscore the importance of clinical practice review during training. First, despite limited evidence, individual physicians around the world are still being judged and paid, to varying degrees, on the quality and safety of the care they provide as part of pay-for-performance programs.[17,18] Second, clinical practice review can help learners improve care and acquire critical competencies for 21st-century practice. Thus learners at a minimum must engage in learning basic quality and safety of care principles and use performance data from medical records and other sources to guide improvement. Before exploring the "what and how" of performance measurement, an overview of systems principles and concepts will be helpful to put this form of assessment in perspective. Clinical performance is always grounded in context and therefore by extension so is the assessment of that care through quality and safety measures and indicators.

A Systems and Quality Primer

The healthcare system is not an abstract entity but the cooperative interaction between people and technology. Moreover, to implement changes in healthcare systems, physicians must become system architects and engineers in helping to transform the systems to cross the quality chasm. The journey to acquire these competencies must begin early in training. As a result, the Accreditation Council for Graduate Medical Education (ACGME) and American Board of Medical Specialties (ABMS) in the United States determined it is essential that physicians-in-training, critical people in the healthcare system, acquire competence in systems-based practice and practice-based learning and improvement[19] (see Chapter 1). The Royal College of Physicians and Surgeons of Canada (RCPSC) recognized the importance of more explicitly incorporating systems and quality improvement by revising the manager role to leader.[20] At the undergraduate level, the 11 original medical schools participating in the American Medical Association's (AMA's) Accelerating Change in Medical Education Consortium have identified health systems science as the critical third science integrated with basic and clinical science in curricular transformation to better prepare students to succeed in our evolving healthcare systems. Health systems science content includes the principles and practice of quality improvement, safety, teamwork, leadership, and other domains relevant to the effective function of physicians in healthcare systems.[21–23]

Commitment to quality improvement, patient safety, and accountability is now established as a core professional value. The Physician Charter on Medical Professionalism, originally developed jointly by the American Board of Internal Medicine Foundation (ABIMF), European Federation of Internal Medicine (EFIM), and American College of Physicians (ACP) Foundation, explicitly listed active involvement in quality improvement as a core principle of professionalism 20 years ago.[24] Others have highlighted quality improvement as not only a professional obligation but also a civic responsibility.[25–30] These authors speak to a new set of beliefs and ethics physicians must embrace to bring about meaningful improvements in healthcare.

• BOX 11.1 Institute of Medicine Core Competencies for all Healthcare Providers

- Provide patient-centered care.
- Employ evidence-based medicine.
- Utilize informatics.
- Work in interdisciplinary teams
- Apply quality improvement.

The NAM created its own competency framework grounded in the two reports on quality and safety problems in US healthcare listing the ability to apply quality improvement methods and to employ evidence-based medicine methods to deliver care through the coordinated effort of interdisciplinary teams as core competencies for all healthcare providers[30] (Box 11.1).

To teach and evaluate these new competencies, educators must understand key concepts and methods of quality improvement science and recognize that multiple healthcare professionals working together within a system deliver care, not just doctors alone. Interprofessional practice should now be the norm for delivering care that is safe, effective, patient centered, timely, efficient, and equitable.[30] Core competencies for interprofessional collaborative practice are now available for training programs, and interprofessional teamwork and communication is a core subcompetency in the US Accreditation Council for Graduate Medical Education Milestone.[31,32] Despite the growing availability of resources to teach quality improvement science, such as the Institute for Healthcare Improvement (IHI) Open School,[33] such concepts remain new to many medical educators and practicing physicians.[22,34] Assessment of ability in QIPS will need to include clinical performance measurement but must also assess knowledge, skills, and attitudes around systems and QIPS.

What Is a System?

When most physicians hear the word *system* they immediately think about large healthcare organizations such as health plans, hospital and physician networks, national health services, or the vague concept of all the people and operations that deliver the elusive service called healthcare. For physicians, the word *system* can carry a pejorative connotation and is referenced as being in opposition to physician-level quality of care. This attitude arises from the professional value of autonomy and responsibility; unfortunately, it also impedes progress in physicians gaining competence in quality improvement and safety science.

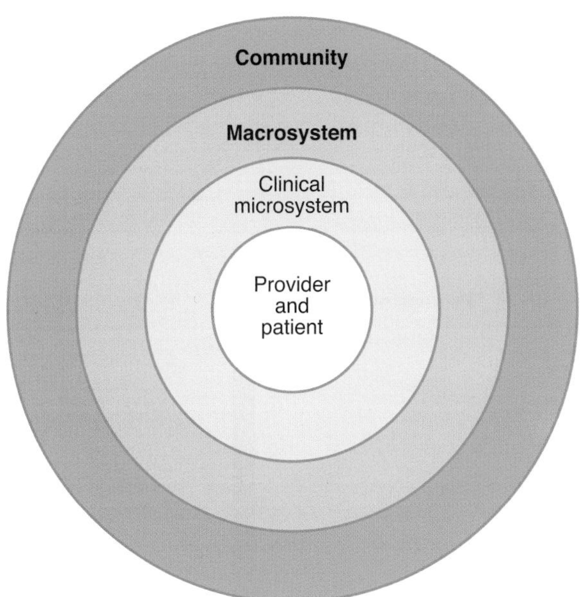

• **Fig. 11.1** Centering the levels of the system around providers and patients.

What we mean by system in this context is the organization of the people, their work processes, and the technical tools, procedures, and therapies they use to accomplish their common goals of good patient care. To get our minds around systems, it is helpful to use the Batalden model of concentric circles or levels of organization or relationship that has stood the test of time (Fig. 11.1).[35]

At the inner circle is the dyadic patient–provider relationship. From the physician perspective, we tend to think of this as only the physician–patient relationship; however, from the patient's perspective it is actually a multitude of patient–other relationships (i.e., other health professionals) that occur in the course of healthcare. In fact, the center circle has increasingly become an interprofessional healthcare team with multiple individual healthcare professionals interacting and working directly with the patient. For purposes of assessment, both the physician–patient dyad and the interprofessional team–patient/family are vital and important.

The next concentric circle Batalden calls the clinical microsystem—this is the unit of the organization where patients receive their care.[35–37] For primary or principle care this unit is now sometimes called the patient-centered medical home."[38–42] A microsystem is the small organization of people and technology who work collaboratively to provide, or coproduce, care with patients and families.[35,37] Education is no different and it is important to recognize that the majority of clinical education occurs in these microsystems.[43] The clinical microsystem is increasingly recognizing health and healthcare is a cocreation and coproduction process in partnership with patients and families.[44–46]

The third circle contains the network of the multiple microsystems that are tied together to provide the range of services needed for care. This circle is called the macrosystem. These third-circle microsystems include laboratories, imaging services, consultation, diagnostic and therapeutic

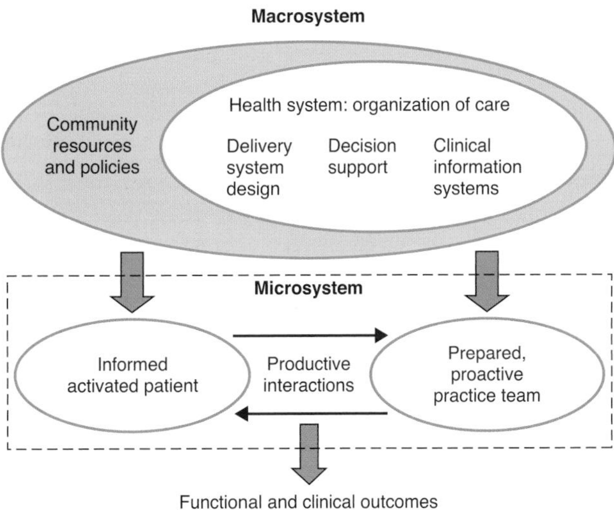

• **Fig. 11.2** The macrosystem in the care of chronic disease.

procedural services, patient education and counseling, pharmacy, and many more. The fourth circle contains the community (Fig. 11.1). Wagner's chronic care model demonstrates how a macrosystem is needed to facilitate high-quality care for patients with chronic illness such as diabetes[44,45] (Fig. 11.2).

Fig. 11.3 from Batalden and colleagues builds on the Wagner model and others through the lens of coproduction.[46] As Batalden and colleagues noted, most patient outcomes are the result of coproduced activities such as when physicians and "patients communicate effectively, develop a shared understanding of the problem and generate a mutually acceptable evaluation and management plan."

For the purposes of discussing systems in the context of training, we will focus on the second level, the clinical microsystem, its functioning, and its relationship to the inner dyadic system and next-level macrosystem that directly affect trainees' acquisition and application of competencies, and the program's ability to assess the competencies of practice-based learning and improvement and systems-based practice. In these systems physicians-in-training must learn to coproduce health and healthcare with patients and families and this requires assessment of clinical practice.

Components of a Clinical Microsystem

Nelson and colleagues defined a microsystem as "a small group of people who work together on a regular basis to provide care to discrete subpopulations of patients and who share clinical and business aims, linked processes of care and information for the purpose of producing meaningful performance outcomes."[35–37] Examples of a clinical microsystem in the training environment would include ambulatory clinics, radiology units, hospital wards, and surgical suites. Trainees must learn how these microsystems should function most efficiently and effectively, and how microsystems relate and interact with one another. Fig. 11.4 shows how the steps doctors use to provide medical care, the clinical

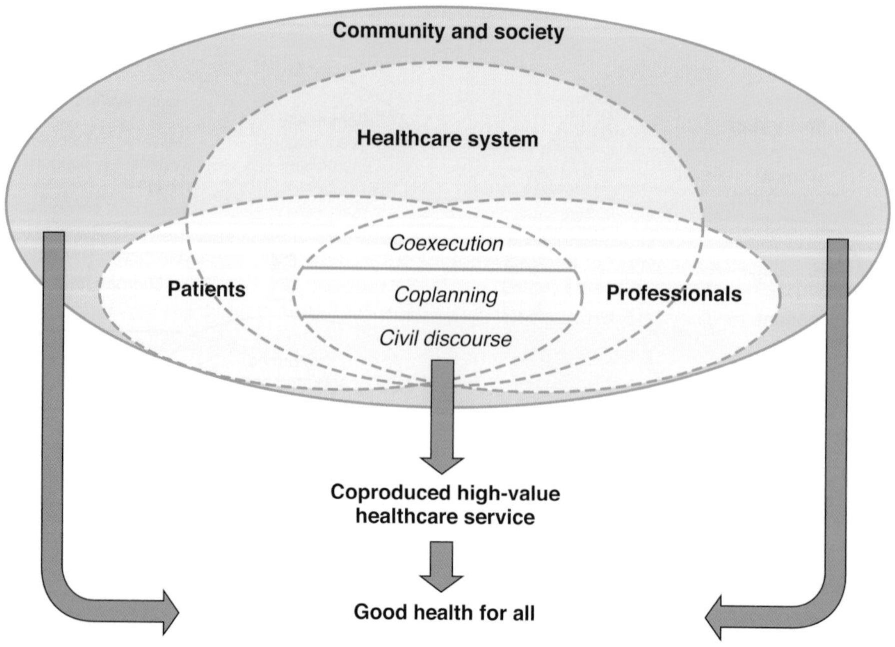

• **Fig. 11.3** Using coproduction to improve care and learning. Reproduced from Batalden M, Batalden P, Margolis P, et al. Coproduction of healthcare service. *BMJ Qual Saf.* 2016;25:509-517. doi:10.1136/bmjqs-2015-004315.

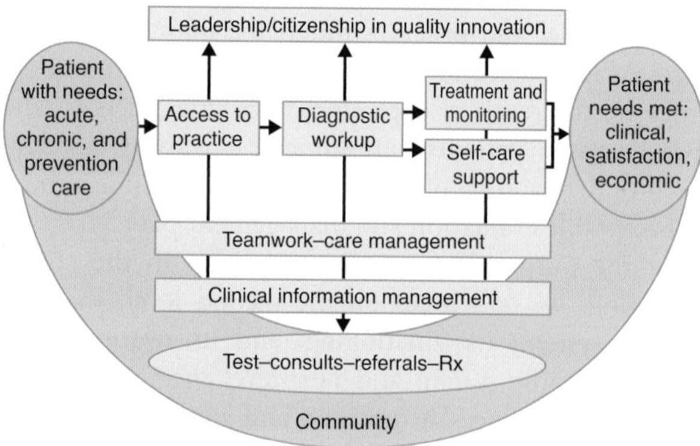

• **Fig. 11.4** An overview of the clinical microsystem.

method, come together in a sequence of work processes and are integrated with supporting processes, people, and technology to create a clinical microsystem. Let's break down these important components and steps further.

Population of patients with need: The circle on the far left of the figure shows the population of patients with specific healthcare needs (acute care, prevention of future disease, management of chronic care, promotion of health) who seek care from the particular microsystem. In primary care microsystems, some patients select a practice because it is convenient to home or work, while others choose a practice for financial reasons or because it has attractive cultural or social features. It is important to understand the needs of the patient population using the microsystem, because the design of the work process must vary to meet the needs efficiently and effectively.

Clinical processes: The sequential steps shown in the rectangles in the middle of the diagram are the familiar components of the clinical method: (1) access to the practice—appointments, telephone or mail contact; (2) workup and diagnosis—the first medical task that requires strong clinical skills (see Chapter 5); (3) treatment and monitoring—the second important medical task; and (4) patient self-care support—the third medical task, which informs the patient about their role in the care process and assists them in carrying it out.

Outcomes of care – patient needs met: The circle on the right shows the outcomes of the care that are of interest to everyone: meeting the needs of the patient population. The obvious goal is to achieve desirable clinical outcomes (e.g., blood pressure control, acceptable A1C levels for those with diabetes) for an individual patient and for the population of patients seeking care from the practice.

In addition to clinical outcomes, other important measures of practice success include patient judgment of and satisfaction with their *experience* of care as well as their reports of outcomes important to them. Equally important is physician and staff satisfaction with their work. The satisfaction of residents with their clinical experience, especially in outpatient microsystems, is an underappreciated factor in their ultimate career choice but also a major factor in health professional well-being. In fact, many now refer to the Quadruple Aim of quality: patient experience as defined by the Institute of Medicine's six aims of healthcare; population health; cost; and health professional wellness.[47,48] Some are now calling for the Quintuple Aim, calling out the need for health equity explicitly.[49] A fourth important measure of the success of the practice is its economic viability and its ability to provide care at an affordable price and achieve its business goals.[50] As a result, an increasing number of measures are targeting measures of overuse (e.g., use of antibiotics in viral infections).[51,52]

Supporting processes: The thin rectangles in the figure represent important processes of the clinical microsystem that make the care directed by clinicians reliable, safe, and efficient. At the top of the diagram is "Leadership/citizenship in quality innovation." This tops the list of supporting processes. In many training program microsystems, residents have a difficult time knowing who has leadership responsibility for quality performance. Moreover, few microsystems explicitly enable resident "citizenship," albeit a temporary role, for contributing to microsystem quality performance. Residents and senior house officers are too often not meaningfully involved in quality improvement or patient safety initiatives within their training institution and the recent COVID-19 pandemic exacerbated the situation.[53–55]

While more GME training programs are now looking at performance measures of the quality of care delivered in their primary microsystems, the penetration of these activities remains insufficient in many programs, with too many trainees not having a good sense of their own performance on important clinical care measures. At the heart of physician-level competence in practice-based learning and quality improvement is the attitude of embracing performance measurement and the personal capacity to use performance measurement to apply quality improvement (QI) practices (such as root cause analysis [RCA] or failure mode and effects analysis [FMEA]) to develop ideas for redesigning a process of care as well as to test its impact on the practice to determine if the change improved performance on the measures.[56]

The rectangle below the clinical method in the figure is labeled "Teamwork and care management." This process, performed by physician and nonphysician healthcare professionals, ensures proactive care of patients with chronic conditions and delivery of appropriate preventive care. The microsystem designs the most efficient sequence of tasks to be performed and assigns appropriate members of the healthcare team to roles and responsibilities to execute them. Each team member has a role and responsibility for the seamless handoff of patients or information along the train of steps in managing their care. When rotating through a microsystem, residents must learn their roles and responsibilities for tasks in the care management process. By experiencing different microsystems, they will learn how teamwork occurs to achieve goals for different patient problems.

The lower rectangle in the figure shows the clinical information management process that ties the entire microsystem together and connects it to the external consultants, laboratories, and pharmacies (shown in the oval at the bottom of the diagram) that are necessary for providing integrated care for the patient. An effective information management system is essential for the reliable execution and coordination of care. Complete interoperability of electronic clinical information systems is still unrealized in many institutions but is slowly improving. A microsystem's success depends in large part on the effectiveness of its information management system. Regardless of the level of computerization of the microsystem's information, its flow can be managed by using a system of templates, flowsheets, order forms, request forms, medical record pages, prescriptions, telephone notes, and others that are passed along, collated, and managed by members of the microsystem.

Supplier microsystems: The oval at the bottom of the figure indicates the external microsystems that supply vital services to patients in the practice. These microsystems include laboratory services, imaging services, pharmacy, the variety of consulting services for hospitalization, and diagnostic and therapeutic services. The practice's clinical information management system must connect clinical data collected within the practice microsystem with these external services; there must be processes for tracking and recording the information returned from these external services. Important interpersonal tasks of any microsystem are managing these external service relationships to ensure quality patient care through reliable coordination and follow-through on care provided by multiple microsystems.

Systems and Adaptation

As we have now learned, a system is a set of interdependent parts sharing a common purpose. Interdependence means the parts of the system work in a coordinated manner and understand their dependency on one another. It is a system and not the individual that ultimately produces results. When the parts lack a common purpose and interdependence, or act with individual autonomy, as so often happens in medicine, the system weakens and ultimately may collapse.

Common purpose is not a platitude to provide "high-quality care," it is a clear statement of goals that are tied to specific quality measures that guide those who work together in intentionally seeking to improve them through changes in the way they work together. Clinical environments continually change; therefore, for a care system of people and methods to thrive, it must have the capacity to adapt. Change and adaptation are essential properties of healthy systems that arise from the capacity of the individuals, whose work comprises the system, to adapt and change.[54,57,58] This does not mean we should ask students and residents to continually devise "workarounds" to get their work done in the dysfunctional systems they too often encounter in the clinical setting. Rather, adaptation here refers to the ability of all individuals to identify when a change in the environment has occurred, the ability to determine the impact of the change in reaching healthcare team and patient quality goals, and the ability to develop a plan for an improved way of working together. Thus quality improvement is not a "science fair project" that is intermittently applied to the system or that takes time out from regular work to make a change. Improving quality and patient safety requires additional competencies that are now reflected in competency frameworks discussed in Chapter 1. Performance data provide the necessary substrate for trainees to engage and learn quality improvement and safety science while concomitantly providing meaningful assessment information about the trainee as part of a program of assessment.

Appendix 11.1 provides a host of resources to learn about quality improvement, systems science, and tools that can be used to judge the operating effectiveness of microsystems and patient-centered medical homes. It is important to understand the overall performance of systems to maximize assessment methods such as medical record audit and multiple source feedback. With this brief background we will now turn our attention to medical record review and clinical performance measures.

Clinical Practice Review to Assess Quality and Safety of Care

Now that the reader hopefully has a fuller understanding of systems, let's next turn our attention to the role of clinical practice review to assess and support training in quality improvement and patient safety (QIPS). Medical records serve a number of important functions: (1) they provide an archive of important patient medical information for use by other healthcare providers *and* patients (especially true with the move toward open notes and online patient portals); (2) they are a source of data to assess performance in practice such as specific chronic medical conditions (e.g., diabetes), postoperative care, or prevention; (3) they enable monitoring of patient safety and complications; and (4) they enable documentation of diagnostic and therapeutic decisions. One can readily see how these patient care functions of the medical record can be used for educational and assessment purposes to support professional development.[43,58]

Practice audits are an essential method in assessment of the competencies of Practice-based Learning and Improvement and Systems-based Practice in the ACGME/ABMS general competency framework and of the Leader role in Canadian Medical Education Directives for Specialists (CanMEDS) model. The ability to effectively design, implement, and evaluate a QIPS intervention is now an explicit, desired outcome in postgraduate training in the United States (see Appendix 11.1). These competencies require that residents be actively involved in monitoring their own clinical practice and improving the quality of care based on a systematic review of the care they provide. Clinical performance metrics that can be gleaned from the medical record based on documentation and ordering practices can also serve an important role in providing information about Patient Care, Medical Knowledge, and Interpersonal and Communication Skills in the ACGME/ABMS general competency framework and about the Medical Expert and Communicator roles in CanMEDS. Finally, practice review can promote self-reflection and support self-regulated learning, important skills needed for lifelong learning.

A Primer on Quality (Performance) Measures

Before getting into the specific types of clinical performance reviews, a quick tutorial on clinical performance measures may be helpful. The US Department of Health and Human Services (HHS) states that performance measures "are designed to measure systems of care and are derived from clinical or practice guidelines. Data that are defined into specific measurable elements provide an organization with a meter to measure the quality of its care."[59] The HHS also highlights that performance measures and clinical guidelines are not the same. Clinical guidelines are systematically designed to guide physicians and patients in making decisions about appropriate healthcare for specific clinical circumstances.[59] Some parts of clinical guidelines focus on standardizing aspects of care that can be easily captured and represented as performance measures. However, other parts and sometimes even entire guidelines are too complex to pull out care standardization that can be reliably expected in most encounters the guideline focuses on.

The HHS categorized performance measures as follows, based on the Donabedian model:[60]

- Structure of care measure: Quantifies a feature of a healthcare organization (or clinician) relevant to its capacity to provide healthcare. Simple examples for an organization would be presence or absence of an electronic medical record (EMR) and its capabilities and having the appropriate instruments in an operating suite or resuscitation room.[61] An example at the individual level would be how many clinicians have been successfully trained to use the essential features of an EMR. While not purely a structural measure, an organization may also want to assess the overall time spent in the EMR by clinicians, time spent in individual aspects of the electronic record, and movement through aspects of the electronic record as proxies for workflow and efficiency.
- Process measure: Quantifies a particular healthcare service provided to, on behalf of, or by a patient, based on scientific evidence of efficacy or effectiveness.[61] An example of a process measure would be what proportion of eligible women in a physician's practice received a mammogram.
- Outcome measure: Quantifies a patient's health status resulting from healthcare. Improving outcome measures is the ultimate goal. Mortality and morbidities (e.g., complications) are common outcome measures. Some outcome measures are classified as "intermediate" outcome measures, such as blood pressure control, as robust scientific evidence demonstrates the clear linkage between blood pressure and stroke, heart disease, et cetera. Other important outcome measures include patient experience with their care and patient-reported outcome measures (PROMs).[62–64] PROMs predominantly target functional status, such as the ability to walk without pain 6 months after a hip replacement.
- Balancing measures: Ensure that changes to improve one part of the system are not causing new problems in other parts of the system.[65]

These different types of measures highlight what Hall and colleagues have detailed as three levels that can be considered: micro, meso, and macro.[66] The micro level focuses on individual clinicians, dyads, or small teams. At this level, process and structure of care measures are most readily useful and outcome and balancing measures may be less applicable depending on the focus of a measure. Moving to the meso (training program or institution) and macro (national organizations and specialties) shifts this balance toward outcome and balancing measures and away from process and structure of care measures.

Hall and colleagues also detail other components of a taxonomy of measures that are useful to consider. First, they note that measures can be educationally focused or clinically focused. However, as this chapter highlights, clinical measures can, and should, be harnessed for education purposes as well. Second, they describe the importance of considering measures that are most useful as three stages of training and practice: training, transition to practice, and practice. Indeed, many existing clinical performance measures focus on clinicians in practice after training. This leaves a gap for ideal measures best fit for those individuals still in training. This has led Schumacher and colleagues to develop resident-sensitive quality measures (RSQMs), which are metrics important to care and also likely attributable to residents. In their original work, RSQMs were developed for three common illnesses in the pediatric emergency department (asthma, bronchiolitis, and closed head injury) and fell into three broad categories:[66–68]

- Appropriate medications, dosing, and timeliness
  - Ex: Use asthma order set in the EMR, time to steroid order, initial treatment matches documented Pediatric Respiratory Assessment Measure (PRAM)
- Appropriate documentation of key history and exam findings
  - Ex: Previous intubation or biphasic positive airway pressure (BiPAP), work of breathing, wheezing, document own PRAM
- Appropriate discharge guidance
  - Ex: Follow-up recommendation, return if needing albuterol more than every 4 hours

While RSQMs focus on residents, similar measures could, and should, be developed for medical students and fellowship trainees. RSQMs are a good example of process measures focused at the micro level and are useful for both education and clinical purposes.

Sources of Data for Practice Review

Electronic Medical Record

Most healthcare systems and practices have moved to EMRs to document visit encounters and track important aspects of care. This record is a vital component of the educational experience and captures a plethora of data about care provision. Clinical data are necessary for performance assessments and quality improvement. Without robust clinical data targeted for specific populations of patients (e.g., those needing preventive services, patients with chronic disease such as diabetes, etc.), it is almost impossible to implement quality improvement.

These data can be accessed through simple chart review (opening a chart to review and discuss it with a peer or supervisor for the purpose of assessment, reflection for learning, or both) or more sophisticated queries and organizations of data contained in them. With the growth of machine learning (ML) and artificial intelligence (AI), even written aspects of the medical record (compared to discrete fields such as orders) can be ascertained and organized through approaches such as natural language processing (NLP).

In addition to giving insights into practice patterns, EMRs can be highly valuable in helping to determine the actual clinical experiences of trainees.[67–72] Learners need to know what types of patients and conditions they are seeing in clinical practice. Electronic systems can provide learners with a much better snapshot of what patients comprise their population panel. The work of informatics scholars such as Mai and Dziorny has spearheaded efforts to use the EMR to give rich insights into the diagnoses trainees are seeing and in what volume based on clinical setting (e.g., inpatient, ambulatory clinic, emergency department).[73]

At the local level, each EMR has its own design and set of limitations, so it is important to discuss with your local quality improvement and information technology department what types of data are available at your institution in your specific specialty and who can best help pull and organize these data in meaningful ways.[74–83] For example, the internal medicine program at the University of Cincinnati has created quality dashboards for all its residents as part of their ambulatory practice.[84]

The majority of clinical care units across the globe now have at least partial access to EMRs, and we encourage the reader to work with their local information specialists to pull data from the EMR as part of the curriculum for teaching QIPS and for assessment of individual learners and the program. However, some sites may not have an EMR, or have one that is very difficult to access data from. In these situations, manual practice reviews (aka medical record audits) are still a useful learning and assessment exercise, and it is important that medical educators in this setting understand how to perform and use a manual audit. Appendix 11.2 provides an example manual abstraction form that may be helpful.[85]

Claims Data

At the residency and fellowship levels, trainees and/or office staff routinely use ICD and CPT codes for patient visits, especially in the outpatient setting in the United States.[86] This can be a valuable source of information about the clinical practice of trainees. For example, claims data can be very helpful in identifying a cohort of patients. Claims data can be used to assess processes of care (such as whether measurement of hemoglobin A1C, lipids, and microalbumin for diabetic patients was ordered and completed). Claims databases can be used to "track" the makeup of each resident's patient panel. Likewise, the claims database can be used to identify a group of patients admitted with conditions such as acute myocardial infarction and pneumonia. This can then facilitate the identification of charts for review. Finally, claims data can be useful to assess efficiency and cost consciousness, such as how many tests or diagnostic studies are ordered.

Several caveats should be noted about using claims data for evaluation. First, the use of claims data to measure "quality" is highly dependent on the quality of the coding. Poor coding practices can limit the value of the claims data. Second, claims data are essentially limited to the process of care and usually cannot provide specific detail about the outcomes of care. Finally, insufficient data and the quality of the claims data can limit analysis when using claims data to examine the relationship between assessment of learners and future practice.[87] EMRs (discussed earlier) possess important advantages over claims data, including examining diagnostics.[88]

Registries

Registries have become more common in a number of countries. For example, in the United States robust, long-standing registries exist for invasive cardiac procedures, vascular surgery, and thoracic surgery.[89–91] In Sweden there are now over 100 registries that cover 80% of the Swedish population, including measures of functional status (i.e., PROMs).[92] Locally developed registries can be very useful in tracking quality and performance within subsets of patients as highlighted in a group of family medicine programs.[71] The use of national registries remains limited in medical education, but investigators used the American College of Surgeons (ACS) National Surgical Quality Improvement Program (NSQIP) registry to examine the experience and complications in surgical residency programs.[70] More recently, a group of researchers used the Vascular Quality Initiative (VQI) registry to examine outcomes among vascular surgery trainees. While it is obviously very difficult to attribute outcomes to a single resident from a registry, the information can be very useful in aggregate for the training program (the meso level discussed previously) and the residents to improve care and acquire needed competencies in quality improvement and patient safety. Recent work by Smith and colleagues found that the VQI registry provided useful findings on outcomes related to both the trainee and program.[91,93] The use of both local and national registries is likely to continue to grow. If your specialty in your country has a registry, we recommend exploring the registry if for no other reason than to help improve curriculum and assessment.

Patient Experience Data

A number of countries now use patient experience surveys and PROMs as part of their quality improvement efforts (see also Chapter 12 on multisource feedback). For example, many hospitals and clinics use one of the Consumer Assessment of Healthcare Providers and Systems (CAHPS) patient experience surveys linked to specific sites of care (e.g., hospital, ambulatory clinic). Patients' experiences with their physicians have been associated with clinical outcomes.[94] As another example, a study using a registry of patient complaints managed by Vanderbilt University across hundreds of hospitals found an association between patient complaints in early clinical practice and resident/fellow Milestone ratings in professionalism and communication skills near graduation.[95] If patient- and family-centered care is a core healthcare outcome (i.e., part of the Quadruple Aim), review of clinical practice must include the patient and family voice as part of the assessment program.

Unannounced Standardized Patients

While not drawn from an existing database or from a medical record, unannounced standardized patients (USPs), sometimes called "secret shoppers," have been used to assess the quality of care by physicians. Ramsey and colleagues in the 1990s used USPs to examine the quality of care by practicing primary care physicians, uncovering a number of deficiencies that may be difficult to detect using a medical record alone.[96] Peabody and Luck also used USPs to judge quality, finding USPs were better than a medical record audit but not as robust as using clinical vignettes[97,98] (discussed further later in the chapter). Zabar and colleagues used USPs to study 11 primary care teams, finding the USPs were particularly good at capturing team and system performance as well as assessing physician–patient centeredness.[99] Another group has found USPs can detect errors in diagnostic reasoning, a serious quality and safety issue.[100,101] The primary challenges in using USPs are the cost and logistics of managing the visits and data feedback, which are significant and a reason why USPs may not represent a cost-effective strategy for routine assessment of physician performance or quality of care. The reader is encouraged to see Chapter 5 on for a more detailed discussion of USPs.

The Review Process

Understanding the basics of the measurement review (audit) process is crucial to maximize the utility of clinical data and medical records as tools for assessment. Because clinical practice reviews can be time consuming, you should not perform an audit until you are clear regarding the educational and assessment purposes. The PDSA (plan-do-study-act) quality improvement cycle was developed by Shewart over 60 years ago and highlights the critical importance of data at the plan and study phases.[102] Without such data, it is nearly impossible to determine "quality" of performance or to measure progress. As mentioned earlier, measuring performance using data from clinical practice, whether from the medical record or the other sources listed, is an essential component of the ACGME/ABMS competencies of Practice-based Learning and Improvement and Systems-based Practice and the CanMEDS Leader role.

The value of the review process is only as good as the information abstracted from the medical record. There are two main approaches: explicit review and implicit review. Medical record review in the past primarily depended on

• BOX 11.2 Example of a Process of Care Quality Measure for Diabetes Patients

Measure	Numerator	Denominator	Exclusions	Data source
Percentage of patients with 1 or more hemoglobin A1C tests	One or more hemoglobin A1C tests conducted during the measurement year identified by the appropriate CPT code, or at a minimum, documentation in the medical record must include a note indicating the date on which the Hgb A1C was performed and the result	A systematic sample of patients age 18-75 who had a diagnosis of either type 1 or 2 diabetes	Exclude patients with a history of polycystic ovaries, gestational diabetes, or steroid-induced diabetes during the measurement year	Visit, lab or pharmacy encounter data or claims; electronic data may be supplemented by medical record data

implicit review. In other words, an individual would review the chart for the quality of care and decisions without explicit criteria or standards ("Is this a good chart?" "Was this good care?"). Reviewers often used gestalt, or a general sense about the quality of the documentation, to judge the quality of a record. In medical education, implicit review without good criteria is still unfortunately commonly used for judging learners. This has gotten more difficult in the era of EMRs.

An explicit review approach uses detailed criteria (i.e., criterion referenced). In explicit reviews, the quality measures are carefully chosen and defined to be sure the measures can be assessed reliability and accurately, are generalizable across clinical sites, and can be aggregated for populations of patients. Likewise, the audit process is also carefully described with well-defined inclusion and exclusion criteria. Criteria for both the numerator and denominator of a measure are well defined. Box 11.2 provides an example of a quality measure from the US National Quality Forum (NQF).[103]

There are now extensive sets of standardized measures for many specialties, yet some specialties still lack sufficient numbers of meaningful measures. In the view of some, there may now be too many quality measures that are not used effectively.[104–106] For training programs, especially postgraduate residency and specialty fellowships, programs should be highly selective in the measures they use. The measures should align with the curriculum and assessment purpose. While quality measures are important, there are other aspects of care they do not capture effectively, such as diagnosis, that are essential to assess and improve in other ways.[104,106] As noted previously, it is also important to consider how well existing measures capture the important work of trainees, potentially opening up the need to develop more measures for this purpose when existing measures fall short.

As an example, primary care physicians will learn to care for patients with multiple chronic conditions such as diabetes, hypertension, asthma, and so on. To enable appropriate development in this important care activity (i.e., Entrustable Professional Activity [EPA]; see Chapter 1), the learner must first work in a clinical system that is functional (such as a patient-centered medical home) and designed to deliver high-value care. The measures chosen for audit must align with the curricular and clinical care goals (e.g., glycemic and blood pressure control; receipt of appropriate vaccines; effective use of asthma medications; etc.) (see Chapter 3). As with any assessment tool, using quality measures misaligned with needed competencies and curricula goals is counterproductive.

Advantages of Clinical Practice Review

As an assessment method, review of the clinical practice has a number of important strengths. Some form of clinical practice review should be part of every training program's assessment system. The specific advantages are described in the following subsections.

Availability

EMRs are available, but pulling out specific aspects of care may be a challenge. Partnership with informaticists and/or quality improvement scientists is likely foundational for most individuals unless they possess these skills. Electronic patient registries are best for creating population-based reports for specific quality process measures (such as for chronic conditions), but even the use of flow sheets and problem lists can greatly facilitate the collection and analysis of the quality of chronic care, prevention, et cetera.

Feedback

Clinical practice review allows for corrective feedback centered on actual clinical care in a timely manner. Too often faculty fail to take advantage of information obtained from the medical record for use in their assessment of and feedback to the trainee. In fact, the medical record can be used as a "guide" to query the resident about why they chose specific diagnostic or therapeutic approaches for the patient. One approach, chart-stimulated recall (CSR), is discussed in greater detail in Chapter 7.

Changing Clinical Behavior

The majority of studies have shown that clinical practice review can change trainee behavior through direct feedback such as report cards on performance of targeted clinical interventions (e.g., prevention), but the effects when using only audit as the intervention are modest.[107–110] One systematic review has also found positive effects of audit and feedback on clinical care for all developmental stages of physicians, but the effects tend to be modest overall.[7] Effects are more pronounced with physicians whose baseline performance is low. There are a number of reasons for the modest effect size of simply providing data only through audit. First and foremost, simply providing data does not equal feedback (see Chapter 14 on feedback). Table 11.1 provides a summary of recommendations on how to maximize the formative impact of medical record audit and quality measures.[110] These are well suited for the training environment.

For example medical record audits appear to be most effective when the data feedback is *resident* (or physician) specific and the data are provided back to the individual resident for their review. Data provided at the group level appear to be less effective; individuals looking at group data often remark, "I wish my colleagues would do a better job because I know I'm doing better than this!"[110,111] Finally, clinical practice review ideally should not be done in isolation from an intervention to improve quality and safety. For example, providing performance data around the quality of care provided to patients with chronic conditions such as diabetes, hypertension, and others should be part of an intervention/effort to improve the care for these patients.

Practicality

Clinical practice reviews can allow for a random or targeted selection of patients to be surveyed, and record reviews can be done without the patient physically being present. Furthermore, audits can be scheduled into clinical activities convenient for the training program and resident. Reviews can, and should, be done by the learners as part of their own self-directed assessment and learning, enhancing practicality for programs and faculty (discussed later in the chapter). Medical record reviews are an unobtrusive assessment tool that may help minimize the Hawthorne effect.

Evaluation of Clinical Reasoning

Depending on the quality of the documentation, evaluation of skills in analysis, interpretation, and management is possible. In addition, evaluations of particular patients or conditions can be performed over time and for many chronic conditions, and good evidence is available to develop key outcome and process metrics. Chapter 7 discusses how to use the medical record to assess clinical reasoning.

Reliability and Validity

When *explicit* criteria are used, a high degree of reliability is attainable. This includes such areas as appropriate use of laboratory studies, preventive health measures, medication and lab orders, cost-effectiveness, care of chronic illnesses such as diabetes, and quality of documentation. Explicit criteria are best suited for process of care measures (such as ordering a hemoglobin A1C on a diabetic patient within a certain time frame), and some outcomes that are easily measured and do not require substantial time (e.g., measuring the level of hemoglobin A1C as an intermediate outcome). Because the information contained in the record relates directly to actual patients, the results of clinical practice reviews are highly authentic. Medical records provide documentation of performance; that is, what a trainee actually does;[112] see Chapter 1). Some studies have found other validity evidence, such as relationship with other variables, indicating that results of quality of care audits modestly correlate with cognitive expertise as measured by a secure examination and/or certification status.[113–117] However, the amount of variance explained by high-stakes testing on clinical performance is quite modest, usually in the range of only 5% to 10%, indicating the critical importance of using work-based methods like clinical practice review to assess actual performance.[117] High-stakes tests are only modest proxies for clinical practice performance at best. Such high-stakes tests also have bias baked into them, whereas clinical performance measures are more objective; either they are performed and captured in the EMR or they are not.

Learning and Assessing by Doing

Medical record audits allow residents to directly participate in the process of peer review. Ashton[118] "made the case" for involving residents in hospital quality improvement programs nearly 30 years ago. Having the residents perform their own review may be even more powerful; one study involving resident self-audit found the majority of trainees were surprised by results demonstrating that they often failed to perform key quality indicators.[111] Studies with practicing physicians who used a web-based tool called a practice improvement module (PIM) that was part of the former maintenance of certification program in the United States, to self-audit their own practice found the process useful and discovered a number of areas where they were unexpectedly not performing well.[119] We call this the chagrin, or "aha" factor. The main power of self-audit is the trainee cannot "hide" from the results and cannot complain about the quality of the data or blame an abstractor for errors since they themselves entered most of the data and performed the audit. Several studies using self-audit as part of quality improvement initiatives did find improved care for patients.[84,110,111]

Teaching effective clinical practice review, such as medical record audit, is increasingly important. Many health systems, insurance companies, and national entities such Ministries of Health or the US Centers for Medicare & Medicaid Services (CMS) are increasingly conducting performance audits and reviews of physicians in their systems. Despite evidence of limited effectiveness, many national health systems provide quality data back to physicians as part of pay-for-performance schemes and learners will need to be prepared for this aspect of practice. Thus involving trainees in the clinical practice review is important for their future success.

TABLE 11.1 Improving the Effectiveness of Clinical Practice Review and Feedback

Suggested Implementation Strategy	Examples
Nature of the desired action/activity	
1. Recommend actions consistent with established goals and priorities in the institution and training program.	Consider feedback interventions that are consistent with existing priorities; investigate perceived need and salience of actions needed for current as well as future practice before providing feedback to learners.
2. Recommend actions or activities that can improve and are under the learner's control.	Measure baseline performance before providing feedback; establish that the action is under the learner's control (e.g., ordering and counseling about starting a new medication).
3. Recommend specific actions and/or activities.	Include functionality for corrective actions (e.g., coaching or other skill building) along with feedback; require learner-generated if-then plans to overcome barriers to target action.
Nature of the data available for feedback	
4. Provide multiple instances of feedback.	Replace one-off feedback with regular feedback. Clinical practice review should be longitudinal and ongoing throughout the entire training program.
5. Provide feedback as soon as possible and at a frequency informed by the number of new patient cases.	Increase frequency/decrease interval of feedback for outcomes with many patient cases. Quality dashboards can be potentially useful here by providing ongoing access to meaningful practice data.
6. Provide individual rather than general data.	Provide learner-specific rather than hospital-specific data. While it may be hard to attribute the quality of care to a single learner, individualized data are more powerful and likely to generate behavior change.
7. Choose comparators that reinforce desired behavior change.	Choose 1 comparator rather than several. For example, using a criterion-referenced standard, such as the achievable benchmark of care, or national norms, can be helpful.
Feedback display	
1. Closely link the visual display and summary message.	Put the summary message in close proximity to the graphical or numerical data supporting it.
2. Provide feedback in more than one way.	Present key messages textually and numerically; provide graphic elements that mirror key recommendations (e.g., clinical guidelines).
3. Minimize extraneous cognitive load for feedback recipients.	Eliminate unnecessary 3D graphical elements, increase white space, clarify instructions, and target fewer outcomes. In other words, "less is more."
Delivering the feedback intervention	
1. Address barriers to feedback use.	Assess barriers before feedback provision, incorporate feedback into care pathway rather than providing it outside of care. See Chapter 14 on feedback.
2. Provide short, actionable messages followed by optional detail.	Put key messages/variables on front page, make additional detail available for users to explore. Providing learners with links to clinical decision support may also be helpful.
3. Address the credibility of the information.	Ensure that feedback comes from a trusted local champion or colleague rather than the research team, increase transparency of data sources, disclose conflicts of interest. This is also where self-review/audit by the learner can be especially helpful as it is hard to "run from your own data" if you have honestly abstracted it.
4. Prevent defensive reactions to feedback.	Guide reflection, include positive messaging along with negative, conduct "feed-forward" discussions. See Chapter 13 on specific strategies for delivering feedback and dealing with the defensive learner.
5. Construct feedback through social interaction.	Encourage self-assessment around target behaviors before receiving feedback, allow user to respond to feedback, engage in dialogue with peers as feedback is provided, engage in facilitated conversations/coaching about the feedback. This can be facilitated when all learners are involved in clinical practice review and use the information collaboratively to improve care within the training setting.

Adapted from Brehaut JC, Colquhoun HL, Eva KW, et al. Practice feedback interventions: 15 suggestions for optimizing effectiveness. *Ann Intern Med*. 2016 Mar 15;164:435-441. doi:10.7326/M15-2248.

Practice-Based Learning and Improvement 2: Reflective Practice and Commitment to Personal Growth				
Level 1	Level 2	Level 3	Level 4	Level 5
Accepts responsibility for personal and professional development by establishing goals	Demonstrates openness to performance data (feedback and other input) to inform goals	Seeks performance data episodically, with adaptability, and humility	Seeks performance data consistently with adaptability, and humility	Models consistently seeking performance data with adaptability and humility
Identifies the factors that contribute to gap(s) between ideal and actual performance, with guidance	Analyzes and reflects on the factors which contribute to gap(s) between ideal and actual performance, with guidance	Institutes behavioral change(s) to narrow the gap(s) between ideal and actual performance	Challenges one's own assumptions and considers alternatives in narrowing the gap(s) between ideal and actual performance	Coaches others on reflective practice
	Actively seeks opportunities to improve	Designs and implements an individualized learning plan, with prompting	Independently creates and implements an individualized learning plan	Uses performance data to measure the effectiveness of the individualized learning plan and when necessary, improves it
Comments:				Not Yet Completed Level 1

• **Fig. 11.5** Example of a reflective practice Subcompetency Milestone.

Self-Assessment and Reflection

When the learner is incorporated into the review process, the result can be a powerful tool to promote self-assessment, self-regulated learning, and reflection. Given what was stated earleir about public reporting and continual assessment, physicians-in-training must be prepared to effectively self-assess their performance using practice data, reflect accurately on the results, and then use the results for continuous professional development and quality improvement.[120–122] Self-directed assessment also aligns well with the important principles from self-regulated learning of maximizing intrinsic motivation and giving the learner more control/autonomy over their own assessment of their clinical practice;[123] see Chapter 14). Reflective practice is now a specific subcompetency for the GME training programs in the United States and several other countries (Fig. 11.5).

Clinical practice review can be a very useful educational tool, can potentially change behavior, and can provide useful information when explicit criteria for review are utilized. Such reviews can be tracked and included as part of a comprehensive clinical competency record and can be easily incorporated into a portfolio (see Chapter 16). Finally, the result of a clinical practice review across multiple learners provides valuable information for the evaluation of program effectiveness. In one national study, substantial deficiencies in care for older adults were found across a large number of quality indicators in internal medicine and family medicine residencies.[124] A recent study within a single US healthcare system found variation in performance using ambulatory preventive care measures in eight primary care residency programs.[125,126] This variation abounds in medical education programs, and a substantial proportion of this variation in care is unwarranted and not grounded in evidence-based practice.[127]

All these studies highlight the importance of a program that understands how effectively it is providing care at the individual learner, program, and institutional levels. Clinical practice reviews can identify strengths and weaknesses in the actual care delivered to patients that should play a major role in program assessment and curriculum design. Some would argue that clinical training is only as good as the quality of the care given to patients. Multiple studies provide compelling evidence that this is true. Asch and colleagues found strong correlations between the quality of care practicing obstetricians provided and the quality of care at the level of the hospital where they had trained. The relative risk difference between the bottom and top quintiles of major obstetrical complications was 32%.[21,22] This association was found to persist for over 15 years after the physician graduated from the residency. Bansal and colleagues found a similar pattern for surgical complications among general surgeons.[23] Chen and colleagues found the same pattern with regard to cost of care and appropriately conservative management: residents who trained in high-cost/high resource-utilizing hospitals became higher physicians in practice even if they work in a lower spending system.[13] Smith and colleagues found an association of major complications in endovascular aneurysm repair (EVAR) among early-career vascular surgeons and where they trained.[93] The bottom line is that training programs need to use quality performance data to help individual learners, the program, and the clinical institution continually improve care. Clinical practice reviews can be used to assess the effectiveness of integrating educational and clinical care interventions in the training setting.

Potential Disadvantages of Clinical Practice Reviews

Despite the tradition of using the medical record as a tool for assessment of clinical competence, the lack of good research using trainees' medical records for education and assessment is still not as robust as needed and much work remains to be done. First, whereas the organizational format used for creating a medical admission or progress note has received a lot of attention in medical school, the same scrutiny seems to evaporate at the residency and fellowship levels. The biggest change has been the introduction of the EMR that has led to documentation akin to deciphering hieroglyphics. Many EMRs use a templating function that allows trainees to simply check a series of boxes (especially common in emergency department notes), which produces a disjointed summary of the patient's history, physical examination, assessment, and management. The thought processes involved in the decisions are very difficult to interpret or infer. Add to this situation the different EMR vendors all using different organizational formats involving various combinations of templates, checklists, and free text. This world has created a whole host of new problems for medical educators. However, this can be curbed moving forward by emphasizing the importance of strong medical decision-making documentation, which is arguably the most important piece of patient care notes and almost certainly the best place to focus for assessing trainee abilities and helping them continue to learn and improve.

Another persistent serious documentation problem is the "cut and paste" syndrome where learners cut and paste previous notes for use in admission and daily progress notes, with or without adequate editing. In one of our previous hospital's internal quality improvement activity, we noted this was a common activity for "efficiently" completing daily progress notes. However, unless we've moved into a new time dimension, it is hard to believe a patient was "post-operation day 1" for 7 consecutive days. In a study examining notes in an intensive care unit, both attendings and residents frequently copied information from previous notes.[128,129] The Joint Commission has recognized this as a safety issue and provided guidance on the risks and appropriate use of "cut and paste."[130] The American Health Information Management Association (AHIMA) has listed the risks of cut and paste:[131]

- Inaccurate or outdated information
- Redundant information, which makes it difficult to identify the current information
- Inability to identify the author or intent of documentation
- Inability to identify when the documentation was first created
- Propagation of false information
- Internally inconsistent progress notes
- Unnecessarily lengthy progress notes

Educators should be particularly sensitive to this practice and should consider the monitoring of cut and paste as a safety and educational issue well suited for review and audit. We posit copy and paste actions are flags for a lack of conscientiousness, raising potential concerns about trustworthiness.[132,133]

Quality of the Documentation

Part of the quality of a medical record audit hinges on the quality of the documentation. When trying to assess more than whether certain processes of care were or were not delivered, important questions to ask yourself (or what the trainee should be asking of themselves) are:

- Does the record accurately reflect what occurred during the visit?
- Was all the pertinent information collected during the patient encounter recorded? Does the EMR effectively and accurately capture key and appropriate aspects of care?
- Are impressions and plans justified in the record? Does the EMR allow for meaningful and efficient entry of free text to better describe the complexity of the patient's condition(s)?
- What facilitating tools (e.g., templates, problem lists, flowcharts, etc.) are provided with the medical record? How do you prepare and train your learners to use these tools?

These considerations underscore findings of Schumacher's RSQM work. These measures often focus on elements of documentation and use of facilitating tools, most notably order sets in the RSQM work.[67,68] While we noted earlier that part of the quality of a medical record audit hinges on the quality of documentation, RSQM work actually highlights the importance of missing documentation that is deemed critical as a measure of performance and feedback from trainees. In fact, clinical competency committee (CCC) members in a study by Schumacher and colleagues found that lack of expected aspects of documentation was "sticky," or adhered to their minds as a red flag, for them.[134]

One study investigated use of the IDEA framework to judge the quality of student admission notes. IDEA stands for interpretive summary, differential diagnosis, explanation of reasoning, and alternatives. Using a 15-item instrument, the investigators found moderate reliability and correlation with final clerkship grades.[135] These types of tools deserve further study given the critical importance of the medical record as a communication between and for interprofessional team members and patients.

While we have highlighted the importance of appropriate and expected documentation, we must also note that a "good chart" does not necessarily equal "good care." For example, the chart may have a checkbox for smoking cessation counseling, but such a "check" does not provide much information about what was covered in the counseling session and how well the counseling was performed—this requires direct observation (see Chapter 5). More work is needed on examining the impact of quality charting with patient outcomes, especially in the era of EMRs. This may be especially important in an era where patient care is often fragmented among a number of doctors who still "communicate" diagnostic and therapeutic choices through written records that include letters and email due to lack of interoperability between EMRs. Lack of continuity is an especially pressing problem for GME training programs that move their learners between multiple training sites. These studies raise questions as to the best combination of methods to measure both learners and program performance regarding quality of care.

Process Versus Outcomes

Clinical practice reviews are a reasonably good method to determine whether specific processes of care have been performed, especially when explicit criteria are defined. However, the utility of using the medical record to determine causation for patient outcomes is very limited. Most often an intermediate outcome is used, such as blood pressure, hemoglobin A1C level, or absence of a postsurgical complication. Systematic approaches to reviewing critical incidents, such as RCAs,[43,102,136] will use information from the medical record. While it is very difficult and in many cases inappropriate to attribute patient outcomes such as infections, complications, functional status, other morbidities, and even death to the actions and decisions of single learners in most circumstances, a more helpful framework is to explore the *contribution* of the learner, especially those in GME programs, to the outcomes in the context of the system and interprofessional team. For example, Graber and colleagues found that most adverse events resulted from a combination of individual errors (e.g., poor data gathering and faulty synthesis of information) and system factors (e.g., interprofessional breakdowns, poor handoffs, lack of appropriate alerts).[137] RCA is an effective method to explore adverse events.

While this focus on the trainee's role in the team and system is important because care is ultimately provided by teams working in systems, we also believe maintaining a focus on individuals and what can be attributed to them is important as well. We graduate, credential, and certify individuals. This is unlikely to change soon, if ever. Therefore we need ways to pull individuals out from teams even if this means the best measures we have for this are process ones that should lead to good outcomes but may not in all instances.[138]

Assessment of Clinical Judgment

Resident analytic and integrative skills can only partially be assessed through record review, especially when one considers the problems in the quality of documentation. Furthermore, is the physician's judgment adequately recorded on the record? Did that judgment translate into an appropriate management plan? Gennis and Gennis[139] found in an older study that when a separate attending physician evaluated a patient independent from the resident, the faculty attending's recommendations for care management were different in nearly 33% of the resident's patients. A similar study in a military outpatient training clinic found a similar frequency of differences between attending and resident management decisions but the differences were less dramatic and the majority of the recommended changes from faculty were minor.[140] These two older studies raise significant questions about the ability to accurately assess the appropriateness of management plans from medical record review. These studies and other chapters in this book (see Chapters 3 and 5) reinforce the importance of direct observation around clinical skills and reasoning and the need to combine different types of assessments to judge clinical competence most effectively.

Time and Quantity of Review

Clinical practice review can be very time consuming, especially if you decide to use medical record reviews for high-stakes decisions, something not supported by existing literature in the medical education space. First and foremost, you can only assign attribution for quality and safety measures to individual learners for some things given supervising physicians and others are involved (or should be). Second, researchers working with practicing physicians have found that at least 25 to 35 patient medical records are required for defensible pass/fail decisions for a single condition (e.g., diabetes) in provider recognition programs[141] and there may often be insufficient numbers of encounters at the level of individual trainees to make such defensible high-stakes decisions, potentially even if taken as part of a complete program of assessment where several types and sources of data are being used. A recent study found that some evidence-based primary care measures were reliable at the level of the individual resident, but functioned better overall at the level of the training program.[126] However, the use of composite measures (composites) has been found to enhance reliability and have validity around individual physician performance.[117,141] The problem is still the number of patients needed with specific conditions, the presence of analysts who can perform the statistical calculations using composite methodology, and whether there is sufficient added value in using composites in the training setting. For those specialties who care for patients with multiple chronic conditions, such as general practice, family medicine, and internal medicine, there may be some value in using composites with residents and senior house officers, especially if they will be held accountable for composite performance in their future practice.

Clinical practice review also requires the development and testing of abstraction instruments, data collection and entry, data analysis, and dissemination of the results to individual residents. If you are fortunate enough to work with a functional EMR, our suggestion is to work with your information technology experts to see how much of this process can be automated. Even if they can only export the data into a spreadsheet, you have at least organized data for basic analyses. It is advisable to use standardized abstraction tools and quality measures already developed and field-tested whenever possible. This is increasingly becoming the standard across the globe for many specialties, but in all honesty much work remains to be done. Several authors have commented on the lack of alignment of many measures in the United States, with too many duplicate measures. In the United States, there is actually a web-based clearinghouse for quality measures supported by the Agency for Healthcare Research and Quality (AHRQ).[142] If you or your hospital/clinic is not currently using quality measures/indicators in your program, this is a good place to start to examine potential measures you might use in your specialty. The NQF systematically endorses quality measures; approved measures can be downloaded from the organization's website.[143] However, these measures often focus on teams and systems, and even when they focus on individuals they often do not apply to trainees very well or at all. Using existing well-defined measures and abstraction tools can save training programs substantial time. Second, strongly consider having the learners perform the actual clinical practice review. Not only does this save time for faculty and programs, but, as previously discussed, the self-audit experience is valuable for the trainee.[68,124,144]

Cost

There may be a cost charged by your institution's information technology department to pull EMR data specific to learners. Cost can also be a factor if you use faculty or other administrative personnel to perform manual abstraction. For faculty, the usual cost is their time. If you use other abstractors, there may be a monetary fee for their services. Because patients will often interact with many learners, especially in the inpatient setting, it can be very difficult to determine who is the patient's primary resident. There are some simple algorithms that can be used (such as the number of encounters with a particular physician), but if the EMR allows for "assignment" of a learner to a patient, that is the ideal situation.[73] Schumacher and colleagues were able to create a reliable algorithm in their program to pull resident-specific EMR data.[145] We recommend talking with your information services department to see what they might be able to do for you locally.[73]

Faculty Development

Few faculty have extensive experience with clinical practice review[19] or knowledge of patient safety and quality improvement science. There are several key issues around faculty development: quality of clinical documentation, abstraction skills (when needed), interpretation of the data, and use of the data for improvement purposes. Many faculty exhibit the same behaviors as learners when documenting the results of their own medical encounters. Your first priority should be to train your faculty in the optimal use of the medical record at your institution. Second, reliable and accurate abstraction is a skill in itself, and most faculty have little experience if a manual abstraction is required. While we do not advocate that faculty be the primary source for abstraction services, faculty do need to understand how to conduct a proper quality review, including how to use an abstraction manual, how to properly interpret the specifications of quality measures, and how to use the data for feedback (see Table 11.1) and quality improvement. Faculty must know how to interpret the results of a clinical practice review to help learners improve. For example, what should a faculty member tell a learner whose "quality report" shows poor compliance with several quality measures? Appendix 11.1 provides a list of resources around quality improvement and patient safety training. In addition, Chapter 13 provides a wonderful feedback model to use with clinical performance data.

Table 11.2 summarizes some of the key limitations of clinical practice review with possible solutions.

Assessing Abilities in Quality Improvement and Patient Safety

Up to this point in the chapter, we have primarily focused on clinical practice performance data as a form of assessment of learners. The strengths of this approach are (1) it targets the "does" level of Miller's pyramid (Chapter 1); (2) it is highly authentic as it represents the quality and safety of care provided to patients; and (3) it is a critical component of acquiring abilities in QIPS. While it is beyond the scope of this chapter and textbook to discuss curricular approaches (see Appendix 11.1 for suggestions), assessing learners' abilities in QIPS is important.

Quality Improvement Knowledge Application Tool

Ogrinc and colleagues produced a useful framework on the abilities needed by graduates of postgraduate training programs that has stood the test of time.[43,56] The key domains of specific abilities in QIPS are (1) describe the issue; (2) build a team; (3) define the problem; (4) choose a target (of the improvement); (5) test the change; and (6) extend improvement efforts.[43,56] Hess and colleagues used this framework to create a self-assessment needs survey training program that can be used with learners prior to initiating a new curriculum or QIPS project.[147] As you will see in the following text, much of this framework is reflected in the various assessment tools discussed in this section. We provide a few tools that can be helpful to medical educators in assessing the QIPS abilities of their learners.

The Quality Improvement Knowledge Application Tool (QIKAT) uses a series of vignettes to assess learners' ability

TABLE 11.2 Summary of Medical Record Audit (MRA) Limitations

Limitation	Possible Solutions
Quality of documentation	▪ Use problem lists and flowcharts for chronic conditions and preventive care. ▪ Use templates for medical history and physical examination. ▪ Use the electronic medical record (may or may not improve documentation; training required in effective use of EMRs). ▪ Combine the MRA with direct observation or patient interviews (to supplement information in the medical record).
Time	▪ Have trainees perform an audit of their own charts and/or their peers. ▪ Seek assistance from the hospital or clinic quality improvement department to generate performance reports, especially if you have an EMR. ▪ Use other healthcare personnel (if available).
Implicit review	▪ In general, avoid unstructured implicit review (i.e., "is this a good chart of not"). ▪ Provide a minimal framework (e.g., IDEA framework) for medical record review and do not rely solely on the judgment of the reviewer. ▪ Use explicit criteria whenever possible as well as auditor training and quality monitoring/feedback.
Cost	▪ Have trainees perform an audit of their own charts and/or their peers'. ▪ Use existing reports, when available, from quality improvement departments.
Assessing clinical judgment	▪ Combine the MRA with chart-stimulated recall.

MRA, medical record audit.

to create an aim statement, choose appropriate measures, and develop a change intervention likely to lead to improvement.[148] The learner writes their responses to these three questions and the responses are assessed using a rubric. This is an excellent tool to assess "knows how" in developing a QI intervention based on the model for improvement.[102]

A3 Problem-Solving Assessment Tool

A3 problem-solving is an important aspect of the Lean approach to quality improvement. Myers and colleagues created a tool to assess a QIPS project before implementation (i.e., "shows how" on Miller's pyramid; see Chapter 1). The tool contains 23 items across six domains: (1) background, (2) current situation, (3) goal, (4) analysis, (5) countermeasures, and (6) action plan. This tool was developed using an iterative process, and reliability (as measured by intraclass correlation) was excellent across all domains.[149] The original article comes with a robust appendix on how to best use the tool and can be downloaded online[149]

Quality Improvement Project Evaluation Rubric

The Quality Improvement Project Evaluation Rubric (QIPER) tool assesses ability in designing ("shows how"), and implementing, analyzing results of, and reporting on a QI/PS project (the "does" level Miller's pyramid). The QIPER contains 19 items across six domains: (1) definition of the problem; (2) project design; (3) QIPS intervention; (4) data collection and analysis; (5) results; and (6) conclusions and implications. One limitation of the tool is the use of a normative scale (below expectations to exceeds expectations). Each gradation on the 4-point scale does come with a brief description, but use of the tool requires understanding and some expertise in QIPS. The primary focus of this instrument is to judge oral presentations of QIPS projects once they are complete.[150]

Multidomain Assessment of Quality Improvement Projects

Multidomain Assessment of Quality Improvement Projects (MAQIP) is a nine-item instrument that can be used to assess QIPS projects at various stages; unlike the QIPER, which is mostly designed to judge a QIPS project at the end. The MAQIP's domains are (1) problem identification, (2) objective, (3) population, (4) stakeholders, (5) change, (6) measures, (7) data analysis, (8) project evaluation, and (9) sustained improvement. Reliability, as measured by intraclass correlation, is reasonable for all but the project evaluation and sustained improvement phases. The MAQIP is probably most useful as a formative tool for learners involved in QIPS projects.[151] Finally, multiple quality improvement tools and resources are available as part of the Institute for Healthcare Improvement QI toolkit.[152]

Conclusion

Clinical practice review, from multiple potential sources such as the medical record, claims data, and registries, can be a valuable tool to assess clinical competence. Given the critical importance of performance data for quality improvement and the competencies of Practice-based Learning and Improvement and Systems-based Practice in the United States and the Leader role in CanMEDS, all learners should receive individual performance data at a minimum during residency training and clinical practice review should be a core part of any learner's program of assessment. Medical records are readily accessible, allow the examination of a potentially large number of clinical encounters, and authentically assess what the learner actually does in caring for patients in a relatively unobtrusive manner. When explicit criteria and endpoints are used, important information about practice habits in specific areas of care (i.e., preventive health) is possible. EMRs, claims databases, and registries can provide a wealth of accessible information in a timely and ongoing manner.

Involving trainees in clinical practice review and QIPS projects and initiatives is imperative. This promotes self-directed assessment and reflection and is highly consistent with the principles of self-regulated learning. Furthermore, physicians will experience substantial scrutiny of the quality of care they provide from multiple organizations and stakeholders over the course of their careers. Physicians will need a good understanding of audit methodology, and clinical practice review remains a cornerstone of most audit programs.

Acknowledgment

The authors wish to thank Dr. Daniel Duffy for his contributions to previous editions of this chapter.

Annotated Bibliography

1. Ivers N, Jamtvedt G, Flottorp S, et al. Audit and feedback: effects on professional practice and healthcare outcomes. *Cochrane Database Syst Rev.* 2012 Jun 13(6):CD000259. doi:10.1002/14651858.CD000259.pub3.
   This Cochrane review is the gold standard of reviews on the impact of audit and feedback. This review shows that the impact of this approach to improve quality is modest. For example, the authors found a 4.3% absolute increase in compliance with desired practice, although physicians with lower quality scores saw higher levels of improvement in their practice after feedback. One hypothesis for the modest outcome is inadequate attention to how audit and feedback are implemented, an important issue for all medical educators. We would recommend educators read the executive summary of this systematic review.
2. Brehaut JC, Colquhoun HL, Eva KW, et al. Practice feedback interventions: 15 suggestions for optimizing effectiveness. *Ann Intern Med.* 2016 Mar 15;164(6):435–441. doi:10.7326/M15-2248.
   This important article addresses the finding that clinical practice review and feedback alone are insufficient to promote substantial practice change. In this article the authors, using educational theory and some empiric evidence, provide 15 recommendations to enhance the effectiveness of clinical practice review that can be useful to medical educators implementing quality and safety reviews.
3. Ogrinc GS, Headrick LA, Barton AJ, et al. *Fundamentals of Health Care Improvement: A Guide to Improving Your Patients' Care.* 4th ed. Joint Commission Resources and Institute for Healthcare Improvement; 2022.
   This is a really useful basic textbook on QIPS and a good place to start for teachers just beginning work on curriculum and assessment.
4. Singh MK, Ogrinc G, Cox KR, et al. The Quality Improvement Knowledge Application Tool Revised (QIKAT-R). *Acad Med.* 2014 Oct;89(10):1386–1391. doi:10.1097/ACM.0000000000000456.
   The QIKAT is a very useful tool to assess the "knows how" and "shows how" levels of Miller's pyramid in developing the initial stages of a quality improvement project. The QIKAT-R uses a series of vignettes as the stimulus to create a project aim statement, choose appropriate measures, and choose an intervention to address the specific quality issue in the vignette.
5. Institute for Healthcare Improvement (IHI). Quality Improvement Essentials Toolkit. Accessed March 21, 2023. https://www.ihi.org/resources/Pages/Tools/Quality-Improvement-Essentials-Toolkit.aspx.
   The IHI is a wonderful resource for QIPS tools and guidance. You will need to create an account to access this Essentials Toolkit.

References

1. Institute of Medicine. *To Err is Human.* National Academy Press; 1991.
2. Institute of Medicine. *Crossing the Quality Chasm.* National Academy Press; 2001.
3. Landrigan CP, Parry GJ, Bones CB, Hackbarth AD, Goldmann DA, Sharek PJ. Temporal trends in rates of patient harm resulting from medical care. *N Engl J Med.* 2010 Nov 25;363(22):2124–2134. doi:10.1056/NEJMsa1004404.
4. National Patient Safety Foundation. Free from Harm: Accelerating Patient Safety Improvement Fifteen Years after To Err Is Human. Accessed March 20, 2023. https://www.ihi.org/resources/Pages/Publications/Free-from-Harm-Accelerating-Patient-Safety-Improvement.aspx.
5. Commonwealth Fund. 2020 International Profiles of Health Care Systems. Tikkanen R, Osborn R, Mossialos E, Djordjevic A, Wharton G, eds. Accessed March 19, 2023. https://www.commonwealthfund.org/sites/default/files/2020-12/International_Profiles_of_Health_Care_Systems_Dec2020.pdf.
6. World Health Organization. *World health statistics 2022: monitoring health for the SDGs, sustainable development goals.* Geneva: World Health Organization; 2022 License: CC BY-NC-SA 3.0 IGO. Accessed March 19, 2023. 9789240051140-eng.pdf.
7. Hill L, Ndugga N, Artiga S. Key data on health and health care by race and ethnicity. Kaiser Family Foundation. Accessed March 19, 2023. https://www.kff.org/racial-equity-and-health-policy/report/key-data-on-health-and-health-care-by-race-and-ethnicity/#:~:text=At%20birth%2C%20AIAN%20and%20Black,people%20between%202019%20and%202021.
8. World Health Organization. Global excess deaths associated with COVID-19, January 2020 to December 2021. Accessed March 19, 2023. https://www.who.int/data/stories/global-excess-deaths-associated-with-covid-19-january-2020-december-2021#:~:text=The%20global%20excess%20mortality%20associated,directly%20attributable%20to%20COVID%2D19.
9. The Economist. The pandemic's true death toll. Accessed March 19, 2023. https://www.economist.com/graphic-detail/coronavirus-excess-deaths-estimates.
10. Asch DA, Nicholson S, Srinivas S, Herrin J, Epstein AJ. Evaluating obstetrical residency programs using patient outcomes. *JAMA.* 2009 Sep 23;302(12):1277–1283. doi:10.1001/jama.2009.1356.

11. Epstein AJ, Srinivas SK, Nicholson S, Herrin J, Asch DA. Association between physicians' experience after training and maternal obstetrical outcomes: Cohort study. *BMJ*. 2013 Mar 28;346:f1596. doi:10.1136/bmj.f1596.
12. Bansal N, Simmons KD, Epstein AJ, Morris JB, Kelz RR. Using patient outcomes to evaluate general surgery residency program performance. *JAMA Surg*. 2016 Feb;151(2):111–119. doi:10.1001/jamasurg.2015.3637.
13. Chen C, Petterson S, Phillips R, Bazemore A, Mullan F. Spending patterns in region of residency training and subsequent expenditures for care provided by practicing physicians for Medicare beneficiaries. *JAMA*. 2014 Dec 10;312(22):2385–2393. doi:10.1001/jama.2014.15973.
14. Crosson FJ, Leu J, Roemer BM, Ross MN. Gaps in residency training should be addressed to better prepare doctors for a twenty-first-century delivery system. *Health Aff (Millwood)*. 2011 Nov;30(11):2412–2418. doi:10.1377/hlthaff.2011.0184.
15. Schumacher DJ, West DC, Schwartz A, et al. Longitudinal assessment of resident performance using Entrustable Professional Activities. *JAMA Netw Open*. 2020 Jan 3;3(1):e1919316. doi:10.1001/jamanetworkopen.2019.19316.
16. Lau BD, Streiff MB, Pronovost PJ, Haider AH, Efron DT, Haut ER. Attending physician performance measure scores and resident physicians' ordering practices. *JAMA Surg*. 2015;150(8):813–814. doi:10.1001/jamasurg.2015.0891.
17. Scott A, Sivey P, Ait Ouakrim D, et al. The effect of financial incentives on the quality of health care provided by primary care physicians. *Cochrane Database Syst Rev*. 2011 Sep 7(9):CD008451. doi:10.1002/14651858.CD008451.pub2.
18. Torgan C. Patient outcomes improved by pay-for-performance. Accessed March 23, 2023. https://www.nih.gov/news-events/nih-research-matters/patient-outcomes-improved-pay-performance#:~:text=One%20new%20health%20care%20model,amount%20regardless%20of%20patient%20outcomes.
19. Batalden P, Leach D, Swing S, Dreyfus H, Dreyfus S. General competencies and accreditation in graduate medical education. *Health Aff*. 2002 Sep-Oct;21(5):103–111. doi:10.1377/hlthaff.21.5.103.
20. Royal College of Physicians and Surgeons of Canada. CanMEDS: Better standards, better physicians, better care. Accessed March 19, 2023. https://www.royalcollege.ca/ca/en/canmeds/canmeds-framework.html
21. Gonzalo JD, Dekhtyar M, Starr SR, et al. Health systems science curricula in undergraduate medical education: identifying and defining a potential curricular framework. *Acad Med*. 2017 Jan;92(1):123–131. doi:10.1097/ACM.0000000000001177.
22. Gonzalo J, Hamilton M, DeWaters AL, et al. Implementation and evaluation of an interprofessional health systems science professional development program. *Acad Med*. 2023 Jun 1;98(6):703–708. doi:10.1097/ACM.0000000000005144.
23. Borkan JM, Hammoud MM, Nelson E, et al. Health systems science education: the new post-Flexner professionalism for the 21st century. *Med Teach*. 2021 Jul;43(sup2):S25–S31. doi:10.1080/0142159X.2021.1924366.
24. Blank L, Kimball H, McDonald W, Merino J. Medical professionalism in the new millennium: a physician charter 15 months later. *Ann Int Med*. 2003 May 20;138(10):839–841. doi:10.7326/0003-4819-138-10-200305200-00012.
25. Becher EC, Chassin MR. taking health care back: the physician's role in quality improvement. *Acad Med*. 2002 Oct;77(10):953–962. doi:10.1097/00001888-200210000-00005.
26. Brennan TA. Physicians' professional responsibility to improve the quality of care. *Acad Med*. 2002 Oct;77(10):973–980. doi:10.1097/00001888-200210000-00008.
27. Goode LD, Clancy CM, Kimball HR, Meyer G, Eisenberg JM. when is "good enough"? The role and responsibility of physicians to improve patient safety. *Acad Med*. 2002 Oct;77(10):947–952. doi:10.1097/00001888-200210000-00004.
28. Gruen RL, Pearson SD, Brennan TA. Physician-citizens-public roles and professional obligations. *JAMA*. 2004 Jan 7;291(1):94–98. doi:10.1001/jama.291.1.94.
29. Holmboe E, Bernabeo E. The 'special obligations' of the modern Hippocratic Oath for 21st century medicine. *Med Educ*. 2014 Jan;48(1):87–94. doi:10.1111/medu.12365.
30. Institute of Medicine. *Educating Health Professionals: A Bridge to Quality*. National Academy Press; 2003.
31. Interprofessional Education Collaborative. Core competencies for interprofessional collaborative practice. 2016. at IPEC Core Competencies (ipecollaborative.org). Accessed March 20, 2023. https://www.ipecollaborative.org/ipec-core-competencies.
32. Edgar L, McLean S, Hogan SO, Hamstra S, Holmboe ES. The Milestones Guidebook. 2020. Accessed March 19, 2023. https://www.acgme.org/globalassets/milestonesguidebook.pdf
33. Institute for Healthcare Improvement. The IHI Open School. Accessed March 20, 2023. www.ihi.org/education/ihiopenschool/Pages/default.aspx
34. Wong BM, Holmboe ES. Transforming the academic faculty perspective in graduate medical education to better align educational and clinical outcomes. *Acad Med*. 2016 Apr;91(4):473–479. doi:10.1097/ACM.0000000000001035.
35. Batalden PB, Nelson EC, Edwards WH, Godfrey MM, Mohr JJ. Microsystems in healthcare. Part 9: developing small clinical units to attain peak performance. *Jt Comm J Qual Safety*. 2003 Nov;29(11):575–585. doi:10.1016/s1549-3741(03)29068-7.
36. Nelson EC, Batalden PB, Huber TP, et al. Microsystems in healthcare. Part 1: learning from high performing front-line clinical units. *Jt Comm J Qual Safety*. 2002 Sep;28(9):472–493. doi:10.1016/s1070-3241(02)28051-7.
37. Nelson EC, Batalden PB, Godfrey MM. *Quality by Design: A Clinical Microsystems Approach*. Jossey-Bass; 2007.
38. Grumbach K, Bodenheimer T. A primary care home for Americans: putting the house in order. *JAMA*. 2002 Aug 21;288(7):889–893. doi:10.1001/jama.288.7.889.
39. Patient Centered Primary Care Collaborative. Defining the medical home. Accessed March 20, 2023. https://www.pcpcc.org/about/medical-home
40. Jackson GL, Powers BJ, Chatterjee R, et al. Improving patient care. The patient centered medical home. A systematic review. *Ann Intern Med*. 2013 Feb 5;158(3):169–178. doi:10.7326/0003-4819-158-3-201302050-00579.
41. Saynisch PA, David G, Ukert B, Agiro A, Scholle SH, Oberlander T. Model homes: evaluating approaches to patient-centered medical home implementation. *Med Care*. 2021 Mar 1;59(3):206–212. doi:10.1097/MLR.0000000000001497.
42. Budgen J, Cantiello J. Advantages and disadvantages of the patient-centered medical home: a critical analysis and lessons learned. *Health Care Manag (Frederick)*. 2017 Oct/Dec;36(4):357–363. doi:10.1097/HCM.0000000000000178.
43. Ogrinc GS, Headrick LA, Barton AJ, et al. *Fundamentals of Health Care Improvement: A Guide to Improving Your Patients' Care*. 4th ed. Joint Commission Resources and Institute for Healthcare Improvement; 2022.

44. Wagner EH, Austin BT, Von Korff M. Organizing care for patients with chronic illness. *Milbank Q.* 1996;74:511–542. PMID: 8941260.
45. Von Korff M, Gruman J, Schaefer J, Curry SJ, Wagner EH. Collaborative management of chronic illness. *Ann Intern Med.* 1997 Dec 15;127(12):1097–1102. doi:10.7326/0003-4819-127-12-199712150-00008.
46. Batalden M, Batalden P, Margolis P, et al. Coproduction of healthcare service. *BMJ Qual Saf.* 2016 Jul;25(7):509–517. doi:10.1136/bmjqs-2015-004315.
47. Berwick DM, Nolan TW, Whittington J. The triple aim: care, health, and cost. *Health Aff.* 2008 May-Jun;27(3):759–769. doi:10.1377/hlthaff.27.3.759.
48. Bodenheimer T, Sinsky C. From triple to quadruple aim: care of the patient requires care of the provider. *Ann Fam Med.* 2014 Nov-Dec;12(6):573–576. doi:10.1370/afm.1713.
49. Nundy S, Cooper LA, Mate KS. The quintuple aim for health care improvement: a new imperative to advance health equity. *JAMA.* 2022 Feb 8;327(6):521–522. doi:10.1001/jama.2021.25181.
50. Demming WE. *The New Economics For Industry, Government, Education.* 2nd ed. MIT Press; 1994:92–115.
51. ABIM Foundation. Choosing Wisely. Accessed March 20, 2023. www.choosingwisely.org/
52. Choosing Wisely Canada. Accessed March 20, 2023. https://choosingwiselycanada.org/
53. Bagian JP, Weiss KB. The overarching themes from the CLER National Report of Findings 2016. *J Grad Med Educ.* 2016 May;8(2 Suppl 1):21–23. doi:10.4300/1949-8349.8.2s1.21.
54. Koh NJ, Wagner R, Newton RC, Kuhn CM, Co JPT, Weiss KB; on behalf of the CLER Evaluation Committee and the CLER Program. *CLER National Report of Findings 2021.* Chicago, IL: Accreditation Council for Graduate Medical Education; 2021. doi:10.35425/ACGME.0008.
55. Koh NJ, Wagner R, Newton RC, Hirsch KW, Kuhn CM, Weiss KB; on behalf of the CLER Evaluation Committee and the CLER Program. *CLER National Report of Findings 2022: The COVID-19 Pandemic and Its Impact on the Clinical Learning Environment.* Chicago, IL: Accreditation Council for Graduate Medical Education; 2022. doi:10.35425/ACGME.0009.
56. Ogrinc G, Headrick LA, Morrison LJ, Foster T. Teaching and assessing resident competence in practice-based learning and improvement. *J Gen Intern Med.* 2004 May;19(5 Pt 2):496–500. doi:10.1111/j.1525-1497.2004.30102.x.
57. Bowen JL. Adapting residency training. Training adaptable residents. *West J Med.* 1998 May;168(5):371–377.
58. Wagner R, Weiss KB, Headrick LA, et al. Program Directors Patient Safety and Quality Educators Network: a learning collaborative to improve resident and fellow physician engagement. *J Grad Med Educ.* 2022 Aug;14(4):505–509. doi:10.4300/JGME-D-22-00490.1.
59. US Department of Health and Human Services Health Resources and Services Administration. Performance measurement and quality improvement. 2023. Accessed March 20, 2023. https://www.hrsa.gov/library/performance-measurement-quality-improvement.
60. Donabedian A. *An Introduction to Quality Assurance in Health Care.* Oxford University Press; 2003.
61. Agency for Healthcare Research and Quality. National Quality Measures Clearinghouse. Last reviewed September 2018. Accessed March 20, 2023. www.qualitymeasures.ahrq.gov.
62. Nelson EC, Eftimovska E, Lind C, Hager A, Wasson JH, Lindblad S. Patient reported outcome measures in practice. *BMJ.* 2015 Feb 10;350:g7818. doi:10.1136/bmj.g7818.
63. Chen J, Ou L, Hollis SJ. A systematic review of the impact of routine collection of patient reported outcome measures on patients, providers and health organisations in an oncologic setting. *BMC Health Serv Res.* 2013 Jun 11;13:211. doi:10.1186/1472-6963-13-211.
64. Churruca K, Pomare C, Ellis LA, et al. Patient-reported outcome measures (PROMs): a review of generic and condition-specific measures and a discussion of trends and issues. *Health Expect.* 2021 Aug;24(4):1015–1024. doi:10.1111/hex.13254.
65. Kaplan RS. Conceptual foundations of the balanced scorecard. *Handbooks Manage Account Res.* 2009;3:1253–1269. doi:10.1016/S1751-3243(07)03003-9.
66. Hall AK, Schumacher DJ, Thoma B, et al. on behalf of the ICBME Collaborators. Outcomes of competency-based medical education: a taxonomy for shared language. *Med Teach.* 2021 July;43(7):788–793. doi:10.1080/0142159X.2021.1925643.
67. Schumacher DJ, Martini A, Holmboe E, et al. Developing resident-sensitive quality measures: engaging stakeholders to inform next steps. *Acad Pediatr.* 2019 Mar;19(2):177–185. doi:10.1016/j.acap.2018.09.013.
68. Schumacher DJ, Holmboe ES, van der Vleuten C, Busari J, Carraccio C. Developing resident-sensitive quality measures: a model from pediatric emergency medicine. *Acad Med.* 2018 Jul;93(7):1071–1078. doi:10.1097/ACM.0000000000002093.
69. Emilsson L, Lindahl B, Köster M, Lambe M, Ludvigsson JF. Review of 103 Swedish healthcare quality registries. *J Intern Med.* 2015 Jan;277(1):94–136. doi:10.1111/joim.12303.
70. Hoffman RL, Bartlett EK, Medbery RL, Sakran JV, Morris JB, Kelz RR. Outcomes registries: an untapped resource for use in surgical education. *J Surg Educ.* 2015 Mar-Apr;72(2):264–270. doi:10.1016/j.jsurg.2014.08.014.
71. Carek PJ, Dickerson LM, Stanek M, et al. Education in quality improvement for practice in primary care during residency training and subsequent activities in practice. *J Grad Med Educ.* 2014 Mar;6(1):50–54. doi:10.4300/JGME-06-01-39.1.
72. Kilo CM, Leavitt M. *Medical Practice Transformation with Information Technology.* Chicago: Healthcare Information and Management Systems Society; 2005.
73. Mai MV, Orenstein EW, Manning JD, Luberti AA, Dziorny AC. Attributing patients to pediatric residents using electronic health record features augmented with audit logs. *Appl Clin Inform.* 2020 May;11(3):442–451. doi:10.1055/s-0040-1713133.
74. Hier DB, Rothschild A, LeMaistre A, Keeler J. Differing faculty and housestaff acceptance of an electronic health record. *Int J Med Inform.* 2005 Aug;74(7-8):657–662. doi:10.1016/j.ijmedinf.2005.03.006.
75. O'Connell RT, Cho C, Shah N, Brown K, Shiffman RN. Take note(s): differential EHR satisfaction with two implementations under one roof. *J Am Med Inform Assoc.* 2004 Jan-Feb;11(1):43–49. doi:10.1197/jamia.M1409.
76. Meeks DW, Smith MW, Taylor L, Sittig DF, Scott JM, Singh H. An analysis of electronic health record-related patient safety concerns. *J Am Med Inform Assoc.* 2014 Nov-Dec;21(6):1053–1059. doi:10.1136/amiajnl-2013-002578.
77. Graber ML, Siegal D, Riah H, Johnston D, Kenyon K. Electronic health record-related events in medical malpractice

claims. *J Patient Saf.* 2019 Jun;15(2):77–85. doi:10.1097/PTS.0000000000000240.
78. Chi J, Verghese A. Clinical education and the electronic health records: the flipped patient. *JAMA.* 2014 Dec 10;312(22):2331–2332. doi:10.1001/jama.2014.12820.
79. Hammoud MH, Margo K, Christner JG, Fisher J, Fischer SH, Pangaro LN. Opportunities and challenges in integrating electronic health records into undergraduate medical education: a national survey of clerkship directors. *Teach Learn Med.* 2012;24(3):219–224. doi:10.1080/10401334.2012.692267.
80. Sequist TD, Singh S, Pereira AG, Rusinak D, Pearson SD. Use of an electronic medical record to profile the continuity clinic experiences of primary care residents. *Acad Med.* 2005 Apr;80(4):390–394. doi:10.1097/00001888-200504000-00017.
81. Kaushal R, Shojania KG, Bates DW. Effects of computerized physician order entry and clinical decision support systems on medication safety: a systematic review. *Arch Int Med.* 2003 Jun 23;163(12):1409–1416. doi:10.1001/archinte.163.12.1409.
82. Bates DW, Gawande AA. Improving safety with information technology. *N Engl J Med.* 2003 Jun 19;348(25):2526–2534. doi:10.1056/NEJMsa020847.
83. Longo DR, Hewett JE, Ge B, Schubert S. The long road to patient safety: a status report on patient safety systems. *JAMA.* 2005 Dec 14;294(22):2858–2865. doi:10.1001/jama.294.22.2858.
84. Zafar MA, Diers T, Schauer DP, Warm EJ. Connecting resident education to patient outcomes: the evolution of a quality improvement curriculum in an internal medicine residency. *Acad Med.* 2014 Oct;89(10):1341–1347. doi:10.1097/ACM.0000000000000424.
85. Wong BM, Etchells EE, Kuper A, Levinson W, Shojania KG. Teaching quality improvement and patient safety to trainees: a systematic review. *Acad Med.* 2010 Sep;85(9):1425–1439. doi:10.1097/ACM.0b013e3181e2d0c6.
86. Hripcsak G, Stetson PD, Gordon PG. Using the Federated Council for Internal Medicine curricular guide and administrative codes to assess IM residents' breadth of experience. *Acad Med.* 2004 Jun;79(6):557–563. doi:10.1097/00001888-200406000-00011.
87. Kendrick DE, Thelen AE, Chen X, et al. Association of surgical resident competency ratings with patient outcomes. *Acad Med.* 2023 Jul 1;98(7):813–820. doi:10.1097/ACM.0000000000005157.
88. HealthIT.gov. Benefits of EHRs: Improved diagnostics and patient outcomes. Last reviewed June 4, 2019. Accessed May 28, 2016. https://www.healthit.gov/providers-professionals/improved-diagnostics-patient-outcomes.
89. American College of Cardiology. National Cardiovascular Data Registry. Accessed March 20, 2023. http://cvquality.acc.org/ncdr-home.aspx.
90. The Society of Thoracic Surgeons. The STS national database. Accessed March 20, 2023. www.sts.org/national-database.
91. The Society for Vascular Surgery. The VQI Registries. Accessed March 20, 2023. https://www.vqi.org/vqi-registries/.
92. Nationella Kvaliteregister. Quality Registries. Published June 15, 2022. Accessed March 20, 2023. https://skr.se/en/kvalitetsregister/omnationellakvalitetsregister.52218.html.
93. Smith B, Yamazaki K, Tekian A, et al. ACGME Milestone ratings during training predict surgeons' early outcomes. Submitted September 2023.
94. Levinson W, Lesser CS, Epstein RM. Developing physician communication skills for patient-centered care. *Health Aff (Millwood).* 2010 Jul;29(7):1310–1318. doi:10.1377/hlthaff.2009.0450. PMID: 20606179.
95. Han M, Hamstra SJ, Hogan SO, et al. Trainee physician milestone ratings and patient complaints in early post-training practice. *JAMA Netw Open.* 2023 Apr 3;6(4):e237588. doi:10.1001/jamanetworkopen.2023.7588.
96. Ramsey PG, Curtis JR, Paauw DS, Carline JD, Wenrich MD. History-taking and preventive medicine skills among primary care physicians: an assessment using standardized patients. *Am J Med.* 1998 Feb;104(2):152–158. doi:10.1016/s0002-9343(97)00310-0.
97. Luck J, Peabody JW, Dresselhaus TR, Lee M, Glassman P. How well does chart abstraction measure quality? A prospective comparison of standardized patients with the medical record. *Am J Med.* 2000 Jun 1;108(8):642–649. doi:10.1016/s0002-9343(00)00363-6.
98. Peabody JW, Luck J, Glassman P, Dresselhaus TR, Lee M. Comparison of vignettes, standardized patients, and chart abstraction. *JAMA.* 2000 Apr 5;283(13):1715–1722. doi:10.1001/jama.283.13.1715.
99. Zabar S, Hanley K, Stevens D, et al. Unannounced standardized patients: a promising method of assessing patient-centered care in your help system. *BMC Health Serv Res.* 2014 Apr 5;14:157. doi:10.1186/1472-6963-14-157.
100. Weiner SJ, Schwartz A. Directly observed care: can unannounced standardized patients address a gap in performance measurement? *J Gen Intern Med.* 2014 Aug;29(8):1183–1187. doi:10.1007/s11606-014-2860-7.
101. Schwartz A, Peskin S, Spiro A, Weiner SJ. Direct observation of depression screening: identifying diagnostic error and improving accuracy through unannounced standardized patients. *Diagnosis (Berl).* 2020 Aug 27;7(3):251–256. doi:10.1515/dx-2019-0110. PMID: 32187012.
102. Langley GJ, Nolan KM, Nolan TW, Norman CL, Provost LP. *The Improvement Guide. A Practical Approach to Enhancing Organizational Performance.* Jossey-Bass; 2009.
103. The National Quality Forum. Accessed March 20, 2023. www.qualityforum.org
104. Berenson RA. If you can't measure performance, can you improve it? *JAMA.* 2016 Feb 16;315(7):645–646. doi:10.1001/jama.2016.0767.
105. Berwick DM. Era 3 for medicine and health care. *JAMA.* 2016 Apr 5;315(13):1329–1330. doi:10.1001/jama.2016.1509.
106. Rosenbaum L. Metric myopia—trading away our clinical judgment. *N Engl J Med.* 2022 May 5;386(18):1759–1763. doi:10.1056/NEJMms2200977.
107. Holmboe ES, Scranton R, Sumption K, Hawkins R. Effect of medical record audit and feedback on residents' compliance with preventive health care guidelines. *Acad Med.* 1998 Aug;73(8):65–67. doi:10.1097/00001888-199808000-00016.
108. Veloski J, Boex JR, Grasberger MJ, Evans A, Wolfson DB. Systematic review of the literature on assessment, feedback and physicians' clinical performance: BEME Guide No. 7. *Med Teach.* 2006 Mar;28(2):117–128. doi:10.1080/01421590600622665.
109. Ivers N, Jamtvedt G, Flottorp S, et al. Audit and feedback: effects on professional practice and healthcare outcomes. *Cochrane Database Syst Rev.* 2012 Jun 13(6):CD000259. doi:10.1002/14651858.CD000259.pub3.

110. Brehaut JC, Colquhoun HL, Eva KW, et al. Practice feedback interventions: 15 suggestions for optimizing effectiveness. *Ann Intern Med.* 2016 Mar 15;164(6):435–441. doi:10.7326/M15-2248.
111. Holmboe ES, Prince L, Green ML. Teaching and improving quality of care in a residency clinic. *Acad Med.* 2005 Jun;80(6):571–577. doi:10.1097/00001888-200506000-00012.
112. Miller G. Invited reviews: the assessment of clinical skills/competence/performance. *Acad Med.* 1990 Sep;65(9 Suppl):S63–S67. doi:10.1097/00001888-199009000-00045.
113. Tamblyn R, Abrahamowicz M, Dauphinee WD, et al. Association between licensure examination scores and practice in primary care. *JAMA.* 2002 Dec 18;2888(23):3019–3026. doi:10.1001/jama.288.23.3019.
114. Tamblyn R, Abrahamowicz M, Brailovsky C, et al. Association between licensing examination scores and resources use and quality of care in primary care practice. *JAMA.* 1998 Sep 16;280(11):989–996. doi:10.1001/jama.280.11.989.
115. Norcini JJ, Lipner RS, Kimball HR. Certifying examination performance and patient outcomes following acute myocardial infarction. *Med Educ.* 2002 Sep;36(9):853–859. doi:10.1046/j.1365-2923.2002.01293.x.
116. Lipner RS, Hess BJ, Phillips Jr RL. Specialty board certification in the United States: issues and evidence. *J Contin Educ Health Prof.* 2013 Fall;33(Suppl 1):S20–S35. doi:10.1002/chp.21203.
117. Holmboe ES, Weng W, Arnold GK, et al. The comprehensive care project: measuring physician performance in ambulatory practice. *Health Serv Res.* 2010 Dec;45(6 Pt 2):1912–1933. doi:10.1111/j.1475-6773.2010.01160.x.
118. Ashton CM. Invisible doctors: making a case for involving medical residents in hospital quality improvement programs. *Acad Med.* 1993 Nov;68(11):823. doi:10.1097/00001888-199311000-00003.
119. Holmboe ES, Meehan TP, Lynn L, Doyle P, Sherwin T, Duffy FD. The ABIM Diabetes Practice Improvement Module: a new method for self assessment. *J Cont Educ Health Prof.* 2006 Spring;26(2):109–119. doi:10.1002/chp.59.
120. Davis DA, Mazmanian PE, Fordis M, Van Harrison R, Thorpe KE, Perrier L. Accuracy of physician self-assessment compared with observed measures of competence. *JAMA.* 2006 Sep 6;296(9):1094–1102. doi:10.1001/jama.296.9.1094.
121. Duffy FD, Holmboe ES. Self-assessment in lifelong learning and improving performance in practice: physician know thyself. *JAMA.* 2006 Sep 6;296(9):1137–1138. doi:10.1001/jama.296.9.1137.
122. Sargeant J, Armson H, Chesluk B, et al. Processes and dimensions of informed self-assessment. *Acad Med.* 2010 Jul;85(7):1212–1220. doi:10.1097/ACM.0b013e3181d85a4e.
123. Artino Jr AR, Dong T, DeZee KJ, et al. Achievement goal structures and self-regulated learning: relationships and changes in medical school. *Acad Med.* 2012 Oct;87(10):1375–1378. doi:10.1097/ACM.0b013e3182676b55.
124. Lynn LA, Hess BJ, Conforti LN, Lipner RS, Holmboe ES. The relationship between clinic systems and quality of care for older adults in residency clinics and in physician practices. *Acad Med.* 2009 Dec;84(12):1732–1740. doi:10.1097/ACM.0b013e3181bf6f38.
125. Kim JG, Mazotti L, McDonald KM, Holmboe E, Kanter MH. Rowing together: publicly reported quality of care measures, us graduate medical education accountability, and patient outcomes. *J Comm J Qual Patient Saf.* 2023 Mar;49(3):174–178. doi:10.1016/j.jcjq.2022.12.005.
126. Kim JG, Rodriguez HP, Holmboe ES, et al. The reliability of graduate medical education quality of care clinical performance measures. *J Grad Med Educ.* 2022 Jun;14(3):281–288. doi:10.4300/JGME-D-21-00706.1.
127. Holmboe ES, Kogan JR. Will any road get you there? Examining warranted and unwarranted variation in medical education. *Acad Med.* 2022 Aug 1;97(8):1128–1136. doi:10.1097/ACM.0000000000004667.
128. Thornton JD, Schold JD, Venkateshaiah L, Lander B. Prevalence of copied information by attendings and residents in critical care progress notes. *Crit Care Med.* 2013 Feb;41(2):382–388. doi:10.1097/CCM.0b013e318271 1a1c.
129. Heiman HL, Rasminsky S, Bierman JA, et al. Medical students' observations, practices, and attitudes regarding electronic health record documentation. *Teach Learn Med.* 2014;26(1):49–55. doi:10.1080/10401334.2013.857337.
130. The Joint Commission. Quick Safety 10: Preventing copy-and-paste errors in EHRs. Updated July 2021. Accessed March 20, 2023. https://www.jointcommission.org/resources/news-and-multimedia/newsletters/newsletters/quick-safety/quick-safety–issue-10-preventing-copy-and-paste-errors-in-ehrs/preventing-copyandpaste-errors-in-ehrs/
131. American Health Information Management Association. Appropriate Use of the Copy and Paste Functionality in Electronic Health Records. Accessed March 20, 2023. http://bok.ahima.org/PdfView?oid=300306
132. Kennedy TJ, Regehr G, Baker GR, Lingard L. Point-of-care assessment of medical trainee competence for independent clinical work. *Acad Med.* 2008 Oct;83(10 Suppl):S89–S92. doi:10.1097/ACM.0b013e318183c8b7.
133. Kennedy TJ, Lingard L, Baker GR, Kitchen L, Regehr G. Clinical oversight: conceptualizing the relationship between supervision and safety. *J Gen Intern Med.* 2007 Aug;22(8):1080–1085. doi:10.1007/s11606-007-0179-3.
134. Schumacher DJ, Martini A, Sobolewski B, et al. Use of resident-sensitive quality measure data in entrustment decision making: a qualitative study of clinical competency committee members at one pediatric residency. *Acad Med.* 2020 Nov;95(11):1726–1735. doi:10.1097/ACM.0000000000003435.
135. Baker EA, Ledford CH, Fogg L, Way DP, Park YS. The IDEA assessment tool: assessing the reporting, diagnostic reasoning, and decision-making skills demonstrated in medical students' hospital admission notes. *Teach Learn Med.* 2015;27(2):163–173. doi:10.1080/10401334.2015.1011654.
136. Battles JB, Shea CE. A system of analyzing medical errors to improve GME curricula and programs. *Acad Med.* 2001 Feb;76(2):125–133. doi:10.1097/00001888-200102000-00008.
137. Graber ML, Franklin N, Gordon R. Diagnostic error in internal medicine. *Arch Intern Med.* 2005 Jul 11;165(13):1493–1499. doi:10.1001/archinte.165.13.1493.
138. Schumacher DJ, Dornoff E, Carraccio C, et al. The power of contribution and attribution in assessing educational outcomes for individuals, teams, and programs. *Acad Med.* 2020 Jul;95(7):1014–1019. doi:10.1097/ACM.0000000000003121.
139. Gennis VM, Gennis MA. Supervision in the outpatient clinic: effects on teaching and patient care. *J Gen Intern Med.* 1993;9:116. doi:10.1007/BF02600077.
140. Omori DM, O'Malley PG, Kroenke K, Landry F. The impact of the bedside visit in the ambulatory clinic. Does it make a difference? *J Gen Intern Med.* 1997;12(S1):96A.
141. Kaplan SH, Griffith JL, Price LL, Pawlson LG, Greenfield S. Improving the reliability of physician performance assessment:

identifying the "physician effect" on quality and creating composite measures. *Med Care.* 2009 Apr;47(4):378–387. doi:10.1097/MLR.0b013e31818dce07.
142. Agency for Healthcare Quality and Research. Quality information and improvement. Page last reviewed December 3033. Accessed March 20, 2023. www.ahrq.gov/qual/qualix.htm.
143. National Quality Forum. ABCs of measurement. Accessed March 20, 2023. https://www.qualityforum.org/Measuring_Performance/ABCs_of_Measurement.aspx.
144. Shunk R, Dulay M, Julian K, et al. Using the American Board of Internal Medicine Practice Improvement Modules to teach internal medicine residents practice improvement. *J Grad Med Educ.* 2010 Mar;2(1):90–95. doi:10.4300/JGME-D-09-00032.1.
145. Schumacher DJ, Wu DTY, Meganathan K, et al. A feasibility study to attribute patients to primary interns on inpatient ward teams using electronic health record data. *Acad Med.* 2019 Sep;94(9):1376–1383. doi:10.1097/ACM.0000000000002748.
146. Levin JC, Hron J. Automated reporting of trainee metrics using electronic clinical systems. *J Grad Med Educ.* 2017 Jun;9(3):361–365. doi:10.4300/JGME-D-16-00469.1.
147. Hess BJ, Johnston MM, Lynn LA, Conforti LN, Holmboe ES. Development of an instrument to evaluate residents' confidence in quality improvement. *Jt Comm J Qual Patient Saf.* 2013 Nov;39(11):502–510. doi:10.1016/s1553-7250(13)39066-7.
148. Singh MK, Ogrinc G, Cox KR, et al. The Quality Improvement Knowledge Application Tool Revised (QIKAT-R). *Acad Med.* 2014 Oct;89(10):1386–1391. doi:10.1097/ACM.0000000000000456.
149. Myers JS, Kin JM, Billi JE, Burke KG, Van Harrison R. Development and validation of an A3 problem-solving assessment tool and self-instructional package for teachers of quality improvement in healthcare. *BMJ Qual Saf.* 2022 Apr;31(4):287–296. doi:10.1136/bmjqs-2020-012105.
150. Steele EM, Butcher R, Carluzzo KL, Watts BV. Development of a tool to assess trainees' ability to design and conduct quality improvement projects. *Am J Med Qual.* 2020 Mar/Apr;35(2):125–132. doi:10.1177/1062860619853880.
151. Rosenbluth G, Burman NJ, Ranji SR, Boscardin CK. Development of a multi-domain assessment tool for quality improvement projects. *J Grad Med Educ.* 2017 Aug;9(4):473–478. doi:10.4300/JGME-D-17-00041.1.
152. Institute for Healthcare Improvement. Quality Improvement Essentials Toolkit. Accessed March 21, 2023. https://www.ihi.org/resources/Pages/Tools/Quality-Improvement-Essentials-Toolkit.aspx.

12

Multisource Feedback

JOCELYN M. LOCKYER, PHD

CHAPTER OUTLINE

Introduction

Multisource feedback (MSF) is a formative assessment tool. Properly executed MSF is a four-stage process whereby (1) data about an individual's observable workplace behaviors are collected through questionnaires from those interacting with the individual; (2) data are aggregated for anonymity and confidentiality; (3) the aggregated data, along with a self-assessment if available, are provided to the individual; and (4) the recipient meets with a facilitator to review the data and develop an action plan.[1–5]

MSF is used along the continuum of medical education for formative feedback to medical students, residents, licensed physicians, and faculty. It may be combined with other assessments or used as a stand-alone assessment. MSF's goal is to provide performance feedback in a manner that allows recipients to reflect upon their data and use the data for ongoing professional development[3] and personal improvement cycles.

This chapter uses a number of terms. Refer to Table 12.1 for terminology.

TABLE 12.1 Terminology

ACGME	Accreditation Council for Graduate Medical Education (US)
Assessee	Learner, resident, or physician being assessed
CBME	Competence-based medical education
CME/CPD	Continuing medical education/Continuing professional development
FD	Faculty development
GMC	General Medical Council
Observer	Professionals, healthcare professionals from other disciplines, patients, and family members/caregivers providing the ratings or assessments
PGME	Postgraduate medical education (i.e., residency program)
RCPSC	Royal College of Physicians and Surgeons of Canada
Source	Type of respondent providing the assessment (e.g., patient, nurse, peer)
UME	Undergraduate medical education

Data and Data Collection

MSF questionnaires comprise sets of items organized within constructs or domains (e.g., communication skills, collaboration, professional). Usually the domains are broad and align with frameworks developed by national professional bodies, such as the competencies developed by the Accreditation Council for Graduate Medical Education (ACGME) in the United States,[6–9] the Canadian Medical Education Directives for Specialists (CanMEDS) roles developed by the Royal College of Physicians and Surgeons of Canada (RCPSC),[10,11] and the Good Medical Practice duties developed by the General Medical Council (GMC) in the United Kingdom.[12,13] MSF domains/items may be designed for a specific discipline or be generic to be used across residency programs or specialty groups. Common domains include communication skills, interpersonal skills, professionalism, teamwork, leadership, and collaboration. Effective MSF draws on those domains to create assessment items that are observable.

Items provide brief, one-idea statements to which observers can respond to capture workplace expectations (e.g., "This physician treats me with respect"; "This physician provides appropriate information at handover"). Different sources, including physician colleagues and patients, can be asked to respond to different items or to the same items provided the items are observable by that source. Items are written at an appropriate language and literacy level, particularly for patients. (See Tables 12.2 and 12.3 for examples of constructs and items.)

In addition to quantitative data, there is space for qualitative or narrative comments as narratives help with data interpretation. (See Table 12.4 for examples of open-ended questions.) Observers provide assessments using a multipoint rating scale with items aligned with the intent of the item. See Table 12.5 for examples of rating scales.)

Observers may be selected by the assessee, or identified by someone in a leadership position such as a program director or department/division head. However, observers must be able to observe and know about the workplace behaviors of the person being assessed. Observers may come from within the same discipline (e.g., physician colleagues, residents, medical students, referring physicians, senior residents) or from other healthcare disciplines (e.g., nurses, pharmacists, psychologists), or may be patients and their family members/caregivers.[6,7,14–16]

Generally, data are collected through a secure and individualized internet link. Sufficient numbers of observers are required to ensure anonymity and confidentiality and to provide sufficient numbers of responses to ensure that the scores are valid and reliable for the decision-making that is required by the assessee or the program.

See Appendix 12.1 for exemplary examples of instruments.

Data Aggregation

The feedback provided to the assessee can vary. However, most often data are aggregated for each source (e.g., peer group, patients), by domain/construct (e.g., communication) and by item. Aggregation occurs through the calculation of means (standard deviation) and ranges. There may be means provided for the domains. Narrative data are generally grouped by question and source.

Data Reporting

Reports can vary. Generally, organizations provide descriptive data (means, standard deviations and ranges) and

TABLE 12.2 Examples of Selected Constructs, Sources, and Items for Emergency Medicine Residents

Construct	Source	Examples of Items
Communication	Patients	I understand what my doctor told me.
		My doctor introduced themselves to me.
	Nonphysician coworkers (e.g., nurses, pharmacists)	Communicates effectively with patients and families.
		Communicates effectively with other health professionals.
	Physician colleagues (peers, referring and referral physicians)	Handoffs are effective.
		Communicates effectively in critical situations.
Professionalism	Patients	My doctor respected me.
		My doctor respected my social and financial situation while treating me.
	Nonphysician coworkers	Demonstrates respect for others regardless of sex, ethnicity, or disability.
		Responsive to concerns raised by other team members.
	Physician colleagues	Maintains patient confidentiality.
		Recognizes limits of expertise.

From LaMantia J, Yarris LM, Sunga K, et al. Developing and implementing a multisource feedback tool to assess competencies of emergency medicine residents in the United States. *AEM Educ Train*. 2017 Jun 15;1(3):243-249. doi:10.1002/aet2.10043.

TABLE 12.3 Examples of Selected Constructs and Items From MSF for Interprofessional Professionalism Assessment

Communication	Works with members of other health professions to coordinate communication with patients/clients and family members.
	Demonstrates active listening with members of other health professions.
Altruism and caring	Offers to help members of other health professions when caring for patients.
Ethics	Discusses with members of other health professions any ethical implications of healthcare decisions.
Accountability	Works with members of other healthcare professions to identify and address errors and potential errors in the delivery of care.

From Frost JS, Hammer DP, Nunez LM, et al. The intersection of professionalism and interprofessional care: development and initial testing of the interprofessional professionalism assessment (IPA). *J Interprof Care*. 2019 Jan-Feb;33(1):102-115. doi:10.1080/13561820.2018.1515733.

TABLE 12.4 Examples of Open-Ended Questions

- Provide comments related to the behaviors associated with communication (ethics, accountability, respect, etc.), including those that are positive and those needing improvement.[a]
- Areas for improvement related to interprofessional professionalism.[a]
- Please feel free to add any other comments you have about this doctor.[b]
- What is one (1) thing the physician does particularly well?[c]
- What is one (1) thing you would have the physician target for action?[c]
- What does this physician do well?[c]
- What might this physician do to enhance their practice?[c]

[a]From Frost JS, Hammer DP, Nunez LM, et al. The intersection of professionalism and interprofessional care: development and initial testing of the interprofessional professionalism assessment (IPA). *J Interprof Care*. 2019 Jan-Feb;33(1):102-115. doi:10.1080/13561820.2018.1515733.

[b]From Richards SH, Campbell JL, Walshaw E, Dickens A, Greco M. A multi-method analysis of free-text comments from the UK General Medical Council Colleague Questionnaires. *Med Educ*. 2009 Aug;43(8):757-766. doi:10.1111/j.1365-2923.2009.03416.x.

[c]From Lockyer JM, Sargeant J, Richards SH, Campbell JL, Rivera LA. Multisource feedback and narrative comments: polarity, specificity, actionability, and CanMEDS roles. *J Contin Educ Health Prof*. 2018 Winter;38(1):32-40. doi:10.1097/CEH.0000000000000183.

graphical data (e.g., bar graphs) for domains as well as individual items. Reports may include comparator data with others who were assessed. If there is a self-assessment, those data are also provided to the individual, often in conjunction with the related items so that comparisons can be made. Responses to open-ended questions will also be provided. Comments are usually verbatim and grouped by the question and the source.

Facilitated Feedback Discussions

While initial work in MSF rarely included facilitated discussions, the opportunity to discuss one's data is seen as critical to good outcomes from MSF[1,2,4,5,17] and thus the facilitated discussion is the fourth stage in MSF processes. This may occur with a colleague using a scripted set of questions,[18,19] a trained facilitator from the discipline,[5,17] or a nonmedical coach.[2,20] This ensures cocreation of an action plan and follow-up. Facilitation encourages reflection and has been shown to increase the potential for implementation.[5]

Optimizing MSF

Considering the research and testing that have taken place broadly, a conceptual model is presented in Fig. 12.1 depicting potential outcomes from the process whereby assessees receive their data from a variety of sources. MSF works best when assessees review and reflect on the data, have a facilitated session with a coach or other trusted individual, and create an action plan that includes follow-up as part of a personal improvement cycle. Both individual factors as well as external factors in the workplace or culture may influence assessees' preparedness to use the data. As will be shown later, careful attention to instrument design, preparation of both assessees and observers, organizational commitment, as well as evaluation will help ensure more successful outcomes.

MSF and Its Role in Learning and Assessment

MSF is a formative assessment. It is an educational tool to guide learning and development. The constructs and the items on the instruments provide a means of educating learners and physicians about workplace behaviors and expectations, as the greatest success will occur when the items focus on the behaviors deemed critical for effective work in clinical environments.

MSF has been used along the continuum of medical education to promote learning and assessment. Tools have been developed for use with undergraduates with promising examples of its use, particularly for the clerkship or clinical phases of education.[14,15,21,22] For postgraduate trainees, experience with MSF is longer with examples going back to the early 1990s and continuing to the present in a number of countries.[6,7,10,23–26] For practicing physicians, MSF has a similar history with examples from the United States[27,28] and Canada,[29] and continuing to the present, worldwide.[30,31] There are also examples of MSF used within faculty development to improve teaching expertise.[32,33]

TABLE 12.5 Selected Examples of Scales

Type						
Agreement[a]	Strongly disagree	Disagree	Neutral	Agree	Strongly agree	No opportunity to observe in this environment
Frequency[b]	Never	Rarely	Sometimes	Usually	Always	
Concerns[c]	No concerns observed	Observed 1 or 2 minor concerns	Observed several minor or 1 major concern			Unable to assess
Expectations[d]	Exceeds expectations		Meets expectations		Below expectations	Don't know/not applicable
Quality[e,f]	Poor (1)				Excellent (5)	Unable to evaluate

[a]From Frost JS, Hammer DP, Nunez LM, et al. The intersection of professionalism and interprofessional care: development and initial testing of the interprofessional professionalism assessment (IPA). J Interprof Care. 2019 Jan-Feb;33(1):102-115. doi:10.1080/13561820.2018.1515733.

[b]From Chesluk BJ, Reddy S, Hess B, Bernabeo E, Lynn L, Holmboe E. Assessing interprofessional teamwork: pilot test of a new assessment module for practicing physicians. *J Contin Educ Health Prof*. 2015 Winter:35(1):3-10. doi:10.1002/chp.21267.

[c]From Dudek N, Duffy MC, Wood TJ, Gofton W. The Ottawa Resident Observation Form for Nurses (O-RON): assessment of resident performance through the eyes of the nurses. *J Surg Educ*. 2021 Sep-Oct;78(5):1666-1675. doi:10.1016/j.jsurg.2021.03.014.

[d]From Goldhamer ME, Baker K, Cohen AP, Weinstein DF. Evaluating the evaluators: implementation of a multi-source evaluation program for graduate medical education program directors. *J Grad Med Educ*. 2016 Oct;8(4):592-596. doi:10.4300/JGME-D-15-00543.1.

[e,f]From Byrd A, Iheagwara K, McMahon P, Bolton M, Roy M. Using multisource feedback to assess resident communication skills: adding a new dimension to milestone data. *Ochsner J*. 2020 Fall;20(3):255-260. doi:10.31486/toj.19.0054; and Carenzo L, Cena T, Carfagna F, et al. Assessing anaesthesiology and intensive care specialty physicians: an Italian language multisource feedback system. *PLoS One*. 2021 Apr 23;16(4):e0250404. doi:10.1371/journal.pone.0250404.

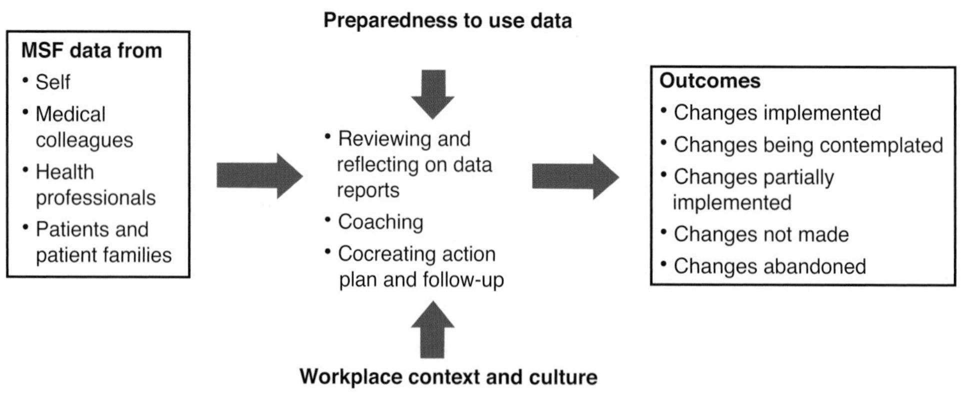

• **Fig. 12.1** Conceptual model for multisource feedback adoption.

Many factors led to MSF becoming an assessment tool to guide performance. Heightened interest in patient safety and the recognition that all healthcare professionals needed to function effectively as part of interdisciplinary teams encouraged the assessment of nonmedical experts' broader competencies. Similarly, the movement toward competency-based medical education (CBME) and the need to assess the broader competencies described within the ACGME, the RCPSC CanMEDS, and the GMC Good Medical Practice framework reinforced the need for MSF and facilitated the development of tools for MSF. Tools traditionally used to assess physicians and learners, such as multiple-choice questions (MCQs), objective structured clinical examinations (OSCEs), and direct observation of procedures, could not provide feedback on the interpersonal workplace behaviors critical to optimal patient-centered care. MSF offered flexibility and a systematic approach and could be adapted for specific foci such as leadership skills[25,26,34] and broadly based competencies.[5,10,13,27,28] MSF was also seen as a way to identify physicians whose behaviors were inappropriate or at risk for dyscompetence.[35,36]

In postgraduate medical education (PGME), MSF may be combined with other assessments to gain a fuller picture of the individual's performance in a holistic way.[6,9,16,37–43] For example, the combination of mini clinical evaluation exercises (mini-CEX) and direct observation of procedures with MSF has been shown to provide a reliable base for judgments about trainees.[37] Similarly, the combination of MSF, case-based discussion, mini-CEX, and direct observation of procedures has been used to assess UK Foundation (PGY 1 and 2) trainees.[44]

In continuing medical education/continuing professional development (CME/CPD), MSF has been used for quality

TABLE 12.6 Critical Steps in Implementing MSF

Communicate	Establish the purpose. Determine the focus. Assess organizational readiness. Determine infrastructure stability. Develop questionnaires. Create the report. Appoint and train facilitators. Determine consequences. Conduct the field test.

improvement of individuals[29] as part of certification program maintenance[5,45] and to provide feedback to physicians about selected competencies.[29] MSF has also been used as part of the decision-making for licensure with international medical graduates seeking to work in a new country.[46–48] An association between malpractice claims and MSF ratings has been noted and it is felt that the identification and modification of negative physician behaviors may mitigate malpractice risk and ultimately result in improved quality of patient care.[49] Its use has been expanded into assessment of supervisors[32,33] and assessment of specific skills such as teamwork.[18]

Getting Started

Introducing MSF into an organization is a major undertaking. It requires the full support of administration and buy-in at all levels of the organization, program, or unit for sustainability. It is relatively easy to develop questionnaires and test them for feasibility and acceptability in a one-time experiment. However, moving into full implementation and a sustainable program requires that attention be paid to the critical steps outlined in Table 12.6.[50,51]

Communicate

Communication is a critical component that needs to be frequent and clear. It needs to occur throughout the process of implementation, from the initial stages that announce the program and its intent, through testing, implementation, and evaluation. Communication vehicles might include email, newsletters, departmental meetings, rounds, and scholarly activities. Messages need to be consistent. Clarity about the nature of the assessment is critical, particularly around any consequences for participants. People must believe that the system is trustworthy and data will be used as intended.

Establish the Purpose of MSF

The intended use of this assessment tool must be determined. As noted earlier, MSF is optimally suited for formative assessment. Nonetheless, decisions need to be made and communicated about whether the purpose is to be used for self-guided reflection and improvement, to monitor progress, or as an adjunct to other assessments for decisions related to progress/promotion or initiate support and remediation. In cases where it may inform key judgment or trigger other assessments or surveillance, communication without ambiguity is required. Knowing how an instrument is going to be used may cause observers to respond differently and assessees to select different observers.

Determine the Focus of MSF

MSF instruments are composed of a series of items. As such, MSF is a flexible tool and can be used to measure almost any behavior in the workplace provided the behavior is observable and can be seen by potential respondents. A key step in development is deciding the constructs/domain(s) that will be measured. While instruments can assess a range of constructs (e.g., communication, professionalism, collaboration, teamwork), they can also be limited to a specific domain (e.g., leadership or teamwork) depending on the roles the physician plays or the length of the instrument. Items must be developed in alignment with the constructs. Selection of items should consider the needs and level of the physician/learner, the environment/setting, the specialty, the criticality of the behavior to the patient and team, and the ability of potential observers who are able to observe the item.

Assess Organizational Readiness

The program's or organization's readiness for MSF requires consideration. There are settings where implementation will be challenging. Considerations include how this type of assessment will meet evaluation needs and complement or replace existing tools, policies, and processes. MSF has to be seen as a value-added program and not another assessment burden. Ideally, MSF will provide data to guide the development of the individual and fit within the value-system of the organization's culture, curricula, and assessment procedures. Given the criticality of the development, execution, and creation of action plans and follow-up, it is important that this be considered in faculty development. Support from the leadership will be needed for sustainability. Creating a "leadership team" will guide and monitor the process and ensure communication with all stakeholders including leaders and participants.

Determine Infrastructure Stability

MSF requires a stable infrastructure. While systems can be developed on an ad hoc or pilot basis, in the longer-term implementation will require a commitment and leadership to obtain full support from people in the organization and ensure that the work can continue beyond an initial or feasibility study. IT, personnel, and other resources are required to ensure that data are collected, reports are generated, facilitated discussions are scheduled and held, and there are follow-up on action plans.

Develop Questionnaires

Determining whether the organization will create its own instruments or adopt existing instruments is necessary and needs to be done in conjunction with information about the validity and reliability of existing tools, congruence between an organization's needs and existing instruments, and work required to create instruments that are specific to the organization's needs. It may be more useful for an organization without expertise in instrument design and testing to select an instrument used in a comparable setting. Several examples of instruments are provided in the appendix.

Identify Assessees and Observers

The team will need to determine the group(s) to be assessed and their observers. Potential data sources—for example, from physicians, nurses, pharmacists, and patients—will vary based on the student or physician group. As MSF is based on behaviors, careful selection of sources requires determining whether the sources can observe the behavior. There can be feasibility and acceptability issues related to asking people from diverse backgrounds to complete questionnaires. For example, surveys may be difficult to collect from patients/family members where care involves acute emergency, psychiatric, or terminal illnesses. Similarly, patients whose literacy and language skills are limited may be difficult to include without translators or the help of family members or caregivers. Decisions will need to be made about whether people will select their own observers or have them assigned by, for instance, a program director or unit administrator. The number of observers will need to be determined based on feasibility and the level of reliability needed. The frequency of administration will be governed by feasibility, survey burden, and importance of providing enough time between administrations so that assessees can reasonably see the results of action plans.

Create the Report

Both the content and mechanism for delivery need to be developed early. Reports may contain numeric, graphical, and narrative data. Numeric data can be presented as mean (standard deviation) scores for constructs and individual items as well as range. For items that have a self-assessment, there may be comparator data providing the assessee's data and data from other sources. Comparator data may also be provided for the larger cohort who are participating in MSF. Graphical data (e.g., bar graphs) may provide a visual depiction of some or all of the data. Narrative data are usually provided verbatim and presented by source. Reports are likely to be made available to participants through a secure website, although paper reports may be generated.

Timing the distribution of reports and subsequent facilitation is important. There needs to be sufficient time to collect data from observers to ensure sufficient responses. When responses are delayed, reminders and even replacement of nonrespondents may be required. Nonetheless, reporting should be timely so that assessees accept the relevance of the data. There should be sufficient time between the delivery of the report and the facilitation session so that participants can reflect on their data, identify areas for improvement, and begin to create an action plan and follow-up.

Appoint and Train Facilitators

Processes for facilitation need to be built into the plan. Facilitation is critical in ensuring that participants understand their data and can use the data to create an action plan for improvement that contains the specific actions that will be undertaken, the resources that will be required and used, when the work will begin and end, and when the participant believes they will start to see results of their behavioral changes. Cocreation of the plan appears to yield better results than either the physician or the facilitator leading the plan.[5] This is likely due to the guidance that a facilitator can provide in ensuring that the assessee understands the data and receives help to create an implementable plan with identifiable results.

Determine Consequences

While MSF is a formative assessment, the data may raise surprises and concerns. Assessees may believe the data are biased or may feel bad about the results. Data may identify assessees whose scores and narrative data are suboptimal or below expectations. It is helpful to have plans in place early in the development of the program to support or provide additional assessments.

Conduct the Field Test

Field-testing with a small subset is recommended prior to full implementation. Understanding how observers respond to items and what they take into consideration in their ratings and narratives can avoid problems later. Pilots can enable item modification. Pilots often examine the acceptability, feasibility, and responses with a small group. This can be done by having observers respond to a questionnaire for someone they might assess and discuss what they understood the question was asking as well as the score or narrative they provided.

Ensuring That Tools Are Fit for Purpose

MSF is a questionnaire-based formative assessment tool. The items and scaling on each MSF are critical to its success and core to ensuring that the assessment meets the standards for a measurement scale. As with other assessment tools described in this book, assessment of validity requires a structured argument to support the use and intended interpretations and decisions that are based on the test scores. Evidence must be collected to construct a coherent argument in support of the intended interpretations.[52] There

are more stringent or lenient than scores provided by those whom the organization selects.[28,36] This has been of particular concern given findings that lower performing individuals have selected more lenient observers.[36]

- Scores provided at different times have been examined to ascertain whether scores change and whether the changes might be indicative of practice improvement, thus providing evidence that MSF had impact.[26,73,74]
- Instruments have been examined with varying numbers of items to determine whether instruments can be shortened without losing information.[75]
- The accuracy of scores has been examined as well as the perceptions of different disciplines to provide ratings.[76]

Qualitative data have been collected as stand-alone analyses or in conjunction with quantitative data has also provided key information about MSF procedures, processes and outcomes. There are multiple examples of how questionnaires,[9] cognitive interviews,[77] interviews[66,78] and focus groups[26,79] have provided data. These data often complement and supplement the quantitative data and help ensure that there is coherence between the objectives of the assessment and the intended inferences about behavior and competence. They also help with theory building[4,80] and provide new insights into the data.[81] Several examples of qualitative studies are presented below.

- Observers' interpretation or understanding of items of questionnaires has been explored through focus groups and talk-aloud interviews to ensure that what is being asked is what is understood.[66,77]
- The ways that observers make decisions about scores provided for items has been examined to identify the high and low scoring behaviors that were being used by family physicians and specialists to score to rate physicians on the items on the questionnaires.[81]
- Surveys have been conducted exploring perceptions of MSF. This has included perceptions of value, feasibility, utility and impact.[9,18,61]
- Changes people have made as a result of MSF have been explored[4,5,45] along with the factors influencing and impacting on changes.[4,5]
- Narrative comments have been analyzed for polarity (positive/negative), specificity, association with item scores, ability to provide constructive direction, as well as by theme.[5,82,83,84]
- The role that facilitators play in ensuring reflection and developing action plans and their implementation has been explored.[1,2,5,85]

It is fairly clear that many approaches have been taken to develop an argument for the use of scores generated from MSF processes. These studies suggest that careful attention is needed to ensure that the instruments and their scores make sense for the individual being assessed as well as the organization. MSF must be a value-add for physician/learner improvement and judgements. Both quantitative and qualitative data can help ascertain the value of MSF. Ultimately, MSF must be feasible, acceptable and lead to measurable change.

Faculty Development

Communication and Training End Users

MSF may be a novel and infrequent form of assessment for learners and physicians. As a result, it is particularly critical that there be open and truthful communication to ensure that everyone understands the intent of the assessment. This includes learning about the purpose and intent of the MSF program, anticipated value-add, obligations related to selection of observers, processes and procedures involved, and most importantly, potential consequences. These approaches will help people gain trust in MSF and its resulting data. For residents and medical students, dedicated training sessions that describe the program and answer questions will be required. For physicians being assessed by their regulatory authority or health system, it will be important to reach them through a variety of approaches including open forum, departmental meetings, newsletters, and email.

While training workshops of all the assessees and their potential observers may be seen as impractical, there is value to ensuring that those most likely to be assessed and their observers have training to gain an understanding of the items and processes involved. This may include faculty and residents. It can be done through synchronous sessions at rounds or online sessions. This type of training should lead to high-quality completion of questionnaires.

If training is not possible, communication through a variety of vehicles, such as newsletters, email with links to critical information, and short presentations at meetings, should be considered to ensure that as many people as possible are aware of the MSF program, its goals and scope, and its consequences. It is also important that healthcare professionals and administrative staff, particularly nonphysicians such as nurses, pharmacists, and therapists, are also informed. Consideration needs to be given to how patients and their caregivers will be informed about MSF when asked to participate.

Assessing Faculty

MSF tools have been developed to assess faculty. The tools have taken different forms. For example, Archer et al.[33] described the development and testing of an instrument created for the London Deanery, which is responsible for training 20% of the UK's physicians. The resulting 18-item instrument focused on several areas including the ability of the supervisor to inspire, challenge, give constructive feedback, and remain up-to-date regarding learners' progress and interests. Educational supervisors identified that the data helped them ensure protected, uninterrupted time for educational supervision sessions and use of a more formal, structured approach to clinical teaching. Goldhamer et al.[32] described a set of three MSF instruments developed to assess program directors from residents/fellows, department chairs, and institutional graduate medical education (GME) leadership. They found that program directors found the data helpful and planned to use the data to make changes. Rourke et al.[34] described the development of a tool to assess leadership performance of Memorial University's discipline chairs, dean, and vice dean to provide these leaders with evaluation results to help them improve their performance.

Facilitator Training

Training facilitators is particularly critical. It is clear from early studies that assessees often don't make full use of their data or that they misunderstand the data without an opportunity for discussion. Several studies attest to the importance of assessees having a discussion with someone related to their own data.[2,5,17,57,64] These discussions increase acceptance and implementation of the feedback and help assessees determine how they can be successful.

Facilitation has taken many forms. For example, researchers have created structured discussion protocols to be used by people selected by the assessee.[18,19] These studies show that assessees chose a range of professionals and others including colleagues, peers, staff, and spouses.[18,19] Assessees found the reflection exercise useful in processing feedback and most indicated they were successful in implementing change, though time, habit, and structures were cited as barriers.[19] Training facilitators may involve a one-day program that includes an explanation of the assessment system, training in basic interview skills, and role-plays.[1] The benefit of trained facilitators has been noted. For example, a comparison of the impact of report only, debriefing only, and debriefing and development on leadership teamwork found that debriefing and development provided the greatest increase in scores.[57] The R2C2 theory and evidence-based model[86,87] has been used to build a relationship with the assessee, query their reactions to the data, confirm content, and coach for a commitment to change.[2,5,11,17] Collectively, it appears that the R2C2 model enhanced perceptions of the utility and effectiveness of MSF.[2,5,17] While most studies have drawn on the expertise of a physician coach, nonmedical coaches have been engaged with residents who noted that having a neutral and objective person afforded an open and safe context to the discussion prior to meeting with a program director.[20] These studies and other publications[1,3,5,31,51,57] have demonstrated the importance of discussion and follow-up and are informing best practices for MSF.

Strengths

The main strength of MSF is in its versatility. It has been used successfully along the continuum of medical education to provide feedback data for those in undergraduate medical education (UME), for PGME, and for physicians who are in practice and those who are serving as faculty or in leadership positions. MSF programs have afforded an examination of a broad array of observable behaviors as well as selected behaviors (e.g., communication skills, leadership). Instruments can be modified as needed to optimize feedback.

MSF also provides data that are uniquely different from the assessments provided by written examinations, OSCEs, direct observation, or clinical audit. The data come from different perspectives and observations regarding performance based on the context in which people interact. By including many observers, bias can be reduced compared to settings in which feedback is only provided by one person (department head, preceptor, program director). This can help reduce accusations of bias based on a bad day or a misinterpretation of a single event.

The process of developing or reviewing instruments for adoption provides an opportunity for the creation of an oversight or steering committee to identify the appropriate constructs and the items that best capture the constructs of concern. As items are considered, the values, policies, and curricula can be considered along with job-relevant criteria for performance. This may provide an opportunity to call into question "rules" in the culture and environment that are often unspoken. MSF might be among the more transparent forms of assessment in linking items and job performance. MSF can then provide an opportunity to make assessees and observers aware of expectations. MSF can create an opportunity to remind professionals that they are responsible for providing constructive, supportive, and professionally presented feedback to peers and others within the system.

For the individual, the completion of the self-assessment component serves as a reminder of expectations but also enables them to reflect on their performance. When the physician receives their report, they can compare how they see themselves to how others see them, further developing awareness and insight. The facilitated discussion helps assessees understand their data and how they can act upon it to create action and follow-up plans and build MSF into personal improvement cycles.

At the organizational level, aggregate data can be used to assess intraorganizational cultures and expectations, particularly if comparisons across sites/programs are available. Aggregated data across individuals can form part of a program evaluation. These data may highlight areas in which there are high levels of performance by all physicians and suggest items that can be eliminated. Conversely, aggregating data across individuals may highlight issues with patient handover, racism, communication within teams, or responsiveness to phone calls. In these settings, it may be possible to get agreement on specific behaviors, develop interventions, and subsequently monitor improvement in behaviors across the organization or program.

Nonetheless, ensuring the quality of MSF initiatives is important to optimize its use. Attention to the evidence for the validity and reliability of the data collected, the scores provided, and overall program effectiveness is essential to ensure a highly functioning program. This does require establishing the appropriate questions for studying efficacy and doing this work in a strategic but programmatic way.

Weaknesses and Overcoming Challenges

Every assessment tool has its challenges. No single tool is the answer to assessing competence or performance in all circumstances. Unlike assessment tools that can be standardized for use across large numbers (e.g., multiple-choice examinations, OSCEs), MSF stimuli are daily, real events during which observations take place. Observers are sampling from their perspectives, drawing on what they see and their interactions. If care isn't taken to ensuring that the items are observable and observers don't have an opportunity to observe the behaviors, there can be concerns about data bias and validity.

The context in which MSF is implemented needs careful consideration. Inattention to the setting, the respondents, and how feedback is delivered can reduce the utility of MSF. Attention should be given to obtaining buy-in at all levels of the organization and to having an appropriate infrastructure to support MSF. For example, the organizational culture must be trusting and must view active participation in feedback as a professional expectation and not another unnecessary administrative burden. Concerns about the use of the data, confidentiality of observers, and legal implications for the use of inaccurate, harmful, or misused information may need to be addressed. There may be work settings that are inappropriate. Where numbers of observers are limited, such as occurs in small residency programs, rural practices, or settings where an individual works in isolation or with very few people, the data may be insufficient, leading to questions about validity and reliability.

Results that assessees receive can cause distress, particularly if the scores are low or lower than the recipient believes are correct. Physicians typically work together for the years of their residency program and into practice. Learning that their physician colleagues and other healthcare professionals feel their performance is suboptimal may come as a surprise and may cause unintended reactions for a considerable time after the feedback has been transmitted. Communication about the process and consequences can be helpful. More importantly, assessees require facilitated discussion and other supports to address areas of concern. MSF needs to be delivered in a timely manner so that the results resonate with the physician/learner and can be acted upon.

As described throughout this chapter, MSF doesn't end when assessees receive scores. Facilitation is critical and facilitators need to be trained to understand both the process and the content of the data to effectively work with the assessee.[88] Feedback sessions should follow a structured format in which the recipient has an opportunity to build a relationship with the facilitator, react to the data, focus on the content of the data, and make the necessary commitments to change as well as providing follow-up on the changes made.[5]

Conclusion

It is clear from several decades of MSF instrument development and evaluation that MSF data, reports, and facilitation can be useful in professional development and can improve care for patients and their families. MSF requires good processes supported by organizational leaders; good communication plans to ensure that participants understand the purpose and goals of the program and how the data will be used; and a steering group to lead and manage the program. The instruments can produce measures that are suitable for low-stakes formative purposes.

Acknowledgment

The author thanks Dr. Stephen G. Clyman, MD, MS for his contributions to previous versions of this chapter.

References

1. Overeem K, Wollersheim H, Driessen E, et al. Doctors' perceptions of why 360-degree feedback does (not) work: a qualitative study. *Med Educ.* 2009 Sep;43(9):874–882. doi:10.1111/j.1365-2923.2009.03439.x.
2. Pooley M, Pizzuti C, Daly M. Optimizing multisource feedback implementation for Australasian physicians. *J Contin Educ Health Prof.* 2019 Fall;39(4):228–235. doi:10.1097/CEH.0000000000000267.
3. Lockyer J, Sargeant J. Multisource feedback: an overview of its use and application as a formative assessment. *Can Med Educ J.* 2022 Aug 26;13(4):30–35. doi:10.36834/cmej.73775.
4. Hennel EK, Trachsel A, Subotic U, Lörwald AC, Harendza S, Huwendiek S. How does multisource feedback influence residency training? A qualitative case study. *Med Educ.* 2022 Jun;56(6):660–669. doi:10.1111/medu.14798.
5. Roy M, Lockyer J, Touchie C. Family Physician Quality Improvement Plans: A Realist Inquiry Into What Works, for Whom, Under What Circumstances. *J Contin Educ Health Prof.* 2023 Summer 01;43(3):155–163. doi:10.1097/CEH.0000000000000454. Epub 2022 Jul 6. PMID: 37638679.
6. Hicks PJ, Margolis M, Poynter SE, et al. The Pediatrics Milestones Assessment Pilot: development of workplace-based assessment content, instruments, and processes. *Acad Med.* 2016 May;91(5):701–709. doi:10.1097/ACM.0000000000001057.
7. Schwartz A, Margolis MJ, Multerer S, Haftel HM, Schumacher DJ. APPD LEARN–NBME Pediatrics Milestones Assessment Group. A multi-source feedback tool for measuring a subset of Pediatrics Milestones. *Med Teach.* 2016 Oct;38(10):995–1002. doi:10.3109/0142159X.2016.1147646.
8. LaMantia J, Yarris LM, Sunga K, et al. Developing and implementing a multisource feedback tool to assess competencies of emergency medicine residents in the United States. *AEM Educ Train.* 2017 Jun 15;1(3):243–249. doi:10.1002/aet2.10043.
9. Byrd A, Iheagwara K, McMahon P, Bolton M, Roy M. Using multisource feedback to assess resident communication skills: adding a new dimension to milestone data. *Ochsner J.* 2020 Fall;20(3):255–260. doi:10.31486/toj.19.0054.
10. Probyn L, Lang C, Tomlinson G, Bandiera G. Multisource feedback and self-assessment of the communicator, collaborator, and professional CanMEDS roles for diagnostic radiology residents. *Can Assoc Radiol J.* 2014 Nov;65(4):379–384. doi:10.1016/j.carj.2014.04.003.
11. Roy M, Kain N, Touchie C. Exploring content relationships among components of a multisource feedback program. *J Cont Educ Health Prof.* 2022 Oct 1;42(4):243–248. doi:10.1097/CEH.0000000000000398.

12. Campbell JL, Richards SH, Dickens A, Greco M, Narayanan A, Brearley S. Assessing the professional performance of UK doctors: an evaluation of the utility of the General Medical Council patient and colleague questionnaires. *Qual Saf Health Care.* 2008 Jun;17(3):187–193. doi:10.1136/qshc.2007.024679.
13. Wright C, Richards SH, Hill JJ, et al. Multisource feedback in evaluating the performance of doctors: the example of the UK General Medical Council Patient and Colleague Questionnaires. *Acad Med.* 2012 Dec;87(12):1662–1678. doi:10.1097/ACM.0b013e3182724cc0.
14. Prediger S, Fürstenberg S, Berberat PO, Kadmon M, Harendza S. Interprofessional assessment of medical students' competences with an instrument suitable for physicians and nurses. *BMC Med Educ.* 2019 Feb 6;19(1):46. doi:10.1186/s12909-019-1473-6.
15. Prediger S, Schick K, Fincke F, et al. Validation of a competence-based assessment of medical students' performance in the physician's role. *BMC Med Educ.* 2020 Jan 7;20(1):6. doi:10.1186/s12909-019-1919-x.
16. Moonen-van Loon JM, Overeem K, Donkers HH, van der Vleuten CP, Driessen EW. Composite reliability of a workplace-based assessment toolbox for postgraduate medical education. *Adv Health Sci Educ Theory Pract.* 2013 Dec;18(5):1087–1102. doi:10.1007/s10459-013-9450-z.
17. Arabsky S, Castro N, Murray M, Bisca I, Eva KW. The influence of relationship-centered coaching on physician perceptions of peer review in the context of mandated regulatory practices. *Acad Med.* 2020 Nov;95(11S Association of American Medical Colleges Learn Serve Lead: Proceedings of the 59th Annual Research in Medical Education Presentations):S14–S19. doi:10.1097/ACM.0000000000003642.
18. Chesluk BJ, Reddy S, Hess B, Bernabeo E, Lynn L, Holmboe E. Assessing interprofessional teamwork: pilot test of a new assessment module for practicing physicians. *J Contin Educ Health Prof.* 2015 Winter;35(1):3–10. doi:10.1002/chp.21267.
19. Francois J, Sisler J, Mowat S. Peer-assisted debriefing of multisource feedback: an exploratory qualitative study. *BMC Med Educ.* 2018 Mar 14;18(1):36. doi:10.1186/s12909-018-1137-y.
20. Buis CAM, Eckenhausen MAW. Ten Cate O. Processing multisource feedback during residency under the guidance of a non-medical coach. *Int J Med Educ.* 2018 Feb 23;9:48–54. doi:10.5116/ijme.5a7f.169d.
21. House JB, Franko LR, Haque F, Cranford JA, Santen SA. Variation in assessment of first-year medical students' interprofessional competencies by rater profession. *J Int Educ Pract.* 2021;24:100424. doi:10.1016/j.xjep.2021.100424.
22. Hsu CM, Hsiao CT, Chang LC, Chang HY. Is there an association between nurse, clinical teacher and peer feedback for trainee doctors' medical specialty choice? An observational study in Taiwan. *BMJ Open.* 2018 Apr 12;8(4):e020769. doi:10.1136/bmjopen-2017-020769.
23. Woolliscroft JO, Howell JD, Patel BP, Swanson DB. Resident-patient interactions: the humanistic qualities of internal medicine residents assessed by patients, attending physicians, program supervisors, and nurses. *Acad Med.* 1994 Mar;69(3):216–224. doi:10.1097/00001888-199403000-00017.
24. Archer JC, Norcini J, Davies HA. Use of SPRAT for peer review of paediatricians in training. *BMJ.* 2005 May 28;330(7502):1251–1253. doi:10.1136/bmj.38447.610451.8F.
25. Lakshminarayana I, Wall D, Bindal T, Goodyear HM. A multisource feedback tool to assess ward round leadership skills of senior paediatric trainees: (1) development of tool. *Postgrad Med J.* 2015 May;91(1075):262–267. doi:10.1136/postgradmedj-2014-132692.
26. Goodyear HM, Lakshminarayana I, Wall D, Bindal T. A multisource feedback tool to assess ward round leadership skills of senior paediatric trainees: (2) testing reliability and practicability. *Postgrad Med J.* 2015 May;91(1075):268–273. doi:10.1136/postgradmedj-2015-133308.
27. Wenrich MD, Carline JD, Giles LM, Ramsey PG. Ratings of the performances of practicing internists by hospital-based registered nurses. *Acad Med.* 1993 Sep;68(9):680–687. doi:10.1097/00001888-199309000-00014.
28. Ramsey PG, Carline JD, Inui TS, Larson EB, LoGerfo JP, Wenrich MD. Use of peer ratings to evaluate physician performance. *JAMA.* 1993 Apr 7;269(13):1655–1660.
29. Hall W, Violato C, Lewkonia R, et al. Assessment of physician performance in Alberta: the Physician Achievement Review Project. *CMAJ.* 1999 Jul 13;161(1):52–57.
30. Stevens S, Read J, Baines R, Chatterjee A, Archer J. Validation of multisource feedback in assessing medical performance: a systematic review. *J Cont Educ Heal Prof.* 2018 Fall;38(4):262–268. doi:10.1097/CEH.0000000000000219.
31. Ashworth N, de Champlain AF, Kain N. A review of multisource feedback focusing on psychometrics, pitfalls and some possible solutions. *SN Soc Sci.* 2021 Jan 21;1(1):24. doi:10.1007/s43545-020-00033-1.
32. Goldhamer ME, Baker K, Cohen AP, Weinstein DF. Evaluating the evaluators: implementation of a multi-source evaluation program for graduate medical education program directors. *J Grad Med Educ.* 2016 Oct;8(4):592–596. doi:10.4300/JGME-D-15-00543.1.
33. Archer J, Swanwick T, Smith D, O'Keeffe C, Cater N. Developing a multisource feedback tool for postgraduate medical educational supervisors. *Med Teach.* 2013;35(2):145–154. doi:10.3109/0142159X.2012.733839.
34. Rourke J, Bornstein S, Vardy C, Speed D, White T, Corbett P. Evaluation of and feedback for academic medicine leaders: developing and implementing the Memorial method. *Acad Med.* 2017 Nov;92(11):1590–1594. doi:10.1097/ACM.0000000000001722.
35. Lewkonia R, Flook N, Donoff M, Lockyer J. Family physician practice visits arising from the Alberta Physician Achievement Review. *BMC Med Educ.* 2013 Sep 9;13:121. doi:10.1186/1472-6920-13-121.
36. Archer JC, McAvoy P. Factors that might undermine the validity of patient and multi-source feedback. *Med Educ.* 2011 Sep;45(9):886–893. doi:10.1111/j.1365-2923.2011.04023.x.
37. Moonen-van Loon JM, Overeem K, Govaerts MJ, Verhoeven BH, van der Vleuten CP, Driessen EW. The reliability of multisource feedback in competency-based assessment programs: the effects of multiple occasions and assessor groups. *Acad Med.* 2015 Aug;90(8):1093–1099. doi:10.1097/ACM.0000000000000763.
38. Castanelli DJ, Moonen-van Loon JMW, Jolly B, Weller JM. The reliability of a portfolio of workplace-based assessments in anesthesia training. *Can J Anaesth.* 2019 Feb;66(2):193–200. doi:10.1007/s12630-018-1251-7.
39. Gennissen L, Stammen L, Bueno-de-Mesquita J, Wieringa S, Busari J. Exploring valid and reliable assessment methods for care management education. *Leadersh Health Serv (Bradf Engl).* 2016 Jul 4;29(3):240–250. doi:10.1108/LHS-09-2015-0029.
40. Leep Hunderfund AN, Park YS, Hafferty FW, Nowicki KM, Altchuler SI, Reed DA. A multifaceted organizational physician assessment program: validity evidence and implications for the use of performance data. *Mayo Clin Proc Innov Qual Outcomes.* 2017 Jul 25;1(2):130–140. doi:10.1016/j.mayocpiqo.2017.05.005.

41. Nair BKR, Moonen-van Loon JM, Parvathy M, Jolly BC, van der Vleuten CP. Composite reliability of workplace-based assessment of international medical graduates. *Med J Aust.* 2017 Nov 20;207(10):453. doi:10.5694/mja17.00130.
42. Parvathy MS, Parab A, R Nair BK, Matheson C, Ingham K, Gunning L. Longitudinal outcome of programmatic assessment of international medical graduates. *Adv Med Educ Pract.* 2021 Sep 23;12:1095–1100. doi:10.2147/AMEP.S324412.
43. van der Meulen MW, Boerebach BC, Smirnova A, et al. Validation of the INCEPT: a multisource feedback tool for capturing different perspectives on physicians' professional performance. *J Cont Educ Heal Prof.* 2017 Winter;37(1):9–18. doi:10.1097/CEH.0000000000000143.
44. Davies H, Archer J, Southgate L, Norcini J. Initial evaluation of the first year of the Foundation Assessment Programme. *Med Educ.* 2009 Jan;43(1):74–81. doi:10.1111/j.1365-2923.2008.03249.x.
45. Lipner RS, Blank LL, Leas BF, Fortna GS. The value of patient and peer ratings in recertification. *Acad Med.* 2002 Oct;77(10 Suppl):S64–S66. doi:10.1097/00001888-200210001-00021.
46. Maudsley RF. Assessment of international medical graduates and their integration into family practice: the Clinician Assessment for Practice Program. *Acad Med.* 2008 Mar;83(3):309–315. doi:10.1097/ACM.0b013e318163710f.
47. Nestel D, Regan M, Vijayakumar P, et al. Implementation of a multi-level evaluation strategy: a case study on a program for international medical graduates. *J Educ Eval Health Prof.* 2011;8:13. doi:10.3352/jeehp.2011.8.13.
48. Vayro C, Narayanan A, Greco M, et al. Colleague appraisal of Australian general practitioners in training: an analysis of multisource feedback data. *BMC Med Educ.* 2022 Jun 24;22(1):494. doi:10.1186/s12909-022-03559-5.
49. Lagoo J, Berry WR, Miller K, et al. Multisource evaluation of surgeon behavior is associated with malpractice claims. *Ann Surg.* 2019 Jul;270(1):84–90. doi:10.1097/SLA.0000000000002742.
50. Lockyer J, Sargeant J. Implementing multisource feedback. In: Boud D, Molloy E, eds. *Feedback in Higher and Professional Education.* Routledge; 2013.
51. Lepsinger R, Lucia A. *The Art and Science of 360° Feedback.* Jossey Bass; 2009.
52. Cook DA, Brydges R, Ginsburg S, Hatala R. A contemporary approach to validity arguments: a practical guide to Kane's framework. *Med Educ.* 2015 Jun;49(6):560–575. doi:10.1111/medu.12678.
53. Al Khalifa K, Al Ansari A, Violato C, Donnon T. Multisource feedback to assess surgical practice: a systematic review. *J Surg Educ.* 2013 Jul-Aug;70(4):475–486. doi:10.1016/j.jsurg.2013.02.002.
54. Donnon T, Al Ansari A, Al Alawi S, Violato C. The reliability, validity, and feasibility of multisource feedback physician assessment: a systematic review. *Acad Med.* 2014 Mar;89(3):511–516. doi:10.1097/ACM.0000000000000147.
55. Al Ansari A, Donnon T, Al Khalifa K, Darwish A, Violato C. The construct and criterion validity of the multi-source feedback process to assess physician performance: a meta-analysis. *Adv Med Educ Pract.* 2014 Feb 27;5:39–51. doi:10.2147/AMEP.S57236.
56. Lockyer J. Multisource feedback: can it meet criteria for good assessment? *J Cont Educ Health Prof.* 2013 Spring;33(2):89–98. doi:10.1002/chp.21171.
57. Hu J, Lee R, Mullin S, et al. How physicians change: multisource feedback driven intervention improves physician leadership and teamwork. *Surgery.* 2020 Oct;168(4):714–723. doi:10.1016/j.surg.2020.06.008.
58. Messick S. Validity of psychological assessment: validation of inferences from persons' responses and performances as scientific inquiry into score meaning. *Am Psychol.* 1995;50(9):741–749.
59. Norcini J, Anderson MB, Bollela V, et al. 2018 Consensus framework for good assessment. *Med Teach.* 2018 Nov;40(11):1102–1109. doi:10.1080/0142159X.2018.1500016.
60. Kane MT. Validating the interpretations and uses of test scores. *J Educ Meas.* 2013;50(1):1–73. doi:10.2307/23353796.
61. Hennel EK, Subotic U, Berendonk C, Stricker D, Harendza S, Huwendiek S. A German-language competency-based multisource feedback instrument for residents: development and validity evidence. *BMC Med Educ.* 2020 Oct 12;20(1):357. doi:10.1186/s12909-020-02259-2.
62. Frost JS, Hammer DP, Nunez LM, et al. The intersection of professionalism and interprofessional care: development and initial testing of the interprofessional professionalism assessment (IPA). *J Interprof Care.* 2019 Jan-Feb;33(1):102–115. doi:10.1080/13561820.2018.1515733.
63. Hicks PJ, Margolis MJ, Carraccio CL, et al. A novel workplace-based assessment for competency-based decisions and learner feedback. *Med Teach.* 2018 Nov;40(11):1143–1150. doi:10.1080/0142159X.2018.1461204.
64. Overeem K, Wollersheim HC, Arah OA, Cruijsberg JK, Grol RP, Lombarts KM. Evaluation of physicians' professional performance: an iterative development and validation study of multisource feedback instruments. *BMC Health Serv Res.* 2012 Mar 26;12:80. doi:10.1186/1472-6963-12-80.
65. Carenzo L, Cena T, Carfagna F, et al. Assessing anaesthesiology and intensive care specialty physicians: an Italian language multisource feedback system. *PLoS One.* 2021 Apr 23;16(4):e0250404. doi:10.1371/journal.pone.0250404.
66. Olsson JE, Ekblad S, Bertilson BC, Toth-Pal E. Swedish adaptation of the General Medical Council's multisource feedback questionnaires: a qualitative study. *Int J Med Educ.* 2018 Jun 15;9:161–169. doi:10.5116/ijme.5af6.c209.
67. Narayanan A, Farmer EA, Greco MJ. Multisource feedback as part of the Medical Board of Australia's Professional Performance Framework: outcomes from a preliminary study. *BMC Med Educ.* 2018 Dec 29;18(1):323. doi:10.1186/s12909-018-1432-7.
68. Roberts MJ, Campbell JL, Richards SH, Wright C. Self-other agreement in multisource feedback: the influence of doctor and rater group characteristics. *J Cont Educ Health Prof.* 2013 Winter;33(1):14–23. doi:10.1002/chp.21162.
69. Naidoo S, Lopes S, Patterson F, Mead HM, MacLeod S. Can colleagues', patients' and supervisors' assessments predict successful completion of postgraduate medical training? *Med Educ.* 2017 Apr;51(4):423–431. doi:10.1111/medu.13128.
70. Gregory PJ, Robbins B, Schwaitzberg SD, Harmon L. Leadership development in a professional medical society using 360-degree survey feedback to assess emotional intelligence. *Surg Endosc.* 2017 Sep;31(9):3565–3573. doi:10.1007/s00464-016-5386-8.
71. Lockyer JM, Violato C, Wright BJ, Fidler HM. An analysis of long-term outcomes of the impact of curriculum: a comparison of the three- and four-year medical school curricula. *Acad Med.* 2009;84(10):1342–1347.
72. Leung C, McGee J, Scallan S. A GP fellowship project looking at whether the multi-source feedback and the educational supervisor's report can be used to identify trainees at risk of difficulty. *Educ Prim Care.* 2022 May;33(3):185–187. doi:10.1080/14739879.2022.2045517.

73. Violato C, Lockyer JM, Fidler H. Changes in performance: a 5-year longitudinal study of participants in a multi-source feedback programme. *Med Educ*. 2008 Oct;42(10):1007–1013. doi:10.1111/j.1365-2923.2008.03127.x.
74. Sureda E, Chacón-Moscoso S, Sanduvete-Chaves S, Sesé A. A training intervention through a 360° multisource feedback model. *Int J Environ Res Public Health*. 2021 Aug 30;18(17):9137. doi:10.3390/ijerph18179137.
75. Corbett H, Pearson K, Karimi L, Lim WK. Improving the utility of multisource feedback for medical consultants in a tertiary hospital: a study of the psychometric properties of a survey tool. *Aust Health Rev*. 2019 Jan;43(6):717–723. doi:10.1071/AH17219.
76. Nurudeen SM, Kwakye G, Berry WR, et al. Can 360-degree reviews help surgeons? evaluation of multisource feedback for surgeons in a multi-institutional quality improvement project. *J Am Coll Surg*. 2015 Oct;221(4):837–844. doi:10.1016/j.jamcollsurg.2015.06.017.
77. Mazor KM, Canavan C, Farrell M, Margolis MJ, Clauser BE. Collecting validity evidence for an assessment of professionalism: findings from think-aloud interviews. *Acad Med*. 2008 Oct;83(10 Suppl):S9–S12. doi:10.1097/ACM.0b013e318183e329.
78. Castonguay V, Lavoie P, Karazivan P, Morris J, Gagnon R. Perceptions of emergency medicine residents of multisource feedback: different, relevant, and useful information. *Ann Emerg Med*. 2019 Nov;74(5):660–669. doi:10.1016/j.annemergmed.2019.05.019.
79. Yama BA, Hodgins M, Boydell K, Schwartz SB. A qualitative exploration: questioning multisource feedback in residency education. *BMC Med Educ*. 2018 Jul 24;18(1):170. doi:10.1186/s12909-018-1270-7.
80. Tariq M, Govaerts M, Afzal A, Ali SA, Zehra T. Ratings of performance in multisource feedback: comparing performance theories of residents and nurses. *BMC Med Educ*. 2020 Oct 12;20(1):355. doi:10.1186/s12909-020-02276-1.
81. Sargeant J, Macleod T, Sinclair D, Power M. How do physicians assess their family physician colleagues' performance? Creating a rubric to inform assessment and feedback. *J Cont Educ Health Prof*. 2011 Spring;31(2):87–94. doi:10.1002/chp.20111.
82. Richards SH, Campbell JL, Walshaw E, Dickens A, Greco M. A multi-method analysis of free-text comments from the UK General Medical Council Colleague Questionnaires. *Med Educ*. 2009 Aug;43(8):757–766. doi:10.1111/j.1365-2923.2009.03416.x.
83. Lockyer JM, Sargeant J, Richards SH, Campbell JL, Rivera LA. Multisource feedback and narrative comments: polarity, specificity, actionability, and CanMEDS roles. *J Contin Educ Health Prof*. 2018 Winter;38(1):32–40. doi:10.1097/CEH.0000000000000183.
84. Holm EA, Al-Bayati SJL, Barfod TS, et al. Feasibility, quality and validity of narrative multisource feedback in postgraduate training: a mixed-method study. *BMJ Open*. 2021 Jul 28;11(7):e047019. doi:10.1136/bmjopen-2020-047019.
85. Bindels E, van den Goor M, Scherpbier A, Lombarts K, Heeneman S. Sharing reflections on multisource feedback in a peer group setting: stimulating physicians' professional performance and development. *Acad Med*. 2021 Oct 1;96(10):1449–1456. doi:10.1097/ACM.0000000000004142.
86. Sargeant J, Lockyer J, Mann K, et al. Facilitated reflective performance feedback: developing an evidence- and theory-based model that builds relationship, explores reactions and content, and coaches for performance change (R2C2). *Acad Med*. 2015 Dec;90(12):1698–1706. doi:10.1097/ACM.0000000000000809.
87. R2C2 feedback and coaching resources. Dalhousie University. Accessed September 17, 2022. https://medicine.dal.ca/departments/core-units/cpd/faculty-development/R2C2.html.
88. Armson H, Lockyer JM, Zetkulic M, Könings KD, Sargeant J. Identifying coaching skills to improve feedback use in postgraduate medical education. *Med Educ*. 2019 May;53(5):477–493. doi:10.1111/medu.13818.
89. Dudek N, Duffy MC, Wood TJ, Gofton W. The Ottawa Resident Observation Form for Nurses (O-RON): assessment of resident performance through the eyes of the nurses. *J Surg Educ*. 2021 Sep-Oct;78(5):1666–1675. doi:10.1016/j.jsurg.2021.03.014.
90. Lockyer J, Lee-Kruger R, Armson H, Hanmore T, Koltz E, Könings K, Mahalik A, Ramani S, Roze des Ordons A, Trier J, Zetkulic M, Sargeant J. Application of the R2C2 model to in-the-moment feedback and coaching. *Academic Medicine*. 2023;98(9):1062–1069. doi:10.1097/ACM.0000000000005237.

13

Simulation Overview

ROSS J. SCALESE, MD

CHAPTER OUTLINE

What Are Medical Simulations and Why Use Them?

Although the seminal articles about simulation in medical education appeared more than 50 years ago,[1,2] it is only in the past two decades or so that we have witnessed a significant increase in the use of simulation technology for teaching and assessment in the health professions (e.g., medicine, nursing, dentistry). This represents a bold departure from the traditional approach, a system that for hundreds of years has centered on real patients for training and testing. Multiple factors have contributed to this evolution. Changes in healthcare delivery have resulted in shorter hospital stays and clinic visits, with greater numbers of patients and higher acuity of illnesses; at academic medical centers this has resulted in reduced availability of patients as learning and assessment opportunities, as well as decreased time for clinical faculty to teach and evaluate trainees.[3,4] Simulators, by contrast, can be readily available at any time and can reproduce a wide variety of clinical conditions and situations on demand. Unlike real patients, simulators are never "off the ward" to undergo diagnostic tests or treatment at the time trainees or examinees arrive to perform their evaluations; simulators are never "too sick," nor do they become tired or embarrassed or behave unpredictably, and therefore they provide a standardized educational experience for all.[5]

In addition, technological advances in diagnosis and treatment, such as newer imaging modalities and minimally invasive procedures, require development of psychomotor and perceptual skills that are different from traditional approaches and therefore require new techniques for teaching, learning, and assessment.[6] Concurrent progress in simulation technology, such as virtual reality simulators that are increasingly realistic, offers advantages for such instruction, skills acquisition, and evaluation.

At the same time, landmark international reports[7-11] have focused increased attention on the problem of medical errors and the need to improve patient safety, not only through prevention of mistakes by individuals, but also through correction of faults in the systems of care. Other fields with high-risk performance environments have long and successfully incorporated simulation technology into their training and assessment programs; examples include flight simulators for pilots and astronauts, technical operations scenarios for nuclear power plant personnel, and war games and training exercises for military personnel. In these examples, simulation technology was used not only to develop and test individual skills and effective collaboration in teams, but also to build a culture of safety.[12-15] By adopting these models in medical education, specialties such as anesthesiology, critical care, and emergency medicine have led the way in using simulation modalities, especially for teaching and testing the skills needed to manage rare or critical incidents.[16,17] Trainees can make mistakes and learn to recognize and correct them in the simulated environment without fear of punishment or harm to real patients.

Closely related to these safety issues are important ethical questions about the appropriateness of "using" real (even standardized) patients as training or assessment resources. Such debate often centers on instructional or evaluation settings that involve sensitive tasks (e.g., pelvic examination) or risk of harm to patients (e.g., endotracheal intubation or other invasive procedures). Uses of patient substitutes, such as cadavers or animals, have attendant ethical concerns of their own; additional challenges, including cost, availability, and maintaining an adequate level of realism, have also limited the role of cadaveric and animal tissue models for clinical skills training and assessment. Simulators, on the other hand, circumvent most of these obstacles and thus have come into widespread use for teaching and evaluation at all levels of healthcare professional education.

Finally, all of these influences driving the increased use of simulation are operating within a broader new context: as described in Chapter 1, recent decades have seen a worldwide shift in focus toward outcomes- or competency-based education throughout the healthcare professions. This paradigm change derives in part from attempts by academic institutions and professional organizations to self-regulate and set quality standards, but chiefly it represents a response to public demand for assurance that doctors are competent.[18] Implicit in the outcomes-based model is the obligation to assess whether specified competencies have actually been achieved: "While student learning is clearly the goal of education, there is a pressing need to provide evidence that learning or mastery actually occurs."[19] Accordingly, medical schools, postgraduate training programs, hospital and healthcare system credentialing committees, and licensing and specialty boards (including their high-stakes certification examinations) have for the past several decades placed greater emphasis on using simulation modalities for the evaluation of clinical competence across multiple domains.[20-27]

So what do we mean by medical simulations? In general terms, medical simulations aim to imitate real patients, anatomic regions, or clinical tasks, and to mirror the real-life situations in which professionals render healthcare services. Such simulations range from static anatomic models and single-task trainers (such as venipuncture arms and intubation mannequin heads) to dynamic computer-enhanced systems that can respond to user actions (such as full-body anesthesia patient simulators); from relatively low-technology standardized patient (SP) encounters to very high-tech virtual reality (VR) surgical simulators; and from individual trainers for evaluating the performance of a single user to interactive role-playing scenarios involving teams of health professionals. The subsequent discussion will employ two variants of the root word: as above, "simula*tion*" refers broadly to any device or set of conditions—including, for example, computer case- and SP-based examinations—that attempts to present evaluation problems authentically, whereas a "simula*tor*," more narrowly defined, is a simulation *device*. Most of our considerations will apply to simulations in general, but because earlier chapters of this textbook (see Chapters 6 and 7) have already explored issues related to SP-based assessments in some depth, this chapter (especially the section on available technologies) will focus more specifically on simulators.

A further clarification of semantics is warranted before proceeding with our discussion. An online dictionary defines *assessment* as follows: "the evaluation or estimation of the nature, quality, or ability of someone or something."[28] This simple but useful definition includes the closely related term *evaluation*, which some distinguish from *assessment* in the educational context by selectively employing the latter to describe methods of obtaining data used to draw inferences about *people*, while reserving *evaluation* to mean similar systematic techniques used to determine characteristics of some unit of instruction or educational *program* (see Chapter 18). For purposes of the ensuing discussion, we will continue to use these terms almost interchangeably, although generally our considerations will focus on the assessment of learning, skills acquisition, or other educational achievement by people, specifically health professionals in training or in practice.

Our analysis will at times center more on simulation-based assessments used for *summative* purposes, rather than *formative* ones. The intention, however, is not to downplay the latter's importance. On the contrary, the provision of individualized feedback plays a role crucial to achieving effective educational outcomes from simulation-based interventions:[29-31] trainees receive guidance directed toward future improvement based on evaluation of their past performance, and thus teaching and learning are intimately related to formative assessment (i.e., assessment *for* learning). Common examples of summative assessments (i.e., assessment *of* learning), on the other hand, include examinations at the end of a clinical clerkship, or after a year of residency training, or prior to specialty certification. These evaluations usually involve higher stakes than tests undertaken for formative purposes; they can determine pass/fail decisions or whether clinical performance meets accepted standards of care for professional licensure.

Finally, one comment as something of a disclaimer: the author will naturally draw on personal educational and clinical experiences to inform the discussion that follows. Therefore examples cited will frequently relate to physician education in the North American context. This is not to discount valuable contributions and lessons learned from experiences in nursing and allied health professions or in other cultures and countries; instead, the intention is to elucidate points that are broadly applicable to simulation-based health professional training and assessment worldwide.

Psychometric Properties and Related Considerations

Before we can discuss utilizing simulations (or, for that matter, any other modality) for the evaluation of clinical competence, we should first establish criteria for appraising the quality and utility of various assessment methods.[32] Traditionally the focus has been on psychometric properties of a given test, especially its validity and reliability evidence, but more recently evaluation experts have proposed additional factors to consider when weighing the pros and cons of different methods and deciding which to utilize for a particular purpose.[33,34] Previous chapters have discussed these criteria for "good assessment," with considerable emphasis appropriately placed on the essential concepts of reliability and validity (see Chapter 2), so we will revisit these topics here in the context of simulation-based evaluations and then return later to explore other criteria good assessments should meet, such as those relating to educational impact and credibility/acceptability of resulting decisions.

To start, although we often speak of reliability and validity as properties intrinsic to an evaluation tool itself, it is important to remember that they actually characterize the test scores—and subsequent interpretations and decisions based on them—obtained using a given assessment method with a certain population under a particular set of circumstances and for a specific purpose.[35] Therefore it is preferable to say "there is validity evidence for a particular use of an assessment tool" versus "a tool is valid." Furthermore, when considering these properties as they pertain to simulation technologies, evaluators must distinguish between the measurement characteristics of the simulator per se and those of the assessment overall. This is because simulators themselves usually do not constitute the entire assessment, but rather serve as tools to complement existing evaluation methods, present clinical findings, and facilitate standardization. For example, simulators often serve effectively as tools used in the examining stations of an objective structured clinical examination (OSCE). In such assessments, examiners often utilize checklists or global rating scales to judge examinee performance in the simulations, and these rating instruments have their own measurement characteristics. Thus we can discuss separately the psychometric properties of a simulation itself versus those of a rating scale versus those of an OSCE in its entirety; at the same time, it is worthwhile to consider the interrelated ways in which, say, the reproducibility of performance metrics obtained from a simulator in one testing station contributes evidence for the reliability of overall examination scores and the validity of decisions based on those assessment results.

Reliability

Viewed in a simplified way, *reliability* in the context of assessments in general refers to the reproducibility of scores obtained using a particular evaluation method and, more specifically applied to medical simulations, involves the ability of the simulator to capture performance data dependably and/or present the same stimulus (clinical findings, task, or scenario) repeatedly and consistently over multiple occasions and to any number of examinees. If we consider that the clinical assessment equation contains three variables—patient, examiner, and examinee—then to devise an evaluation from which the score obtained represents a true measure of an examinee's clinical competence, we must control for the first two variables.[5] Examiner training and the reliable use of other evaluation tools (checklists, rating scales, etc.) allow for standardization of the "examiner" component. Simulators, on the other hand, by virtue of their programmability, can standardize many aspects of the "patient" variable, offering a uniform, reproducible experience to multiple examinees. Thus an inherent advantage of simulations for assessment is that there is generally strong reliability evidence to support their use, which is especially important for high-stakes examinations. Reliability coefficients for scores obtained using a simulator in a particular assessment setting are relatively straightforward to calculate.[36]

Validity

By contrast, we cannot directly measure *validity* or calculate a "validity coefficient"; instead, we must accumulate evidence from various analyses and empirical studies to support (or refute) the validity of interpretations and uses we make of test results.[37,38] Whereas reliability relates to reproducibility and consistency—and is a property of the data collected in an assessment—validity refers to accuracy and defensibility and is a characteristic of the interpretations, uses, and decisions we make based on those data. Thus the two concepts are very closely interrelated: without reliable measurements, valid interpretations and uses of resulting data are nearly impossible to make. As stated earlier, validity is not an intrinsic attribute of certain rating instruments or assessment methods per se, but rather is critically dependent on the context in which an evaluation takes place (i.e., a particular test is administered for a particular purpose at a particular time with a particular group of examinees).[35] Moreover, validity evidence presented to support the interpretation of scores obtained in one assessment context might not be appropriate to defend decisions based upon data derived under different testing conditions or with a different population.[37,38]

Now, historically the educational literature has discussed different facets of validity. For instance, we can speak of "construct validity" as it pertains to a simulator used for assessment: if it is a valid test of, say, endoscopic skills, experts with the most experience in real endoscopy should perform best on the simulated task, novices with no real-life endoscopy experience should perform least well on the simulator, and a group with some experience in actual endoscopy should perform at a level somewhere between that of the other two groups. Alternatively, we might infer "predictive validity" of a certain VR catheterization simulator if the same radiology residents who perform better on simulator-based skills testing later perform better, as rated by trained expert examiners, during actual interventional radiology (IR) procedures. Consensus opinion of a panel of experts can provide evidence of "content validity":

experienced cardiologists agree that the findings on a cardiology patient simulator are representative of those in patients with actual cardiac diseases, or surgeons with expertise in a particular procedure determine that skills assessed on a surgical simulator represent the key steps in performing the real task.

Our contemporary concept of validity has evolved significantly over the past 40 to 50 years, and experts in educational measurement today tend to avoid such terminology that distinguishes different facets of validity, maintaining that all validity arguments aim to present evidence of *construct validity*.[37,38] Messick[39] first proposed this unifying framework—which leading educational and psychological testing organizations subsequently adopted and which remains the current standard[40]—describing five main sources of validity evidence: content, response process, internal structure, relationship to other variables, and consequences.[37-40] The preceding paragraph offered examples of different sources of validity evidence that could potentially be used to argue in favor of (or against) proposed interpretations of assessment data: the endoscopy and catheterization simulator–based evaluations could provide evidence from relationships to other variables (e.g., correlation with practitioners' level of experience in endoscopy and with ratings during performance of actual IR procedures, respectively), and descriptions of convening expert panels to create simulation scenarios and scoring rubrics could contribute to content evidence. These latter two sources of validity evidence, as well as internal structure evidence (often supported by reliability data or item analyses), are by far the most frequently reported—versus a paucity of evidence about response process and consequences—for simulation-based assessments.[41]

Kane[42-44] proposed another approach to validity that structures the evidence from these various sources into a cohesive overall argument intended to justify proposed interpretations or uses of test results. He contends that we draw multiple inferences, each underpinned by various assumptions, when we make the leap from observations of performance in a given assessment to some downstream decision based on those observations. He describes four main links in this "chain of inferences": (1) scoring—we assume that observations made and data collected during an assessment have been accurately translated into a score that represents examinee performance/competence in a given domain (i.e., the construct of interest); (2) generalization—we assume that performance and resulting scores in one examination, one "snapshot in time," accurately predict performance in the "universe" of possible testing situations that purport to assess the same competencies; (3) extrapolation—we assume that performance in such testing situations accurately predicts performance under real-world conditions; and (4) decision/interpretation—we assume that final interpretations of scores, and that rules applied to make decisions based on those scores (e.g., that an examinee passes or fails), are justifiable and credible to multiple stakeholders in the assessment process.

Characteristics of various assessment methods will impact which components of the validity argument are usually most sound and which typically constitute "the weakest link" in the chain of inferences.[45] For simulator-based assessments, for example, evidence to support the scoring component of the validity argument is often readily obtainable: if simulators contain built-in sensors that record performance data which are used to determine scores, documentation that the devices are periodically checked and calibrated to guarantee proper functioning and data capture would reinforce this piece of the argument. Additional substantiating evidence for this element could include descriptions of how specific scoring criteria are developed and how raters are trained to apply those criteria. The generalization component of the validity argument, on the other hand, is often more problematic: by contrast with, say, written exams, most simulation-based evaluations have a relatively small number of items (i.e., testing scenarios), which limits the generalizability of results from one exam administration to another. In fact, the potential for such "construct underrepresentation" (which can lead to sampling error) and related problems with content specificity are significant threats to validity for most performance-based evaluations.[38] However, unlike workplace-based assessments (where test observations are limited to the actual patients, conditions, or procedures encountered in the clinic or hospital on a given day), simulations are programmable and therefore permit as many additional testing scenarios to be created and carried out as needed (within the constraints of available resources). Increasing the number of exam items in this manner and utilizing sampling procedures that determine case mix according to a blueprint broadly representative of the domain under consideration are effective ways to reinforce this weak (generalization) link in the validity argument for simulation-based assessments. The extrapolation component of the argument usually relies on the assumption that the more realistic the simulation, the stronger the link between performance in the testing environment and performance under real-world conditions. Of course, we must still provide evidence that this assumption is valid before we can justify interpretations of assessment results and uses of those judgments to make final decisions.

Fidelity

Thus any discussion about simulation validity eventually entails use of another important term, *fidelity*, which describes some aspect of the authenticity of the experience, or the likeness of the simulation to the real-world circumstances it was designed to duplicate. As was just alluded to in the preceding section, the fidelity of a simulation used for assessment purposes is important principally as it relates to the *extrapolation* component of the validity argument in support of using simulation-based test results to make certain decisions. (The older assessment literature refers to the related concept of *face validity*, a term that most educational measurement professionals now discourage.[38]) Of course, despite technological advances that result in ever more lifelike systems, the fidelity of a simulation is never completely identical to "the real thing." Some reasons are obvious: engineering limitations, psychometric requirements, ethical and safety considerations, and time and cost constraints.[46]

Again, fidelity describes the extent to which the appearance and behavior of the simulation imitate the appearance and behavior of the real system, but several authors have offered clarification of past inconsistency and imprecision in use of the term, highlighting important distinctions between physical (or engineering) fidelity and functional (or psychological) fidelity.[47] Some even suggest abandoning the term *fidelity* altogether and using instead more intuitive and useful expressions such as "physical resemblance" and "functional task alignment."[48] The latter (or psychological fidelity) refers to the degree to which the simulated task duplicates the skills or behaviors in the real task. Engineering or physical fidelity, on the other hand, refers to the degree to which the simulation device or training environment reproduces the physical characteristics or appearance of the real clinical situation. Simulators with high-level engineering fidelity often employ high-tech components (e.g., full-body computerized mannequins or VR simulators), thus inappropriately leading some to equate "high-tech" with "high-fidelity" simulation. However, simulations can achieve high-level psychological fidelity with relatively low-technology methods (e.g., SP scenarios). Conversely, the use of high-tech computerized mannequins to test interpersonal communication skills would be less authentic than using SPs as the simulation modality, and this lower fidelity would be a threat to validity (of the extrapolation component) in the argument to defend decisions based on such an assessment. Therefore, as with choosing simulators for training purposes, evaluators must match the fidelity of a simulation with its intended use as an assessment tool. "The highest possible fidelity may be unnecessary or even introduce undesired complexity for teaching [or evaluating] a particular skill and may result in unacceptably expensive simulations, making the methodology an unfeasible teaching [or assessment] tool."[4]

Feasibility

Therefore another important consideration when discussing the use of simulators for assessment is *feasibility*, which generally relates to the practicality and cost-effectiveness of employing a particular device or method as an evaluation tool. A later section of this chapter addresses the various costs (for the device, training, personnel, maintenance, etc.) to be tallied. In addition, the reckoning of a simulation's feasibility for assessment must include not only whether we *can* afford a simulator in terms of resources required, but also whether we *should* acquire and implement it for a particular evaluation—that is to say, are any demonstrable improvements in testing with the simulator compared with a traditional method worth the expenditure of money, time, and so forth?

Scoring and Rating Instruments

Finally, there are important considerations relevant to developing scoring rubrics for simulation-based assessments. Several criteria are available for generating scores for performance during trainee evaluations, and the optimal choice generally depends on whether the competency tested relates more to a *process* (such as completing an orderly and thorough "code blue" resuscitation) or an *outcome* (such as the status of the [simulated] patient after said cardiopulmonary resuscitation). In some cases, such as summative assessments to determine if examinee performance meets a minimum acceptable level or standard of care, process criteria form a more appropriate basis for the evaluation, with measurement against a checklist of explicit steps being the most commonly employed technique. In other instances, we might deem the final result or "bottom line"—Did the examinee make the right diagnosis? Is the patient alive?—more important than the method of achieving that result, in which case outcome criteria may be more relevant.[35,49] Tables 13.1 to 13.3 illustrate how we might assess processes and/or outcomes with simulators.[50]

As mentioned briefly earlier in this section and detailed in previous chapters (see Chapters 2 and 4), the checklists and global rating scales based on such criteria and used along with simulators in performance-based clinical examinations have their own reliability and validity characteristics, which depend (among other factors) on rater training, the specific skill under evaluation, and the purpose of the particular assessment. For example, if evaluation is undertaken as a formative exercise, particularly with novice learners, process criteria assessed via checklists can provide specific and actionable feedback: trainees can see exactly which key questions they failed to ask when taking a history during simulated patient encounters, or which critical steps they skipped when performing a certain procedure on a simulator, and thus they can focus their remediation efforts on those areas. By contrast, seeing the results of an evaluation that utilized global rating scales—for instance, that an individual received a 4 on a 7-point Likert scale in one assessment domain, especially if the numeric ratings lack corresponding specific behavioral anchors—may not provide as useful feedback toward future improvement for that learner. On the other hand, when used for summative assessment, including that of more advanced trainees, outcome criteria judged by expert examiners using well-constructed rating scales can produce more reliable scores than checklists, leading to decisions (e.g., about promotion to the next phase of training or specialist certification) with reasonable validity evidence.[49,51]

TABLE 13.1 Scoring Criteria and Examples

Criteria Type	Example
Explicit process (measurement)	A case-specific checklist to record action steps during suturing on a skin wound simulator (see Table 13.2)
Implicit process (judgment)	A global rating scale (with well-defined anchor points) that allows an evaluator to observe and judge the quality of suturing performed on a skin wound simulator (see Table 13.3)
Explicit outcome (measurement)	Observing and recording specific indicators of patient (simulator) status—alive, cardiac rhythm, blood pressure—after an Advanced Cardiac Life Support "code blue" resuscitation
Implicit outcome (judgment)	A global rating scale (with well-defined anchor points) that allows an evaluator to observe and judge the quality of the overall patient status after an Advanced Cardiac Life Support "code blue" resuscitation
Combined (explicit process and outcome)	A task-specific checklist for performing a bedside cardiac examination and observation/recording of correct identification and interpretation of physical findings

TABLE 13.2 Explicit Process Criteria: Suturing

Process	Not Done or Incorrect	Done Correctly
Held instruments correctly		X
Spaced sutures 3–5 mm	X	
Tied square knots		X
Cut suture to correct length		X
Apposed skin without excessive tension on sutures	X	

Adapted from Kalu PU, Atkins J, Baker D, Green CJ, Butler PEM. How do we assess microsurgical skill? *Microsurgery*. 2005;25(1):25-29. doi:10.1002/micr.20078.

Strengths and Best Applications

Earlier we highlighted the reliability of simulations as one of the principal advantages of their use for assessment: because they are programmable, simulators are usually highly standardized, thereby minimizing the variability inherent in actual clinical encounters. This reproducibility and consistency in presenting evaluation problems in the same manner for every examinee is extremely important, especially when high-stakes decisions hinge on these assessments. We also mentioned previously an additional strength of simulators as evaluation tools: namely, the ability of some devices to simulate a wide range of patients or clinical problems, and to do so on demand. In addition to increasing the number of observations in a test sample and thereby improving the generalizability of exam results, this transforms assessment planning from an opportunistic process (dependent on finding patients with specific conditions of interest) to a proactive scheme with great flexibility for evaluators. Add to these benefits the avoidance of problems when performing assessments in actual clinical settings related to patients' acuity of illness, modesty, or safety, and multiple advantages of simulation-based evaluations become apparent.

Now, in considering the best applications of simulation technology (or any modality) for assessment purposes, we should examine multiple dimensions of an evaluation system and look for optimal alignment with the testing methods. As described in Chapter 1, the core dimensions of an assessment framework include (1) the outcomes that need to be assessed; (2) the level of assessment that is most appropriate; and (3) the developmental stage of those undergoing assessment; additional dimensions that merit careful consideration encompass the overall context, especially the purpose(s), of the assessment (Fig. 13.1).[52]

TABLE 13.3 Implicit Process Criteria: Suturing

1	2	3	4	5
Time and motion				
Many unnecessary or repetitive movements		Efficient time/motion, but some unnecessary and repetitive movements		Clear economy of movements and maximum efficiency
Instrument handling				
1	2	3	4	5
Repeatedly makes tentative or awkward moves with instruments through inappropriate use		Consistent use of instruments, but occasionally appears stiff or awkward		Fluid movement with instruments

Adapted from Kalu PU, Atkins J, Baker D, Green CJ, Butler PEM. How do we assess microsurgical skill? *Microsurgery*. 2005;25(1):25-29. doi:10.1002/micr.20078.

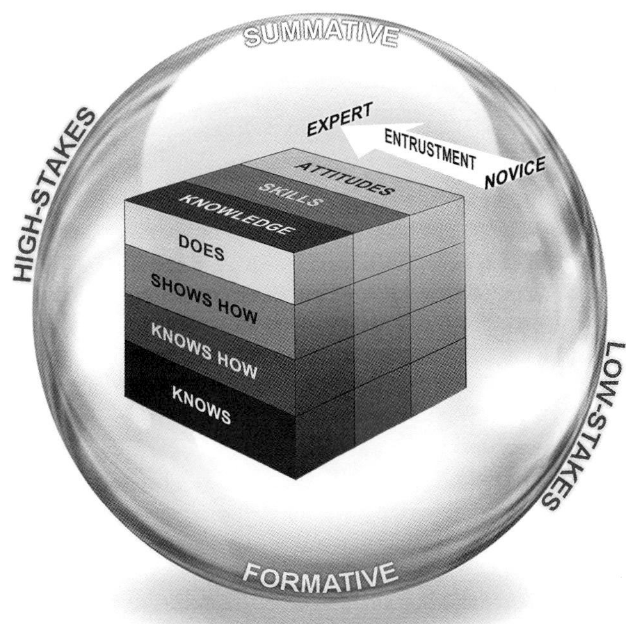

• **Fig. 13.1** Multidimensional assessment framework.

For our discussion of the outcomes to be assessed, we can use the framework established by the Accreditation Council for Graduate Medical Education (ACGME), which describes six general domains constituting the core competencies that all postgraduate trainees in the United States must demonstrate: (1) Professionalism, (2) Patient Care and Procedural Skills, (3) Medical Knowledge, (4) Practice-based Learning and Improvement, (5) Interpersonal and Communication Skills, and (6) Systems-based Practice.[53] (Other international accreditation bodies have outlined analogous core roles of a physician and standards of good medical practice.[54,55]) Evaluators may use simulations to assess various knowledge, skills, and attitudes within these domains. During a ward rotation for internal medicine residents, for example, faculty may test aspects of trainees' *patient care* (using a cardiology patient simulator, demonstrate the ability to perform a focused cardiac examination and identify the presence of a third heart sound in a "patient" presenting with dyspnea); *medical knowledge* (using a full-body simulator during a simulated case of sudden cardiac death, verbalize the correct steps in the algorithm for treatment of ventricular fibrillation); or *interpersonal and communication skills* and *professionalism* (during a simulation integrating an SP with a plastic mannequin arm, demonstrate how to draw blood cultures while explaining to the patient the indications for the procedure). This last example highlights the fact that real clinical encounters often require practitioners to bring to bear their abilities in multiple competency domains simultaneously. Formal assessments traditionally focused on isolated clinical skills (e.g., perform a procedure on a simulator at one station in an OSCE, obtain a history or deliver bad news with an SP at another station). More recently, innovative work has featured evaluations more reflective of actual clinical practice by integrating simulation modalities—for instance, a trainee must interact (gather some history, obtain consent, explain the procedure) with a male SP who is draped below the waist *while* inserting a urinary bladder catheter into a task trainer placed beneath the drape—for simultaneous assessment of technical and nontechnical (communication) skills.[56]

When the ACGME promulgated the six general competencies (as well as certain "required skills" within each of these domains), it also provided a Toolbox of Assessment Methods that can help to align "suggested best methods for evaluation" with competencies along the outcomes dimension of our assessment framework.[57] For example, in the *Patient Care* domain, the toolbox ranked simulations among "the most desirable" methods for evaluating ability to perform medical procedures and "the next best method" for demonstrating how to develop and carry out patient management plans; within the *Medical Knowledge* competency, evaluators can devise simulations to assess trainees' investigatory/analytic thinking or knowledge/application of basic sciences; simulations are "a potentially applicable method" to evaluate how clinicians analyze their own practice for needed improvements (*Practice-based Learning and Improvement* domain); and in the realm of *Professionalism*, simulations are among the methods listed for assessing ethically sound practice.[57] More recently, the ACGME has updated this resource in the form of an Assessment Guidebook,[58] with one section devoted to simulation methods for assessing the ACGME general competencies; this includes summary descriptions of best uses and features of simulations for assessment, as well as suggested references that provide further information. (Comparable international bodies have published similar guidance for assessments aligned with their outcomes frameworks.[59,60])

The next dimension of an evaluation system to consider relates to the level of assessment required. Accordingly, within any of the domains of competence just described, we can assess learners at four different levels, according to the pyramid model conceptualized by Miller:[61]

1. *Knows* (knowledge)—recall of basic facts, principles, and theories
2. *Knows how* (application of knowledge)—ability to solve problems, make decisions, and describe procedures
3. *Shows how* (performance)—demonstration of skills in a controlled setting
4. *Does* (action)—behavior in real practice

Recently some have argued that Miller's pyramid framework does not go far enough, suggesting there are other considerations or levels of assessment beyond what a clinician "does" in practice.[62,63] After all, the ultimate purpose of the assessment system for health professions education programs is to ensure that graduates can be entrusted to provide high-quality and safe care in unsupervised practice (see Chapter 1). In other words, we can try to assess the real-world *behaviors* of health professionals, but in the end we are most interested in the *results* of those behaviors (i.e., individual patient outcomes as well as population health effects). Later we will discuss a parallel model with different levels—elaborated in terms of translational science—that encompass these aspirational patient care and public health outcomes.[64,65]

Returning for the moment to Miller's pyramid, various assessment methods are more (or less) suitable for evaluation at the different levels of competence. For instance, written instruments, such as examinations consisting of multiple-choice questions (MCQs), are efficient tools for assessing what a student "knows." Similarly, other types of written formats (e.g., constructed-response items, such as short-answer or essay questions) are effective methods to evaluate problem-solving; alternatively, an oral examination might require a trainee to verbally describe the steps for, say, intravenous (IV) cannulation to assess whether the trainee "knows how" to perform that procedure. However, it's another thing entirely for the same trainee to "show how" to place an IV catheter, so assessment at this level requires performance-based/observational methods, either in simulated settings (e.g., stations of an OSCE) or in the actual workplace. Indeed, it is at this "shows how" level that the ACGME Assessment Guidebook suggests simulations are most appropriately employed to evaluate a range of competencies.[58] Assessment at the highest level of the pyramid, though, can be more challenging: simulations are generally suboptimal methods to evaluate what a health professional "does" in actual practice, because providers might alter their behavior as soon as they become aware that a clinical encounter is, in fact, a simulation. However, interesting research employing unannounced or "incognito SPs" represents a promising (but underused) simulation-based technique to assess practitioners' attitudes and behaviors under real-world conditions.[66-71]

Thus far we have considered dimensions of an assessment system separately and attempted to find the best alignment of various evaluation methods with either the competencies being assessed or the level of assessment. Obviously, though, the area of interaction between these two dimensions circumscribes a smaller set of evaluation tools that are best suited for a given purpose: from the foregoing analysis, then, we see that the optimal uses of simulation-based methods are for assessment of technical (i.e., clinical or procedural) skills and nontechnical (i.e., behavioral or affective) competencies at the "shows how" level in Miller's model.[52]

Revisiting the ACGME competency framework, it is no accident that the Toolbox of Assessment Methods rates simulations most highly for the evaluation of just such performance-based outcomes.[57] Extending the metaphor, we can graphically depict this "toolbox": various assessment methods are the tools stored inside its many "drawers," which are organized in columns corresponding to outcomes—distilling core competencies from any framework into just three categories that encompass all cognitive ("knowledge"), psychomotor ("skills"), and affective ("attitudes") domains—and in rows according to assessment levels. Accordingly, Fig. 13.2 illustrates the best places (assessment settings) in which to keep (use) our simulation tools.[52]

Careful consideration of this construct highlights a fundamental threat to the validity of using current assessment

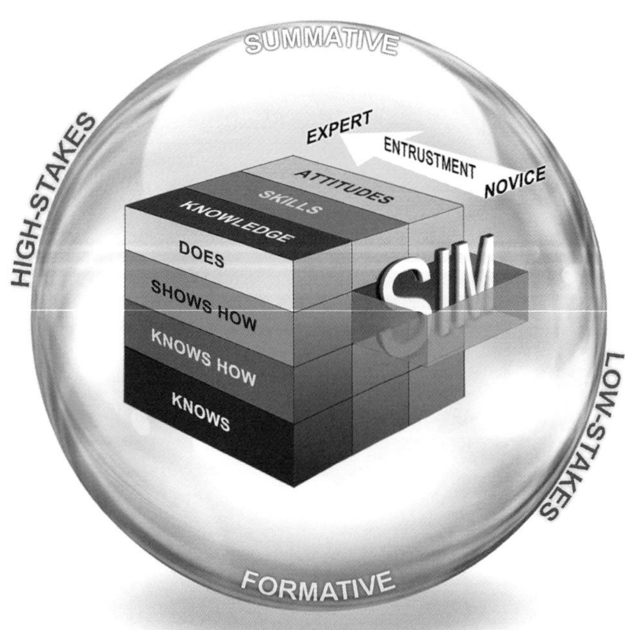

• **Fig. 13.2** Simulation uses within a multidimensional assessment framework.

methods—principally *written* (MCQ) and, in some cases, *oral* exams—for the purpose of initial board certification of surgeons and other procedural specialists in the United States. While these methods are well suited to evaluating clinicians' factual knowledge and ability to apply that knowledge for problem-solving and so forth, the competencies that actually distinguish these procedural medical specialties from others comprise mainly psychomotor skills and behaviors that, as just discussed, are best assessed at the "shows how" level using *performance-based* methods. While these might include direct observations of performance in real-world settings with patients, such assessments would lack standardization if attempts were made to implement them at a national scale. Simulation-based methods, on the other hand, facilitate to a much greater degree the standardization of exam stimuli, response processes, and so forth that are especially important in high-stakes examination settings such as this. We will further explore the uses of simulation for specialty board certification in the final section of the chapter, when we attempt to predict future trends in the application of these modalities for assessment.

Yet another section (on available technologies) will describe just how many simulation options are available in various compartments of the toolbox. In choosing from among the multiple simulation-based methods at our disposal, we should next consider which tools are best suited to assess learners at different stages of development. Here the level of simulation fidelity becomes important. For example, devices with low to medium physical and psychological fidelity (such as simple anatomic models and part-task trainers) that test single competencies of an individual are more appropriate for novices, who might otherwise become overwhelmed by full-blown team-based scenarios in immersive simulation environments. Beginners may find this level of cognitive and psychological load unmanageable and, especially if the assessment is undertaken for formative purposes, this could have negative effects on learning outcomes. Experts, on the other hand, are expected to cope with the many stressors encountered in actual clinical practice, so highly realistic simulations—often incorporating multiple participants and computerized mannequins or VR devices—would be required to replicate real-life clinical situations and thereby test several competencies simultaneously. Otherwise, lack of authenticity in simulation-based assessments could weaken the extrapolation component of the argument and threaten the validity of decisions based on such evaluations of performance by experts.

Therefore the developmental stage of those undergoing assessment is another dimension to which we must pay attention in any evaluation system. These stages can be described in multiple ways: the terms used earlier (novice and expert) represent opposite ends of a five-stage continuum of skill acquisition—with several intermediate (advanced beginner–competent–proficient) stages—in the model proposed by the Dreyfus brothers.[72] In the ACGME outcomes framework, similar concepts (also described in a five-stage model) have been elaborated in terms of specialty-specific developmental "milestones" such that, for any of the required skills within the six core ACGME domains, a resident's progress toward readiness for unsupervised practice can be assessed.[73] However, because some of the general competencies—such as Practice-based Learning and Improvement and Systems-based Practice—are relatively abstract (and often very broad), they have proven difficult to understand (and to assess).[74] (Also see Chapters 10 and 11.) In response to these challenges, educators have recently focused their attention on Entrustable Professional Activities (EPAs), which are those skills and behaviors that comprise the critical day-to-day activities of a practitioner in a given discipline.[75,76] EPAs often encompass elements from several different general competency domains, which, while difficult to evaluate in isolation, can be directly observed in aggregate during such activities, allowing judgments to be made about the degree to which a trainee can be trusted to carry out those clinical tasks. Levels of entrustment in this rating scheme include (1) not trusted to perform at all (even with supervision), (2) trusted to perform only with direct supervision, (3) trusted to perform with indirect supervision/backup nearby, (4) trusted to perform independently, and (5) trusted to perform at aspirational level (i.e., equivalent to an attending physician, trusted to supervise and teach others to perform).[77] Such entrustment decisions can be aligned in parallel with developmental milestones/stages along the same dimension of an assessment system (Figs. 13.1 and 13.2). At first thought, because the EPAs constitute mainly skills and behaviors that can be directly observed—versus knowledge outcomes that can only be inferred—simulation-based assessments should be well suited to assist in making these entrustment decisions. However, EPAs (by definition) capture the essential things a health professional *does* in daily practice, so the level of assessment here should be at the highest tier of Miller's pyramid where, as already mentioned, applicable simulation-based assessment modalities are limited (to those employing incognito SPs). Nonetheless, simulations can still play a role in evaluating EPAs: because of patient safety and ethical concerns with novices at the lower levels of entrustment (see further discussion later in this chapter), simulator-based assessments can provide a safe context for trainees to *show* that they have acquired certain competencies and can aid in decisions about whether/when they are ready to be awarded greater clinical responsibilities.

For at least 20 years, clinical educators have called for greater use of simulations in health professions training as "an ethical imperative."[78] Unfortunately, some of the same obstacles to wider implementation cited then still exist today: "Health care has lagged behind in simulation applications for a number of reasons, including cost, lack of rigorous proof of effect, and resistance to change."[78,p.783] There are costs associated with simulation assessment programs (which we will discuss in the next section); in addition, the challenges posed by the legacy of conservatism in medicine historically have been difficult to overcome. There has been progress, however, in the form of translational science research that provides solid evidence linking learning in the simulation context to improved patient care practices and outcomes.[79] Reports citing impacts at these higher translational (so-called T2 and T3[64]) levels have focused primarily on simulation-based formative assessment as an essential component of educational interventions that feature mastery learning with deliberate practice.[80-84] Both of these training models set very high standards that go beyond "competent" performance, instead aspiring to "mastery" or "expert" levels of achievement in a particular domain; such rigorous expectations are entirely appropriate in the healthcare context given the implications for patient safety. Attainment of these high standards is guided by individualized feedback derived from ongoing assessments of performance that may employ simulators. Given mounting evidence that demonstrates effectiveness for the acquisition of various (especially procedural) skills across multiple discipli nes,[82,83,85-92] simulation-based mastery learning and performance assessment should be standard practice in health professions training programs today.

To continue exploring the topic of simulation-based evaluation of EPAs: moving the location of such exercises from a simulation lab or dedicated testing center to the actual clinical environments in which trainees or practitioners work (so-called "in situ" simulation) can enhance the authenticity of examination scenarios,[93] thus further justifying entrustment decisions by strengthening inferences that performance in the assessment setting is likely to predict real-world behavior. Physical location and testing environment are just two of many interrelated contextual dimensions that are important to consider in any assessment framework; others include availability of resources and sociocultural norms as they exist in the local setting. Sensitivity to such factors when designing simulation scenarios for evaluation is critical to achieving buy-in from stakeholders in the process.

Of course, the most essential element of context surrounding any assessment is its purpose: are we trying to make summative determinations, or provide formative feedback to individuals/teams, or obtain information for program evaluation? Do we intend to make decisions based on the assessment that have high-stakes implications for individual examinees/clinicians, or for teachers/training programs, or for patients/society? Educators must remain cognizant of the fact that tests, no matter their purpose (i.e., whether summative or formative), will have some educational impact on examinees—"assessment drives learning"—and evaluators must try to use this phenomenon to best advantage by developing assessment programs that will guide learners' educational efforts in a positive direction.[94] Moreover, both Messick's[37-40] and Kane's[42-44] frameworks recognize that consideration of the consequences of an examination, whether high or low stakes, is an important (but sometimes overlooked[41]) source of evidence when making an argument that the use of a given assessment for a particular purpose is valid.

The best applications, then, of simulation-based evaluation tools will be those that align possible testing methods along different axes of an assessment framework: such analysis must encompass the specification of outcomes, assessment levels, and learner developmental stages, as well as consider the overall purpose of an evaluation and other contextual layers that surround and influence dimensions at the core of the assessment system (see Fig. 13.2).

Weaknesses and Challenges

Some of the same features that make simulations an asset in the context of competency evaluation can also become liabilities. For example, we began the preceding section (about strengths of simulation-based methods) by talking about the reliability of sensor data from simulators and the reproducibility of scenario presentations, which are ordinarily quite high. But what if a device malfunctions or a standardized patient deviates from the script? This would represent a threat to the validity of assumptions in the scoring phase of the argument to defend the use of such simulation-based assessment results.

We also highlighted versatility—that is, the capability of some simulators to reproduce a wide array of clinical problems or situations on demand—as another strength of these methods for testing competencies across many disciplines and professions. However, despite the availability of an ever-growing assortment of technologies (detailed in the next section), several subject areas remain for which realistic simulations scarcely exist. Notably, in the realm of basic clinical skills evaluation: until as recently as five years ago there were very few commercially available anatomic models that authentically replicate the look, feel, and sounds of the human abdomen for testing ability to perform relevant portions of the physical exam. Similarly, although some computer-enhanced simulators feature isolated neurologic findings (pupils that react to light, or arm drift on upper-extremity strength testing), currently no mannequin can reproduce a range of lifelike motor, sensory, or deep-tendon reflex findings during neurologic examination. Although actors might be able to feign abdominal tenderness or focal weakness, there are many other physical exam abnormalities (e.g., organomegaly, certain cranial neuropathies, etc.) that SPs simply cannot mimic unless they happen to have such pathologic findings.

Another major gap in simulator technology pertains to the assessment of surgical skills: although the advent of minimally invasive techniques has spurred the invention of numerous VR systems to evaluate competencies unique to those "keyhole" procedures, good simulations for replicating open surgical procedures remain difficult to find. Currently cadaveric/fresh-frozen human tissue and animal models are utilized to practice and assess operative surgical skills, but these face significant challenges in terms of cost, realism, and ethical concerns (with animal welfare issues in particular receiving much public scrutiny). However, obstacles such as these—related to unavailability of simulations in certain domains and disciplines—hardly seem insurmountable: already the educators of today are creatively leveraging technologies and expertise from arenas outside medicine (e.g., materials science and engineering, even television and film prosthetics) to develop new simulations that can meet the training and evaluation needs of tomorrow.[95-97]

On the other hand, challenges related to psychometric and feasibility considerations can prove more difficult to overcome. As touched upon previously, costs are often among the most significant roadblocks to implementation of a simulation program, whether for teaching or for assessment. Simulators—especially those utilizing sophisticated technologies, such as computer-enhanced mannequins or VR systems—can be expensive: beyond the initial purchase price, we must also factor in ongoing costs to operate, store, maintain, and update the devices. For example, high-fidelity patient simulators can range in price from around $30,000 to more than $250,000, and service agreements for the most full-featured models can exceed an additional $10,000 per year. Beyond these obvious direct financial expenditures, assessment planners should not underestimate the human resources (and associated indirect costs) required for any evaluation program, including those employing simulation-based methods. Even for relatively low-tech modalities (e.g., those utilizing SPs), there are costs associated with recruiting, training, and utilizing various personnel for role-playing, supervision, and evaluation (see Chapter 6). This is not to say, however, that simulation-based training and assessment programs will always yield negative returns on investment; on the contrary, especially if simulation interventions can be linked to downstream improvements in patient care, the anticipated positive benefits should easily justify the funding required to develop, implement, and sustain such programs. The difficulty lies in demonstrating such causal links, given the many confounding contributors to ultimate patient outcomes in complex clinical settings. These challenges notwithstanding, there is (limited) research to suggest that simulation-based training and assessment programs can be cost-effective.[98,99]

The ability to save faculty time is an often-touted advantage of simulation technology as an instructional tool (i.e., when trainees can use the devices for self-directed learning). When simulation methods are used for testing, however, often the same does not hold true. Although some simulators have built-in measurement/recording functions that can provide assessment data, we noted earlier that most tests use simulators in conjunction with other evaluation instruments, such as checklists or rating scales, and these require human scoring. Thus we may not save faculty or staff time; in fact, for such assessments to be reliable, examiners must receive adequate training, and even raters with expertise in the domains under evaluation—who presumably need less training than, say, nonmedical personnel employed for the purposes of a given examination—will require time for familiarization with a particular measurement tool and for standardization of ratings. Their time is a valuable commodity. Development of scenarios for use in simulator-based examinations can also be time and resource intensive. Ideally, pilot testing of these evaluation schemes should occur, and this has associated costs that accrue even before final implementation of the assessment. All of these factors pose even greater challenges for large-scale (e.g., national) testing programs and high-stakes (e.g., professional licensure) examinations.

Another drawback of some simulators for assessment is lack of portability: they may be bulky, and their computer or other hardware components may be delicate, limiting testing to dedicated centers and controlled environments. This imposes significant disadvantages if we are trying to assess, say, the skills of paramedics or military personnel in a realistic field setting. Along similar lines, many devices simulate only specific conditions or procedures; although such models may have very high fidelity within their limited domains, the lack of flexibility to design tests for a wide range of clinical contexts or skills limits the use of some simulators as evaluation tools.

These considerations lead again to questions raised earlier about feasibility: can we design tests with strong validity and reliability evidence for a desired outcome using a particular device? Can (or should) we justify the expense of a simulator for a given assessment? High-tech devices have a certain allure—we all want to have "the latest and greatest" gadget—but program planners must consider the cost-effectiveness of any method and, ultimately, whether the decisions based on such evaluations will better identify those healthcare providers who are competent for safe practice with patients. Rational allocation of resources for assessment programs—whether at the level of medical schools, residency training programs, credentialing bodies, or certification boards—demands *evidence* that the investment will yield valuable results.

In this respect, systematic reviews[29,30,100,101] of the extant research on medical simulations have demonstrated significant shortcomings: (1) many publications in the field (especially early reports) are descriptive in nature rather than experimental designs; (2) many studies predominantly measure the effects of simulation versus traditional training or nonsimulation methods (rather than direct simulation-to-simulation comparisons)[102]; and (3) most research is discipline specific, limited to a single institution, and statistically underpowered—all contributing to a lack of scientific rigor sufficient to support meaningful analysis.[103] In addition, much of the research on simulation-based assessment per se, including the good earlier work on evaluations utilizing SPs,[104,105] focuses on psychometric properties and scoring. Although issues such as a test's validity evidence are certainly important, most of these studies offer evidence of (using older terminology) face, construct, or content validity, while not addressing the perhaps more important question of predictive validity—that is, will performance on a given assessment predict future performance in actual practice? Only relatively recently have reports of newer simulation devices for testing (e.g., VR systems for minimally invasive procedures) spoken to such important considerations.[106,107] (We will continue to explore this topic when discussing particular simulation technologies in the next section of this chapter.) Translational validation studies such as these, however, pose dilemmas of their own: in trying to gather evidence (e.g., from relationship to other variables) to support inferences in the extrapolation phase of the validity argument, is it ethical to let subpar performers identified in a simulation exercise later carry out tasks, especially invasive procedures, on live patients?

Available Technologies

As mentioned several times already, there are numerous medical simulators commercially available today and, keeping pace with remarkable technological and engineering advances that allow creation of higher fidelity devices, that number is increasing rapidly. Therefore this chapter cannot provide a comprehensive listing of all the technologies available to educators and evaluators; any such compendium would quickly become outdated. Rather, we will attempt to provide an overview of the range and types of simulators currently available, as well as some references for those seeking to obtain more detailed information about particular systems (see Appendix 13.1 and the disclosure at the end of this chapter). To organize our approach to the large number of simulators available, we will discuss current technologies for various medical disciplines broadly grouped into three categories (each briefly introduced here and then detailed in the sections that follow): part-task trainers, computer-enhanced mannequin simulators, and VR devices.[108]

Part-task trainers consist of representations of body parts/regions with functional anatomy for teaching and evaluating particular skills, such as plastic arms for venipuncture or suturing, or head/neck/torso mannequins for central line placement or endotracheal intubation. In most cases, the interface with the user is passive: that is to say, the (typically single) operator performs some examination or procedure on the model with no (or only rudimentary) response from the simulator. These task trainers generally have lower engineering fidelity and usually don't incorporate sophisticated technological components, making them less expensive, yet they can reproduce the tasks to be assessed with moderate to high degrees of psychological fidelity.

Computer-enhanced mannequins (CEMs) consist of life-sized (often full-body) simulators connected to and controlled by computers, which reproduce not only the anatomy but also normal and pathophysiologic functions. The interface with the user can be active or even interactive. In the former case, the simulator responds in a preprogrammed way to user actions (e.g., if in ventricular fibrillation, the heart rhythm will change to sinus rhythm whenever the user shocks the mannequin). With interactive programming, the simulator response will vary according to user actions (for the previous example, the heart rhythm will return to sinus rhythm only if an adequate energy level is used for defibrillation; for another example, heart rate and blood pressure will change appropriately, depending on the specific dose of a particular drug administered intravenously). Because they feature high-tech components—making them more costly than simple anatomic models—the term *high-fidelity simulators* has (at times inappropriately) become synonymous with this category. CEMs, however, can vary considerably in their degree of physical fidelity and, more importantly, functional task alignment vis-à-vis real patients and actual clinical duties. Assessments using CEMs can focus on individual skills (e.g., ability of a paramedic to intubate) or the effectiveness of teams (e.g., an emergency department resuscitation scenario). Championed initially by anesthesiologists, the advent of these CEMs led the expansion in use of simulation technologies in medical education.

VR simulations are even newer innovations in which a computer-generated display simulates the physical world, and user interactions are with the computer (or some extension thereof) within that simulated (virtual) world. Existing technologies now allow for simulations that are highly realistic, ranging from desktop computer environments (much like those in video games) to immersive VR systems (e.g., CAVE simulations where the user employs new visualization and interaction techniques, such as stereoscopic goggles and handheld tracking tools, to interface with a specially designed three-dimensional [3D] display).[109] Sound and visual feedback in these simulations are often very lifelike, with recent progress in haptic (touch and pressure feedback) technology improving the tactile experience as well; the (usually high) cost is commensurate with the level of technological sophistication in these VR systems. Like assessments with CEMs, we can use VR simulations to evaluate both individual and collaborative skills. Moreover, one potential advantage of assessment in the virtual environment, especially for programs in remote locations[110] or those with restricted resources,[111,112] is that examinees need not be collocated with team members or even with examiners. Most recently, the need for social distancing in response to the COVID-19 pandemic has further accelerated the adoption of distance learning; similarly, "distance testing" in realistic (virtual) clinical contexts is now possible via "telesimulation."[113,114]

Part-Task Trainers

Simulators that reproduce nearly every anatomic region or clinical task are available today to assess numerous competencies across various medical specialties and different healthcare professions.[115] The simplest of these consist of foam pads that simulate soft tissue and overlying skin for learning and evaluating venipuncture or injection technique. Slightly more sophisticated models include vessels filled with mock blood for practice and assessment of cannulation techniques; simulations of various anatomic regions allow testing of skills ranging from peripheral to central intravenous line placement,[116,117] as well as arterial catheter insertion. The simulated tissues/structures in some of these task trainers are even ultrasound compatible, yielding sonographically realistic images that facilitate skills assessment for procedures ordinarily carried out under ultrasound guidance.

There are numerous simulators for evaluation of general examination skills. For example, ocular examination simulators consist of a mannequin head whose eyes have variable pupil sizes for testing funduscopic technique, permitting examinees to use a real ophthalmoscope for diagnosis of normal eye grounds, as well as many pathologic retinal findings of common diseases (demonstrated via changeable funduscopic slides).[118] In similar fashion, ear examination simulators test trainees with actual otoscopes and realistic interchangeable plastic auricles, requiring identification of normal and pathologic middle ear findings, in addition to allowing procedures such as foreign body removal.[119] Breast trainers simulate realistic anatomy for assessing examination technique and ability to diagnose pathologic findings (cyst, lipoma, fibroadenoma, carcinoma, lymphadenopathy); some even allow evaluation of procedural skills, such as cyst aspiration.[120]

For assessment of surgical skills, there are multilayered pads for suturing techniques, some even with filled veins for cut-down procedures. Various trainers exist for performance of minor skin and other procedures, including local anesthetic injection, shave biopsy, linear and elliptical incision/closure, cyst and lipoma removal, subcuticular suturing, and ingrown toenail removal. Still other models allow testing of more advanced surgical skills, such as incision/closure of the abdominal wall, and bowel or vascular anastomosis. Other simulators provide the anatomy of the lower abdomen and perineum for performing diagnostic peritoneal lavage.

For anesthesiology, emergency medicine, critical care, or other specialties, there are numerous airway trainers, usually consisting of representations of the head and neck (with or without torso/lungs attached) for assessing airway management skills;[121] many of these task trainers can simulate variations in tongue, dentition, and other upper airway anatomy and vary conditions under which examinees can perform bag-valve-mask ventilation, placement of oral-pharyngeal or laryngeal mask airways, nasal or oral endotracheal intubation, and needle cricothyroidotomy.

For related skills, Laerdal Medical created Resusci Anne,[122] one of the earliest medical simulators of the modern era,[123] for teaching and practicing cardiopulmonary resuscitation (CPR), and this is still widely used for assessment of these critical life-saving techniques. Although it mimics a full-sized adult, rather than just one body part or region, it is still essentially a task trainer, with functional anatomy for performing ventilation and chest compressions, but (at least in earlier models) no interactive features or (patho) physiologic functions. Child, infant, and even premature neonate-sized mannequins are now available for analogous pediatric skills assessment.

For evaluating general examination skills as well as more specialized orthopedics, sports medicine, or rheumatologic examinations and procedures, part trainers that mimic accurate anatomy and landmarks for nearly every joint area (e.g., shoulder, elbow, wrist and hand, knee) allow assessment of examination technique, as well as joint and soft tissue injections; specially wired needles for these procedures provide indicators of proper placement.

For internal medicine, pediatrics, neurology, and anesthesia skills assessment, there are part-task trainers scaled to both adult and infant sizes for evaluation of lumbar puncture and various epidural/spinal injection techniques.[124,125]

In the realm of obstetric skills testing, there are several birthing simulators for assessment of vaginal delivery technique. Some are extremely simple trainers that strap onto the operator, who plays the role of the mother and manually controls how the delivery proceeds during a scenario.[126] These are inexpensive and require relatively little training to use effectively—making them ideal for teaching and evaluating the skills of midwives and birth assistants in low-resource countries—but nonetheless create compelling simulations of normal or complex birthing scenarios: for example, a reservoir in the unit can be filled with artificial blood and used to simulate maternal postpartum hemorrhage. Related task trainers allow assessment of technique for episiotomy suturing or umbilical vein cannulation/cord blood sampling.[127] Other birthing simulators are slightly more realistic in appearance, consisting of partial (pelvis/perineum/thighs) maternal anatomy, as well as neonate models with umbilical cord/placenta, that can re-create a variety of scenarios, including normal delivery in various maternal positions, shoulder dystocia, breech presentation, and forceps- and vacuum-assisted deliveries.[128]

For evaluation of urologic and gynecologic skills, trainers exist that simulate the pelvis/perineum of both male and female patients. These can assess technique for digital rectal examination and insertion of a proctoscope, as well as the ability to identify abnormal findings, such as rectal polyp or carcinoma and various prostate or scrotal/testicular pathologies.[129] Some trainers mimic anatomy for procedures such as bladder catheterization, while others focus on assessment of female pelvic examination technique, allowing both bimanual and speculum examinations, and requiring identification of normal and abnormal uterine/ovarian findings.[130]

Besides permitting examination by inspection and palpation, some of these models incorporate built-in "phantoms" with "tissue" properties that realistically mimic the sonographic appearance of organs, blood vessels, and other structures when imaged using real ultrasound machines.[131,132] Recent trends toward increased teaching and assessment of ultrasonography skills—beginning in medical school and continuing into postgraduate training in multiple specialties[133-138]—have prompted the development and proliferation of such simulations with added features like ultrasound compatibility, which facilitate evaluation of healthcare providers' abilities to perform many diagnostic and therapeutic procedures under ultrasound guidance.[85-88]

Other enhancements to simulations employing part-task trainers may augment their overall level of realism. We have already mentioned briefly how so-called "hybrid" simulations that combine simple anatomic models with standardized patients can significantly improve the authenticity of assessment scenarios by leveraging the best features of each type of simulation:[56] placing a female pelvic model beneath a drape allows examinees to perform sensitive or even invasive procedures (without risk of embarrassment or physical harm to the patient, or violation of cultural mores) and to identify pathologic findings (that a simulated patient cannot mimic), while attaching the task trainer to a draped female SP permits evaluation of interpersonal/communication skills and professional behaviors that would be impossible (or at least highly unrealistic) to evaluate using a plastic mannequin alone.

We can find additional examples of enhancements to simple anatomic models that are even more sophisticated and of a technological nature: for instance, clinician-educators have added to one gynecologic simulator haptic sensors that record performance metrics during female pelvic examination, including time to complete the exam, number of critical locations palpated, maximum pressure used, and frequency with which these areas were touched during the exam.[139-141] Task trainers like this have incorporated computer elements to capture data from which indicators of performance quality can be derived that may aid in assessment. For other examples, some airway trainers measure amount of cricoid pressure used during rapid sequence induction of anesthesia,[142] while later-generation Resusci Anne models and similar Laerdal trainers have optional built-in systems to assess and provide feedback on frequency/volume of ventilations, frequency/depth of chest compressions, and hand placement during CPR.[143] Despite their computerized components, these simulators are still classified as part-task trainers, as the device–user interface is still essentially passive. Moreover, although these technological enhancements have the potential to provide more detailed analysis of examinee performance, determining which outcome measures are most meaningful among the plethora of assessment data some simulators can provide remains a challenge and the focus of ongoing research.[30,141,144,145]

Harvey, the Cardiopulmonary Patient Simulator,[146] is perhaps the most sophisticated example of such computerized task trainers: among the very earliest CEM simulators[147] and still in production after several "generations" of further development and refinement, Harvey is the longest continuous high-fidelity simulation project in health professions education. However, unlike some of the other life-sized computer-enhanced mannequins described in the section that follows, Harvey is not interactive and does not permit performing interventions like defibrillation, intubation, CPR, and so forth. Rather, it was designed to teach and evaluate bedside physical examination and diagnostic reasoning skills. As such, Harvey features blood pressure, arterial and venous pulses, precordial movements, as well as heart and lung sounds—all synchronized realistically to simulate 50 different cardiac conditions. The mannequin is portable, and an operator can speak for Harvey via a wireless microphone; otherwise, no outside personnel or programming are required, as the computer is self-contained within the unit and digitally coordinates all the findings once a specific disease code is entered on the control keypad. As the bedside examination of heart and lungs represents a fundamental skill set irrespective of discipline, educators have employed Harvey for evaluation across many medical specialties[148,149] and healthcare professions,[150,151] and at multiple levels of training, from medical students at the end of rotations[152] to residents each academic year[153] to fellows sitting for high-stakes certification exams.[27] Numerous studies have validated the use of Harvey as an assessment tool.[3,154,155]

Computer-Enhanced Mannequin (CEM) Simulators

The previously described static models reproduce specific anatomy or a particular clinical task (and therefore are most germane to a few focused disciplines), whereas other devices use computer technology with programming that enables the simulators to present a wide range of (patho)physiology and to respond dynamically to user actions. These CEMs are adaptable to a host of simulation scenarios, and thus are more generally applicable to multiple clinical domains. As mentioned previously, those specialties with high-risk performance environments (particularly anesthesiology) led the expansion in use of medical simulations by incorporating these technologies into their training and evaluation programs: following the example of flight simulators in commercial aviation, the focus has been on emergency or crisis management skills—both of individuals and teams—and most of the simulators described in this section can facilitate assessment of these competencies. Thanks to the flexibility of CEMs in simulating numerous and varied conditions on demand, other medical specialties, plus many nursing and allied health professions education programs, have also adopted these methods for training and testing. Among the various types of simulators, CEMs have perhaps the most rigorous validity evidence to support their use in assessment.[123,156-158]

Sim One was the earliest such CEM: introduced in 1967 (only one year before Harvey), it was a full-sized mannequin with computer controls that interfaced with an anesthesia machine and simulated hemodynamic, cardiac, and airway problems.[2] This prototypical simulator no longer exists, but—despite computer and other technological advancements that have allowed significant improvements in later systems—the general concept and design of Sim One still serve as a template for current human patient simulators.

A present-day "descendant" of the high-fidelity anesthesia simulators, and arguably among the most sophisticated of CEMs, is the Human Patient Simulator (HPS)[159] first developed and marketed by Medical Education Technologies, Inc. (METI), and later acquired/now distributed by CAE Healthcare. This adult-sized mannequin simulates not only blood pressure, multiple peripheral arterial pulses, and breath and heart sounds, but also muscle twitch from nerve stimulation, pupillary reflexes, salivation, lacrimation, and urine output. A system included with the simulator (or conventional external monitors) can display vital signs, electrocardiogram, oxygen saturation, and other physiologic parameters in real time; these recordings are particularly useful when the HPS is used for assessment. Other distinguishing features include: true gas exchange, such that users can administer volatile anesthetics/medical gases and perform real capnography and pulse oximetry; sophisticated modeling of pharmacology coupled with a drug recognition system that allows administration of more than 50 intravenous and inhaled medications and automatic/appropriate patient responses to drugs; and realistic lung mechanics that simulate complex surgical, anesthetic, and critical care scenarios. In addition, the simulator responds appropriately to a host of procedures, including intubation and ventilation, chest compressions, defibrillation/cardioversion/pacing, needle or tube thoracostomy, and arterial and venous cannulation. The HPS contains multiple preprogrammed patient profiles and can simulate numerous scenarios involving these patients; educators and evaluators have developed many more customized programs for use in particular settings, and these are often shared freely online or are available from simulation user networks and other special interest groups. A pediatric version, PediaSIM HPS, scaled to the size and physiology of a 6-year-old (17-kg) child, offers capabilities for high-fidelity simulations analogous to its adult-sized counterpart.[159]

The comprehensive and realistic simulations possible with the HPS make the system relatively expensive. In addition, the accompanying hardware limits portability or use of the mannequin outside controlled environments (e.g., simulating military or emergency medical services in the field). For this reason, CAE produces other simulators[160,161] that are wireless/tetherless and therefore more portable, allowing an examiner to operate them remotely from a laptop or tablet

PC. More rugged components also make these devices more suitable for use in simulated or real-world field settings, such as might be desired for the assessment of military or prehospital medical personnel. A "family" of related simulators[162] with less complex hardware and software—including child[163] and newborn infant[164] mannequins that accurately model the corresponding pediatric physiology—have fewer preprogrammed patient scenarios and respond automatically to a smaller range of interventions. These systems are commensurately less expensive than the full-featured HPS and may actually have better functional task alignment for the assessment of health professionals in disciplines other than anesthesiology.

Building on its earlier task trainers, Laerdal Medical has likewise developed a number of CEM simulators with varying degrees of fidelity for teaching and assessing a broad range of life-saving skills related to airway, resuscitation, trauma, and other emergency care.[165] The SimMan series[166-170] comprises full-sized adult mannequins featuring realistic airways with variable anatomy that can reproduce different conditions for assessing ventilation, supraglottic device placement, and intubation techniques. They possess a full complement of physical exam findings (e.g., heart, lung, and bowel sounds; cyanosis, bleeding, lacrimation, and diaphoresis; blood pressure and peripheral arterial pulses), along with oxygen saturation and electrocardiographic and other monitoring capabilities that allow assessment of various patient evaluation and management skills, particularly those related to advanced cardiac and trauma life support. In addition to intubation, chest compressions and defibrillation, various SimMan models permit testing of other invasive procedures, ranging from peripheral venipuncture and (tibial/sternal) intraosseous access techniques to needle or tube thoracostomy and cricothyroidotomy. Special sensors in the mannequins record precise timing of user interventions (e.g., administration of oxygen or initiation of CPR), and such data can be very useful for providing formative feedback and/or for summative assessment decisions.

No longer in production, the original ("Classic") version of SimMan required a physical connection to both a computer (to run the programming that controlled the simulator) and an external air compressor (that drove respiratory movements and caused swelling of various upper airway structures for difficult ventilation/intubation scenarios). Later generation ("3G") models possess the same capabilities but are untethered: a miniature compressor is built into the mannequin itself and the simulator will run on rechargeable batteries for several hours. These wireless units can be remotely operated via a computer, tablet, or handheld control pad that communicates with the mannequin over its own local Wi-Fi network. By employing webcams and other secure audio-visual transmission systems (which already exist for clinical telemedicine applications) to observe and rate examinee performance and conduct debriefings, evaluators are leveraging the wireless connectivity of such CEMs to permit long-distance control of the simulators and further facilitate assessment via telesimulation.[171,172]

Although perhaps not as comprehensive as CAE's HPS systems, at least in terms of physiologic/pharmacologic modeling and the ability to administer inhaled anesthetic agents and medical gases—functionality that is rather narrowly focused in the realm of anesthesiology practice—SimMan models are generally less expensive; nonetheless, some come equipped with a system that recognizes multiple medications administered by various routes and triggers automatic and realistic responses from the simulator, as reflected in vital signs and other patient status indicators. Perhaps because of familiarity with the simpler Laerdal mannequins (such as Resusci Anne), and because they seem to strike a good balance between versatile functionality and affordability, a unit from the SimMan line is often the initial high-fidelity CEM system acquired by new simulation or clinical skills centers, and consequently they have come into widespread use at many institutions worldwide.

SimMom[173] combines features of the birthing task trainers described in the previous section—multiple anatomic variants, and normal or complex delivery scenarios with various fetal presentations and maternal complications—with the computer-enhanced capabilities of SimMan, such as wireless operation, full respiratory and hemodynamic monitoring, and the ability to perform a host of critical interventions and life-saving procedures with appropriate physiologic responses from the simulator. The accompanying neonate model can be delivered manually or in fully automated fashion via an optional module inserted into the maternal simulator; this baby is a realistic appearing but static task trainer without computerized elements. Rounding out this "Sim family," however, are other CEMs scaled to (6-year-old) child,[174] infant,[175] neonate,[176] and now even premature newborn[177] sizes that possess general functionality analogous to their adult-sized counterparts—plus capabilities to simulate findings and tasks specific to patients in these age groups, such as a bulging fontanel and umbilical pulse/vascular access—for assessing pediatric emergency skills.

Gaumard[178] is another company that produces a line of pediatric CEMs: these have a different range of child-sized mannequins (both 1- and 5-year-old), in addition to neonate and preemie models, and are notable for having been the first completely tetherless/wireless simulators in the pediatrics space.[179-182] This feature would be advantageous for scenarios involving, say, resuscitation while carrying a newborn from the labor and delivery room to the neonatal intensive care unit, especially in situ simulations conducted in actual clinical or field settings. In fact, with its introduction of the HAL[183] family of simulators (which are similar in functional capabilities to various mannequins in the SimMan series), Gaumard actually pioneered such fully tetherless technology, with long-range simulator control (from up to 300 meters away) via a wireless tablet/monitor system; these simulators were also some of the first to permit attachment of real pulse oximetry probes, ECG leads, and defibrillation pads. Most recently, Gaumard has developed (first pediatric,[184] then adult[185]) mannequins that simulate lifelike emotions through dynamic facial expressions, movement, and speech—which can create highly realistic assessment scenarios. These CEMs track examiner movement around the patient by following with their head and eyes, and they can follow (currently limited) commands with preprogrammed automatic responses. This functionality—plus the ability to simulate nystagmus, ptosis, unilateral facial droop, and arm drift—begins to fill the gap noted earlier in the realm of neurologic exam (e.g., stroke) assessment.[185]

Gaumard was probably best known originally for its NOELLE[186] line of simulators, and newer generations that constitute the VICTORIA[187] brand are probably the most sophisticated/full-featured CEMs in the obstetrics domain: these consist of life-sized female adult and neonate mannequins that, unlike previously described obstetric care simulators, feature computer-enhanced components in both mother and child models, thus enabling simulation of a wide range of scenarios involving emergency care and management of complications in pregnancy and childbirth. Users can assess maternal and fetal/neonatal vital signs and oxygenation status, uterine activity, and so forth via two separate monitors; implement emergency procedures such as intubation, CPR, or defibrillation/cardioversion of mother and baby; administer medications via (peripheral or umbilical) intravenous or intraosseous routes; and perform a very wide range of delivery procedures. The most advanced models have additional features, including realistic pelvic landmarks and natural feel of the amniotic sac while determining fetal position; palpable contractions that peak and subside in real time throughout a scenario; two different fetuses for increased realism when simulating vertex versus breech presentations and corresponding device-assisted deliveries; optional separate task trainers (e.g., for epidural procedures and episiotomy repair) that insert into the maternal mannequin; and a highly realistic and precisely controllable automated delivery system that reproducibly moves the fetus through the stages of labor. The latter functionality—along with built-in sensors that track user actions and record parameters such as force experienced by the fetus during delivery maneuvers—facilitates the provision of formative feedback, as well as the collection of performance data for summative assessment.

Various hybrid simulations exist that combine CEMs with other forms of simulation. We just mentioned that certain NOELLE models allow insertion of task trainers into the maternal mannequin to assess particular competencies related to obstetric care (such as injection of epidural anesthetics or surgical repair of perineal lacerations). Alternatively, some simulations integrate SPs with patient mannequins (like the examples cited earlier with part-task trainers) to assess both nontechnical and technical skills. Many human patient simulators have built-in microphones that allow operators to speak remotely for the mannequin—providing salient details about the chief complaint, asking the provider to "help me," coughing or retching frequently, or simply moaning in pain—to test trainees' history-taking/communication skills or empathetic attitudes. A variation of this approach involves having the SP in the same room with the examinee (usually seated/lying right next to the mannequin) for a more realistic "human element" in the evaluation of nontechnical skills, while also allowing performance of physical exam maneuvers or invasive procedures on the simulator to assess technical abilities. Still other hybrids integrate VR simulations with CEMs: for example, some patient simulators incorporate technological components under the mannequins' skin that enable performance of (virtual) ultrasound examinations to reveal findings consistent with a given testing scenario.[188] The same technology can be combined with SPs to simulate internal pathology that actors obviously cannot mimic.[189] (See more detailed discussion in the section on VR simulators that follows.)

The preceding discussion has focused chiefly on the assessment of *individual* competencies in both technical (i.e., psychomotor skills) and nontechnical (i.e., attitudes or behavioral) domains, and mention of the latter has mostly addressed ethical/professional conduct, compassionate care, and interpersonal communication with patients. Another major area of attention in health professions education (and consequently competency assessment) of a nontechnical nature is that of *team* skills. Simulations involving computer-enhanced mannequins most frequently form the basis for assessment of competencies such as communication, leadership, situation monitoring, and mutual support within teams.[190,191] Because CEMs can simulate a vast array of patient conditions and permit performance of numerous interventions including invasive procedures, resuscitations, and other critical incident scenarios (conducted in laboratory or in situ settings), these simulators most often provide the context for such simulations designed to evaluate interdisciplinary and interprofessional teamwork skills among healthcare providers, both in training[192] and in practice.[193,194]

Virtual Reality (VR) Simulators

Rather than demonstrating skills only on simple task trainers or more complex patient simulator mannequins, examinees can also perform required techniques now on "virtual" patients. VR systems have been available for some time; the earliest were computer screen–based simulators with only keyboard or rudimentary "joystick" controls. Today systems are being developed that employ sophisticated interfaces capable of simulating a wide variety of procedures, ranging from relatively simple nonoperative techniques such as intravenous cannulation[195] to more complex surgeries like laparoscopic cholecystectomy,[196] and from percutaneous catheter–based approaches such as carotid artery stenting[197] to endoscopic methods like flexible sigmoidoscopy.[198] Beyond these applications for assessment of procedural skills, VR simulations can facilitate evaluation of patient management and communication skills for both individuals and teams: for instance, in a virtual emergency department for trauma resuscitation scenarios[199] or a virtual delivery room for neonatal examinations,[200] we can remotely and simultaneously assess multiple participants as they cooperate in the treatment of virtual patients within a computer-generated environment.

Nevertheless, the most common uses of VR simulators for testing purposes are for evaluating competence in performing procedures, including medical examinations, nonoperative invasive techniques, and surgeries. Among the latter two categories, percutaneous catheter–based and endoscopic interventions and minimally invasive or limited-access surgical procedures share common characteristics that not only make them difficult to learn, but also render them particularly adaptable to VR simulation.[201] These techniques require psychomotor and perceptual skills that are quite different from traditional open surgical approaches, because practitioners must (1) perform complex invasive procedures based on indirect and limited viewing of 2D images representing the 3D task; (2) overcome reduced depth perception and sometimes poor quality of such imaging, especially the grayscale fluoroscopic displays used in some procedures; (3) manipulate delicate instruments at a distance from the operative site, with consequent limitations in tactile feedback and degree of movement; and (4) compensate for the "fulcrum effect" of handling instruments in this way, whereby proprioceptive and visual feedback often conflict.[202] The same limitations that pose challenges for learners of these real procedures, however, actually simplify modeling of the simulated task: for example, the circumscribed field of view and restricted degree of movement when performing endoscopy require less comprehensive visual and tactile simulation in the corresponding virtual procedure.

This is not to say that incredibly lifelike simulations are not already possible with current VR technology. Indeed, recent advances—many led by the video gaming industry—in computer processing speed, 3D rendering, and other technologies have significantly improved the authenticity of these simulations. In addition to their increasingly realistic audiovisual content, the most sophisticated VR systems for assessing procedural skills also feature haptic (touch and proprioceptive feedback) technology to convey "the feel" of the procedure, instruments, or anatomic structure under examination. As examples of such technology, 3D Systems' Phantom Premium and other haptic devices[203] allow users to palpate and manipulate virtual objects via mechanical jointed arms that provide force feedback with up to six degrees of freedom: a thimble, stylus, or actual surgical instruments affixed to the end of the apparatus allow simulation of the tactile sensation (pressure, resistance, contour, etc.) involved, for instance, in palpating internal organs or making incisions and suturing. The haptic mechanism interfaces with a computer that generates the visual components of the experience; 3D glasses are sometimes required for the most realistic effect, but remarkably, modern systems have such sensitive and accurate motion detection that essentially no lag occurs between the physical movement of the haptic device and the visible response displayed on the monitor. VR haptic simulators such as these already have applications in multiple medical disciplines,[204-209] as well as in other health professions such as dentistry[210-213] and veterinary medicine.[214-217]

In addition to haptic technologies, VR simulation developers have created head-mounted and other wearable tracking devices[218] with sensors that detect position and follow movement of the participant's head and/or hands,[219] thereby enhancing the realism of the user's interaction with the virtual world. Some systems also include built-in recording functions that allow measurement of certain parameters such as economy of movement and instrument handling, which may be important in technical assessments of surgical skill.[106,220]

Consequently, as first predicted three decades ago,[221] nearly all branches of surgery now utilize various forms of VR technology for teaching, learning, and assessing various competencies. In neurosurgery, for instance, applications of VR methods to simulate ventricular shunt placement encompass simple web-based visual models[222] as well as more complex devices incorporating haptic feedback.[219,223-225] VR simulations for evaluating other important neurosurgical skills (e.g., tumor resection) already exist.[226-230] Rapid advances in this field were anticipated some time ago,[231] and the trend toward development of more systems in related areas is likely to continue. Examples include virtual temporal bone dissection simulations, which not only neurosurgeons but also otolaryngologists can use to assess their trainees' technique.[206,232-236] VR haptic devices are available that simulate a spectrum of additional ENT procedures,[237] ranging from noninvasive examinations such as palpation of head and neck malignancies,[205] to endoscopic approaches for sinus surgery,[238-241] to myringotomy procedures[242,243]—with one of the latter simulators even incorporating an optical tracking system to follow users' navigation and targeting with a real blade.[244]

Plastic and reconstructive surgeons have utilized virtual patients for some time now,[245-247] but mostly to plan the surgical approach and model intended cosmetic results, rather than to assess the skills of, say, a novice prior to performing a procedure for the first time on real patients. Some VR applications for testing, however, do exist in this domain: one haptic system generates scores for user technique during simulated cleft lip repair.[248] Other VR tools can be useful for assessing performance of various osteotomy and fusion procedures employed in multiple specialties, including not only plastics but also oral-maxillofacial surgery and orthopedics.[249-251]

The minimally invasive analogue among orthopedic surgery procedures is arthroscopy. Accordingly, VR platforms exist that simulate diagnostic and therapeutic arthroscopic techniques:[252] several simulators are already commercially available,[253,254] with modules for arthroscopic knee,[208,255,256] shoulder,[257-259] and to a lesser extent, hip[260] procedures. These systems track data for performance assessment, including time to complete tasks, efficiency of instrument movement, number of collisions with any tissue, and force applied to joint structures.[261,262] Still other VR systems simulate various open orthopedic (especially hip) procedures, including arthroplasty, reduction of fractures, and amputation.[263-265]

More than 25 years ago ophthalmologists developed a VR device with haptic feedback mechanisms as well as stereo views of the operation—a key component in eye surgery—to simulate a cataract extraction procedure; the system design included capability for playback of the surgery and analysis of operative technique from multiple viewpoints (including from inside the eye).[266] Further work with VR technology has created other ophthalmic simulators that can facilitate assessment of a number of skills, ranging from simple ocular examination[267] to more complex procedures such as phacoemulsification,[268-270] capsulorhexis,[271-273] retinal photocoagulation,[274] and vitreoretinal surgery.[275,276] Among the few ophthalmologic VR simulators commercially available today,[277,278] almost all of the published validation research has been conducted using the Eyesi Surgical simulator. This system consists of a stylized mannequin head with artificial eyes, realistic foot pedals for equipment control, various handheld instruments that are wired for position tracking but still freely moveable, and a surgical microscope to which the computer transmits appropriate stereo images of the operative field. Several different procedure modules permit evaluation of a range of intraocular surgical skills. For example, the platform can simulate anterior segment procedures (especially the critical steps in cataract surgeries) and, using a vitreoretinal eye interface and instrument set (including a vitrectomy machine and endolaser), can also reproduce posterior segment surgeries. The system records various parameters, such as microscope and instrument handling, surgical efficiency, and tissue treatment, that facilitate feedback and objective skills assessment. Another ophthalmic surgery simulator—developed by a nonprofit foundation[279] and therefore not commercially available at present—is used to train providers to perform manual small-incision cataract surgery in resource-constrained settings. Among current eye surgery simulators, HelpMeSee's VR device is unique, because it incorporates high-end graphics with an extremely realistic haptic feedback system based on sophisticated modeling from precise force measurements obtained during actual eye surgeries. The system provides metrics obtained during simulated procedures that can be used for objective assessment of the microsurgical skills required to safely perform such ophthalmic surgeries.[280,281]

For general surgery, VR systems can simulate performance of procedures ranging in difficulty from simple suturing[282] to diagnostic peritoneal lavage,[283] and from other trauma evaluations/treatments[284-286] to a range of laparoscopic surgeries including cholecystectomy.[287] One of the earlier (and probably most extensively studied) systems is the Procedicus Minimally Invasive Surgical Trainer-Virtual Reality (MIST-VR). Formerly marketed by Mentice[288] (but now retired; see Appendix 13.1), this simulator consists of a structural frame supporting two mechanical arms that hold standard laparoscopic instruments and links to a computer whose monitor displays the movement of these instruments in real time. Although the graphics are 3D, some of the basic training modules utilize simple geometric shapes rather than more realistic representations of the anatomy or tissues involved. Nonetheless, the user can perform tasks of progressive complexity that represent key skills employed in laparoscopic surgery, including withdrawal and insertion of instruments, stretching and clipping of soft tissues, use of diathermy, intracorporeal knot tying, manipulating needles, and continuous or interrupted suturing. The system records data that enable evaluation of performance, comprising scores for time to complete the task, number of errors, efficiency of instrument movements, and economy in the use of diathermy; the computer can also separately analyze right- and left-hand performance to assess ambidextrous skills. Scores for task completion on the MIST correlate with expert ratings during laparoscopic cholecystectomy carried out on live animals.[220] Moreover, well-designed (so-called "VR to OR") studies using this system were among the first to demonstrate transfer of skills from the simulated task to the actual operation performed on real patients, offering important evidence of (predictive) validity for assessments employing such VR simulators.[107,287] Currently several other VR platforms for evaluation of laparoscopic skills are commercially available.[289-291] These trainers feature designs and functionality (with or without haptic hardware) similar to the MIST—many of the latest models also incorporate VR goggles/headsets—but can simulate and assess a wider range of surgeries, including appendectomy, sigmoidectomy,[292] inguinal/incisional hernia repair, and bariatric procedures such as gastric bypass.[293] Validation research has likewise demonstrated that assessments based on metrics obtained with these VR systems during performance of simulated colectomy and cholecystectomy extrapolate to performance during actual surgeries, not only in experimental settings with live animals,[294] but also in the OR with real patients.[295]

Surgeons utilize many of these same skills to perform minimally invasive procedures other than intra-abdominal surgeries. Not surprisingly, then, these same (and comparable) simulators—using (optional) additional software modules and/or interchangeable instrument handles—have found applications for the assessment of competence in performing many other techniques, including lobectomy through video-assisted thoracoscopic surgery (VATS), nephrectomy, and a range of gynecologic procedures such as tubal occlusion,[296] ectopic pregnancy,[297,298] salpingo-oophorectomy, and hysterectomy. Still other VR devices create realistic simulations that permit evaluation of different procedural skills in gynecology, such as hysteroscopy.[299] For the latter, commercially available platforms[300] provide modules to assess general skills such as navigation through the cervical canal, uterine visualization, and fluid management,[301] as well as performance of specific procedures, including placement of tubal sterilization implants,[302,303] uterine polypectomy, and myomectomy.[304] These simulators track time and precision in completing psychomotor tasks and generate metrics that can aid in performance evaluations.

Other VR devices can accurately model genitourinary procedures, ranging from prostate examination[204] and cystoscopy/ureteroscopy[305-307] to transurethral resection of the prostate (TURP)[308] and bladder (TURB).[309,310] The URO Mentor, one of a series of "Mentor" VR simulators developed by Simbionix (now part of Surgical Science),[311] probably has the most validity evidence to support its use as an assessment tool in this domain,[312,313] including a large VR to OR study demonstrating that evaluation of skills in the simulation setting correlates with ratings of performance during actual urologic procedures.[314] All of these systems are quite versatile in the range of diagnostic and therapeutic endourologic techniques they are capable of reproducing, including cystoscopic bladder biopsy and tumor resection; TURP and laser therapy for benign prostatic hypertrophy; ureteroscopic treatment of strictures/obstructions via balloon dilation or catheter or stent placement; and stone extraction or intracorporeal lithotripsy.[315] These simulators support the use of actual flexible and rigid endoscopes with working channels for insertion of original tools; the user can control these instruments (e.g., catheters, guidewires, baskets, forceps, lithotripters, electrodes, stents, balloons) with real handles, while the computer displays a virtual representation of the operating end of these devices interacting with photorealistic graphics of the genitourinary anatomy. Haptic technology provides a lifelike feel during scope insertion and instrument manipulation. Examinees can demonstrate endoscopy skills with direct visualization and treatment of pathologic lesions or show their ability to perform real-time fluoroscopy with correct C-arm positioning and simulated injection of contrast agents. Built-in systems track multiple parameters to aid in performance assessment, including time to complete key steps in the procedure, X-ray exposure time, and number of errors (such as perforations or laser misfires).

The PERC Mentor—first designed by Simbionix as a stand-alone system and later combined with the URO Mentor (in which one unit comprised both devices)—originally simulated related urologic techniques for performing percutaneous renal access procedures.[316,317] The former platform consisted of a stylized partial mannequin representing the patient's back and bilateral flanks: cartridges with layers to simulate the feel of skin, subcutaneous tissues, and ribs—interchangeable for practice on normal weight or obese patients—enabled the user to carry out percutaneous punctures using various real needles, while simultaneously manipulating a virtual C-arm and following fluoroscopic images to pass guidewires and access the proper renal calyx. The simulator had built-in capabilities to record data for use in assessment exercises, such as time to perform important steps in the procedure, total X-ray exposure time and amount of contrast used, number of attempts to puncture the collecting system, and number of complications (e.g., extravasation, infundibular tears, and vessel injury). Although validation studies have accumulated some evidence to support using such metrics for competency assessment, experts rated several items pertaining to fidelity and "overall realism" of this VR simulation lower than that of a live animal model; at the same time, they acknowledged advantages of the virtual system in terms of feasibility and ability to perform procedures repetitively on the simulator, and they found "overall usefulness" of the PERC Mentor to be equivalent to the porcine model for training percutaneous renal access procedures.[316,318] One might envision adapting the same hardware platform to simulate related procedures such as percutaneous transhepatic cholangiography[319,320] by developing additional software modules, but because different diagnostic/therapeutic methodologies provide unique evaluation contexts, further research would be needed to judge the validity of using this technology as an assessment tool in different settings.

Obviously, evaluation of skills required to carry out such image-guided percutaneous techniques is germane to fields other than urology, so the PERC Mentor Suite (now developed/marketed by Surgical Science[321]) has been redesigned as a single VR platform supporting a library of different modules that comprise task trainers and corresponding software to simulate other image-guided percutaneous interventions, including thoracentesis, central line placement, pericardiocentesis, and upper extremity nerve blocks, which are performed by practitioners from multiple specialties.

Along similar lines, VR simulators exist that can facilitate the assessment of competence in performing angiography and endovascular techniques performed by vascular surgeons and other specialists carrying out interventional radiology, nephrology, neurology/neurosurgery, and cardiology procedures.[322-324] For instance, ANGIO Mentor[322] is another Simbionix simulator that typifies the capabilities of most VR systems in this domain: it can simulate an expansive range of carotid/intracerebral, coronary/cardiac, aortic, renal, and lower extremity artery diagnostic and therapeutic interventions, including cine and digital subtraction angiography, angioplasty and stenting, and aneurysm rep air.[207,325,326] High-end haptic mechanisms realistically mimic use of guidewires, catheters, balloons, stents, grafts, and other devices. Advanced features can facilitate rehearsal before performing actual procedures by creating 3D models of a patient's particular anatomy based on real images scanned into the system. The simulation includes dynamic indicators of patient status (e.g., vital signs, ECG, oxygen saturation, intra-arterial pressure gradients, and even virtual neurologic exam findings) that change appropriately with drug administration and procedural maneuvers, thereby allowing assessment of trainees' medical decision-making and ability to manage complications. The simulator tracks a set of parameters and generates statistical reports to aid in evaluations of individual or group performance.

The Vascular Intervention Simulation Trainer (VIST)[324] is another system for assessing endovascular procedure skills. Like the VR platforms referenced previously, the VIST simulates not only a spectrum of aortic, renal, and peripheral artery techniques, but also a wide range of interventional cardiology procedures, including cardiac catheterization with coronary angiography, angioplasty, and stenting; pacemaker placement, electrophysiology studies, and cardiac rhythm management; transseptal puncture and septal defect/left atrial appendage occlusion; and transcatheter aortic valve implantation/replacement (TAVI/TAVR).[327] For all of these simulated procedures, the user manipulates real tools and devices passed through an introducer in the simulator; haptic mechanisms reproduce the tactile feedback, while simulated fluoroscopic images display the anatomy and results of interventions in real time. Studies have demonstrated reliability[202] and validity[328-332] evidence for use of this system as a test of ability to perform various endovascular techniques, supporting the landmark decision by the US Food and Drug Administration (FDA), when it approved a clinical carotid stenting system, to require would-be practitioners of this high-risk procedure to document adequate proficiency through participation in a training/evaluation program involving VR simulation.[197] The professional societies representing physicians who perform these endovascular procedures subsequently issued a consensus statement supporting the use of VR simulation for training and assessment of clinical competence in this domain.[333]

Other nonoperative but nonetheless invasive procedures amenable to VR simulation include various endoscopic techniques. Employed chiefly by surgeons and interventional medicine subspecialists, such as pulmonologists and gastroenterologists, these procedures include bronchoscopy, esophagogastroduodenoscopy (EGD), sigmoidoscopy, and colonoscopy.[334-337] Haptic VR devices are commercially available that simulate a very wide range of endoscopic procedures: some comprise all-in-one systems,[338] whereas others consist of separate bronchoscopy[339] and gastrointestinal (GI) endoscopy[340] simulators with the option to configure as stand-alone units or combine on a single platform. (The latest Simbionix "Mentor" endoscopy system[341] combines capabilities of both the bronchoscopy and GI devices with those of the endourologic simulator described earlier.) In all of these simulators, users deploy authentic endoscopes with ports through which various real instruments can be passed, while haptic technology replicates the tactile experience of scope insertion and manipulation. Lifelike 3D graphic displays reproduce variations in patient anatomy and tissue responses to interventions (e.g., bleeding). Bronchoscopy modules allow assessment of basic endoscopic and inspection skills,[342] as well as various techniques for specimen collection (endobronchial sampling, transbronchial needle aspiration, and bronchoalveolar lavage); an additional program simulates the more difficult navigation through pediatric airways. Similarly, upper and lower GI modules permit evaluation of basic endoscopic skills (instrument handling, navigation, and inspection of mucosa for lesions),[343,344] as well as performance of more complex techniques, ranging from biopsies and polypectomy to endoscopic retrograde cholangiopancreatography (ERCP).[345,346] Recently these VR simulation systems have added programs to teach and assess skills related to using ultrasound guidance for diagnostic and therapeutic interventions during endobronchial and GI endoscopy procedures.[347-349]

Techniques for performing transesophageal echocardiography (TEE) are obviously very similar to those involved with other endoscopic ultrasound approaches, so developers have created VR simulations[350-352] that can likewise be used to teach and evaluate proficiency in carrying out this procedure.[353] The same systems can be used to assess skills required to perform echocardiography from a transthoracic approach.[354] Some ultrasound simulators focus exclusively on cardiovascular imaging techniques,[350] whereas others[351,352] are also capable of reproducing a wide range of transthoracic, transabdominal, and—with separate male and female mannequins plus additional mock ultrasound probes—transvaginal ultrasound examinations, thereby permitting assessment of many procedural skills for trauma and emergency medicine,[135,355] as well as obstetrics and gynecology.[356-358]

We have previously discussed the recent rise in clinical use of bedside or point of care ultrasound (POCUS) and the resulting development and employment of ultrasound simulators for teaching and assessing relevant skills. However, unlike the devices mentioned earlier—which comprise part-task trainers with embedded tissue phantoms and fluid-filled vessels that can actually be scanned using real ultrasound machines—the VR systems here consist of computerized (typically life-sized) mannequins representing the patient's head, neck and torso, or other anatomic regions, with sensors that track the position and orientation of emulated (handheld or endoscopic) ultrasound probes, and computer programming that displays corresponding lifelike sonographic images (often obtained from real patients with various pathologies). Simulations such as these—which combine physical components (the mannequin and ultrasound probe) with computer-generated/virtual elements (the ultrasound images)—are sometimes classified as "augmented reality" (AR) systems.[359] Because they are not purely virtual (i.e., not entirely computer screen–based) simulations, many of the haptic devices described thus far might technically fall under the category of augmented reality as well; however, because the physical interface with these simulators is via tangible components bearing little resemblance to actual body parts or patients (e.g., a "black box" with openings for insertion of scopes/instruments), we usually apply the more general term *virtual reality* (*VR*) and reserve "augmented reality" for simulations containing virtual elements interacting with (or superimposed on) realistic physical representations of the human body or real world. Thus we would likely characterize the VIST[324] endovascular simulator described earlier, by itself, as a VR system, while integration of that device into one of the Laerdal acute care CEMs mentioned in the previous section[360] would probably be classified as an AR or—without delving into the evolving semantics too much—a "mixed reality" (MR) simulator, depending on the degree of interactivity of the user with the virtual and real-world components of the experience. Although used primarily for training rather than assessment, another new simulator incorporates MR technology with Gaumard obstetrical CEMs:[361] wearing special 3D headsets that provide holographic visualization, users gain "X-ray vision" to see the underlying maternal anatomy and position of the fetus while performing the hands-on delivery using the mannequins. Because the latter two systems combine different forms of simulation, we can also consider them to be "hybrid" simulations.

Returning to the discussion of ultrasound simulators, we previously referenced another hybrid simulation[189] that combines a VR platform with CEMs (or even SPs) and offers unique advantages for teaching and assessing ultrasonography skills. Whereas other systems require proprietary mannequins with embedded sensors that track position and orientation of the emulated ultrasound probe, SonoSim LiveScan[189] utilizes a special probe plus radio frequency identification (RFID) tags that can be placed on any mannequin (including part-task trainers and CEMs) or live humans, instantly transforming even healthy SPs into cases for evaluating, say, trainees' ability to correctly identify various pathologic findings (drawn from an extensive library of actual ultrasound scans obtained from real patients). The RFID tags intended for humans are hypoallergenic and designed for one-time use, while mannequin tags are reusable and can even be pre-installed under the skin of certain CEM simulators.[188] Although this system permits only external (not endoscopic or transvaginal) ultrasound examinations, the integration of SonoSim technology with mannequins or live humans can enable the development of very realistic hybrid simulation testing scenarios: for example, an SP relates a history of sudden, colicky, right upper quadrant pain after a fatty meal and mimics a positive Murphy's sign, while virtual ultrasound images reveal corresponding sonographic findings of acute cholecystitis. An optional system allows immediate or longitudinal tracking of performance metrics that can facilitate summative evaluation or formative assessment programs.

One more area amenable to simulation using VR devices is robotic surgery, the use of which has increased significantly in recent years across multiple surgical specialties. Robotic procedures require psychomotor skills that are different from both open surgical techniques and laparoscopic approaches, and which are particularly challenging for novice practitioners to acquire. Like keyhole procedures, however, many of the characteristics of robotic surgeries that make them difficult to learn also make them relatively easy to replicate using VR technology. The da Vinci system[362] was the first commercially available robotic surgery platform and it remains the system most widely used in clinical practice; the same company manufactures a proprietary simulator for training would-be robotic surgeons,[363] and validation research using this system has demonstrated transfer of skills from the simulation setting to the performance of (hysterectomy) procedures on real patients.[364] Several other VR simulators have been developed to assess skill proficiency in operating surgical robots,[365,366] and a growing body of research provides additional validity evidence supporting use of these devices for the evaluation of competence in the domain of robotic surgery.[367-371]

As mentioned at the beginning of this section, we have provided only a sampling here of the numerous simulation devices currently available or under development. The technology continues to advance at such a pace that future progress and applications seem limited only by the bounds of imagination.

Practical Suggestions for Use Now and Future Directions

The task of implementing simulation-based assessment methods, then, can be a daunting one for evaluation program planners: faced with choosing from among simulators that range so widely in terms of fidelity, features, and cost, how do we decide whether to use CEMs versus task trainers or VR simulators for a given assessment? Ultimately, the decision to use simulations for testing depends on local circumstances, the needs and purpose of the particular examination, and the competencies under evaluation. Wherever possible, we have tried to couch the foregoing discussion in terms that are broadly applicable, irrespective of particular healthcare disciplines or level of training of examinees. Clearly, however, many of the existing simulators are more relevant to specific specialties and to education or evaluation at the postgraduate and continuing professional development levels. In this final portion of the chapter, we raise several important points for consideration by program directors wishing to implement simulation methods within their curricula now. In addition, we offer thoughts on what the future may hold for simulation-based assessment and suggest areas for ongoing research in this field.

First and foremost, in keeping with principles of curricular alignment, defined learning outcomes should drive the use of simulators for assessment, rather than the other way around. Any good curricular "blueprint" *begins* with the enumeration of competencies or learning objectives, which *then* determine the optimal instructional strategies to attain those goals and best assessment tools to document achievement of outcomes. Sometimes, however, programs acquire simulators without careful advance planning for their use—as stated earlier, high technology can be alluring—and then curriculum directors end up looking for ways to make them fit into their educational and evaluation schemes. Having a simulator that *can* be used to assess certain competencies does not mean that we *should* use it in this way, if these outcomes are beyond the scope of a particular course or inappropriate for our trainees' level.

Along similar lines, evaluators must match the features and fidelity of the simulator to the competencies under examination. For example, insertion of a bladder catheter is one skill that can be assessed on the Human Patient Simulator (HPS);[159] if the *only* competency to evaluate is bladder catheterization, however, it makes little sense to purchase the very expensive HPS if testing on a far less costly anatomic (pelvic) model accomplishes the same goal. On the other hand, acquiring one full-featured device such as the HPS may be more economical than buying multiple single-task trainers to assess, say, endotracheal intubation, administration and pharmacology of intravenous medications, and induction of anesthesia, if all of those are outcomes to be assessed. Additional factors to balance include costs to maintain the equipment (HPS usually requires an annual service contract, whereas plastic models need little upkeep); value added in terms of higher fidelity (realism) and presentation/assessment of a wider variety of clinical conditions or scenarios with multifeature simulators; and savings in rater time if the mannequin features built-in recording functions to capture objective assessment data.

Similar considerations around other feasibility issues, as discussed earlier, include the time and costs involved with training personnel and developing simulation scenarios. One way to surmount some of these challenges is to avoid reinventing the wheel. Simulation societies and other user groups publish guidelines, host online discussions, and convene meetings for the sharing of ideas, lessons learned, and actual resources, which can save considerable effort and expense. For example, members of the Society for Simulation in Healthcare (SSH)[372] can access a listserv that facilitates networking with other simulation educators; share experiences using and troubleshooting particular simulators; and explore a library of resources that include evaluation tools such as checklists and rating scales to be used in simulation-based assessments, scenario scripts, and so forth.[373] SSH members can also attend online webinars in a Live Learning Center[374] and view presentations and courses recorded from international simulation meetings. The SSH journal, *Simulation in Healthcare*,[375] publishes peer-reviewed research and commentaries on this area of health professions education, as well as best practice recommendations that can prove very useful to directors of new programs utilizing simulation modalities. International conferences feature special tracks for those interested in establishing and operating simulation centers, dealing with issues ranging from construction and space planning to personnel recruitment and resource procurement.

Such "special interest" sessions arose because numerous institutions worldwide are now constructing dedicated clinical skills or simulation centers, but the notion that such facilities are required for a successful simulation program, whether for training or assessment, is sometimes intimidating to those with limited resources. We can make a persuasive argument, however, against conducting tests in such artificial or in vitro settings: more authentic (and therefore perhaps more valid) assessments of clinical competence may entail evaluation in the environments in which practitioners actually work (in vivo, if you will: in the operating room, emergency department, or clinic examination room). As already discussed, assessments that utilize integrated simulations (e.g., a part-task trainer—like a skin suturing pad—strapped to the arm of an SP) in such settings are probably our best approximations of real patient encounters;[93] because in situ hybrid simulations facilitate simultaneous evaluation of both technical skills and nontechnical competencies in authentic contexts, these may become the clinical assessment methods of choice in the future.[376] Additionally, because such "testing centers" already exist (in the hospitals and clinics where trainees and practitioners work) and some of the task trainers involved are relatively inexpensive, programs with limited resources may still enter the arena of simulation-based evaluations. As mentioned earlier, in situ observations such as these will likely become important components of ongoing programs to assess and document the achievement of milestones and mastery of EPAs that are required by accreditation bodies.

Other innovative ways of integrating simulation modalities are already on the horizon. In addition to coupling task trainers with humans, we have already discussed methods of combining VR systems with SPs or mannequins. Other promising applications of such AR technology will allow simulation designers to customize and alter the appearance of simulated patients on demand: beyond displaying cyanosis, rashes, or other physical hallmarks of disease, assessment developers can change a patient's apparent gender, age, race, or ethnicity, depending on the particular scenario. The latter capabilities are especially important when attempting to present diverse, inclusive, and authentic simulations reflective of clinical practice environments today. While still manipulating a physical mannequin or examining a live human, the user's visual experience will be mediated via special stereoscopic (3D) display headsets. Additionally, by programming actual patient data (radiographic imaging, physiologic parameters, etc.) into simulations, VR technology will also allow rehearsal and evaluation of complex or rare procedures in advance of performing them on real patients.[377-379]

As suggested earlier in this chapter, to correct the mismatch between current testing methods and levels of assessment, future trends in the application of simulation technologies for evaluating health professionals are also likely to include greater use for high-stakes testing (e.g., exams for licensure, specialty board certification and maintenance of certification).[380] Some simulation-based assessments were already well accepted in these settings: for instance, long experience using SPs for national examinations in the United States and Canada—and robust research substantiating the psychometric properties of these simulation-based methods—had provided validity evidence for utilizing SPs in such evaluations.[381,382] However, although initially planned as only temporary suspensions because these in-person exams could not be conducted during the height of the COVID-19 pandemic, both the United States Medical Licensing Examination (USMLE) Step 2 Clinical Skills (CS) exam and the Medical Council of Canada Qualifying Exam (MCCQE) Part II have now been permanently discontinued over concerns about costs (especially to examinees) and the paucity of consequential (or predictive) validity evidence.[383,384] It is interesting to note that, prior to the pandemic, authorities in other countries were following and even moving beyond the North American lead by adopting simulation-based clinical skills performance assessments of medical students that employed not only SPs but also part-task trainers, and in some instances, computerized mannequin simulators. In China this took the form of a national clinical skills "competition" rather than an exam per se,[385,386] whereas in Russia medical students from across that vast country were required to pass a simulation-based OSCE-format accreditation examination prior to entering residency training.[387]

For the assessment of US postgraduate trainees, computer- (i.e., purely screen-) based patient case simulations continue to comprise one component of the final Step in the USMLE sequence.[388-390] Taken together, these three exams constitute high-stakes settings because satisfactory performance during such evaluations is required both for selection into residency/fellowship training and for physician licensure to practice in the United States. On the other hand, compared to computer- or SP-based exams, uses of mannequin-based or VR simulations are still quite limited for assessments implemented at the national level, especially for the initial certification of medical specialists. With only one very recent exception—discussed in detail toward the end of this section—all of the (few) other examples come from countries outside the United States. For instance, for more than a decade the Royal College of Physicians and Surgeons of Canada (RCPSC) utilized a CEM cardiac patient simulator[146] (in addition to SPs and computer-based audio-visual simulations) for the oral (OSCE-format) component of their national internal medicine certification examinations.[27] In Israel, experts from that country's Center for Medical Simulation[391] and the National Institute for Testing and Evaluation have collaborated with the Israeli Board of Anesthesiology to incorporate several different CEM simulators (as well as SPs) into that specialty's certification exams.[392,393] Finally, the Brazilian Society of Nephrology requires candidates seeking certification in that specialty to undergo evaluations, which since 2011 have included a practical component utilizing mannequin simulators to assess procedural skills.[394,395]

While barely utilized yet in US board exams per se, several simulation-based assessments currently constitute *prerequisites* for specialty certification—for example, through the American Board of Surgery (ABS)[396]: applicants must document successful completion of both Advanced Cardiac Life Support (ACLS) and Advanced Trauma Life Support (ATLS) programs, which usually employ CEM simulators for skills evaluation. In addition, formal assessment is required via the Fundamentals of Laparoscopic Surgery (FLS™)[397] exam, which includes a psychomotor skills component that tests manual dexterity through measures of efficiency and precision. Only designated testing centers and certified proctors can administer this exam, but interestingly, the simulation modality utilized in the skills assessment is a relatively simple task trainer without sophisticated computer, VR, or haptic technology elements.[398] Advantages of such a system include portability, as well as relative ease and low cost of production and dissemination. During the timed assessment, examinees insert various instruments through covered openings in the FLS Laparoscopic Trainer Box and must demonstrate five basic psychomotor skills—transferring small (physical, not virtual) objects stacked on pegs inside the trainer, precision cutting, loop ligation, and two suturing tasks—while viewing the "operative field" through a television camera. The model was intentionally designed to test fundamental skills applicable to a broad range of laparoscopic surgeries, rather than procedure-specific techniques; as a result, the American Board of Obstetrics and Gynecology (ABOG) recently added completion of the FLS program to the eligibility requirements to sit for its Certifying Exam as well.[399] Evaluations for the manual skills component of the FLS are based chiefly on speed and accuracy of task completion,[397,400] and a robust validation process preceded formal adoption of this prerequisite to board certification.[401,402] Similarly, successful completion of the Fundamentals of Endoscopic Surgery (FES)[403] program is also required now for applicants seeking ABS certification.[396] Much like the laparoscopic surgery program, FES certification requires examinees to undergo assessments that include a simulator-based manual skills component, but this time the simulation modality employs VR and haptic technologies.[340] The skills exam again consists of five timed tasks requiring psychomotor skills that are not procedure-specific but are necessary to perform a range of basic endoscopic surgical techniques;[403] here, too, validation research has provided adequate evidence to support judgments about examinees' competence in this domain based on the simulation-based assessment.[404] Even more recently, clinician-educators have created the Fundamentals of Endovascular Surgery (FEVS) model to assess comparable skills with catheter-based techniques:[405] following a rigorous development process, they first fabricated a silicone task trainer that is a non-anatomic representation of branching "vessels" with various structural features designed to test basic endovascular skills through a series of eight tasks. Preliminary validation studies demonstrated that assessment of proficiency using this simulation model could discriminate between interventionalists with different levels of experience.[405] In collaboration with industry, this research group subsequently replicated an identical (but virtual) version of the simulation on a commercially available VR-haptic platform.[322] Several other simulations for assessing vascular surgery skills—both open and endovascular techniques—have been developed, but further research will be needed to establish validity evidence for applications of these models, especially if they are to be implemented in future high-stakes assessment settings.[405,406]

Of course, constructing a validity argument to support proposed uses of data obtained during simulation-based evaluations entails gathering evidence about the simulator itself and about any additional tools used in the course of the assessment. As was stated previously, although some simulators have built-in functionality to measure and record objective performance data, almost all clinical examinations also include ratings made by human judges (often experts in the domain of interest), and the use of such scoring instruments and raters must undergo validation as well. For example, before studies were undertaken to validate use of the simulators per se in the FLS and FES assessment programs, antecedent research outside the simulation setting (usually in the context of actual procedures performed on live animals or patients) needed to demonstrate reliability and validity evidence for using various rating tools (e.g., the Global Operative Assessment of Laparoscopic Skills [GOALS][407] and Global Assessment of Gastrointestinal Endoscopic Skills [GAGES][408,409] instruments, respectively), which trained observers would later employ in simulation-based evaluations. An analogous tool called the Global Rating Assessment Device for Endovascular Skill (GRADES) was used with the FEVS model.[405]

Despite reasonable evidence for the reliability of scores obtained by trained observers using such instruments, the inherent subjectivity of these ratings always prompts evaluators to search for more objective measurements of performance, especially when important decisions depend on the assessments. Many of the newer high-tech simulators can capture large amounts of data while the operator is performing various techniques; the challenge is determining what metrics correlate meaningfully with procedural "skill." As mentioned throughout the section on available technologies, the VR simulators, especially those featuring haptic elements, can measure many parameters (e.g., time to complete various steps in a procedure and efficiency of instrument handling) that are thought to indicate level of proficiency. In particular, "manual dexterity" as gauged by motion analysis (i.e., kinematic movement of the instrument/scope/catheter/guidewire/etc. tracked via sensors within the simulator) has received much attention and, for most of the minimally invasive procedures under discussion here, has been shown to correlate with progressive levels of operator experience.[410,411] Surprisingly, other parameters thought to be useful for determining skill level display variable psychometrics depending on the specific procedure under evaluation: for instance, time to task completion did *not* correlate (inversely as expected) with increasing level of expertise in performing endovascular techniques as it *did* with laparoscopic procedures.[405] This underlines—as emphasized early on—the importance of understanding that validity is highly dependent on context: "Investigators must also be aware that, depending on the purpose of the assessment and administration conditions, evidence to support the use of various scoring tools may be idiosyncratic to the cohort being measured. Therefore it is rarely appropriate to justify the use of a particular scoring tool based solely on previous validation studies."[412,p.S51] Even when such research does support the use of a particular simulator-based metric, interpretations of scores in that domain will vary depending on the examinee level(s) that the assessment aims to differentiate (e.g., "competence" vs. "proficiency" vs. "expertise"). Finally, with all simulator-based evaluations one must ensure that the construct of interest (i.e., some clinical skill) is actually what is being measured, as opposed to some confounding variable such as familiarity with the particular technology or hardware: for example, one study employing a VR system demonstrated that the number of task repetitions needed to reach "minimal proficiency" (determined through scores automatically recorded by the computer) was significantly higher among experienced laparoscopists than those who had little or no experience.[413] Obviously this represents a fundamental threat to the validity of using such scores to make any judgments about clinical competence, and it highlights the ongoing challenge to determine meaningful outcome measures for simulation-based assessments. Several consensus conferences have acknowledged this state of affairs and listed the need for further studies in the area of outcome measurement among their recommended priorities for simulation-based assessment research going forward.[144,145]

Once meaningful performance metrics have been more clearly defined, residency program directors may increasingly rely on simulation methods to evaluate achievement of milestones and document proficiency for entrustment decisions. In doing so, they will have to integrate use of simulations with other assessment instruments in the toolbox to create a system of required, periodic evaluations that will be ongoing throughout the entire postgraduate education program. In fact, there is some suggestion now of employing simulation-based testing even earlier in the process of specialty training, namely when students are applying for residency positions: according to kinesiologic theory, individual learning curves for certain psychomotor skills follow a logarithmic trajectory, such that a few attempts at performing a given technique (say, on a VR surgical simulator) can be extrapolated to allow "quantification of a person's innate abilities to develop task-specific skills."[414] Program directors could potentially use this approach to screen student candidates' aptitude for performing certain skills and to guide selection decisions for further training, especially in highly competitive specialties.[415-417] Imagine future interview days including simulation-based skills testing! The idea—actually, the practice—is not without precedent: in lieu of traditional interviews, the Israel Center for Medical Simulation has for many years conducted simulation (SP-based) scenarios to assess the personal qualities and interpersonal skills of candidates for admission to medical school in that country.[418]

In light of the numerous advantages of simulation-based methods, many experts feel that there is already a sufficient body of evidence to justify expanding the use of simulation modalities to assessment processes required by regulatory agencies.[380] The programmability and consequent reproducibility of simulations make them ideally suited to such testing situations where high-stakes decisions will be made and therefore where high reliability is essential; as more and more studies also demonstrate validity evidence for these evaluation methods (especially correlation with real-world variables of interest, such as patient outcomes), they will gain wider acceptance by certification boards and credentialing organizations. Just as they were early adopters of simulation-based methods for training, anesthesiologists have led the way by becoming the first specialty board in the United States to incorporate a performance-based (OSCE) component including simulation scenarios into their *initial* certification exams.[419,420] The American Board of Anesthesiology (ABA) administers this APPLIED Exam at its Assessment Center in Raleigh, N.C., for which the OSCE component consists of seven 8-minute stations designed to assess communication and professionalism, as well as technical skills related to patient care.[421] The published content outline and example OSCE scenarios suggest that various simulations (including SPs, task trainers, and perhaps ultrasound simulators) will likely constitute important elements in the assessment scenarios.[422,423] The ABA has begun to accumulate validity evidence that argues in favor of using the simulation OSCE components of its APPLIED examination for initial board certification of anesthesiologists.[424]

Driven chiefly by concerns for patient safety, other procedure-based disciplines (surgery, interventional subspecialties of internal medicine and radiology, etc.) will probably follow suit: if not implemented as part of their initial board certification processes, they will likely—as with the case of carotid stenting described earlier[197]—require simulation-based assessments to certify proficiency for users of new medical devices and practitioners of high-risk procedures. Similar patient safety issues have motivated critical care and procedural specialty organizations to develop continuing professional development (CPD) and Maintenance of Certification (MOC) activities in which simulation modalities figure prominently. Not surprisingly, the ABA has once again been in the vanguard of this movement, this time by providing diplomates several opportunities to earn points through simulation activities—both online virtual clinical scenarios and in-person activities conducted at officially endorsed training and assessment centers throughout the country—that will satisfy requirements for the Quality Improvement (QI) portion of its Maintenance of Certification in Anesthesia (MOCA) program.[425] Another early adopter of simulation methods for training, the American Board of Emergency Medicine (ABEM) had previously developed and piloted MOC processes that permitted simulation-based courses to satisfy the requirement to demonstrate participation in Improvement in Medical Practice (IMP) activities, but these have been discontinued. Similarly, the American Board of Internal Medicine (ABIM) had utilized a network of education centers to house VR SimSuites that replicated actual cardiac catheterization labs, where interventional cardiologists could earn MOC points by completing up to five case scenarios that tested their management of common problems faced in clinical practice.[426] Like the USMLE Step 2 CS and MCCQE Part II exams, reasons for discontinuation of these programs likely included the cost (for both administrators and individual participants) and other feasibility issues.

Finally, simulation-based assessment methods are also being utilized in programs to identify practitioners with suspected lapsed competence, offering evaluations of performance against peer-reviewed standards and providing opportunities for remediation and reexamination through simulation. Such programs are receiving increasing support and, in some jurisdictions, legislative mandates.[427,428]

Conclusion

Simulations are increasingly finding a place among our tools for assessment. Technological advances have created a diverse range of simulators that can facilitate testing in numerous areas of healthcare education. In general, simulators are most appropriate for the evaluation of competence in performing clinical skills or procedures; demonstrating interpersonal, communication, and team skills; and displaying attitudes of professionalism. Simulators provide standardization of the patient variable in clinical examinations and contribute to more reliable assessments of performance in these domains. Simulators complement other testing methods, such as the OSCE, and allow us to measure and judge the wide range of processes and outcomes encountered in clinical training. Furthermore, a growing body of translational research strongly suggests, at least for some procedural skills, that simulation-based mastery learning should now be the standard approach for training healthcare professionals. When we have evidence that simulation-based training and assessment improve care and outcomes for patients, we have an ethical obligation to use these methods in our educational programs.

Consideration of the multiple dimensions of an assessment system can inform not only the choice of an evaluation strategy in general (e.g., whether to use a performance-based vs. written exam) and adoption of particular methods within a given category (e.g., simulation-based test vs. direct observation of clinical skills), but also selection of a specific type of simulation technology from among the many modalities available. Notably, the different dimensions of an assessment system are interrelated, and thinking about areas where they intersect will aid in identifying best applications to favor and potential challenges to offset. Enumeration of the competencies to be assessed is the first step in the current outcomes-based educational model. These must then be considered in the context of required level of assessment, developmental stage of examinees, and overall purpose of the assessment. Alignment of these various factors will increase the likelihood that more quality criteria will be satisfied from the viewpoint of multiple stakeholders in the assessment process, including individuals undergoing evaluation, teachers and schools, accreditation organizations, and ultimately the patients whose care has been entrusted to us as health professionals.

Acknowledgment

The author wishes to express his gratitude to several colleagues at the University of Miami Gordon Center for Simulation and Innovation in Medical Education for their assistance during the update of this chapter for the third edition. In particular, thanks go to S. Barry Issenberg, MD, for co-authoring the first edition chapter and providing valuable guidance for subsequent revisions; and to Diego Waisman for his graphic design expertise and refining the author's conception of the figures created for the chapter.

Disclosure

The author has no significant financial relationships with any of the commercial manufacturers or products referenced in this chapter. In particular, although the author holds a faculty appointment at the University of Miami Miller School of Medicine, which manufactures Harvey, the Cardiopulmonary Patient Simulator, he receives no compensation directly related to the distribution of Harvey or other simulation systems. Mention in this chapter of specific simulators does not constitute endorsement by the author, editors, or publisher. Particular companies or technologies are cited when, in the opinion of the author, they have historical significance or represent common or exemplary models used in health professions education today. Some company/simulator names referenced herein may have changed as products/business enterprises have evolved over the years since publication of the cited articles; every attempt has been made to reference names that are current at the time of chapter manuscript submission.

References

1. Barrows HS, Abrahamson S. The programmed patient: a technique for appraising student performance in clinical neurology. *J Med Educ.* 1964 Aug;39:802–805.
2. Abrahamson S, Denson JS, Wolf RM. Effectiveness of a simulator in training anesthesiology residents. *J Med Educ.* 1969 Jun;44(6):515–519. doi:10.1097/00001888-196906000-00006.
3. Issenberg SB, McGaghie WC, Hart IR, et al. Simulation technology for health care professional skills training and assessment. *JAMA.* 1999 Sep 1;282(9):861–866. doi:10.1001/jama.282.9.861.
4. Fincher R-ME, Lewis LA. Simulations used to teach clinical skills. In: Norman GR, van der Vleuten CPM, Newble DI, eds. *International Handbook of Research in Medical Education.* Kluwer Academic; 2002:499–535.
5. Collins JP, Harden RM. AMEE Medical Education Guide No. 13: real patients, simulated patients and simulators in clinical examinations. *Med Teach.* 1998;20(6):508–521. doi:10.1080/01421599880210.
6. Haluck RS, Marshall RL, Krummel TM, Melkonian MG. Are surgery training programs ready for virtual reality? A survey of program directors in general surgery. *J Am Coll Surg.* 2001 Dec;193(6):660–665. doi:10.1016/s1072-7515(01)01066-3.
7. Institute of Medicine Committee on Quality of Health Care in America. *To Err is Human: Building a Safer Health System.* National Academies Press; 2000.
8. Institute of Medicine. *Crossing the Quality Chasm: A New Health System for the 21st Century.* National Academies Press; 2001.
9. Department of Health. *An Organisation With a Memory: Report of an Expert Group on Learning from Adverse Events in the NHS Chaired by the Chief Medical Officer.* The Stationery Office; 2000.
10. Department of Health. *Building a Safer NHS for Patients: Implementing an Organisation With a Memory.* The Stationery Office; 2001.
11. Baker GR, Norton PG. Adverse events and patient safety in Canadian health care. *CMAJ.* 2004 Feb 3;170(3):353–354.
12. Goodman W. The world of civil simulators. *Flight International Magazine.* 1978:435.
13. Kanki B, Helmreich R, Anca J. *Crew Resource Management.* 2nd ed. Elsevier; 2010.
14. Wachtel J, Walton DG. The future of nuclear power plant simulation in the United States. In: Walton DG, ed. *Simulation for Nuclear Reactor Technology.* Cambridge University Press; 1985.
15. Ressler EK, Armstrong JE, Forsythe GB. Military mission rehearsal: from sandtable to virtual reality. In: Tekian A, McGuire CH, McGaghie WC, eds. *Innovative Simulations for Assessing Professional Competence.* Department of Medical Education, University of Illinois at Chicago; 1999:157–174.
16. Gaba D. Improving anesthesiologists' performance by simulating reality. *Anesthesiology.* 1992 Apr;76(4):491–494. doi:10.1097/00000542-199204000-00001.
17. Gaba D, Howard S, Fish K, et al. Simulation-based training in anesthesia crisis resource management (ACRM): a decade of experience. *Simul Gaming.* 2001;32(2):175–193. doi:10.1177/104687810103200206.
18. Scalese RJ, Issenberg SB. Effective use of simulations for the teaching and acquisition of veterinary professional and clinical skills. *J Vet Med Educ.* 2005 Winter;32(4):461–467. doi:10.3138/jvme.32.4.461.
19. Kochevar DT. The critical role of outcomes assessment in veterinary medical accreditation. *J Vet Med Educ.* 2004 Summer;31(2):116–119. doi:10.3138/jvme.31.2.116.
20. Langsley DG. Medical competence and performance assessment. A new era. *JAMA.* 1991 Aug 21;266(7):977–980.
21. Dauphinee D, Norcini J. Introduction: assessing health care professionals in the new millenium. *Adv Health Sci Educ Theory Pract.* 1999 Jan;4(1):3–7. doi:10.1023/A:1009810219564.
22. Kassebaum DG, Eaglen RH. Shortcomings in the evaluation of students' clinical skills and behaviors in medical school. *Acad Med.* 1999 Jul;74(7):842–849. doi:10.1097/00001888-199907000-00020.
23. Edelstein RA, Reid HM, Usatine R, Wilkes MS. A comparative study of measures to evaluate medical students' performance. *Acad Med.* 2000 Aug;75(8):825–833. doi:10.1097/00001888-200008000-00016.
24. Medical Council of Canada Qualifying Examination Part II: Information Pamphlet. Medical Council of Canada; 2002.
25. Swing SR. Assessing the ACGME general competencies: general considerations and assessment methods. *Acad Emerg Med.* 2002 Nov;9(11):1278–1288. doi:10.1111/j.1553-2712.2002.tb01588.x.
26. Ben-David MF, Klass DJ, Boulet J, et al. The performance of foreign medical graduates on the National Board of Medical Examiners (NBME) standardized patient examination prototype: a collaborative study of the NBME and the Educational Commission for Foreign Medical Graduates (ECFMG). *Med Educ.* 1999 Jun;33(6):439–446. doi:10.1046/j.1365-2923.1999.00368.x.
27. Hatala R, Kassen BO, Nishikawa J, et al. Incorporating simulation technology in a Canadian internal medicine specialty examination: a descriptive report. *Acad Med.* 2005 Jun;80(6):554–556. doi:10.1097/00001888-200506000-00007.
28. Oxford University Press. Assessment. In: *New Oxford American Dictionary.* Accessed October 28, 2023. https://www.oxfordreference.com/search/search?source=%2F10.1093%2Facref%2F9780195392883.001.0001%2Facref-9780195392883&q=assessment.
29. Issenberg SB, McGaghie WC, Petrusa ER, Gordon DL, Scalese RJ. Features and uses of high-fidelity medical simulations that lead to effective learning: a BEME systematic review. *Med Teach.* 2005 Jan;27(1):10–28. doi:10.1080/01421590500046924.

30. McGaghie WC, Issenberg SB, Petrusa ER, Scalese RJ. A critical review of simulation-based medical education research: 2003-2009. *Med Educ.* 2010 Jan;44(1):50–63. doi:10.1111/j.1365-2923.2009.03547.x.
31. Motola I, Devine LA, Chung HS, Sullivan JE, Issenberg SB. Simulation in healthcare education: a best evidence practical guide. AMEE Guide No. 82. *Med Teach.* 2013 Oct;35(10):e1511–e1530. doi:10.3109/0142159X.2013.818632.
32. van der Vleuten CPM. The assessment of professional competence: developments, research and practical implications. *Adv Health Sci Educ Theory Pract.* 1996 Jan;1(1):41–67. doi:10.1007/BF00596229.
33. van der Vleuten CPM, Schuwirth LWT. Assessing professional competence: from methods to programmes. *Med Educ.* 2005 Mar;39(3):309–317. doi:10.1111/j.1365-2929.2005.02094.x.
34. Norcini J, Anderson B, Bollela V, et al. Criteria for good assessment: consensus statement and recommendations from the Ottawa 2010 Conference. *Med Teach.* 2011;33(3):206–214. doi:10.3109/0142159X.2011.551559.
35. Boulet JR, Swanson DB. Psychometric challenges of using simulations for high-stakes testing. In: Dunn WF, ed. *Simulators in Critical Care and Beyond.* Society of Critical Care Medicine; 2004:119–130.
36. Streiner DL, Norman GR, Cairney J. Reliability. In: Streiner DL, Norman GR, Cairney J, eds. *Health Measurement Scales: A Practical Guide to their Development and Use.* 5th ed. Oxford University Press; 2015:159–199.
37. Downing SM. Validity: on meaningful interpretation of assessment data. *Med Educ.* 2003 Sep;37(9):830–837. doi:10.1046/j.1365-2923.2003.01594.x.
38. Downing SM, Haladyna TM. Validity and its threats. In: Downing SM, Yudkowsky R, eds. *Assessment in Health Professions Education.* Routledge; 2009:21–56.
39. Messick S. Validity. In: Linn RL, ed. *Educational Measurement.* 3rd ed. American Council on Education and Macmillan; 1989:13–103.
40. American Educational Research Association, American Psychological Association, National Council on Measurement in Education. *Standards for Educational and Psychological Testing.* American Educational Research Association; 2014.
41. Cook DA, Zendejas B, Hamstra SJ, Hatala R, Brydges R. What counts as validity evidence? Examples and prevalence in a systematic review of simulation-based assessment. *Adv Health Sci Educ Theory Pract.* 2014 May;19(2):233–250. doi:10.1007/s10459-013-9458-4.
42. Kane MT. An argument-based approach to validity. *Psychol Bull.* 1992;112(3):527–535. doi:10.1037/0033-2909.112.3.527.
43. Kane MT. Validation. In: Brennan RL, ed. *Educational Measurement.* Praeger; 2006:17–64.
44. Kane MT. Validating the interpretations and uses of test scores. *J Educ Meas.* 2013 Spring;50(1):1–73. doi:10.1111/jedm.12000.
45. Kane MT. The assessment of professional competence. *Eval Health Prof.* 1992 Jun;15(2):163–182. doi:10.1177/016327879201500203.
46. McGaghie WC. Simulation in professional competence assessment: basic considerations. In: Tekian A, McGuire CH, McGaghie WC, eds. *Innovative Simulations for Assessing Professional Competence.* Department of Medical Education, University of Illinois at Chicago; 1999:7–22.
47. Maran NJ, Glavin RJ. Low- to high-fidelity simulation—a continuum of medical education? *Med Educ.* 2003 Nov;37(Suppl 1):22–28. doi:10.1046/j.1365-2923.37.s1.9.x.
48. Hamstra SJ, Brydges R, Hatala R, Zendejas B, Cook DA. Reconsidering fidelity in simulation-based training. *Acad Med.* 2014 Mar;89(3):387–392. doi:10.1097/ACM.0000000000000130.
49. Regehr G, MacRae H, Reznick RK, Szalay D. Comparing the psychometric properties of checklists and global rating scales for assessing performance on an OSCE-format examination. *Acad Med.* 1998 Sep;73(9):993–997. doi:10.1097/00001888-199809000-00020.
50. Kalu PU, Atkins J, Baker D, Green CJ, Butler PEM. How do we assess microsurgical skill? *Microsurgery.* 2005;25(1):25–29. doi:10.1002/micr.20078.
51. Hodges B, McIlroy JH. Analytic global OSCE ratings are sensitive to level of training. *Med Educ.* 2003 Nov;37(11):1012–1016. doi:10.1046/j.1365-2923.2003.01674.x.
52. Scalese RJ, Hatala R. Competency assessment. In: Levine AI, DeMaria S Jr, Schwartz AD, Sim AJ, eds. *The Comprehensive Textbook of Healthcare Simulation.* Springer; 2013:135–160.
53. Accreditation Council for Graduate Medical Education (ACGME). Common Program Requirements (Residency) Updated June 13, 2021, effective July 1, 2022. Accessed April 22, 2023. https://www.acgme.org/globalassets/pfassets/programrequirements/cprresidency_2022v3.pdf.
54. Frank JR, Snell L, Sherbino J. *CanMEDS 2015 Physician Competency Framework.* Royal College of Physicians and Surgeons of Canada; 2015.
55. General Medical Council. *Good Medical Practice.* General Medical Council; 2020.
56. Kneebone R, Kidd J, Nestel D, Asvall S, Paraskeva P, Darzi A. An innovative model for teaching and learning clinical procedures. *Med Educ.* 2002 Jul;36(7):628–634. doi:10.1046/j.1365-2923.2002.01261.x.
57. Accreditation Council for Graduate Medical Education/American Board of Medical Specialties (ACGME/ABMS) Joint Initiative. Toolbox of Assessment Methods. Accessed April 22, 2023. https://www.partners.org/Assets/Documents/Graduate-Medical-Education/ToolTable.pdf.
58. Holmboe ES, Iobst WF. *ACGME Assessment Guidebook.* Accreditation Council for Graduate Medical Education; 2020. Accessed April 22, 2023. https://www.acgme.org/globalassets/pdfs/milestones/guidebooks/assessmentguidebook.pdf.
59. Bandiera G, Sherbino J, Frank JR. *The CanMEDS Assessment Tools Handbook: An Introductory Guide to Assessment Methods for the CanMEDS Competencies.* Royal College of Physicians and Surgeons of Canada; 2006.
60. Glover Takahashi S, Abbott C, Oswald A, Frank JR. *CanMEDS Teaching and Assessment Tools Guide.* Royal College of Physicians and Surgeons of Canada; 2015.
61. Miller GE. The assessment of clinical skills/competence/performance. *Acad Med.* 1990 Sep;65(9 Suppl):S63–S67. doi:10.1097/00001888-199009000-00045.
62. Wijnen-Meijer M, Van der Schaaf M, Booij E, et al. An argument-based approach to the validation of UHTRUST: can we measure how recent graduates can be trusted with unfamiliar tasks? *Adv Health Sci Educ Theory Pract.* 2013 Dec;18(5):1009–1027. doi:10.1007/s10459-013-9444-x.
63. Cruess RL, Cruess SR, Steinert Y. Amending Miller's pyramid to include professional identity formation. *Acad Med.* 2016 Feb;91(2):180–185. doi:10.1097/ACM.0000000000000913.
64. McGaghie WC. Medical education research as translational science. *Sci Transl Med.* 2010 Feb 17;2(19):19cm8. doi:10.1126/scitranslmed.3000679.
65. McGaghie WC, Issenberg SB, Cohen ER, Barsuk JH, Wayne DB. Translational educational research: a necessity for effective health-care improvement. *Chest.* 2012 Nov;142(5):1097–1103. doi:10.1378/chest.12-0148.

66. Gorter SL, Rethans JJ, Scherpbier AJJA, et al. How to introduce incognito standardized patients into outpatient clinics of specialists in rheumatology. *Med Teach*. 2001 Mar;23(2):138–144. doi:10.1080/014215931048.
67. Gorter S, Rethans JJ, van der Heijde D, et al. Reproducibility of clinical performance assessment in practice using incognito standardized patients. *Med Educ*. 2002 Sep;36(9):827–832. doi:10.1046/j.1365-2923.2002.01296.x.
68. Maiburg BHJ, Rethans JJE, van Erk IM, Mathus-Vliegen LMH, van Ree JW. Fielding incognito standardised patients as 'known' patients in a controlled trial in general practice. *Med Educ*. 2004 Dec;38(12):1229–1235. doi:10.1111/j.1365-2929.2004.02015.x.
69. Derkx H, Rethans JJ, Maiburg B, Winkens R, Knottnerus A. New methodology for using incognito standardised patients for telephone consultation in primary care. *Med Educ*. 2009 Jan;43(1):82–88. doi:10.1111/j.1365-2923.2008.03177.x.
70. Borrell-Carrio F, Poveda BF, Seco EM, Castillejo JAP, González MP, Rodríguez EP. Family physicians' ability to detect a physical sign (hepatomegaly) from an unannounced standardized patient (incognito SP). *Eur J Gen Pract*. 2011 Jun;17(2):95–102. doi:10.3109/13814788.2010.549223.
71. Nie J, Zhang L, Gao J, et al. Using incognito standardised patients to evaluate quality of eye care in China. *Br J Ophthalmol*. 2021 Mar;105(3):311–316. doi:10.1136/bjophthalmol-2019-315103.
72. Dreyfus SE. The five-stage model of adult skill acquisition. *Bull Sci Tech Soc*. 2004 Jun;24(3):177–181. doi:10.1177/0270467604264992.
73. Edgar L, McLean S, Hogan SO, Hamstra S, Holmboe ES. *The Milestones Guidebook*. Accreditation Council on Graduate Medical Education; 2020. https://www.acgme.org/globalassets/milestonesguidebook.pdf.
74. Duffy FD, Holmboe ES. Competence in improving systems of care through practice-based learning and improvement. In: Holmboe ES, Hawkins RE, eds. *Practical Guide to the Evaluation of Clinical Competence*. 1st ed. Elsevier; 2008:149–178.
75. ten Cate O. Trust, competence, and the supervisor's role in postgraduate training. *BMJ*. 2006 Oct 7;333:748–751. doi:10.1136/bmj.38938.407569.94.
76. ten Cate O, Scheele F. Competency-based postgraduate training: can we bridge the gap between theory and clinical practice? *Acad Med*. 2007 Jun;82(6):542–547. doi:10.1097/ACM.0b013e31805559c7.
77. Warm EJ, Mathis BR, Held JD, et al. Entrustment and mapping of observable practice activities for resident assessment. *J Gen Intern Med*. 2014 Aug;29(8):1177–1182. doi:10.1007/s11606-014-2801-5.
78. Ziv A, Wolpe PR, Small SD, Glick S. Simulation-based medical education: an ethical imperative. *Acad Med*. 2003 Aug;78(8):783–788. doi:10.1097/00001888-200308000-00006.
79. McGaghie WC, Draycott TJ, Dunn WF, Lopez CM, Stefanidis D. Evaluating the impact of simulation on translational patient outcomes. *Simul Healthc*. 2011 Aug;6(7):S42–S47. doi:10.1097/SIH.0b013e318222fde9.
80. Ericsson KA. Deliberate practice and the acquisition and maintenance of expert performance in medicine and related domains. *Acad Med*. 2004 Oct;79(10 Suppl):S70–S81. doi:10.1097/00001888-200410001-00022.
81. Ericsson KA. Acquisition and maintenance of medical expertise: a perspective from the expert-performance approach with deliberate practice. *Acad Med*. 2015 Nov;90(11):1471–1486. doi:10.1097/ACM.0000000000000939.
82. McGaghie WC, Issenberg SB, Cohen ER, Barsuk JH, Wayne DB. Medical education featuring mastery learning with deliberate practice can lead to better health for individuals and populations. *Acad Med*. 2011 Nov;86(11):e8–e9. doi:10.1097/ACM.0b013e3182308d37.
83. McGaghie WC, Issenberg SB, Barsuk JH, Wayne DB. A critical review of simulation-based mastery learning with translational outcomes. *Med Educ*. 2014 Apr;48(4):375–385. doi:10.1111/medu.12391.
84. McGaghie WC, Barsuk JH, Wayne DB, eds. *Comprehensive Healthcare Simulation: Mastery Learning in Health Professions Education*. Springer; 2020.
85. Wayne DB, Barsuk JH, O'Leary KJ, Fudala MJ, McGaghie WC. Mastery learning of thoracentesis skills by internal medicine residents using simulation technology and deliberate practice. *J Hosp Med*. 2008 Jan;3(1):48–54. doi:10.1002/jhm.268.
86. Barsuk JH, McGaghie WC, Cohen ER, Balachandran JS, Wayne DB. Use of simulation-based mastery learning to improve the quality of central venous catheter placement in a medical intensive care unit. *J Hosp Med*. 2009 Sep;4(7):397–403. doi:10.1002/jhm.468.
87. Barsuk JH, Cohen ER, Vozenilek JA, O'Connor LM, McGaghie WC, Wayne DB. Simulation-based education with mastery learning improves paracentesis skills. *J Grad Med Educ*. 2012 Mar;4(1):23–27. doi:10.4300/JGME-D-11-00161.1.
88. McQuillan RF, Clark E, Zahirieh A, et al. Performance of temporary hemodialysis catheter insertion by nephrology fellows and attending nephrologists. *Clin J Am Soc Nephrol*. 2015 Oct;10(10):1767–1772. doi:10.2215/CJN.01720215.
89. Ault MJ, Rosen BT, Scher J, Feinglass J, Barsuk JH. Thoracentesis outcomes: a 12-year experience. *Thorax*. 2015 Feb;70(2):127–132. doi:10.1136/thoraxjnl-2014-206114.
90. Barsuk JH, Cohen ER, Williams MV, et al. The effect of simulation-based mastery learning on thoracentesis referral patterns. *J Hosp Med*. 2016 Nov;11(11):792–795. doi:10.1002/jhm.2623.
91. Barsuk JH, Cohen ER, Williams MV, et al. Simulation-based mastery learning for thoracentesis skills improves patient outcomes: a randomized trial. *Acad Med*. 2018 May;93(5):729–735. doi:10.1097/ACM.0000000000001965.
92. Vitale KM, Barsuk JH, Cohen ER, et al. Simulation-based mastery learning improves critical care skills of advanced practice providers. *ATS Sch*. 2023 Mar;4(1):48–60. doi:10.34197/ats-scholar.2022-0065OC.
93. Kneebone RL, Kidd J, Nestel D, et al. Blurring the boundaries: scenario-based simulation in a clinical setting. *Med Educ*. 2005 Jun;39(6):580–587. doi:10.1111/j.1365-2929.2005.02110.x.
94. Schuwirth LWT, van der Vleuten CPM. Changing education, changing assessment, changing research? *Med Educ*. 2004 Aug;38(8):805–812. doi:10.1111/j.1365-2929.2004.01851.x.
95. Mahaboob S, Lim LK, Ng CL, Ho QY, Leow MEL, Lim ECH. Developing the "NUS Tummy Dummy", a low-cost simulator to teach medical students to perform the abdominal examination. *Ann Acad Med Singap*. 2010 Feb;39(2):150–151. doi:10.47102/annals-acadmedsg.V39N2p150.
96. Hamm RM, Kelley DM, Medina JA, Syed NS, Harris GA, Papa FJ. Effects of using an abdominal simulator to develop palpatory competencies in 3rd year medical students. *BMC Med Educ*. 2022 Jan 26;22(1):63. doi:10.1186/s12909-022-03126-y.
97. Kneebone R, Arora S, King D, et al. Distributed simulation—accessible immersive training. *Med Teach*. 2010 Jan;32(1):65–70. doi:10.3109/01421590903419749.
98. Cohen ER, Feinglass J, Barsuk JH, et al. Cost savings from reduced catheter-related bloodstream infection after simulation-based education for residents in a medical intensive care unit.

Simul Healthc. 2010 Apr;5(2):98–102. doi:10.1097/SIH.0b013e3181bc8304.

99. Barsuk JH, Cohen ER, Feinglass J, et al. Cost savings of performing paracentesis procedures at the bedside after simulation-based education. *Simul Healthc.* 2014 Oct;9(5):312–318. doi:10.1097/SIH.0000000000000040.
100. Cook DA, Hatala R, Brydges R, et al. Technology-enhanced simulation for health professions education: a systematic review and meta-analysis. *JAMA.* 2011 Sep 7;306(9):978–988. doi:10.1001/jama.2011.1234.
101. Cook DA, Brydges R, Zendejas B, Hamstra SJ, Hatala R. Technology-enhanced simulation to assess health professionals: a systematic review of validity evidence, research methods, and reporting quality. *Acad Med.* 2013 Jun;88(6):872–883. doi:10.1097/ACM.0b013e31828ffdcf.
102. Cook DA. One drop at a time: research to advance the science of simulation. *Simul Healthc.* 2010 Feb;5(1):1–4. doi:10.1097/SIH.0b013e3181c82aaa.
103. McGaghie WC, Issenberg SB, Petrusa ER, Scalese RJ. Effect of practice on standardised learning outcomes in simulation-based medical education. *Med Educ.* 2006 Aug;40(8):792–797. doi:10.1111/j.1365-2929.2006.02528.x.
104. Swanson DB. A measurement framework for performance-based tests. In: Hart I, Harden RM, eds. *Further Developments in Assessing Clinical Competence.* Can-Heal Publications; 1987:13–45.
105. Whelan GP, Boulet JR, McKinley DW, et al. Scoring standardized patient examinations: lessons learned from the development and administration of the ECFMG Clinical Skills Assessment (CSA). *Med Teach.* 2005 May;27(3):200–206. doi:10.1080/01421590500126296.
106. Gallagher AG, Richie K, McClure N, McGuigan J. Objective psychomotor skills assessment of experienced, junior, and novice laparoscopists with virtual reality. *World J Surg.* 2001 Nov;25(11):1478–1483. doi:10.1007/s00268-001-0133-1.
107. Seymour NE, Gallagher AG, Roman SA, et al. Virtual reality training improves operating room performance: results of a randomized, double-blinded study. *Ann Surg.* 2002 Oct; 236(4):458–463; discussion 463–464. doi:10.1097/00000658-200210000-00008.
108. Reznek MA. Current status of simulation in education and research. In: Lloyd GE, Lake CL, Greenberg RB, eds. *Practical Health Care Simulations.* Mosby; 2004:27–47.
109. Demiralp C, Jackson CD, Karelitz DB, Zhang S, Laidlaw DH. CAVE and fishtank virtual-reality displays: a qualitative and quantitative comparison. *IEEE Trans Vis Comput Graph.* 2006 May-Jun;12(3):323–330. doi:10.1109/TVCG.2006.42.
110. Henao O, Escallon J, Green J, et al. [Fundamentals of laparoscopic surgery in Colombia using telesimulation: an effective educational tool for distance learning]. *Biomedica.* 2013 May;33(1): 107–114. doi:10.1590/S0120-41572013000100013.
111. Okrainec A, Henao O, Azzie G. Telesimulation: an effective method for teaching the fundamentals of laparoscopic surgery in resource-restricted countries. *Surg Endosc.* 2010 Feb;24(2):417–422. doi:10.1007/s00464-009-0572-6.
112. Mikrogianakis A, Kam A, Silver S, et al. Telesimulation: an innovative and effective tool for teaching novel intraosseous insertion techniques in developing countries. *Acad Emerg Med.* 2011 Apr;18(4):420–427. doi:10.1111/j.1553-2712.2011.01038.x.
113. Choy I, Fecso A, Kwong J, Jackson T, Okrainec A. Remote evaluation of laparoscopic performance using the global operative assessment of laparoscopic skills. *Surg Endosc.* 2013 Feb;27(2):378–383. doi:10.1007/s00464-012-2456-4.
114. Okrainec A, Vassiliou M, Kapoor A, et al. Feasibility of remote administration of the Fundamentals of Laparoscopic Surgery (FLS) skills test. Surg Endosc. 2013 Nov;27(11):4033-4037. doi:10.1007/s00464-013-3048-7.
115. Limbs & Things. Products by specialty. Accessed April 22, 2023. https://limbsandthings.com/global/specialties.
116. Limbs & Things. Cannulation. Accessed April 22, 2023. https://limbsandthings.com/global/procedures/cannulation?filters=tasktrainers,packs,addons.
117. Kyoto Kagaku. CVC Insertion Simulator II. Accessed April 22, 2023. https://www.kyotokagaku.com/en/products_data/m93ub/.
118. Kyoto Kagaku. EYE Examination Simulator. Accessed April 22, 2023. https://www.kyotokagaku.com/en/products_data/m82m82a/.
119. Kyoto Kagaku. EAR Examination Simulator II. Accessed April 22, 2023. https://www.kyotokagaku.com/en/products_data/mw12/.
120. Limbs & Things. Breast Examination. Accessed April 22, 2023. https://limbsandthings.com/global/procedures/breast-examination-cbe-sbe?filters=tasktrainers,packs,addons.
121. Laerdal Medical. Airway Management Trainers. Accessed April 22, 2023. https://laerdal.com/us/products/skills-proficiency/airway-management-trainers/.
122. Laerdal Medical. Resusci Anne Simulator. Accessed April 22, 2023. https://laerdal.com/products/simulation-training/emergency-care-trauma/resusci-anne-simulator/.
123. Cooper JB, Taqueti VR. A brief history of the development of mannequin simulators for clinical education and training. *Qual Saf Health Care.* 2004 Oct;13(Suppl 1):i11–i18. doi:10.1136/qshc.13.suppl_1.i11.
124. Limbs & Things. Lumbar Puncture. Accessed April 22, 2023. https://limbsandthings.com/global/procedures/lumbar-puncture?filters=tasktrainers,packs,addons.
125. Kyoto Kagaku. Pediatric Lumbar Puncture Simulator II. Accessed April 22, 2023. https://www.kyotokagaku.com/en/products_data/m43d/.
126. Laerdal Medical. MamaNatalie Birthing Simulator. Accessed April 22, 2023. https://laerdal.com/products/simulation-training/obstetrics-paediatrics/mamanatalie.
127. Limbs & Things. Obstetrics & Midwifery. Accessed April 22, 2023. https://limbsandthings.com/global/specialties/obstetrics-midwifery?filters=tasktrainers,packs,addons.
128. Limbs & Things. Birthing Simulator PROMPT Flex - Standard. Accessed April 22, 2023. https://limbsandthings.com/global/products/80100/80100-birthing-simulator-prompt-flex-standard-light-skin-tone#tab2.
129. Limbs & Things. Male Rectal Examination Trainer - Advanced. Accessed April 22, 2023. https://limbsandthings.com/global/products/60187/60187-male-rectal-examination-trainer-advanced-dark-skin-tone.
130. Limbs & Things. Clinical Female Pelvic Trainer Mk3 - Advanced. Accessed October 1, 2022. https://limbsandthings.com/global/products/60935/60935-clinical-female-pelvic-trainer-mk-3-cfpt-advanced-dark-skin-tone.
131. CAE Healthcare. CAE Blue Phantom. Accessed April 22, 2023. https://medicalskillstrainers.cae.com/blue-phantom.
132. Simulab. Ultrasound Procedure. Accessed April 22, 2023. https://simulab.com/collections/ultrasound-procedure.
133. Angtuaco TL, Hopkins RH, DuBose TJ, Bursac Z, Angtuaco MJ, Ferris EJ. Sonographic physical diagnosis 101: teaching senior medical students basic ultrasound scanning skills using a compact ultrasound system. *Ultrasound Q.* 2007 Jun;23(2): 157–160. doi:10.1097/01.ruq.0000263847.00185.28.

134. Webb EM, Cotton JB, Kane K, Straus CM, Topp KS, Naeger DM. Teaching point of care ultrasound skills in medical school: keeping radiology in the driver's seat. *Acad Radiol.* 2014 Jul;21(7):893–901. doi:10.1016/j.acra.2014.03.001.
135. Knudson MM, Sisley AC. Training residents using simulation technology: experience with ultrasound for trauma. *J Trauma.* 2000 Apr;48(4):659–665. doi:10.1097/00005373-200004000-00013.
136. Terkamp C, Kirchner G, Wedemeyer J, et al. Simulation of abdomen sonography. Evaluation of a new ultrasound simulator. *Ultraschall Med.* 2003 Aug;24(4):239–244. doi:10.1055/s-2003-41713.
137. Counselman FL, Sanders A, Slovis CM, Danzl D, Binder LS, Perina DG. The status of bedside ultrasonography training in emergency medicine residency programs. *Acad Emerg Med.* 2003 Jan;10(1):37–42. doi:10.1111/j.1553-2712.2003.tb01974.x.
138. Maul H, Scharf A, Baier P, et al. Ultrasound simulators: experience with the SonoTrainer and comparative review of other training systems. *Ultrasound Obstet Gynecol.* 2004 Oct;24(5):581–585. doi:10.1002/uog.1119.
139. Pelvic ExamSIM. 2004. Accessed April 22, 2023. https://baes.com.ar/catalogos/PelvicExamSim.pdf.
140. Pugh C, Heinrichs WL, Dev P, Srivastava S, Krummel TM. Use of a mechanical simulator to assess pelvic examination skills. *JAMA.* 2001 Sep 5;286(9):1021–1023. doi:10.1001/jama.286.9.1021-a.
141. Pugh CM, Youngblood P. Development and validation of assessment measures for a newly developed physical examination simulator. *J Am Med Inform Assoc.* 2002 Sep-Oct;9(5):448–460. doi:10.1197/jamia.m1107.
142. Ashurst N, Rout CC, Rocke DA, Gouws E. Use of a mechanical simulator for training in applying cricoid pressure. *Br J Anaesth.* 1996 Oct;77(4):468–472. doi:10.1093/bja/77.4.468.
143. Laerdal Medical. Resusci Anne QCPR. Accessed April 22, 2023. https://laerdal.com/products/simulation-training/resuscitation-training/resusci-anne-qcpr.
144. Dieckmann P, Phero JC, Issenberg SB, Kardong-Edgren S, Ostergaard D, Ringsted C. The first Research Consensus Summit of the Society for Simulation in Healthcare: conduction and a synthesis of the results. *Simul Healthc.* 2011 Aug;6(7):S1–S9. doi:10.1097/SIH.0b013e31822238fc.
145. Issenberg SB, Ringsted C, Ostergaard D, Dieckmann P. Setting a research agenda for simulation-based healthcare education: a synthesis of the outcome from an Utstein style meeting. *Simul Healthc.* 2011 Jun;6(3):155–167. doi:10.1097/SIH.0b013e3182207c24.
146. Michael S. Gordon Center for Simulation and Innovation in Medical Education. Harvey. Accessed April 22, 2023. https://gordoncenter.miami.edu/harvey/.
147. Gordon MS. Cardiology patient simulator. Development of an animated manikin to teach cardiovascular disease. *Am J Cardiol.* 1974 Sep;34(3):350–355. doi:10.1016/0002-9149(74)90038-1.
148. Gordon MS, Ewy GA, Felner JM, et al. A cardiology patient simulator for continuing education of family physicians. *J Fam Pract.* 1981 Sep;13(3):353–356.
149. Jones JS, Hunt SJ, Carlson SA, Seamon JP. Assessing bedside cardiologic examination skills using "Harvey," a cardiology patient simulator. *Acad Emerg Med.* 1997 Oct;4(10):980–985. doi:10.1111/j.1553-2712.1997.tb03664.x.
150. Jeffries PR, Beach M, Decker SI, et al. Multi-center development and testing of a simulation-based cardiovascular assessment curriculum for advanced practice nurses. *Nurs Educ Perspect.* 2011 Sep-Oct;32(5):316–322. doi:10.5480/1536-5026-32.5.316.
151. Multak N, Newell K, Spear S, Scalese RJ, Issenberg SB. A multi-institutional study using simulation to teach cardiopulmonary physical examination and diagnosis skills to physician assistant students. *J Physician Assist Educ.* 2015 Jun;26(2):70–76. doi:10.1097/JPA.0000000000000021.
152. Ewy GA, Felner JM, Juul D, Mayer JW, Sajid AW, Waugh RA. Test of a cardiology patient simulator with students in fourth-year electives. *J Med Educ.* 1987 Sep;62(9):738–743. doi:10.1097/00001888-198709000-00005.
153. St Clair EW, Oddone EZ, Waugh RA, Corey GR, Feussner JR. Assessing housestaff diagnostic skills using a cardiology patient simulator. *Ann Intern Med.* 1992 Nov 1;117(9):751–756. doi:10.7326/0003-4819-117-9-751.
154. Hatala R, Issenberg SB, Kassen B, Cole G, Bacchus CM, Scalese RJ. Assessing cardiac physical examination skills using simulation technology and real patients: a comparison study. *Med Educ.* 2008 Jun;42(6):628–636. doi:10.1111/j.1365-2923.2007.02953.x.
155. Hatala R, Scalese RJ, Cole G, Bacchus M, Kassen B, Issenberg SB. Development and validation of a cardiac findings checklist for use with simulator-based assessments of cardiac physical examination competence. *Simul Healthc.* 2009 Spring;4(1):17–21. doi:10.1097/SIH.0b013e318183142b.
156. Devitt JH, Kurrek MM, Cohen MM, et al. Testing the raters: inter-rater reliability of standardized anaesthesia simulator performance. *Can J Anaesth.* 1997 Sep;44(9):924–928. doi:10.1007/BF03011962.
157. Devitt JH, Kurrek MM, Cohen MM, et al. Testing internal consistency and construct validity during evaluation of performance in a patient simulator. *Anesth Analg.* 1998 Jun;86(6):1160–1164. doi:10.1097/00000539-199806000-00004.
158. Devitt JH, Kurrek MM, Cohen MM, Cleave-Hogg D. The validity of performance assessments using simulation. *Anesthesiology.* 2001 Jul;95(1):36–42. doi:10.1097/00000542-200107000-00011.
159. CAE Healthcare. CAE HPS: The Human Patient Simulator. Accessed April 22, 2023. https://www.caehealthcare.com/patient-simulation/hps.
160. CAE Healthcare. CAE Apollo. Accessed April 22, 2023. https://www.caehealthcare.com/patient-simulation/apollo.
161. CAE Healthcare. CAE Ares. Accessed April 22, 2023. https://www.caehealthcare.com/patient-simulation/ares.
162. CAE Healthcare. Patient Simulation. Accessed April 22, 2023. https://www.caehealthcare.com/patient-simulation/.
163. CAE Healthcare. CAE Aria. Accessed April 22, 2023. https://www.caehealthcare.com/patient-simulation/cae-aria.
164. CAE Healthcare. CAE Luna. Accessed April 22, 2023. https://www.caehealthcare.com/patient-simulation/luna.
165. Laerdal Medical. Emergency Care & Trauma. Accessed April 22, 2023. https://laerdal.com/products/simulation-training/emergency-care-trauma/.
166. Laerdal Medical. SimMan 3G. Accessed April 22, 2023. https://laerdal.com/ca/products/simulation-training/emergency-care-trauma/simman/.
167. Laerdal Medical. SimMan 3G Plus. Accessed April 22, 2023. https://laerdal.com/ca/products/simulation-training/emergency-care-trauma/simman/.
168. Laerdal Medical. SimMan 3G Trauma. Accessed April 11, 2023. https://laerdal.com/products/simulation-training/emergency-care-trauma/simman-3g-trauma/.

169. Laerdal Medical. SimMan ALS. Accessed April 22, 2023. https://laerdal.com/products/simulation-training/emergency-care-trauma/simman-als/.
170. Laerdal Medical. SimMan Essential. Accessed April 22, 2023. https://laerdal.com/products/simulation-training/emergency-care-trauma/simman-essential/.
171. Torgeirsen K, Lutnaes DE, Heimvik L, et al. Telemedicine: a new but useful multi-tool in simulation. In: Proceedings of the 21st Annual Meeting of the Society in Europe for Simulation Applied to Medicine (SESAM) 2015. Belfast: SESAM; 2015.
172. Torgeirsen K, Lutnaes DE, Heimvik L, et al. Telemedicine and CRM/human factors challenges. In: Proceedings of the 21st Annual Meeting of the Society in Europe for Simulation Applied to Medicine (SESAM) 2015. Belfast: SESAM; 2015:
173. Laerdal Medical. Obstetric Solution-SimMom and MamaBirthie. Accessed April 22, 2023. https://laerdal.com/products/simulation-training/obstetrics-paediatrics/obstetric-solution-simmom-and-mamabirthie.
174. Laerdal Medical. SimJunior. Accessed April 22, 2023. https://laerdal.com/products/simulation-training/obstetrics-paediatrics/simjunior/.
175. Laerdal Medical. SimBaby. Accessed April 22, 2023. https://laerdal.com/products/simulation-training/obstetrics-paediatrics/simbaby/.
176. Laerdal Medical. SimNewB. Accessed April 22, 2023. https://laerdal.com/products/simulation-training/obstetrics-paediatrics/simnewb/.
177. Laerdal Medical. Premature Anne. Accessed April 22, 2023. https://laerdal.com/products/simulation-training/obstetrics-paediatrics/premature-anne.
178. Gaumard. Gaumard. Accessed April 22, 2023. https://www.gaumard.com/.
179. Gaumard. Pediatric HAL S3005 - Wireless and Tetherless, Five-Year-Old Patient Simulator. Accessed April 22, 2023. https://www.gaumard.com/s3005.
180. Gaumard. Pediatric HAL S3004 - Wireless and Tetherless One-Year-Old Pediatric Simulator. Accessed April 22, 2023. https://www.gaumard.com/s3004.
181. Gaumard. Newborn HAL S3010 - Wireless and Tetherless, Neonate at 40-Weeks Gestational Age. Accessed April 22, 2023. https://www.gaumard.com/s3010.
182. Gaumard. Premie HAL S2209 - 30-Week Premature Infant Patient Simulator. Accessed April 22, 2023. https://www.gaumard.com/hal-s2209.
183. Gaumard. Gaumard Products - Our Brands: HAL. Accessed April 22, 2023. https://www.gaumard.com/gaumard-products/shop-all-products?gs_gaumard_brands=448.
184. Gaumard. Pediatric HAL S2225. Accessed April 22, 2023. https://www.gaumard.com/s2225.
185. Gaumard. HAL S5301. Accessed April 22, 2023. https://www.gaumard.com/hal-s5301.
186. Gaumard. Gaumard Products - Our Brands: NOELLE. Accessed April 22, 2023. https://www.gaumard.com/gaumard-products/shop-all-products?gs_gaumard_brands=450.
187. Gaumard. Gaumard Products - Our Brands: VICTORIA. Accessed April 22, 2023. https://www.gaumard.com/gaumard-products/shop-all-products?gs_gaumard_brands=451.
188. Laerdal Medical. Laerdal-SonoSim Ultrasound Solution 2.0. Accessed April 22, 2023. https://laerdal.com/products/skills-proficiency/ultrasound/laerdal-sonosim-ultrasound-solution/.
189. SonoSim. SonoSim LiveScan. Accessed October 30, 2023. https://sonosim.com/simulation-healthcare-ultrasound-simulator-sonosim-livescan.
190. Agency for Healthcare Research and Quality (AHRQ). *TeamSTEPPS 3.0 Pocket Guide: Team Strategies & Tools to Enhance Performance and Patient Safety.* Updated 2023. Accessed October 28, 2023. https://www.ahrq.gov/sites/default/files/wysiwyg/teamstepps-program/teamstepps-pocket-guide.pdf.
191. Agency for Healthcare Research and Quality (AHRQ). TeamSTEPPS Training Simulation Videos. Updated 2023. Accessed October 28, 2023. https://www.ahrq.gov/teamstepps-program/resources/videos/index.html.
192. Baker VO, Cuzzola R, Knox C, et al. Teamwork education improves trauma team performance in undergraduate health professional students. *J Educ Eval Health Prof.* 2015 Jun 25;12:36. doi:10.3352/jeehp.2015.12.36.
193. Capella J, Smith S, Philp A, et al. Teamwork training improves the clinical care of trauma patients. *J Surg Educ.* 2010 Nov-Dec;67(6):439–443. doi:10.1016/j.jsurg.2010.06.006.
194. Steinemann S, Berg B, Skinner A, et al. In situ, multidisciplinary, simulation-based teamwork training improves early trauma care. *J Surg Educ.* 2011 Nov-Dec;68(6):472–477. doi:10.1016/j.jsurg.2011.05.009.
195. Ursino M, Tasto JL, Nguyen BH, Cunningham R, Merril GL. CathSim: an intravascular catheterization simulator on a PC. *Stud Health Technol Inform.* 1999;62:360–366.
196. Tseng CS, Lee YY, Chan YP, Wu SS, Chiu AW. A PC-based surgical simulator for laparoscopic surgery. *Stud Health Technol Inform.* 1998;50:155–160.
197. Gallagher AG, Cates CU. Approval of virtual reality training for carotid stenting: what this means for procedural-based medicine. *JAMA.* 2004 Dec 22;292(24):3024–3026. doi:10.1001/jama.292.24.3024.
198. Tuggy ML. Virtual reality flexible sigmoidoscopy simulator training: impact on resident performance. *J Am Board Fam Pract.* 1998 Nov-Dec;11(6):426–433. doi:10.3122/jabfm.11.6.426.
199. Halvorsrud R, Hagen S, Fagernes S, Mjelstad S, Romundstad L. Trauma team training in a distributed virtual emergency room. *Stud Health Technol Inform.* 2003;94:100–102.
200. Korocsec D, Holobar A, Divjak M, Zazula D. Building interactive virtual environments for simulated training in medicine using VRML and Java/JavaScript. *Comput Methods Programs Biomed.* 2005 Dec;80(Suppl 1):S61–S70. doi:10.1016/s0169-2607(05)80007-0.
201. Gallagher AG, Cates CU. Virtual reality training for the operating room and cardiac catheterisation laboratory. *Lancet.* 2004 Oct;364(9444):1538–1540. doi:10.1016/S0140-6736(04)17278-4.
202. Patel AD, Gallagher AG, Nicholson WJ, Cates CU. Learning curves and reliability measures for virtual reality simulation in the performance assessment of carotid angiography. *J Am Coll Cardiol.* 2006 May 2;47(9):1796–1802. doi:10.1016/j.jacc.2005.12.053.
203. 3D Systems. Phantom Premium - Haptic Devices. Accessed April 22, 2023. https://www.3dsystems.com/haptics-devices/3d-systems-phantom-premium.
204. Burdea G, Patounakis G, Popescu V, Weiss RE. Virtual reality-based training for the diagnosis of prostate cancer. *IEEE Trans Biomed Eng.* 1999 Oct;46(10):1253–1260. doi:10.1109/10.790503.
205. Stalfors J, Kling-Petersen T, Rydmark M, Westin T. Haptic palpation of head and neck cancer patients—implication for education and telemedicine. *Stud Health Technol Inform.* 2001;81:471–474.
206. Linke R, Leichtle A, Sheikh F, et al. Assessment of skills using a virtual reality temporal bone surgery simulator. *Acta Otorhinolaryngol Ital.* 2013 Aug;33(4):273–281.

207. Weisz G, Smilowitz NR, Parise H, et al. Objective simulator-based evaluation of carotid artery stenting proficiency (from Assessment of Operator Performance by the Carotid Stenting Simulator Study [ASSESS]). *Am J Cardiol.* 2013 Jul;112(2): 299–306. doi:10.1016/j.amjcard.2013.02.069.
208. Jacobsen ME, Andersen MJ, Hansen CO, Konge L. Testing basic competency in knee arthroscopy using a virtual reality simulator: exploring validity and reliability. *J Bone Joint Surg Am.* 2015 May 6;97(9):775–781. doi:10.2106/JBJS.N.00747.
209. Mueller CL, Kaneva P, Fried GM, et al. Validity evidence for a new portable, lower-cost platform for the fundamentals of endoscopic surgery skills test. *Surg Endosc.* 2016 Mar;30(3):1107–1112. doi:10.1007/s00464-015-4307-6.
210. Yoshida Y, Yamaguchi S, Wakabayashi K, et al. Virtual reality simulation training for dental surgery. *Stud Health Technol Inform.* 2009;142:435–437.
211. Pohlenz P, Grobe A, Petersik A, et al. Virtual dental surgery as a new educational tool in dental school. *J Craniomaxillofac Surg.* 2010 Dec;38(8):560–564. doi:10.1016/j.jcms.2010.02.011.
212. Suebnukarn S, Chaisombat M, Kongpunwijit T, Rhienmora P. Construct validity and expert benchmarking of the haptic virtual reality dental simulator. *J Dent Educ.* 2014 Oct;78(10):1442–1450.
213. Farag A, Hashem D. Impact of the haptic virtual reality simulator on dental students' psychomotor skills in preclinical operative dentistry. *Clin Pract.* 2022 Dec 28;12(1):17–26. doi:10.3390/clinpract12010003.
214. Crossan A, Brewster S, Reid S, Mellor D. Comparison of simulated ovary training over different skill levels. *Proceedings of Eurohaptics.* 2001:17–21.
215. Baillie S, Crossan A, Brewster S, Mellor D, Reid S. Validation of a bovine rectal palpation simulator for training veterinary students. *Stud Health Technol Inform.* 2005;111:33–36.
216. Parkes R, Forrest N, Baillie S. A mixed reality simulator for feline abdominal palpation training in veterinary medicine. *Stud Health Technol Inform.* 2009;142:244–246.
217. Baillie S, Crossan A, Brewster SA, May SA, Mellor DJ. Evaluating an automated haptic simulator designed for veterinary students to learn bovine rectal palpation. *Simul Healthc.* 2010 Oct;5(5):261–266. doi:10.1097/SIH.0b013e3181e369bf.
218. CyberGlove Systems. CyberGloves Systems. Accessed April 22, 2023. http://www.cyberglovesystems.com/.
219. Banerjee PP, Luciano CJ, Lemole Jr GM, Charbel FT, Oh MY. Accuracy of ventriculostomy catheter placement using a head- and hand-tracked high-resolution virtual reality simulator with haptic feedback. *J Neurosurg.* 2007 Sep;107(3):515–521. doi:10.3171/JNS-07/09/0515.
220. Grantcharov TP, Rosenberg J, Pahle E, Funch-Jensen P. Virtual reality computer simulation. *Surg Endosc.* 2001 May;15:242–244. doi:10.1007/s004640090008.
221. Satava RM. Virtual reality surgical simulator. The first steps. *Surg Endosc.* 1993 May-Jun;7(3):203–205. doi:10.1007/BF00594110.
222. Phillips NI, John NW. Web-based surgical simulation for ventricular catheterization. *Neurosurgery.* 2000 Apr;46(4):933–936; discussion 936–937. doi:10.1097/00006123-200004000-00031.
223. Larsen OV, Haase J, Ostergaard LR, Hansen KV, Nielsen H. The Virtual Brain Project—development of a neurosurgical simulator. *Stud Health Technol Inform.* 2001;81:256–262.
224. Goncharenko I, Emotob H, Matsumoto S, et al. Realistic virtual endoscopy of the ventricle system and haptic-based surgical simulator of hydrocephalus treatment. *Stud Health Technol Inform.* 2003;94:93–95.
225. Lemole M, Banerjee PP, Luciano C, Charbel F, Oh M. Virtual ventriculostomy with 'shifted ventricle': neurosurgery resident surgical skill assessment using a high-fidelity haptic/graphic virtual reality simulator. *Neurol Res.* 2009 May;31(4):430–431. doi:10.1179/174313208X353695.
226. CAE Healthcare. NeuroVR–User Guide. 2016. Accessed October 30, 2023. https://www.caehealthcare.com/media/legacy/NeuroVR-User-Guide.pdf.
227. Larsen OV, Haase J, Hansen KV, Brix L, Pedersen CF. Training brain retraction in a virtual reality environment. *Stud Health Technol Inform.* 2003;94:174–180.
228. Alotaibi FE, AlZhrani GA, Mullah MAS, et al. Assessing bimanual performance in brain tumor resection with NeuroTouch, a virtual reality simulator. *Neurosurgery.* 2015 Mar;11(1):89–98; discussion 98. doi:10.1227/NEU.0000000000000631.
229. Alotaibi FE, AlZhrani GA, Sabbagh AJ, Azarnoush H, Winkler-Schwartz A, Del Maestro RF. Neurosurgical assessment of metrics including judgment and dexterity using the virtual reality simulator NeuroTouch (NAJD Metrics). *Surg Innov.* 2015 Dec;22(6):636–642. doi:10.1177/1553350615579729.
230. AlZhrani G, Alotaibi F, Azarnoush H, et al. Proficiency performance benchmarks for removal of simulated brain tumors using a virtual reality simulator NeuroTouch. *J Surg Educ.* 2015 Jul-Aug;72(4):685–696. doi:10.1016/j.jsurg.2014.12.014.
231. Spicer MA, Apuzzo ML. Virtual reality surgery: neurosurgery and the contemporary landscape. *Neurosurgery.* 2003 Mar;52(3):489–497; discussion 496–497. doi:10.1227/01.neu.0000047812.42726.56.
232. Arora A, Khemani S, Tolley N, et al. Face and content validation of a virtual reality temporal bone simulator. *Otolaryngol Head Neck Surg.* 2012 Mar;146(3):497–503. doi:10.1177/0194599811427385.
233. Khemani S, Arora A, Singh A, Tolley N, Darzi A. Objective skills assessment and construct validation of a virtual reality temporal bone simulator. *Otol Neurotol.* 2012 Sep;33(7):1225–1231. doi:10.1097/MAO.0b013e31825e7977.
234. Nash R, Sykes R, Majithia A, Arora A, Singh A, Khemani S. Objective assessment of learning curves for the Voxel-Man TempoSurg temporal bone surgery computer simulator. *J Laryngol Otol.* 2012 Jul;126(7):663–669. doi:10.1017/S0022215112000734.
235. Zhao YC, Kennedy G, Hall R, O'Leary S. Differentiating levels of surgical experience on a virtual reality temporal bone simulator. *Otolaryngol Head Neck Surg.* 2010 Nov;143(5 Suppl 3):S30–S35. doi:10.1016/j.otohns.2010.03.008.
236. Wiet GJ, Stredney D, Kerwin T, et al. Virtual temporal bone dissection system: OSU virtual temporal bone system: development and testing. *Laryngoscope.* 2012 Mar;122(Suppl 1):S1–S12. doi:10.1002/lary.22499.
237. Arora A, Lau LYM, Awad Z, Darzi A, Singh A, Tolley N. Virtual reality simulation training in otolaryngology. *Int J Surg.* 2014 Feb;12(2):87–94. doi:10.1016/j.ijsu.2013.11.007.
238. Satava RM, Fried MP. A methodology for objective assessment of errors: an example using an endoscopic sinus surgery simulator. *Otolaryngol Clin North Am.* 2002 Dec;35(6):1289–1301. doi:10.1016/s0030-6665(02)00090-7.
239. Arora H, Uribe J, Ralph W, et al. Assessment of construct validity of the endoscopic sinus surgery simulator. *Arch Otolaryngol Head Neck Surg.* 2005 Mar;131(3):217–221. doi:10.1001/archotol.131.3.217.

240. Fried MP, Sadoughi B, Gibber MJ, et al. From virtual reality to the operating room: the endoscopic sinus surgery simulator experiment. *Otolaryngol Head Neck Surg.* 2010 Feb;142(2):202–207. doi:10.1016/j.otohns.2009.11.023.
241. Fried MP, Kaye RJ, Gibber MJ, et al. Criterion-based (proficiency) training to improve surgical performance. *Arch Otolaryngol Head Neck Surg.* 2012 Nov 1;138(11):1024–1029. doi:10.1001/2013.jamaoto.377.
242. Sowerby LJ, Rehal G, Husein M, Doyle PC, Agrawal S, Ladak HM. Development and face validity testing of a three-dimensional myringotomy simulator with haptic feedback. *J Otolaryngol Head Neck Surg.* 2010 Apr;39(2):122–129. doi:10.2310/7070.2009.090079.
243. Ho AK, Alsaffar H, Doyle PC, Ladak HM, Agrawal SK. Virtual reality myringotomy simulation with real-time deformation: development and validity testing. *Laryngoscope.* 2012 Aug;122(8):1844–1851. doi:10.1002/lary.23361.
244. Wheeler B, Doyle PC, Chandarana S, Agrawal S, Husein M, Ladak HM. Interactive computer-based simulator for training in blade navigation and targeting in myringotomy. *Comput Methods Programs Biomed.* 2010 May;98(2):130–139. doi:10.1016/j.cmpb.2009.09.010.
245. Grunwald T, Krummel T, Sherman R. Advanced technologies in plastic surgery: how new innovations can improve our training and practice. *Plast Reconstr Surg.* 2004 Nov;114(6):1556–1567. doi:10.1097/01.prs.0000138242.60324.1d.
246. Smith DM, Aston SJ, Cutting CB, Oliker A. Applications of virtual reality in aesthetic surgery. *Plast Reconstr Surg.* 2005 Sep;116(3):898–904; discussion 905–906. doi:10.1097/01.prs.0000176901.37684.8a.
247. Pfaff MJ, Steinbacher DM. Plastic surgery resident understanding and education using virtual surgical planning. *Plast Reconstr Surg.* 2016 Jan;137(1):258e–259e. doi:10.1097/PRS.0000000000001853.
248. Montgomery K, Sorokin A, Lionetti G, Schendel S. A surgical simulator for cleft lip planning and repair. *Stud Health Technol Inform.* 2003;94:204–209.
249. Sohmura T, Hojo H, Nakajima M, et al. Prototype of simulation of orthognathic surgery using a virtual reality haptic device. *Int J Oral Maxillofac Surg.* 2004 Dec;33(8):740–750. doi:10.1016/j.ijom.2004.03.003.
250. Kusumoto N, Sohmura T, Yamada S, Wakabayashi K, Nakamura T, Yatani H. Application of virtual reality force feedback haptic device for oral implant surgery. *Clin Oral Implants Res.* 2006 Dec;17(6):708–713. doi:10.1111/j.1600-0501.2006.01218.x.
251. Hsieh MS, Tsai MD, Chang WC. Virtual reality simulator for osteotomy and fusion involving the musculoskeletal system. *Comput Med Imaging Graph.* 2002 Mar-Apr;26(2):91–101. doi:10.1016/s0895-6111(01)00034-9.
252. Tay C, Khajuria A, Gupte C. Simulation training: a systematic review of simulation in arthroscopy and proposal of a new competency-based training framework. *Int J Surg.* 2014 Jun;12(6):626–633. doi:10.1016/j.ijsu.2014.04.005.
253. Surgical Science. Simbionix Simulators: ARTHRO Mentor. Accessed April 22, 2023. https://simbionix.com/simulators/arthro-mentor/.
254. VirtaMed. VirtaMed ArthroS. Accessed April 22, 2023. https://www.virtamed.com/en/medical-training-simulators/arthros/.
255. Howells NR, Gill HS, Carr AJ, Price AJ, Rees JL. Transferring simulated arthroscopic skills to the operating theatre: a randomised blinded study. *J Bone Joint Surg Br.* 2008 Apr;90-B(4):494–499. doi:10.1302/0301-620X.90B4.20414.
256. Alvand A, Logishetty K, Middleton R, et al. Validating a global rating scale to monitor individual resident learning curves during arthroscopic knee meniscal repair. *Arthroscopy.* 2013 May;29(5):906–912. doi:10.1016/j.arthro.2013.01.026.
257. Henn 3rd RF, Shah N, Warner JJP, Gomoll AH. Shoulder arthroscopy simulator training improves shoulder arthroscopy performance in a cadaveric model. *Arthroscopy.* 2013 Jun;29(6):982–985. doi:10.1016/j.arthro.2013.02.013.
258. Rahm S, Germann M, Hingsammer A, Wieser K, Gerber C. Validation of a virtual reality-based simulator for shoulder arthroscopy. *Knee Surg Sports Traumatol Arthrosc.* 2016 May;24(5):1730–1737. doi:10.1007/s00167-016-4022-4.
259. Waterman BR, Martin KD, Cameron KL, Owens BD, Belmont Jr PJ. Simulation training improves surgical proficiency and safety during diagnostic shoulder arthroscopy performed by residents. *Orthopedics.* 2016 May 1;39(3):e479–e485. doi:10.3928/01477447-20160427-02.
260. Pollard TC, Khan T, Price AJ, Gill HS, Glyn-Jones S, Rees JL. Simulated hip arthroscopy skills: learning curves with the lateral and supine patient positions: a randomized trial. *J Bone Joint Surg Am.* 2012 May 16;94(10):e68. doi:10.2106/JBJS.K.00690.
261. Smith S, Wan A, Taffinder N, Read S, Emery R, Darzi A. Early experience and validation work with Procedicus VA—the Prosolvia virtual reality shoulder arthroscopy trainer. *Stud Health Technol Inform.* 1999;62:337–343.
262. Tashiro Y, Miura H, Nakanishi Y, Okazaki K, Iwamoto Y. Evaluation of skills in arthroscopic training based on trajectory and force data. *Clin Orthop Relat Res.* 2009 Feb;467(2):546–552. doi:10.1007/s11999-008-0497-8.
263. Tsai MD, Hsieh MS, Jou SB. Virtual reality orthopedic surgery simulator. *Comput Biol Med.* 2001 Sep;31(5):333–351. doi:10.1016/s0010-4825(01)00014-2.
264. Pedersen P, Palm H, Ringsted C, Konge L. Virtual-reality simulation to assess performance in hip fracture surgery. *Acta Orthop.* 2014 Aug;85(4):403–407. doi:10.3109/17453674.2014.917502.
265. Akhtar K, Sugand K, Sperrin M, Cobb J, Standfield N, Gupte C. Training safer orthopedic surgeons. *Acta Orthop.* 2015 Sep;86(5):616–621. doi:10.3109/17453674.2015.1041083.
266. Sinclair MJ, Peifer JW, Haleblian R, Luxenberg NM, Green K, Hull DS. Computer-simulated eye surgery: A novel teaching method for residents and practitioners. *Ophthalmology.* 1995 Mar;102(3):517–521. doi:10.1016/s0161-6420(95)30992-x.
267. Kaufman DM, Bell W. Teaching and assessing clinical skills using virtual reality. *Stud Health Technol Inform.* 1997;39:467–472.
268. Belyea DA, Brown SE, Rajjoub LZ. Influence of surgery simulator training on ophthalmology resident phacoemulsification performance. *J Cataract Refract Surg.* 2011 Oct;37(10):1756–1761. doi:10.1016/j.jcrs.2011.04.032.
269. Lam CK, Sundaraj K, Sulaiman MN. A systematic review of phacoemulsification cataract surgery in virtual reality simulators. *Medicina (Kaunas).* 2013;49(1):1–8.
270. Lam CK, Sundaraj K, Sulaiman MN, Qamarruddin FA. Virtual phacoemulsification surgical simulation using visual guidance and performance parameters as a feasible proficiency assessment tool. *BMC Ophthalmol.* 2016 Jun 14;16:88. doi:10.1186/s12886-016-0269-2.
271. Privett B, Greenlee E, Rogers G, Oetting TA. Construct validity of a surgical simulator as a valid model for capsulorhexis training. *J Cataract Refract Surg.* 2010 Nov;36(11):1835–1838. doi:10.1016/j.jcrs.2010.05.020.

272. Daly MK, Gonzalez E, Siracuse-Lee D, Legutko PA. Efficacy of surgical simulator training versus traditional wet-lab training on operating room performance of ophthalmology residents during the capsulorhexis in cataract surgery. *J Cataract Refract Surg.* 2013 Nov;39(11):1734–1741. doi:10.1016/j.jcrs.2013.05.044.
273. McCannel CA, Reed DC, Goldman DR. Ophthalmic surgery simulator training improves resident performance of capsulorhexis in the operating room. *Ophthalmology.* 2013 Dec;120(12):2456–2461. doi:10.1016/j.ophtha.2013.05.003.
274. Dubois P, Rouland JF, Meseure P, Karpf S, Chaillou C. Simulator for laser photocoagulation in ophthalmology. *IEEE Trans Biomed Eng.* 1995 Jul;42(7):688–693. doi:10.1109/10.391167.
275. Rossi JV, Verma D, Fujii GY, et al. Virtual vitreoretinal surgical simulator as a training tool. *Retina.* 2004 Apr;24(2):231–236. doi:10.1097/00006982-200404000-00007.
276. Kozak I, Banerjee P, Luo J, Luciano C. Virtual reality simulator for vitreoretinal surgery using integrated OCT data. *Clin Ophthalmol.* 2014 Mar;8:669–672. doi:10.2147/OPTH.S58614.
277. Haag-Streit Simulation. Eyesi Surgical. Accessed April 22, 2023. https://www.vrmagic.com/medical-simulators/eyesi-surgical.
278. Melerit PhacoVision. Accessed April 22, 2023. http://melerit.se/html/pdf/new/MeleritPhacoVision.pdf.
279. HelpMeSee. HelpMeSee. Accessed April 22, 2023. https://helpmesee.org/.
280. Nair AG, Ahiwalay C, Bacchav AE, Sheth T, Lansingh VC. Assessment of a high-fidelity, virtual reality-based, manual small-incision cataract surgery simulator: A face and content validity study. *Indian J Ophthalmol.* 2022 Nov;70(11):4010–4015. doi:10.4103/ijo.IJO_1593_22.
281. Sankarananthan R, Prasad RS, Koshy TA, et al. An objective evaluation of simulated surgical outcomes among surgical trainees using manual small-incision cataract surgery virtual reality simulator. *Indian J Ophthalmol.* 2022 Nov;70(11):4018–4025. doi:10.4103/ijo.IJO_1600_22.
282. Webster RW, Zimmerman DI, Mohler BJ, Melkonian MG, Haluck RS. A prototype haptic suturing simulator. *Stud Health Technol Inform.* 2001;81:567–569.
283. Liu A, Kaufmann C, Ritchie T. A computer-based simulator for diagnostic peritoneal lavage. *Stud Health Technol Inform.* 2001;81:279–285.
284. Kaufmann C, Liu A. Trauma training: virtual reality applications. *Stud Health Technol Inform.* 2001;81:236–241.
285. Tillander B, Ledin T, Nordqvist P, Skarman E, Wahlström O. A virtual reality trauma simulator. *Med Teach.* 2004 Mar;26(2):189–191. doi:10.1080/0142159042000192037.
286. Vergara VM, Panaiotis Kingsley D, et al. The use of virtual reality simulation of head trauma in a surgical boot camp. *Stud Health Technol Inform.* 2009;142:395–397.
287. Grantcharov TP, Kristiansen VB, Bendix J, Bardram L, Rosenberg J, Funch-Jensen P. Randomized clinical trial of virtual reality simulation for laparoscopic skills training. *Br J Surg.* 2004 Feb;91(2):146–150. doi:10.1002/bjs.4407.
288. Mentice. Mentice. Accessed April 22, 2023. https://www.mentice.com/.
289. Surgical Science. LAPSIM. Accessed April 22, 2023. https://surgicalscience.com/simulators/lapsim/.
290. CAE. CAELapVR–User's Guide. 2018. Accessed October 31, 2023. https://www.caehealthcare.com/media/legacy/LapVR-User-Guide.pdf.
291. 3D Systems. LAP Mentor VR. Accessed April 22, 2023. https://www.3dsystems.com/node/53226.
292. Shanmugan S, Leblanc F, Senagore AJ, et al. Virtual reality simulator training for laparoscopic colectomy: what metrics have construct validity? *Dis Colon Rectum.* 2014 Feb;57(2):210–214. doi:10.1097/DCR.0000000000000031.
293. Giannotti D, Patrizi G, Casella G, et al. Can virtual reality simulators be a certification tool for bariatric surgeons? *Surg Endosc.* 2014 Jan;28(1):242–248. doi:10.1007/s00464-013-3179-x.
294. Araujo SEA, Delaney CP, Seid VE, et al. Short-duration virtual reality simulation training positively impacts performance during laparoscopic colectomy in animal model: results of a single-blinded randomized trial: VR warm-up for laparoscopic colectomy. *Surg Endosc.* 2014 Sep;28(9):2547–2554. doi:10.1007/s00464-014-3500-3.
295. Ahlberg G, Enochsson L, Gallagher AG, et al. Proficiency-based virtual reality training significantly reduces the error rate for residents during their first 10 laparoscopic cholecystectomies. *Am J Surg.* 2007 Jun;193(6):797–804. doi:10.1016/j.amjsurg.2006.06.050.
296. Akdemir A, Sendag F, Oztekin MK. Laparoscopic virtual reality simulator and box trainer in gynecology. *Int J Gynaecol Obstet.* 2014 May;125(2):181–185. doi:10.1016/j.ijgo.2013.10.018.
297. Larsen CR, Grantcharov T, Aggarwal R, et al. Objective assessment of gynecologic laparoscopic skills using the LapSimGyn virtual reality simulator. *Surg Endosc.* 2006 Sep;20(9):1460–1466. doi:10.1007/s00464-005-0745-x.
298. Bharathan R, Vali S, Setchell T, Miskry T, Darzi A, Aggarwal R. Psychomotor skills and cognitive load training on a virtual reality laparoscopic simulator for tubal surgery is effective. *Eur J Obstet Gynecol Reprod Biol.* 2013 Jul;169(2):347–352. doi:10.1016/j.ejogrb.2013.03.017.
299. Harders M, Bajka M, Spaelter U, Tuchschmid S, Bleuler H, Szekely G. Highly-realistic, immersive training environment for hysteroscopy. *Stud Health Technol Inform.* 2005;119:176–181.
300. VirtaMed. VirtaMed GynoS. Accessed April 22, 2023. https://www.virtamed.com/en/medical-training-simulators/gynos/.
301. Bajka M, Tuchschmid S, Fink D, Székely G, Harders M. Establishing construct validity of a virtual-reality training simulator for hysteroscopy via a multimetric scoring system. *Surg Endosc.* 2010 Jan;24(1):79–88. doi:10.1007/s00464-009-0582-4.
302. Panel P, Bajka M, Le Tohic A, El Ghoneimi A, Chis C, Cotin S. Hysteroscopic placement of tubal sterilization implants: virtual reality simulator training. *Surg Endosc.* 2012 Jul;26(7):1986–1996. doi:10.1007/s00464-011-2139-6.
303. Janse JA, Goedegebuure RSA, Veersema S, Broekmans FJM, Schreuder HWR. Hysteroscopic sterilization using a virtual reality simulator: assessment of learning curve. *J Minim Invasive Gynecol.* 2013 Nov-Dec;20(6):775–782. doi:10.1016/j.jmig.2013.04.016.
304. Neis F, Brucker S, Henes M, et al. Evaluation of the HystSim-virtual reality trainer: an essential additional tool to train hysteroscopic skills outside the operation theater. *Surg Endosc.* 2016 Nov;30(11):4954–4961. doi:10.1007/s00464-016-4837-6.
305. Schout BMA, Muijtjens AMM, Hendrikx AJM, et al. Acquisition of flexible cystoscopy skills on a virtual reality simulator by experts and novices. *BJU Int.* 2010 Jan;105(2):234–239. doi:10.1111/j.1464-410X.2009.08733.x.
306. Zhang Y, Liu JS, Wang G, Yu CF, Zhu H, Na YQ. Effectiveness of the UroMentor virtual reality simulator in the skill acquisition of flexible cystoscopy. *Chin Med J (Engl).* 2013;126(11):2079–2082.
307. Matsumoto ED, Pace KT, D'A Honey RJ. Virtual reality ureteroscopy simulator as a valid tool for assessing endourological

skills. *Int J Urol.* 2006 Jul;13(7):896–901. doi:10.1111/j.1442-2042.2006.01436.x.

308. Bright E, Vine SJ, Dutton T, Wilson MR, McGrath JS. Visual control strategies of surgeons: a novel method of establishing the construct validity of a transurethral resection of the prostate surgical simulator. *J Surg Educ.* 2014 May-Jun;71(3):434–439. doi:10.1016/j.jsurg.2013.11.006.
309. Surgical Science. Simbionix Simulators: URO MENTOR. Accessed April 22, 2023. https://simbionix.com/simulators/uro-mentor/.
310. VirtaMed. VirtaMed UroS. Accessed October 1, 2022. https://www.virtamed.com/en/medical-training-simulators/uros/.
311. Surgical Science. Simbionix Simulators: Simulators. Accessed April 22, 2023. https://simbionix.com/simulators/.
312. Brunckhorst O, Aydin A, Abboudi H, et al. Simulation-based ureteroscopy training: a systematic review. *J Surg Educ.* 2015 Jan-Feb;72(1):135–143. doi:10.1016/j.jsurg.2014.07.003.
313. Kozan AA, Chan LH, Biyani CS. Current status of simulation training in urology: a non-systematic review. *Res Rep Urol.* 2020 Mar 17;12:111–128. doi:10.2147/RRU.S237808.
314. Schout BMA, Ananias HJK, Bemelmans BLH, et al. Transfer of cysto-urethroscopy skills from a virtual-reality simulator to the operating room: a randomized controlled trial. *BJU Int.* 2010 Jul;106(2):226–231. doi:10.1111/j.1464-410X.2009.09049.x discussion 231.
315. Michel MS, Knoll T, Kohrmann KU, Alken P. The URO Mentor: development and evaluation of a new computer-based interactive training system for virtual life-like simulation of diagnostic and therapeutic endourological procedures. *BJU Int.* 2002 Feb;89(3):174–177. doi:10.1046/j.1464-4096.2001.01644.x.
316. Mishra S, Kurien A, Patel R, et al. Validation of virtual reality simulation for percutaneous renal access training. *J Endourol.* 2010 Apr;24(4):635–640. doi:10.1089/end.2009.0166.
317. Noureldin YA, Elkoushy MA, Andonian S. Assessment of percutaneous renal access skills during urology objective structured clinical examinations (OSCE). *Can Urol Assoc J.* 2015 Mar-Apr;9(3-4):E104–E108. doi:10.5489/cuaj.2482.
318. Mishra S, Kurien A, Ganpule A, Muthu V, Sabnis R, Desai M. Percutaneous renal access training: content validation comparison between a live porcine and a virtual reality (VR) simulation model. *BJU Int.* 2010 Dec;106(11):1753–1756. doi:10.1111/j.1464-410X.2010.09753.x.
319. Villard PF, Vidal FP, Hunt C, et al. A prototype percutaneous transhepatic cholangiography training simulator with real-time breathing motion. *Int J Comput Assist Radiol Surg.* 2009 Nov;4(6):571–578. doi:10.1007/s11548-009-0367-1.
320. Fortmeier D, Mastmeyer A, Schroder J, Handels H. A virtual reality system for PTCD simulation using direct visuo-haptic rendering of partially segmented image data. *IEEE J Biomed Health Inform.* 2016 Jan;20(1):355–366. doi:10.1109/JBHI.2014.2381772.
321. Surgical Science. Simbionix Simulators: PERC Mentor Suite. Accessed April 22, 2023. https://simbionix.com/simulators/perc-mentor-suite/.
322. Surgical Science. Simbionix Simulators: ANGIO Mentor. Accessed April 22, 2023. https://simbionix.com/simulators/angio-mentor/.
323. CAE Healthcare. CAE CathLabVR. Accessed October 31, 2023. https://www.caehealthcare.com/solutions/brands/cae-cathlabvr/.
324. Mentice. Virtual Reality simulators for image-guided interventional therapies. Accessed April 22, 2023. https://www.mentice.com/simulators.
325. Nguyen N, Eagleson R, Boulton M, de Ribaupierre S. Realism, criterion validity, and training capability of simulated diagnostic cerebral angiography. *Stud Health Technol Inform.* 2014;196:297–303.
326. Kim AH, Kendrick DE, Moorehead PA, et al. Endovascular aneurysm repair simulation can lead to decreased fluoroscopy time and accurately delineate the proximal seal zone. *J Vasc Surg.* 2016 Jul;64(1):251–258. doi:10.1016/j.jvs.2016.01.050.
327. Cates CU, Gallagher AG. The future of simulation technologies for complex cardiovascular procedures. *Eur Heart J.* 2012 Sep;33(17):2127–2134. doi:10.1093/eurheartj/ehs155.
328. Hsu JH, Younan D, Pandalai S, et al. Use of computer simulation for determining endovascular skill levels in a carotid stenting model. *J Vasc Surg.* 2004 Dec;40(6):1118–1125. doi:10.1016/j.jvs.2004.08.026.
329. Winder J, Zheng H, Hughes S, Kelly B, Wilson C, Gallagher A. Increasing face validity of a vascular interventional training system. *Stud Health Technol Inform.* 2004;98:410–415.
330. Jensen UJ, Jensen J, Olivecrona GK, Ahlberg G, Tornvall P. Technical skills assessment in a coronary angiography simulator for construct validation. *Simul Healthc.* 2013 Oct;8(5):324–328. doi:10.1097/SIH.0b013e31828fdedc.
331. Rudarakanchana N, Van Herzeele I, Bicknell CD, et al. Endovascular repair of ruptured abdominal aortic aneurysm: technical and team training in an immersive virtual reality environment. *Cardiovasc Intervent Radiol.* 2014 Aug;37(4):920–927. doi:10.1007/s00270-013-0765-1.
332. Jensen UJ, Jensen J, Ahlberg G, Tornvall P. Virtual reality training in coronary angiography and its transfer effect to real-life catheterisation lab. *EuroIntervention.* 2016 Apr 20;11(13):1503–1510. doi:10.4244/EIJY15M06_05.
333. Rosenfield K, Babb JD, Cates CU, et al. Clinical competence statement on carotid stenting: training and credentialing for carotid stenting—multispecialty consensus recommendations: a report of the SCAI/SVMB/SVS Writing Committee to develop a clinical competence statement on carotid interventions. *J Am Coll Cardiol.* 2005 Jan 4;45(1):165–174. doi:10.1016/j.jacc.2004.11.016.
334. Stather DR, Lamb CR, Tremblay A. Simulation in flexible bronchoscopy and endobronchial ultrasound: a review. *J Bronchology Interv Pulmonol.* 2011 Jul;18(3):247–256. doi:10.1097/LBR.0b013e3182296588.
335. Kennedy CC, Maldonado F, Cook DA. Simulation-based bronchoscopy training: systematic review and meta-analysis. *Chest.* 2013 Jul;144(1):183–192. doi:10.1378/chest.12-1786.
336. Triantafyllou K, Lazaridis LD, Dimitriadis GD. Virtual reality simulators for gastrointestinal endoscopy training. *World J Gastrointest Endosc.* 2014 Jan 16;6(1):6–12. doi:10.4253/wjge.v6.i1.6.
337. Singh S, Sedlack RE, Cook DA. Effects of simulation-based training in gastrointestinal endoscopy: a systematic review and meta-analysis. *Clin Gastroenterol Hepatol.* 2014 Oct;12(10):1611–1623.e4. doi:10.1016/j.cgh.2014.01.037.
338. CAE. CAE EndoVR–User Guide. 2018. Accessed October 31, 2023. https://www.caehealthcare.com/media/legacy/EndoVR-User-Guide.pdf.
339. Surgical Science. Simbionix Simulators: BRONCH Mentor. Accessed April 22, 2023. https://simbionix.com/simulators/bronch-mentor/.
340. Surgical Science. Simbionix Simulators: GI Mentor. Accessed April 22, 2023. https://simbionix.com/simulators/gi-mentor/.
341. Surgical Science. Simbionix Simulators: ENDO Mentor Suite. Accessed April 22, 2023. https://simbionix.com/endo-mentor-suite/.

342. Colella S, Sondergaard Svendsen MB, Konge L, Svendsen LB, Sivapalan P, Clementsen P. Assessment of competence in simulated flexible bronchoscopy using motion analysis. *Respiration.* 2015 Feb;89(2):155–161. doi:10.1159/000369471.
343. Grantcharov TP, Carstensen L, Schulze S. Objective assessment of gastrointestinal endoscopy skills using a virtual reality simulator. *JSLS.* 2005 Apr-Jun;9(2):130–133.
344. Gomez PP, Willis RE, Van Sickle K. Evaluation of two flexible colonoscopy simulators and transfer of skills into clinical practice. *J Surg Educ.* 2015 Mar-Apr;72(2):220–227. doi:10.1016/j.jsurg.2014.08.010.
345. Ansell J, Mason J, Warren N, et al. Systematic review of validity testing in colonoscopy simulation. *Surg Endosc.* 2012 Nov;26(11):3040–3052. doi:10.1007/s00464-012-2332-2.
346. Bittner 4th JG, Mellinger JD, Imam T, Schade RR, Macfadyen Jr BV. Face and construct validity of a computer-based virtual reality simulator for ERCP. *Gastrointest Endosc.* 2010 Feb;71(2):357–364. doi:10.1016/j.gie.2009.08.033.
347. Stather DR, MacEachern P, Rimmer K, Hergott CA, Tremblay A. Validation of an endobronchial ultrasound simulator: differentiating operator skill level. *Respiration.* 2011;81(4):325–332. doi:10.1159/000323520.
348. Kefalides PT, Gress F. Simulator training for endoscopic ultrasound. *Gastrointest Endosc Clin N Am.* 2006 Jul;16(3):543–552, viii. doi:10.1016/j.giec.2006.03.018.
349. Barthet M. Endoscopic ultrasound teaching and learning. *Minerva Med.* 2007 Aug;98(4):247–251.
350. Inventive Medical Ltd. HeartWorks. Accessed April 22, 2023. https://www.inventivemedical.com//.
351. Surgical Science. Simbionix Simulators: Ultrasound Mentor. Accessed April 22, 2023. https://simbionix.com/simulators/us-mentor/.
352. CAE Healthcare. CAE Vimedix. Accessed April 22, 2023. https://www.caehealthcare.com/ultrasound-simulation/vimedix/.
353. Jelacic S, Bowdle A, Togashi K, VonHomeyer P. The use of TEE simulation in teaching basic echocardiography skills to senior anesthesiology residents. *J Cardiothorac Vasc Anesth.* 2013 Aug;27(4):670–675. doi:10.1053/j.jvca.2013.01.016.
354. Nanda NC, Kapur KK, Kapoor PM. Simulation for transthoracic echocardiography of aortic valve. *Ann Card Anaesth.* 2016 Jul-Sep;19(3):498–504. doi:10.4103/0971-9784.185541.
355. Paddock MT, Bailitz J, Horowitz R, Khishfe B, Cosby K, Sergel MJ. Disaster response team FAST skills training with a portable ultrasound simulator compared to traditional training: pilot study. *West J Emerg Med.* 2015 Mar;16(2):325–330. doi:10.5811/westjem.2015.1.23720.
356. Staboulidou I, Wustemann M, Vaske B, Elsässer M, Hillemanns P, Scharf A. Quality assured ultrasound simulator training for the detection of fetal malformations. *Acta Obstet Gynecol Scand.* 2010 Mar;89(3):350–354. doi:10.3109/00016340903280941.
357. Madsen ME, Konge L, Norgaard LN, et al. Assessment of performance measures and learning curves for use of a virtual-reality ultrasound simulator in transvaginal ultrasound examination. *Ultrasound Obstet Gynecol.* 2014 Dec;44(6):693–699. doi:10.1002/uog.13400.
358. Chao C, Chalouhi GE, Bouhanna P, Ville Y, Dommergues M. Randomized clinical trial of virtual reality simulation training for transvaginal gynecologic ultrasound skills. *J Ultrasound Med.* 2015 Sep;34(9):1663–1667. doi:10.7863/ultra.15.14.09063.
359. Magee D, Zhu Y, Ratnalingam R, Gardner P, Kessel D. An augmented reality simulator for ultrasound guided needle placement training. *Med Biol Eng Comput.* 2007 Oct;45(10):957–967. doi:10.1007/s11517-007-0231-9.
360. Laerdal Medical. SimMan Vascular. Accessed April 22, 2023. https://laerdal.com/products/simulation-training/emergency-care-trauma/simman-vascular/.
361. Gaumard. Obstetric MR. Accessed April 22, 2023. https://www.gaumard.com/obstetricmr.
362. Intuitive. Da Vinci. Accessed April 22, 2023. https://www.intuitive.com/en-us/products-and-services/da-vinci.
363. Intuitive. SimNow. Accessed April 22, 2023. https://www.intuitive.com/en-us/products-and-services/da-vinci/education/simnow.
364. Culligan P, Gurshumov E, Lewis C, Priestley J, Komar J, Salamon C. Predictive validity of a training protocol using a robotic surgery simulator. *Female Pelvic Med Reconstr Surg.* 2014 Jan-Feb;20(1):48–51. doi:10.1097/SPV.0000000000000045.
365. Simulated Surgical Systems, LLC. ROSS: Robotic Surgery Simulator. Accessed April 22, 2023. http://simulatedsurgicals.com/ross2.html.
366. Surgical Science. Simbionix Simulators: RobotiX Mentor. Accessed April 22, 2023. https://simbionix.com/simulators/robotix-mentor/.
367. Kesavadas T, Stegemann A, Sathyaseelan G, et al. Validation of Robotic Surgery Simulator (RoSS). *Stud Health Technol Inform.* 2011;163:274–276.
368. Seixas-Mikelus SA, Stegemann AP, Kesavadas T, et al. Content validation of a novel robotic surgical simulator. *BJU Int.* 2011 Apr;107(7):1130–1135. doi:10.1111/j.1464-410X.2010.09694.x.
369. Gavazzi A, Bahsoun AN, Van Haute W, et al. Face, content and construct validity of a virtual reality simulator for robotic surgery (SEP Robot). *Ann R Coll Surg Engl.* 2011 Mar;93(2):152–156. doi:10.1308/003588411X12851639108358.
370. Bric JD, Lumbard DC, Frelich MJ, Gould JC. Current state of virtual reality simulation in robotic surgery training: a review. *Surg Endosc.* 2016 Jun;30(6):2169–2178. doi:10.1007/s00464-015-4517-y.
371. Hertz AM, George EI, Vaccaro CM, Brand TC. Head-to-head comparison of three virtual-reality robotic surgery simulators. *JSLS.* 2018 Jan-Mar;22(1):e2017–00081. doi:10.4293/JSLS.2017.00081.
372. Society for Simulation in Healthcare. SSH: Society for Simulation in Healthcare. Accessed April 22, 2023. https://www.ssih.org/.
373. Society for Simulation in Healthcare. SimConnect. Accessed April 22, 2023. https://www.ssih.org/simconnect.
374. Society for Simulation in Healthcare. Live Learning Center. Accessed April 22, 2023. https://www.ssih.org/Professional-Development/Online-Learning/Live-Learning-Center.
375. Wolters Kluwer. Simulation in Healthcare: Journal of the Society for Simulation in Healthcare. Accessed April 22, 2023. https://journals.lww.com/simulationinhealthcare/pages/default.aspx.
376. Amiel I, Simon D, Merin O, Ziv A. Mobile in situ simulation as a tool for evaluation and improvement of trauma treatment in the emergency department. *J Surg Educ.* 2016 Jan-Feb;73(1):121–128. doi:10.1016/j.jsurg.2015.08.013.
377. Cates CU, Patel AD, Nicholson WJ. Use of virtual reality simulation for mission rehearsal for carotid stenting. *JAMA.* 2007 Jan 17;297(3):265–266. doi:10.1001/jama.297.3.265-b.
378. Clarke DB, D'Arcy RCN, Delorme S, et al. Virtual reality simulator: demonstrated use in neurosurgical oncology. *Surg Innov.* 2013 Apr;20(2):190–197. doi:10.1177/1553350612451354.
379. Arora A, Swords C, Khemani S, et al. Virtual reality case-specific rehearsal in temporal bone surgery: a preliminary evaluation. *Int J Surg.* 2014 Feb;12(2):141–145. doi:10.1016/j.ijsu.2013.11.019.

380. Holmboe E, Rizzolo MA, Sachdeva AK, Rosenberg M, Ziv A. Simulation-based assessment and the regulation of healthcare professionals. *Simul Healthc.* 2011 Aug 6;(7):S58–S62. doi:10.1097/SIH.0b013e3182283bd7.
381. Ziv A, Ben-David MF, Sutnick AI, Gary NE. Lessons learned from six years of international administrations of the ECFMG's SP-based clinical skills assessment. *Acad Med.* 1998 Jan;73(1):84–91. doi:10.1097/00001888-199801000-00017.
382. Papadakis MA. The Step 2 clinical-skills examination. *N Engl J Med.* 2004 Apr 22;350(17):1703–1705. doi:10.1056/NEJMp038246.
383. Katsufrakis PJ, Chaudhry HJ. Evolution of clinical skills assessment in the USMLE: looking to the future after Step 2 CS discontinuation. *Acad Med.* 2021 Sep 1;96(9):1236–1238. doi:10.1097/ACM.0000000000004214.
384. Smirnova A. Licensing exams in Canada: a closer look at the validity of the MCCQE Part II. *Can Med Educ J.* 2022 Aug 27;13(4):23–29. doi:10.36834/cmej.73894.
385. Jiang G, Chen H, Wang Q, et al. National Clinical Skills Competition: an effective simulation-based method to improve undergraduate medical education in China. *Med Educ Online.* 2016 Feb 16;21:29889. doi:10.3402/meo.v21.29889.
386. Liu J, Jiang G, Zhou Q, et al. National Clinical Skills Competition for medical students in China. *Simul Healthc.* 2017 Apr;12(2):132–133. doi:10.1097/SIH.0000000000000183.
387. VirtaMed. Stories by VirtaMed — Simulation for nation-wide accreditation of medical proficiency: an example from Russia. Accessed April 22, 2023. https://stories.virtamed.com/simulation-for-nation-wide-accreditation-of-medical-proficiency-an-example-from-russia-0
388. United States Medical Licensing Examination (USMLE). Step 3 Test Question Formats: Computer-based Case Simulations. Accessed April 22, 2023. https://www.usmle.org/step-3-test-question-formats/computer-based-case-simulations.
389. Dillon GF, Clyman SG, Clauser BE, Margolis MJ. The introduction of computer-based case simulations into the United States Medical Licensing Examination. *Academic Medicine.* 2002 Oct;77(10 Suppl):S94–S96. doi:10.1097/00001888-200210001-00029.
390. Clauser BE, Margolis MJ, Swanson DB. An examination of the contribution of computer-based case simulations to the USMLE Step 3 examination. *Acad Med.* 2002 Oct;77(10 Suppl):S80–S82. doi:10.1097/00001888-200210001-00026.
391. Ziv A, Erez D, Munz Y, et al. The Israel Center for Medical Simulation: a paradigm for cultural change in medical education. *Acad Med.* 2006 Dec;81(12):1091–1097. doi:10.1097/01.ACM.0000246756.55626.1b.
392. Berkenstadt H, Ziv A, Gafni N, Sidi A. Incorporating simulation-based objective structured clinical examination into the Israeli National Board Examination in Anesthesiology. *Anesth Analg.* 2006 Mar;102(3):853–858. doi:10.1213/01.ane.0000194934.34552.ab.
393. Ziv A, Berkenstadt H, Eisenberg O. Simulation for licensure and certification. In: Levine AI, DeMaria S Jr, Schwartz AD, Sim AJ, eds. *The Comprehensive Textbook of Healthcare Simulation.* Springer; 2013:161–170.
394. Brazilian Society of Nephrology. [Nephrologists take exam to obtain specialist title]. *Sociedade Brasileira de Nefrologia (SBN) Informa.* 2011:8–9.
395. Pecoits Filho Jr. RFS. *Brazilian Society of Nephrology exam.* Personal Communication; 2016.
396. American Board of Surgery. Training & Certification. Accessed April 22, 2023. https://www.absurgery.org/default.jsp?certgsqe_training.
397. Fundamentals of Laparoscopic Surgery (FLS). Fundamentals of Laparoscopic Surgery (FLS) Program Description. Accessed April 22, 2023. https://www.flsprogram.org/index/fls-program-description/.
398. Limbs & Things FLS. FLS Trainers. Accessed April 22, 2023. https://limbsandthings.com/fls.
399. American Board of Obstetrics & Gynecology (ABOG). Specialty Certification: Eligibility Requirements. Accessed April 22, 2023. https://www.abog.org/specialty-certification/qualifying-exam/eligibility.
400. Ritter EM, Scott DJ. Design of a proficiency-based skills training curriculum for the fundamentals of laparoscopic surgery. *Surg Innov.* 2007 Jun;14(2):107–112. doi:10.1177/1553350607302329.
401. Peters JH, Fried GM, Swanstrom LL, et al. Development and validation of a comprehensive program of education and assessment of the basic fundamentals of laparoscopic surgery. *Surgery.* 2004 Jan;135(1):21–27. doi:10.1016/s0039-6060(03)00156-9.
402. Sroka G, Feldman LS, Vassiliou MC, Kaneva PA, Fayez R, Fried GM. Fundamentals of laparoscopic surgery simulator training to proficiency improves laparoscopic performance in the operating room-a randomized controlled trial. *Am J Surg.* 2010 Jan;199(1):115–120. doi:10.1016/j.amjsurg.2009.07.035.
403. Society of American Gastrointestinal and Endoscopic Surgeons (SAGES). About — The Fundamentals of Endoscopic Surgery (FES). Accessed April 22, 2023. https://www.fesprogram.org/about/.
404. Vassiliou MC, Dunkin BJ, Fried GM, et al. Fundamentals of endoscopic surgery: creation and validation of the hands-on test. *Surg Endosc.* 2014 Mar;28(3):704–711. doi:10.1007/s00464-013-3298-4.
405. Duran C, Estrada S, O'Malley M, et al. The model for Fundamentals of Endovascular Surgery (FEVS) successfully defines the competent endovascular surgeon. *J Vasc Surg.* 2015 Dec;62(6):1660–1666.e3. doi:10.1016/j.jvs.2015.09.026.
406. Irfan W, Sheahan C, Mitchell EL, Sheahan 3rd MG. The pathway to a national vascular skills examination and the role of simulation-based training in an increasingly complex specialty. *Semin Vasc Surg.* 2019 Mar-Jun;32(1-2):48–67. doi:10.1053/j.semvascsurg.2018.12.006.
407. Vassiliou MC, Feldman LS, Andrew CG, et al. A global assessment tool for evaluation of intraoperative laparoscopic skills. *Am J Surg.* 2005 Jul;190(1):107–113. doi:10.1016/j.amjsurg.2005.04.004.
408. Vassiliou MC, Kaneva PA, Poulose BK, et al. Global Assessment of Gastrointestinal Endoscopic Skills (GAGES): a valid measurement tool for technical skills in flexible endoscopy. *Surg Endosc.* 2010 Aug;24(8):1834–1841. doi:10.1007/s00464-010-0882-8.
409. Fried GM, Marks JM, Mellinger JD, Trus TL, Vassiliou MC, Dunkin BJ. ASGE's assessment of competency in endoscopy evaluation tools for colonoscopy and EGD. *Gastrointest Endosc.* 2014 Aug;80(2):366–367. doi:10.1016/j.gie.2014.03.019.
410. Rosen J, Brown JD, Barreca M, Chang L, Hannaford B, Sinanan M. The Blue DRAGON—a system for monitoring the kinematics and the dynamics of endoscopic tools in minimally invasive surgery for objective laparoscopic skill assessment. *Stud Health Technol Inform.* 2002;85:412–418.
411. Hofstad EF, Vapenstad C, Chmarra MK, Langø T, Kuhry E, Mårvik R. A study of psychomotor skills in minimally invasive surgery: what differentiates expert and nonexpert performance. Surg Endosc. 2013 Mar;27(3):854-863. doi:10.1007/s00464-012-2524-9.

412. Boulet JR, Jeffries PR, Hatala RA, Korndorffer JR Jr, Feinstein DM, Roche JP. Research regarding methods of assessing learning outcomes. *Simul Healthc.* 2011 Aug;6(7):S48–S51. doi:10.1097/SIH.0b013e31822237d0.
413. Moore AK, Grow DR, Bush RW, Seymour NE. Novices outperform experienced laparoscopists on virtual reality laparoscopy simulator. *JSLS.* 2008 Oct-Dec;12(4):358–362.
414. Rosenthal R, Gantert WA, Scheidegger D, Oertli D. Can skills assessment on a virtual reality trainer predict a surgical trainee's talent in laparoscopic surgery? *Surg Endosc.* 2006 Aug;20(8):1286–1290. doi:10.1007/s00464-005-0635-2.
415. Roitberg B, Banerjee P, Luciano C, et al. Sensory and motor skill testing in neurosurgery applicants: a pilot study using a virtual reality haptic neurosurgical simulator. *Neurosurgery.* 2013 Oct;73(Suppl 1):116–121. doi:10.1227/NEU.0000000000000089.
416. Roitberg BZ, Kania P, Luciano C, Dharmavaram N, Banerjee P. Evaluation of sensory and motor skills in neurosurgery applicants using a virtual reality neurosurgical simulator: the sensory-motor quotient. *J Surg Educ.* 2015 Nov-Dec;72(6):1165–1171. doi:10.1016/j.jsurg.2015.04.030.
417. Winkler-Schwartz A, Bajunaid K, Mullah MAS, et al. Bimanual psychomotor performance in neurosurgical resident applicants assessed using NeuroTouch, a virtual reality simulator. *J Surg Educ.* 2016 Nov-Dec;73(6):942–953. doi:10.1016/j.jsurg.2016.04.013.
418. Ziv A, Rubin O, Moshinsky A, et al. MOR: a simulation-based assessment centre for evaluating the personal and interpersonal qualities of medical school candidates. *Med Educ.* 2008 Oct;42(10):991–998. doi:10.1111/j.1365-2923.2008.03161.x.
419. American Board of Anesthesiology (ABA). Get Certified. Accessed April 22, 2023. https://www.theaba.org/certifications%20and%20exms.html.
420. Warner DO, Isaak RS, Peterson-Layne C, et al. Development of an objective structured clinical examination as a component of assessment for initial board certification in anesthesiology. *Anesth Analg.* 2020 Jan;130(1):258–264. doi:10.1213/ANE.0000000000004496.
421. American Board of Anesthesiology (ABA). The Applied Exam. Accessed April 22, 2023. https://www.theaba.org/certification-exam-type/applied-exam/.
422. American Board of Anesthesiology (ABA). APPLIED EXAM Objective Structured Clinical Examination (OSCE) Content Outline. Accessed April 22, 2023. https://www.theaba.org/pdfs/OSCE_Content_Outline.pdf.
423. American Board of Anesthesiology (ABA). OSCE Example Scenarios. 2023. Accessed April 22, 2023. https://www.theaba.org/wp-content/uploads/2023/01/Public-Sample-OSCE-all-stations-2023.pdf.
424. Wang T, Sun H, Zhou Y, et al. Construct validation of the American Board of Anesthesiology's APPLIED examination for initial certification. *Anesth Analg.* 2021 Jul 1;133(1):226–232. doi:10.1213/ANE.0000000000005364.
425. American Board of Anesthesiology (ABA). MOCA 2.0 Quality Improvement (QI) Activities. Accessed April 22, 2023. https://theaba.org/pdfs/MOCA_QI_Activities.pdf.
426. American Board of Internal Medicine (ABIM). ABIM to use medical simulation technology to evaluate physician competence. January 29, 2008. Accessed April 22, 2023. https://www.abim.org/media-center/press-releases/medical-simulation-technology-evaluate-physician-competence/.
427. Cregan P, Watterson L. High stakes assessment using simulation—an Australian experience. *Stud Health Technol Inform.* 2005;111:99–104.
428. Levine AI, Schwartz AD, Bryson EO, DeMaria S Jr. Role of simulation in US physician licensure and certification. *Mt Sinai J Med.* 2012 Jan-Feb;79(1):140–153. doi:10.1002/msj.21291.

14

Feedback and Coaching

JOAN M. SARGEANT, PHD, AND ERIC S. HOLMBOE, MD

CHAPTER OUTLINE

Introduction

Feedback has long been linked with summative assessment or assessment of learning in medical education; in fact, the two were often directly connected as "feedback and assessment." However, thanks to much scholarly work over the past 20 years, we now know that feedback is required for ongoing learner development and progress. We also recognize that feedback alone is often not enough to promote learner growth and development and that coaching, as it is known in sports and music, can contribute much to ongoing clinical learning and professional development. This chapter explores recent developments in understanding and using feedback and coaching in health professionals education, with a particular focus on medical education, and offers practical suggestions for their use.

Objectives of the chapter are to:

1. Describe the evolution of feedback and introduction of coaching within medical education.
2. Review recent cultural shifts and strategies in medical education that support these changes.
3. Describe the philosophy and skills of coaching in education.
4. Propose a theoretical framework that positions feedback and coaching as central activities in clinical teaching and learning.
5. Discuss individual and system factors that influence effective feedback and coaching.
6. Offer practical strategies for engaging in effective feedback and coaching conversations and promoting a positive feedback culture.

Evolution of Feedback and Introduction of Coaching in Medical Education

Evolution of Feedback

Feedback traditionally has been depicted as the unidirectional delivery of communication from a supervisor to a learner. In 2008 Van de Ridder et al. defined feedback as a unidirectional process that offers "specific information about the comparison between a trainee's observed performance and a standard, given with the intent to improve the trainee's performance."[1] Archer in a review of feedback approaches challenged this definition as too simplistic and stressed the need for learner engagement and active participation, facilitation of learner reflection upon their performance, and fostering of self-direction.[2] These requirements also speak to the need for a supportive culture including faculty and learner preparation in feedback.

More recently, Lefroy et al.[3] elaborated upon these notions: "Helpful feedback is a supportive conversation that clarifies the trainee's awareness of their developing competencies, enhances their self-efficacy for making progress, challenges them to set objectives for improvement, and facilitates their development of strategies to enable that improvement to occur." The authors continue to provide a comprehensive list of "do's", "don'ts," and "don't knows" when providing feedback, which is a valuable resource. Similarly with regard to definitions, Ajjawi and Regehr[4] offer that "when we say feedback we are referring to a dynamic and co-constructive interaction in the context of a safe and mutually respectful relationship for the purpose of challenging a learner's (and educator's) ways of thinking, acting or being to support growth." More recently, Tavares et al. in comparing feedback and debriefing refer to them both as "learning conversations" in which the supervisor fosters the learner's reflection upon their learning experience and through this reflective conversation, promotes their learning and growth.[5]

Progressive thinking and inquiry in other disciplines also shed light on modern interpretations of feedback. Boud and Molloy in exploring feedback in higher and professional education point out that learners are not passive in the feedback transaction; they are active and volitional.[6] Hence providing information or "telling" is not enough; and the outcome of the feedback interaction, meaning what the learner does with the feedback, is an equally critical component of the feedback interaction. Stone and Heen[7] in the field of human resources also draw attention to the feedback recipient's role, demonstrating that how feedback is received is more important than how it is given, and reminding us that the recipient is in charge of what they attend to in the feedback interaction and whether and how they use it.

While notions of feedback have evolved, so has scholarly work in related domains. Insights have arisen from the field of motivation and development, particularly with research into mindset.[8,9] Dweck[8] describes two core mindsets: fixed and growth. Individuals with a fixed mindset believe success results from innate traits such as intelligence, focus on their competence, view failure as an insult (thus to be avoided at all costs), and hence do not seek feedback or see it as helpful. Individuals with a growth mindset believe abilities are developed through hard work and continuous learning, and hence seek and accept constructive feedback and view limitations and failure as opportunities for growth. Of note, conditions that promote a growth mindset in education are consistent with those outlined above in promoting effective feedback.

Related to growth mindset are the notions of informed self-assessment and self-regulated learning. Studies of self-assessment of the past 20 years have shown that assessment based on one's own perceptions and uninformed by feedback and other external sources is often flawed. Our self-assessments need to be informed or guided by ongoing and relevant feedback to be more accurate in assessing how we are doing.[10–13] Promoting informed self-assessment can also nurture a growth mindset and foster acceptance of feedback. Similarly, self-regulated learning is demonstrated by individuals who effectively assess their learning and performance needs in an ongoing, reflective manner and use this process for continuous learning and improvement.[14,15] Self-regulated learning involves a cyclical process where learners create learning plans and goals, use specific learning strategies, monitor performance, and then reflect and adapt before entering another cycle. All of this requires self-motivation (i.e., is intrinsic) on the part of the learner. Understandably, self-regulated learning is dependent upon accurate and informed self-assessment and strengthened by a growth mindset. Yet self-regulation does not mean having to conduct the process by oneself; external support and facilitation can enhance the process. Notably, reflection upon one's practice and learning and how to further develop and improve is embedded in both informed self-assessment and self-regulation.

Appreciating on the one hand that self-assessment and self-regulation are not solitary activities contributing to growth but benefit from external facilitation and on the other that feedback is an interactive process with the learner and faculty as equal participants to plan future learning has contributed to the introduction of an additional innovation in medical education, that of coproduction[16] or cocreation.[17] Both describe processes by which faculty and learners collaboratively, through shared discussion as equal partners, identify learning needs and create plans to meet them. Each participant also reflects and brings their own experience, expertise, thoughts, and reflections to the process. However, for coproduction/cocreation to succeed, faculty must (1) ensure a psychologically safe environment in which the power differential between them and the learner is reduced, and (2) build trust. Often, faculty also may need to use facilitative skills to encourage the learner's open and equal participation. See "Theoretical Framework" and Figs. 14.2 and 14.3 for further elaboration on coproduction.

Introduction of Coaching

Such transitions in thinking around feedback and practice in medical education have led to exploration of coaching as a potentially helpful strategy. Coaching, long used in sports and music and more recently in leadership development to promote performance improvement, focuses on "getting better." On this note, Heen and Stone in an earlier publication highlighted an important difference at that time between feedback and coaching: that is, feedback is about what is going wrong and hence feels negative, whereas coaching focuses on what to do to get better and be the best one can be, and hence is forward moving and feels positive.[18] Similarly, newer definitions of feedback discussed earlier in this chapter also emphasize this active forward motion of feedback, as do conceptualizations of growth mindset, informed self-assessment, self-regulated learning, and coproduction of learning. All focus on learning and growth.

One of the first people to make the need for coaching explicit in medical practice and education was Atul Gawande, in a personal reflection printed in *The New Yorker* in 2011.[19] As a surgeon, he recounted that he had never been observed in practice or coached, and as a result he selected a trusted mentor to observe him and provide coaching. He details how and why this was a reflective, insightful, positive learning experience and one that he should repeat at regular intervals. He emphasized how being observed in one's practice by a trusted mentor and coached to improve based on those observations is a rare occurrence, adding that it should occur regularly to ensure continuing competence and improvement.

Since that time, definitions of academic coaching have emerged. In one definition, the role of coach is to "facilitate learners' achieving their fullest potential,"[20] A more detailed definition within education describes coaching as "a one-to-one conversation focused on the enhancement of learning and development through increasing self-awareness and a sense of personal responsibility, where the coach facilitates the self-directed learning of the coachee through questioning, active listening, and appropriate challenge in a supportive and encouraging climate.[21] Coaching builds on feedback by promoting informed self-awareness, self-regulation, a growth mindset, and coproduction of learning activities.

While current definitions demonstrate that feedback and coaching have distinct similarities, discriminating between the two can also be helpful. Coaching engages the learner in active planning for improvement following a feedback conversation that shares and discusses both the supervisor's and learner's observations and reflections on performance. Ekpenyong et al.[22] suggest a simple approach to aid the distinction: "While feedback cultivates insight into current performance, coaching focuses on promoting future improved performance" (p. 109). Both are required.

Before exploring feedback and coaching more extensively, we will consider broader transitions within medical education that are influencing clinical teaching and learning.

Recent Cultural Shifts and Strategies Supporting Innovation in Feedback and Coaching

Viewing transitions in feedback and coaching within the context of recent cultural shifts and strategies in medical education enables clearer appreciation of their evolution. Two overarching approaches have been and continue to be integrated into medical education with the intent of improving learning, assessment, and feedback: competency-based medical education (CBME) and programmatic assessment. Both are grounded in theoretical principles and evidence informing effective teaching and learning. While CBME has recently been more fully discussed and adopted in residency education, programmatic assessment actually lays the foundation for CBME.

Programmatic Assessment

Programmatic assessment is a systematic approach to assessment that focuses upon two overarching goals: maximize assessment for learning, and maximize the robustness of high-stakes decisions about learners' progress.[23] Assessment of learners has traditionally focused on assessment *of* their learning and less on assessment *for* their learning. The introduction of CBME offers the opportunity to transition the focus of assessment to assessment *for* learning as well as *of* learning (i.e., to an assessment system that provides rich information and feedback to enable learners to achieve specific competencies or milestones and to advance). CBME is an example of programmatic assessment.

While not a new concept, the notion of "assessment for learning" is now explicit within medical education. As a cultural shift, it requires us to see the roles of assessment and feedback differently, and to think about how we can shape feedback as a way of enabling use of assessment data for learning. In other words, how can we use assessment data and the feedback conversation to guide and enhance learning, professional development, and performance improvement?

To ensure that assessment "for" drives learning requires reconsideration and rethinking of the role of feedback in relation to the learning and assessment activities. Feedback is the activity that connects assessment and learning. With each assessment, the role of the supervisor is to provide information that is as rich, accurate, and specific as possible to guide learning and development. Feedback conversations are seen to perform multiple roles focused upon helping the learner learn and progress by encouraging self-assessment of their own performance based on the data at hand; fostering reflection upon their performance and performance goals; promoting self-directed learning; and coaching. Hence the feedback discussion has a much broader role than just transmitting information. Of course, not all of these activities can be achieved in the informal, "in the moment" feedback interactions in busy clinical settings. However, adopting the belief that the role of feedback and coaching is to promote learning and then scheduling times for fuller feedback discussions with learners throughout their assigned rotations can be a way to achieve broader discussions to enhance learning.

For more information on programmatic assessment, see Chapter 3.

Competency-Based Medical Education

CBME is defined as an educational approach focused on performance outcomes that manifest themselves as abilities of the graduates.[24–27] It focuses attention upon what the learner is expected to be able to do; that is, (1) have specific abilities to support the Quadruple Aim (see Chapter 1) and (2) strive to ensure that their patients receive the best care possible. Within CBME, educational programs are designed to ensure that learners attain prespecified performance outcomes in their discipline. The Accreditation Council for Graduate Medical Education (ACGME) in the United States,[25] Royal College of Physicians and Surgeons of Canada (RCPSC),[26] and College of Family Physicians of Canada (CFPC)[27] have in recent years adopted CBME for their residency programs (see Chapter 1). The basic tenets of CBME underscore the importance of learner observation, followed by feedback and formative assessment conversations to promote development. For example, learners require regular and frequent performance data and feedback to enable them to move efficiently from one milestone to the next in graduate medical education (GME) programs to develop competence in the various domains of practice.

Central to CBME is an understanding of the terms *competencies* and *milestones*.[25,26,28] A competency is defined as an observable ability of a healthcare professional that develops through stages of expertise from novice to master clinician. A milestone is defined as the expected ability at a particular stage of development or a significant point in development. In the United States, milestones are integrated, competency-based, developmental narrative descriptions of educational outcomes (e.g., knowledge, skills, attitudes, and behaviors) that can be demonstrated progressively by residents and fellows from the beginning of their education through graduation to the unsupervised practice of their specialties.[29]

Within CBME, ongoing formative assessment/feedback and coaching is critical for learners' continued progression from novice in a particular competency to expert or master. Both feedback discussions about performance, strengths, and opportunities and coaching to develop improvement plans are central to learners' ability to progress from one level or milestone to the next in an effective manner.

The CFPC residency program is one of the early adopters of CBME and has developed a well-designed assessment system based on the principles of programmatic assessment.[27] Initiatives address the need for frequent observation and feedback conversations. To enable daily specific performance observations and feedback, the CFPC has nationally implemented a daily field note in which supervisors record an observation of a learner's performance in a particular domain of practice and discuss that observation with the learner daily. Field notes are accumulated into summary assessments discussed at regular intervals and enable interim summary discussion of progress and creation of a learning plan as needed.

The introduction of milestones, Entrustable Professional Activities (EPAs), and clinical competency committees (CCCs) has also led to the implementation of individualized learning plans as part of the educational process. In the United States, residency and fellowship programs are required to review resident and fellow performance at least twice yearly, judging where the learner is developmentally across the five Milestone levels. Some programs also ask the resident and fellow to complete a self-assessment of their own progress toward the specialty Milestones, which the supervisor and learner discuss in their feedback conversation and integrate into the learning plan.

Philosophy and Skills of Coaching in Education

CBME and programmatic assessment are cultural shifts that are changing our thinking about learning, assessment, and feedback and how they are linked. They emphasize the formative nature of assessment; that is, that the basic purpose of feedback in the workplace is to foster learning and improvement. As noted earlier, coaching is the practice of observing a learner's or colleague's performance, having a reflective feedback conversation with that person about their performance, and codeveloping a plan to improve.[20,21] Coaching, while borrowed from the sports world primarily, is, in education, central to learning and progression, achieving competence and expertise and fostering deliberate and mindful practice.[30]

Coaching by nature is competency based. Learners' performance is observed, and coaches use the data pertaining to their performance to drive conversations with the learners about how the data can guide improvement. In fact, current thinking suggests the need to consistently integrate coaching with feedback. While the word *feedback* can conjure an image of being told where one stands and how one measures up and hence can feel intimidating and evoke negative emotions, coaching evokes more positive emotions in that it helps one see how to improve and how to consistently improve.[18] It is learner centered, is outcome oriented, supports success, and guides progression from one competency level to the next. Coaching, then, is a way to enable our learners to be "the best that they can be."

Coaching requires a shift from the more traditional directive role of clinical teachers. Coaching in medical education means less direct "telling" of learners what to do and more "facilitating"; that is, engaging, activating, and supporting learners as they strengthen and develop their self-assessment and clinical skills. It also means using the performance data to codevelop plans for improving and fine-tuning their performance.[31] Similar to the activities of sports and music coaches, essential activities for medical education coaches are (1) observing performance, (2) engaging the learner in a feedback conversation about that performance data, (3) enabling reflection, (4) codeveloping a plan for further improvement, and (5) putting the plan in place. It is a continuing cycle of observation, feedback, reflection, and practice. Coaching fits with the notions of progressive competence and expertise[32] and deliberate practice.[33] Deliberate practice is a cyclical activity that includes being observed, receiving data and feedback on that performance, reflecting upon the feedback, practicing again incorporating that feedback, and being observed again, as the cycle continues.

Lovell[34] in a 2018 review of the coaching literature in medical education describes coaching as encompassing four features:

1. The coach provides individualized real-time feedback.
2. The coach and coachee collaboratively set individualized goals.
3. The coach facilitates reflection and development of new behaviors, insights, and approaches.
4. The coach has an analytic understanding of the "game" and the ability to motivate the coachee toward excellence.

Recent research confirms that the culture in medical education has traditionally been more paternalistic in which preceptors tell learners what to do. Coaching, along with other influences discussed earlier, is shifting that culture to a more collaborative one in which preceptors "engage" learners and "facilitate" their self-reflection and improvement.[35–37] Preceptors report that coaching and facilitative skills are generally new to them, are not intuitive, and hence are challenging to put into practice.

In response and in an effort to make explicit the skills required for coaching, Armson et al[38] conducted an analysis of specific coaching skills used by clinical preceptors while engaging in feedback and coaching interactions with residents. They reemphasize that "Coaching moves a step beyond providing feedback and focuses upon identifying performance goals in response to feedback and developing plans to address them." They identified two sets of coaching skills: process and content. Process skills are generic and enable the flow of the coaching interaction while content skills guide the addressing of the specific focus for change. Skills are used iteratively and dynamically in response to the learner and the context; they are not meant to suggest a linear process.

Process skills include preparation, relationship development, exploring the learner's reactions, promoting reflection and self-assessment using microfacilitation and communication skills, and supervisor flexibility. Content skills relate to the specific feedback content and include engaging the resident in its discussion, collaboratively identifying priority gaps and specific goals to address those gaps, codeveloping an action or learning change plan, ensuring resident commitment, and following up on the plan.

Table 14.1 provides contrasting examples of each of these skills done well and done poorly. Of note, the microcommunication or facilitative skills is required throughout the interaction to engage the learner and foster reflection. Box 14.1 provides a list of microcommunication skills and Appendix 14.1 provides a sample action/learning change plan.

Also, in response to increasing interest in coaching and the need to use it in addition to feedback, excellent resources are now available for preceptors, learners, and organizations. One is the American Medical Association's (AMA) extensive online workbook, which includes valuable definitions, tips, and strategies for understanding and implementing coaching and establishing a coaching program.[39] Another is the R2C2 feedback and coaching model[40] (discussed further in this chapter) resource website, which includes the feedback model, handouts to aid its use, research to date, and video demonstrations.

Theoretical Framework Positioning Feedback and Coaching as Central Activities in Clinical Teaching and Learning

Workplace or clinical learning requires learning from experience; that is, learners learn from their experiences of providing patient care. While cognitive learning is foundational for clinical learning, learners further their learning by applying that knowledge in their clinical experiences. Feedback and coaching strengthen that learning.

Hence an early framework of experiential learning (Kolb, 1984)[41] is helpful to guide feedback, coaching, and learning. First, Kolb identified four cyclical steps in learning from an experience (see Fig. 14.1):

1. Participation in a concrete experience—for example, taking a patient history, formulating a treatment plan, communicating bad news to a family, performing a procedure, or leading a team meeting
2. Reflective observation—both observing while participating in the experience and reflecting upon that experience once completed
3. Abstract conceptualization—in other words, making sense of what happened and one's reactions and, based on that, formulating a plan for the next time
4. Active experimentation—trying the new approach and following through to evaluate it, then continuing the cycle

Boud et al.[42] noted that Kolb gave only a rudimentary explanation of the role of reflection in learning from experience. He proposed that in addition to reflecting on their actions, learners also need to reflect on their ideas and feelings related to the experience, and consider them when conceptualizing what happened and why, and their impact and influence upon the new plan.

Importantly, the role of the preceptor or faculty as coach is to collaboratively guide the learner through 4 phases and in this way be an active participant (see Fig. 14.2):

1. Concrete experience—observing the learner in a clinical experience, ideally having discussed it, if only briefly, with them ahead of time and their purpose
2. Observation and reflection—seeking the learner's observations about and reactions, including emotions, to their performance of the activity, promoting their reflection upon the activity and their self-assessment, sharing their own observations, and engaging the learner in a reflective discussion
3. Abstract conceptualization—engaging the learner in a discussion of what this means for learning and improving, identifying a priority, and coproducing a plan
4. Active experimentation—supporting the learner in implementing their plan and in follow-up to assess improvement

While feedback may be more often thought of as occurring "in the moment" following a clinical encounter or at the end of the day, coaching is more often considered as longitudinal, extending over a longer term. However, experience with programmatic assessment and CBME demonstrates that both situations require coaching.[43] The experiential learning model above is more applicable to the provision of feedback and coaching "in the moment" in the workplace.

Longitudinal coaching lends itself naturally to the CBME environment where outcome and milestone goals are clearly stated for the learner, and steady progression toward those goals is the focus. Many UME and PME programs identify program coaches or advisors whose job is to collaboratively review learners' cumulative feedback and assessment data

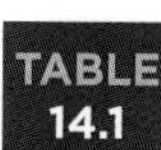

TABLE 14.1 **Process and Content Coaching Skills**

Done well (coach asks, does not tell; consistently uses microcommunication skills)	Done poorly (coach tells, does not ask; does not use microcommunication skills)
Process-Oriented Coaching Skills	
Preparation of the Coach	
Understands the context, assessment process, and learning expectations	Is unfamiliar with the assessment process or requirements of specific levels of learners
Prepared to guide a plan	Demonstrates no need to complete a plan
Relationship Development	
Asks trainee about prior experiences and their understanding of their performance	Omits this altogether or presents a formulaic approach that appears forced and insincere
Enhances engagement through discussing current experiences	
Explore Reactions, Clarify Understanding, and Provide Encouragement	
Explores the resident's interpretation of their experiences and asks for further details and clarification as needed	Talks for majority of the time, overly directive
Summarizes learner's response with additional analysis	Does not recognize or respond to trainee's comments and persists with own agenda
Promote Reflection and Self-Assessment	
Uses open questions to stimulate reflection, self-assessment, and next steps and to clarify learner's thinking, with goal of promoting insight and understanding	Does not ask open questions or the learner's perspective
	Provides feedback without space for reflection, promotes own agenda
	Gives advice without asking for a response
Flexibility	
Identifies when the learner can lead the discussion or when more guidance is required	Discussion is directed entirely by either the coach or the trainee
Refocuses the discussion when something needs to be immediately addressed	If all coach: not sure if trainee is just acquiescing
	If all learner: not sure of trajectory for success
Content-Oriented Coaching Skills	
Done well (coach asks, does not tell; consistently uses microcommunication skills)	**Done poorly (coach tells, does not ask; does not use microcommunication skills)**
Discusses feedback regarding performance by engaging trainee in discussion	
Engages the learner in a discussion about the specific observations to understand what it means to the learner	Is unable to engage the learner in discussion, possibly due to resident resistance or coach's approach of telling, not asking
Collaboratively Identify Priority Performance Gaps and Areas for Improvement	
Draws on the observation data or assessment report to help the resident identify the gaps and priority areas	Identifies the gaps and priority areas for the learner
May push learner out of comfort zone	As the learner acquiesces or does not respond, continues the conversation without attention to resident lack of engagement
May be more directive if a trainee lacks insight	
Collaborative Focus on Goal Setting	
Coach and resident: identify and confirm the specific change or outcome they wish to achieve related to the identified gap	Coach and resident: do not identify a specific change or outcome, and hence do not identify a goal for improvement
Together, identify specific goals related to that change that are achievable and measurable	
Collaboratively Develop a Coaching Plan	
Collaboratively use coaching plan in an orderly manner to cocreate a specific action plan to meet the goal/s	Does not use the coaching plan in a consistent way, skips steps, allows changes that are too broad or not assessable
Collaboratively determine whether each proposed change has the potential to be adopted	Does not consider barriers that might affect outcomes.
	Does not collaborate with the learner, and instead "tells"
Collaboratively Establish and Ensure Follow-up	
Collaboratively ensure a follow-up plan, which may mean including the learner's next preceptor as a preestablished person to review, if they are no longer working together	No planning for follow-up
If they continue working together, collaboratively plan review details	Does not refer back or recalls previous discussions, if continuing to work together

From Armson H, Lockyer JM, Zetkulic M, Könings KD, Sargeant J. Identifying coaching skills to improve feedback use in postgraduate medical education. *Med Educ*. 2019;53(5):477-493.

• BOX 14.1 Microcommunication and Facilitation Skills

- Open-ended questions
- Active listening
- Promoting self-reflection
- Clarifying questions that bring a blind spot into focus

From Armson H, Lockyer JM, Zetkulic M, Könings KD, Sargeant J. Identifying coaching skills to improve feedback use in postgraduate medical education. *Med Educ*. 2019;53(5):477-493.

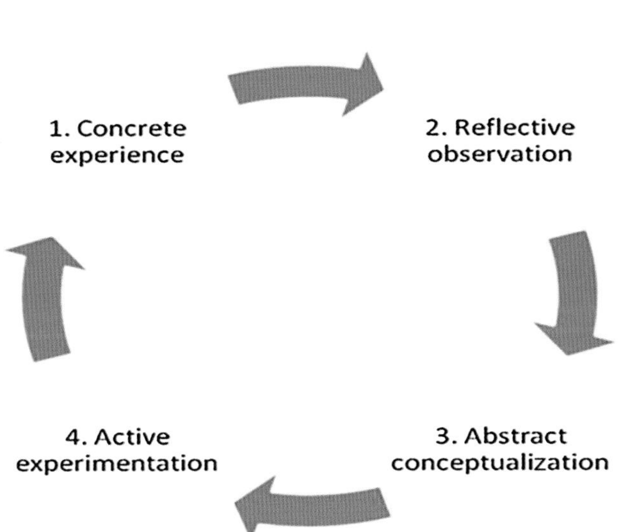

• **Fig. 14.1** Kolb model of experiential learning, the learner's perspective. From Kolb DA. *Experiential Learning: Experience as the Source of Learning and Development*. Prentice-Hall; 1984.

with them, identify opportunities for improvement, and codevelop a plan. Fig. 14.3 outlines the cycle proposed for longitudinal coaching.[44] The AMA[39] offers a comprehensive guide for establishing and maintaining a longitudinal coaching program.

Individual and System Factors Influencing Effective Feedback and Coaching

Understanding the characteristics of effective feedback and coaching and the factors that influence their acceptance and use by learners promotes good practice. In addition to culture, research has identified a number of other factors[45–47] (see Table 14.2 for a summary):

1. The degree to which supervisors have directly observed the performance for which they are providing feedback
2. Characteristics of the performance data and feedback
3. Supervisor–learner relationship
4. Faculty skill in engaging in feedback interactions and learner expectations
5. The nature or sign of the feedback (is it seen as confirming or corrective?)
6. The learner's emotional response to the feedback
7. The learner's own self-assessment or self-perceptions of their performance
8. Systems and culture
   1. **The quality of supervisor observation.** Learners are hesitant to accept feedback from supervisors who have not directly observed them performing the specific activities for which they are receiving feedback. They see feedback on unobserved performance as lacking credibility and not being evidence based, and hence

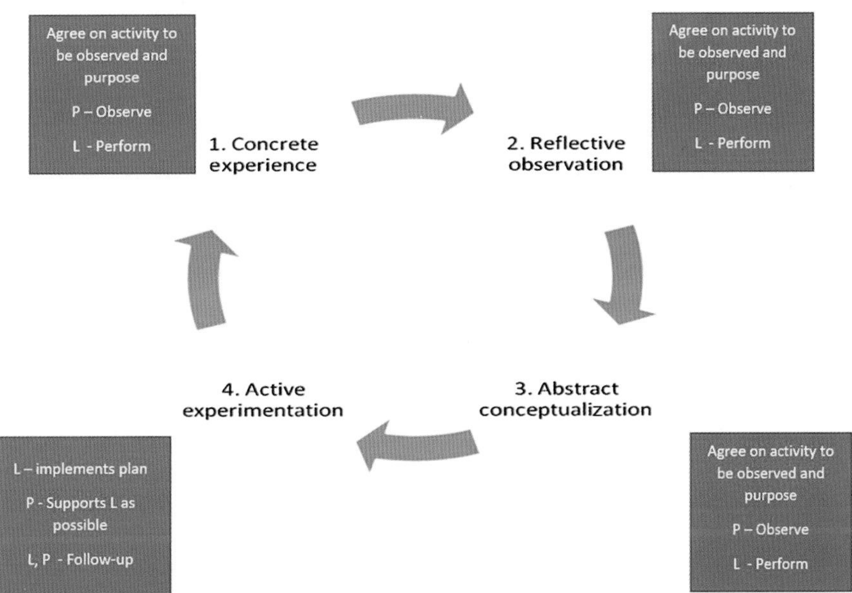

• **Fig. 14.2** Modified Kolb learning cycle for feedback, coaching and coproduction, for preceptors (P) and learners (L). From Boud D, Keogh R, Walker D. Promoting reflection in learning: a model. In: Boud D, Keogh R, Walker D, eds. *Reflection: Turning Experience into Learning*. Routledge Falmer; 1985:19-40.

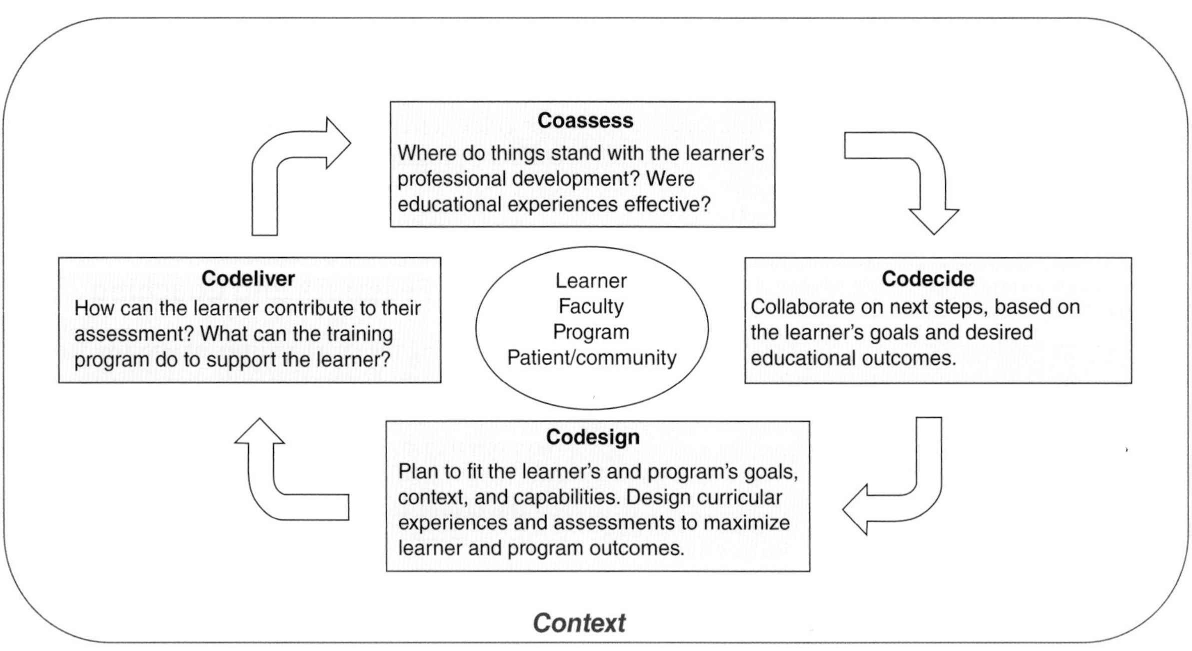

• **Fig. 14.3** Coproduction learning cycle using programmatic assessment. Adapted from Elwyn G, Nelson E, Hager A, Price A. Coproduction: when users define quality. *BMJ Qual Saf*. 2020;29(9):711-16.

TABLE 14.2 **Factors Influencing Learners' Acceptance and Use of Feedback**

Factors	Notes
1. Degree to which the supervisor observes the learner's performance	Only through observation of performance can the feedback and performance data meet the characteristics listed in #2 below.
2. Characteristics of the feedback	Feedback characteristics that promote acceptance and use: Specificity Objectivity Accuracy Credibility Relevance Timeliness
3. Supervisor's relationship with the learner	A respectful, trusting relationship is one that demonstrates engagement in the resident's progress and development and promotes engagement with feedback, acceptance, and use.
4. Supervisor skill in sharing feedback and coaching	Sharing feedback, engaging learners in feedback conversations, and coaching are skills that require development and practice.
5. Nature of the feedback	Feedback that is perceived as disconfirming the learner's own perceptions of how they are doing may be more challenging for the supervisor to share effectively and for the learner to accept.
6. The learner's own self-assessment of their performance	Performance data and feedback that disconfirm the learner's own self-assessment of how they are doing can be a surprise and disappointment for the learner.
7. The learner's emotional response to the performance data	Surprise and disappointment can evoke a negative emotional response (anger, sadness, frustration) that can get in the way of accepting and using the feedback. Supervisors too may have emotional reactions (anxiety, uncertainty) to sharing disconfirming feedback.
8. Education and workplace systems and culture	Cultures and systems that explicitly value learning and development foster and promote the sharing, accepting, and use of feedback.

often actually discount it. Taking the time to observe learners in patient care performing specific skills and to collect specific performance data through observation is critical.[48] (See Chapter 5 for an in-depth discussion about observation.)

2. **Characteristics of the feedback (i.e., the performance data).** The characteristics of the data and feedback are determined by the feedback provider—that is, the supervisor who observes the performance—and they influence the learner's acceptance and use of the feedback. Positive features of good feedback and coaching include being specific, accurate, timely, objective, credible, and relevant.[47] However, it is in fact the learners' perceptions of these characteristics that influence whether they will accept the data and feedback and use them. For example, if they perceive that the feedback is not accurate (e.g., because the supervisor did not actually observe their performance) or is based on an incorrect inference by the supervisor (e.g., the supervisor describing the learner as unempathetic when the learner was instead uncomfortable with the skill being assessed), they are less likely to attend to it.
3. **The supervisor–learner relationship.** The supervisor–learner relationship is pivotal in learning in general and in the ability to have meaningful conversations about a learner's performance and feedback.[49] Learner perceptions of the relationship, and particularly of the supervisors' authenticity, interest, and sincerity in engaging with learners, have a strong impact on the willingness of learners to engage in meaningful conversations about their performance and to accept and use their feedback. The acceptability and impact of feedback can be increased if it relates to personally meaningful goals set by the recipient.[29,39]

   Similar to the doctor–patient relationship that influences patient experience and health outcomes, the supervisor–learner relationship influences learner satisfaction and can influence education outcomes. The positive influence of an educational alliance between supervisors and learners in which learners' best interests are explicitly pursued is now recognized.[49] Also of note, similar to the doctor–patient relationship, longitudinal relationships can be perceived as more beneficial yet are not always possible. It is the quality of that relationship which seems paramount. For example, a supervisor who only has a learner for a short time can build an effective learning relationship using communication and feedback techniques in a very efficient yet sincere and engaged manner. These include:
   - Having a brief conversation at the beginning of the learner's clinical assignment to express their interest in the learner and their learning and to describe what they/their unit can offer given their level of learning; and asking the learner what they need to learn and what they would like to have observed (see Exercise and video 1, "Building the relationship and planning with a new learner," at the end of this chapter)
   - Making arrangements as needed for the learner to meet their learning goal (e.g., a specific patient assignment or opportunity to observe or do a skill)
   - Arranging regular, brief times to observe the learner and have feedback and coaching discussions on those observations and their learning goals

   Refer to Table 14.3 for more practical suggestions on creating a positive learning relationship.
4. **Faculty skill in engaging in feedback and coaching interactions, and learner expectations.** Observing and assessing learners' performance and using those data to engage them in reflective conversations about improving their performance are specialized skills.[50] Many busy clinical supervisors have not received instruction in or had the opportunity to practice these skills. This contributes to discomfort in sharing feedback and coaching.

   As noted elsewhere, faculty development generally remains a significant challenge in clinical teaching. This is especially true for what are considered the "nonmedical expert skills"; or in Canada, under the RCPSC Canadian Medical Education Directives for Specialists (CanMEDS) model, the "intrinsic skills": doctor–patient communication, team collaboration, professionalism, and leadership.[26] Each has its own discrete body of knowledge, skill set, and competencies. Many clinicians lack this specialized information, hence further limiting the ability to teach, assess, and coach in these domains (see Chapter 5 for more on direct observation).

   Recent research has also highlighted the need for learners to be familiarized with the recent shift in the philosophy and practice of feedback and coaching, and with the changing roles expected of them. These require much more active learner participation than traditional top-down feedback. Orienting them to the critical need for being observed, and for their engagement in feedback conversations, self-reflection, being coached, and codevelopment of action plans, will enable them to participate more fully and use their feedback more successfully.[35,51]
5. **The nature of the feedback.** Whether the data and feedback are seen as positive/confirming or negative/disconfirming the learner's performance influences how they are perceived and received by the learner. Sharing observations that disconfirm a learner's self-assessment or that point out a gap in a manner that engages the learner and their acceptance of them can be challenging and requires skilled facilitation. (See also items 6 and 7.) Of note, in many cases it also influences whether and how supervisors share that feedback.[52] (Also refer to Exercises and Videos 2, Addressing sensitive issues: a learner with a professionalism issue (Parts 1 and 3). Coaching: a learner

TABLE 14.3 **Tips for Fostering a Culture of Effective Feedback for Faculty and Learners**

Faculty	Learners
Establishing a Culture of Effective Feedback	**Establishing a Culture of Effective Feedback**
When learners begin to work with you: • Ask for their goals and where they need help (specific area of focus). • Share your goals for them and specifically how you can help. • Describe to the learner when and how you will have feedback conversations. • Ask learners to give you feedback. • Role-model effective feedback seeking and giving with colleagues.	When beginning a new rotation: • Meet with your supervisor and identify your learning goals and where you need help (specific area of focus). • Ask how this fits with their plans. • Ask when and how you might expect feedback. • Ask for feedback when needed.
Observe Before Giving Feedback	**Being Observed**
• Plan with the learner what you will observe (e.g., may not need to observe the full procedure). • Ask for their goals and focus (i.e., know what you and they are looking for). • Confirm time and include it in your schedule. • Share how you'll observe, intervene, and give feedback.	• Plan with your attending your goals and whether you need to be observed for the whole procedure or just a segment. • Be clear on the time and location; be patient. • Provide the attending with relevant information. • Ask how they would like to observe, intervene, and give feedback.
Engaging in and Sharing Feedback	**Engaging in and Receiving Feedback**
• Schedule regular times for feedback. • Seek a private location. • Ask for their self-assessment first. • Prepare for an emotional response if the feedback is disconfirming; explore this response. • Ensure that feedback is timely, specific, objective, and for the observed performance. • Engage the learner and ensure their receptiveness and understanding. • Coach and collaboratively plan for learning and improvement.	• Seek a private location. • Objectively self-assess (i.e., reflect on your own performance). • Provide your own self-assessment and rationale. • Recognize that disconfirming feedback can be emotional; this is normal. • Discuss and reflect upon emotions and feedback content. • Ask for clarification. • Ask for help and collaboration in developing an action plan.
Supporting Feedback Seeking	**Seeking Feedback**
• Ask the learner for goals for the experience. • Ask to identify specific area of focus. • Match these with your expectations for the experience. • Book time in your schedule for planning, observing, and discussing feedback. • Coach the learner and actively engage in developing a plan to use the feedback.	• Identify goals for the experience. • Identify specific area of focus. • Share your goals and area of focus you're your supervisor. • Prepare for all input/ feedback. • Clarify the details. • Actively engage in developing a plan to use the feedback.

with a professionalism issue (Part 2). See discussion at the end of this chapter for an example of sharing sensitive feedback and coaching.)

6. **The learner's own self-assessment or self-perception of their performance.** Noting whether the data and feedback confirm or disconfirm one's self-perceptions about one's performance is generally the first response of the feedback receiver. Feedback that disconfirms one's own beliefs can be surprising and can elicit an emotional response such as disappointment or anger. We have all probably received feedback ourselves that disconfirmed our perceptions of how we thought we were doing and led to our feeling disappointed, angry, or misunderstood. And we have probably also provided disconfirming data and feedback to learners who have responded emotionally as their self-perceptions were not being supported. The reason for the emotional response is that one's professional performance is core to who one is (i.e., professional identity), and assessment of that performance is highly sensitive.[53] Hence an emotional response to disconfirming feedback is understandable and even to be expected in some cases.
7. **Emotional response to the feedback.** The important point is that this emotional response to the feedback can get in the way of the learner accepting and using the feedback. Supervisors too may have some degree of emotional response to sharing corrective data and feedback. Fear of eliciting such an emotional response and of not being able to respond appropriately is frequently cited as a reason for not providing disconfirming feedback.[52] Hence the situation can result in a scenario in which the learner is apprehensive or fearful of receiving disconfirming feedback and the supervisor is apprehensive and fearful of providing that feedback, creating a less than ideal setting for having a

TABLE 14.4 R2C2 Phases, Goals, and Suggested Phrases

Phase	Goal	Suggested Phrases
Phase 1: Build relationships	To engage the resident, build relationship, build respect and trust, understand their context	• How has the rotation gone for you? Tell me about what you enjoyed and what challenged you. • Tell me about your assessment and feedback experiences. What's has and hasn't been helpful? • How do you think you're doing? What are your strengths and opportunities to improve? • What would you hope to get out of this session?
Phase 2: Explore reactions and reflections	For residents to feel understood and that their views are heard and respected	• What were your initial reactions? Anything particularly striking? • Did anything in the report surprise you? Tell me more about that. • How do these data compare with how you think you were doing? Any surprises? • It's difficult to hear feedback that disconfirms how we see ourselves.
Phase 3: Explore understanding of the content	For the resident to be clear about what the assessment data mean for their practice and the opportunities identified for change and development	• Was there anything in the report that didn't make sense to you? • Was there anything you're unclear about? • Let's go through it section by section. • Did anything strike you as something to focus on?
Phase 4: Coach for performance change	For the resident to engage in developing an achievable learning and change plan	• What 1 or 2 priorities for change do the assessment data suggest to you? • What would be your goal? • What actions will you have to take? • What resources do you need? • What might get in the way of you achieving your goal? • Do you think the goal is achievable?

constructive, developmental conversation. In this light, it is similar to a "breaking bad news" communication. Like many such conversations, follow-up meetings may be necessary as the learner processes the information. The challenge for the supervisor is to intervene and have a feedback conversation in a constructive way while appropriately recognizing and integrating the emotional responses to giving and receiving feedback. Using communication and facilitation microskills as discussed earlier in this chapter enables such a conversation (see Table 14.4).

8. **Systems and culture.** Traditional medical and medical education cultures influence the willingness of learners to accept and use performance data and feedback. Appearing competent is generally highly valued and, by default, receiving feedback can be seen as an indicator that one is not competent. Feedback in this case is perceived as a criticism or a failing rather than an opportunity to further develop, improve, and excel. The contrasting perceptions create a tension for learners between wanting feedback to help them improve and feeling reticent in seeking, accepting, and using the feedback.[11,36,54–57] Creating a safe learning climate where feedback is explicitly valued, shared, and used is a way to maximize its positive value. (See Table 14.3 for tips on creating a positive feedback culture.)

In addition to culture, the systems created in medical education and healthcare also can negatively influence the ability to observe learners and provide performance data and feedback to them in ways that can positively influence its uptake and use[58] (see Box 14.2). System issues such as shorter clinical rotations and others limit opportunities for supervisors to observe learners' performance over time and provide feedback. Some accreditation and assessment systems impose requirements for electronic documentation of feedback without necessarily requiring a face-to-face meeting with the learner, which can negatively influence the frequency of those feedback discussions while the electronic nature of the feedback can also reduce its sense of

• BOX 14.2 System Factors That Influence Feedback and Coaching

- Short resident clinical rotations
- Short faculty rotations in their clinical setting
- Limited opportunities for observation
- Limited opportunities for longitudinal observation
- Demand for increased faculty clinical productivity and outcomes
- Legislated shorter resident work week
- Assessment and observation forms and protocols that promote rote instead of authentic, thoughtful feedback
- Assessment databases with rigid structures that interfere with having timely feedback conversations
- Legal and other challenges that can prevent sharing residents' progress and development with supervisors of their subsequent rotations

authenticity and its usefulness. Some clinician educators speak anecdotally of this and its repercussions upon learning as "the fractured clinical environment." While a few undergraduate medical education (UME) and GME programs are beginning to address these negative features, much more collective energy is required to change a decades-old system.

More broadly within Western society, generations of learners and workers over the years perceive learning, being assessed, and receiving feedback in different ways. They see and understand these roles differently. These differences create gaps in understanding on both sides, adding generational mix to the various factors influencing the sharing of feedback. Providing cross-generational training for all groups can help address these differences.

Practical Strategies for Engaging in Effective Feedback and Coaching Conversations and for Changing the Feedback Culture

Drawing on the discussions above, we offer two feedback and coaching models as practical strategies for effective feedback and coaching conversations and two initiatives for promoting change in the feedback culture.

Models for Feedback and Coaching: Prepare to ADAPT and R2C2

Applying the principles of experiential learning, two evidence-based models[59] of feedback and coaching have been developed and used extensively: Prepare to ADAPT and R2C2. The R2C2 model, discussed shortly, is the most extensively researched feedback model (see Appendix 14.4 for a list of R2C2 research publications). Prepare to ADAPT, while less studied, aligns well with the R2C2 model and connects with the robust R2C2 evidence base. Both require that (1) the learner participates in an experience or patient encounter that is observed by the preceptor/coach; (2) the learner and the preceptor reflect upon the experience/observations and have a conversation to share their reflections and reactions; and (3) the learner and the preceptor discuss what it means as a priority for learning and change and codevelop a plan to meet that goal. The following subsections provide specifics of each model and tips for using them.

Prepare to ADAPT Model

Prepare to ADAPT was developed at the University of Washington.[60] It includes six phases and provides actions for learners and coaches for each phase (see Appendix 14.2 for the model, and refer to the website for more details on using it):

1. Prepare. Notably, the first step is preparation, reminding us that feedback and coaching need to be intentional and consistent with a learner's level of education and goals.
2. Perform. The activity is performed and the learner engages in the experience.
3. **A**sk (A). The learner asks for feedback and the preceptor shares their feedback and asks for the learner's reactions to it. This phase can (and should) include the preceptor asking for the learner's self-assessment.
4. **D**iscuss (D). The coach engages the learner in a discussion about their shared observations and reflections and the specific behaviors that were observed.
5. **A**sk (A). The learner asks for clarification and the preceptor asks for confirmation of clarity.
6. **P**lan **T**ogether (PT). The learner and preceptor collaboratively plan next steps.

R2C2 Feedback and Coaching Model

In response to the need to enhance assessment *for* learning and support coaching, the R2C2 research team, through multiple multisite qualitative studies, developed an evidence- and theory-informed reflective model for facilitating performance feedback and coaching conversations to enhance acceptance and practice improvement.[35,40] The model has since been tested by other research teams (see Appendix 14.4). Please refer to the R2C2 resource website (https://medicine.dal.ca/departments/core-units/cpd/faculty-development/R2C2.html) for teaching and practice aids, video demonstrations, and research papers, and to Appendix 14.3 for the R2C2 trifold handout.

The model includes four phases: (1) **R**elationship building; (2) exploring **R**eactions to the feedback; (3) exploring understanding of feedback **C**ontent; and (4) **C**oaching for performance change (Fig. 14.4).

The R2C2 model has been tested with physicians and learners and found to be helpful in various ways. It provides a structure for facilitators and supervisors for engaging learners in the feedback conversation and in their performance data, and it enhances their understanding, acceptance, and use of feedback. Learners and supervisors report

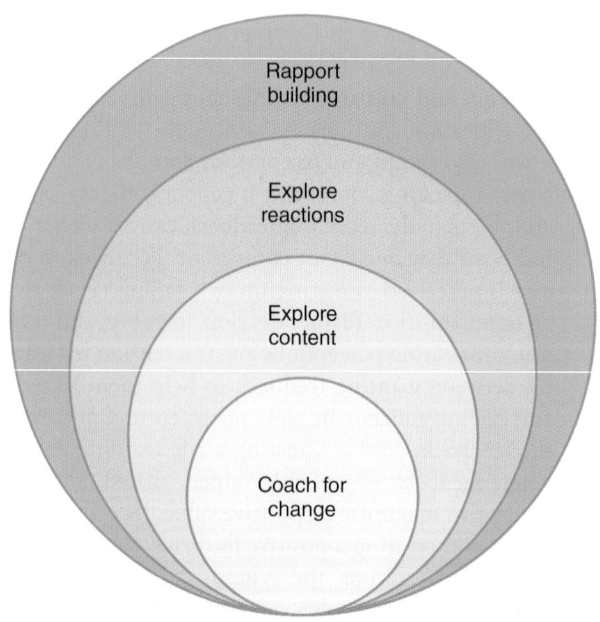

• **Fig. 14.4** Graphic of the R2C2 model.

that the overall model and coaching phase in particular are valuable in a CBME environment to support progression from one level to the next.

The R2C2 feedback model is informed by three theoretical and evidence-based approaches for facilitating acceptance and use of assessment data: (1) humanism and person centeredness, (2) informed or guided self-assessment, and (3) behavior change and the factors influencing change.[40] Each of the four phases in the model has a particular goal guided by the three theoretical perspectives above:

1. **R**elationship building: to engage the learner, build a relationship, build respect and trust, understand their context (humanism)
2. exploring **R**eactions to and reflections upon the feedback: for the learner to reflect and to feel understood and that their views are heard and respected
3. exploring understanding of feedback **C**ontent: for the learner to be clear about what the assessment data mean for their practice, and the priority opportunities identified for change and development
4. **C**oaching for performance change: for the learner to engage collaboratively with the coach in developing an achievable goal and learning and change plan (also see coproduction cycle above)

Specific phrases have been found to be helpful for each phase of R2C2; examples are provided in Table 14.4, in Appendix 14.3, and on the R2C2 website. Links to annotated videos demonstrating the four phases and communication techniques for both "in the moment" and longitudinal coaching are also available on the R2C2 website, and in the exercises at the end of this chapter.

Of note, while the phases are presented in a linear way, the model is iterative and earlier phases can be revisited as required based on how the conversation is unfolding. For example, a reaction or emotion may arise during coaching, and when that happens the faculty should "loop back up" to further explore the reaction or emotion before coaching further.

An overall goal of the model is to promote *reflection* at each phase.[61] The purpose of the microcommunication skills identified earlier in this chapter is to promote reflection, as well as to build a relationship. Facilitating reflection is central to success in feedback and coaching. Note that the phrases are open-ended questions to promote learners' reflection upon their performance data, the feedback they are receiving, their reactions to the feedback, clinical learning, and their goals for using the feedback.

When the external data and feedback disconfirm one's own self-assessment, it is often harder to accept them and take them on. In Phase 2, exploring reactions, facilitating learners' reflection upon why the external data may differ from their own self-assessments and upon the personal impact of receiving disconfirming feedback can enable acceptance of that feedback and prevent defensive reactions. In Phase 3, exploring understanding of feedback content, encouraging specific reflection upon the opportunities for change and development that the performance data may offer can help the learner see the positive value and usefulness of the data for improvement. Finally, in Phase 4, coaching, reflection guides the learner in identifying an achievable performance goal to fill that gap and in identifying a specific plan to achieve that goal. More broadly, a goal of facilitated reflection is to build the learner's skills in critical self-examination and informed self-assessment as a lifelong self-directed learning strategy.

Coaching for change (Phase 4) is a skill that many supervisors report as novel and hence are unclear how to begin. As mentioned earlier, using a template or form to cocreate a learning/change plan with the learner is useful. Talking about each step in the plan and writing the learner's response make the plan concrete and explicit. An example template for such an action plan is included in Appendix 14.1. Steps include identifying the specific goal to be achieved, timeline, barriers and enablers, and strategies for measuring progress, and then following up. Developing the plan involves identifying each step, including the factors that will enable the learner to reach the goal and those that may be barriers. Equally important to developing the plan is follow-up planning; that is, setting a time to return to it and determine with the learner whether they were successful in completing it and what the next steps are. In this way the model fits with the cycles for experiential learning (Fig. 14.2) and quality improvement (Fig. 14.3); the goal is constant improvement. It is also comparable to sports coaching where the goal is constant improvement to enable players to become the best that they can be.

The overarching goal of the R2C2 model, in terms drawn from psychology, is to transition the locus of control for the performance data from external to internal. This means that instead of learners seeing themselves as lacking control and the external data and feedback as being imposed on them, they take ownership of their own performance data, seek out the data, and use them for their development and performance improvement. Notably, it is now recognized in professional practice that seeing oneself as being in control and having agency is protective against burnout. Other burnout protective factors are supportive relationships and having a realistic sense of one's competence, both of which can also be nurtured by coaching strategies.[62,63]

Finally, medical regulatory organizations and healthcare authorities are increasingly providing longitudinal coaching for physicians to enable them to review their performance data and work with their coach to develop an action plan for improvement based on those data.[49,64,65] Similar to residents' experiences, physicians report that supportive relationships and facilitated engagement in reflection and planning are positive features of such programs.

Prepare to ADAPT and R2C2 Comparison

The R2C2 and Prepare to ADAPT models are based on similar principles and employ similar strategies. Fig. 14.5

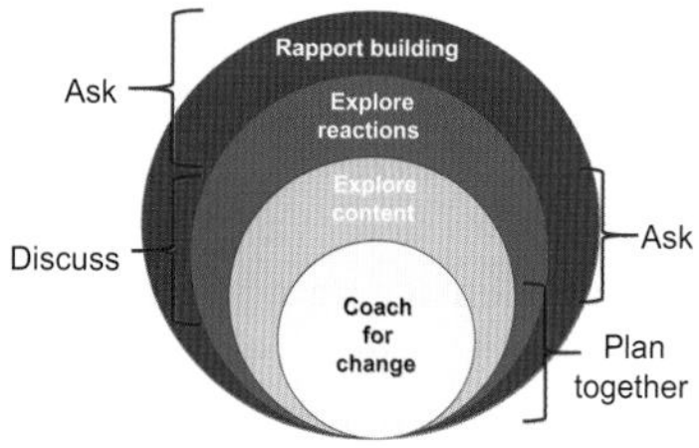

Ask
Rapport building
Explore reactions
Explore content
Coach for change
Discuss
Ask
Plan together

• **Fig. 14.5** Comparison of R2C2 and Prepare to ADAPT models.

provides a comparison of the two. A notable difference is that the R2C2 model does not include a separate preparation phase, although this is inherent in the "Relationship" phase. However, we're learning that preparation by both the preceptor and learner aids the process and we recommend that it be made explicit as in the Prepare to ADAPT model. Additionally, R2C2 does not specifically include the "Perform the observation" phase; instead it is taken for granted that this occurs. Again, making it more explicit would add clarity.

The Prepare to ADAPT model was designed for providing feedback in the moment. Further research on the R2C2 model, originally developed for longitudinal coaching, explores modifications required to be effective for "in the moment" feedback and coaching. Results show that the four phases of the model continue to provide structure for the interaction and can be adapted to meet the time constraints of "in the moment feedback" while still engaging the learner in a collaborative manner.[51,66]

In summary, the Prepare to ADAPT and R2C2 models are similar and complementary, and together provide a comprehensive yet practical guide for undertaking feedback and coaching for both preceptors and learners. Table 14.5 provides tips and strategies for each model, each phase, and both learners and preceptors. The phases or steps of the combined models are:

1. Prepare
2. Perform/observe
3. Reflect on performance and observations; be specific
4. Discuss shared reflections and reactions
5. Agree on priority for improvement
6. Codevelop an action plan
7. Follow up

TABLE 14.5 Practical Tips for "in the Moment" Feedback and Coaching, Adapted from the Prepare to ADAPT and R2C2 Models

Steps/Phases	Tips for Learners	Tips for Preceptors
1. Prepare	General:" What are my goals for this rotation?" Specific: "What specifically am I working on? What would I like coaching on today/this week?" Share with preceptor and plan together for the activity (e.g., time, clinical encounter)	General: Share interest in observing and providing feedback Be familiar with goals of program and ask learner for their goals for your rotation Specific: Ask learner what specifically they are working on today/this week and would like coaching on Plan with learner for the activity
Prepare: note:	The activity/observation may be "spur of the moment"; if so, agree on its purpose and what coaching will help the learner.	
2. Perform/observe	Perform activity naturally	Observe neutrally; if going to intervene, try to prepare learner ahead of time May not need to observe the complete activity; just the portion for which coaching is requested/needed
3. Reflect on performance and observations[a]	Take a minute and reflect on your performance; e.g., what went well, not so well; what you were worried about, what you were thinking	Take a minute and reflect on what you objectively observed; e.g., what went well, not so well; why this might have happened
4. Ask, share, and discuss reflections and reactions[a]	Ask for feedback Share your reflection, reactions to your preceptor's thoughts If views differ, discuss; determine potential reasons Ask for/provide clarification	Ask for their reflections and self-assessment; use open questions, prompts Share yours; ask for their reactions If views differ, explore why this may be the case Ask for/provide clarification
5. Agree on priority for improvement[a]	Discuss and agree	
6. Codevelop an action plan[a]	Collaboratively: • Identify the goal • Make a plan: what needs to be done, timeline, resources needed/available, barriers, success measures • Identify follow-up process (who, when), especially if moving to a different preceptor or rotation	
7. Follow-up	Implement follow-up plan Assess improvement, next steps	Follow up as efficiently as possible

[a]Refer to Appendix 14.3 for sample phrases and questions to use for these phases.

Practical Tips for Changing the Feedback Culture

Encourage Learners to Seek Feedback

Encouraging learners to seek feedback is receiving increasing attention as a strategy to enable them to take more responsibility for their learning and receive more specific guidance and coaching. This represents another shift in our learning and teaching culture, away from a hierarchical, expert-directed model to one in which the learner is expected to be an active, motivated, and self-directed learner. An effective feedback exchange requires learners to be active recipients and seekers of feedback.[55] Seeking feedback is in keeping with the tenets of programmatic assessment in which the learner seeks assessment feedback for learning, and of CBME in which the learner is interested in receiving assessment data and feedback that will enable advancement to the next level (see Chapters 1 and 3).

Studies identify a number of factors that influence whether or not learners will seek feedback. Foremost among these are learners' perceptions of seeking feedback as being a risky activity. They mediate this risk by balancing the costs (e.g., appearing incompetent) and benefits (e.g., receiving needed guidance) of the feedback.[67–69] Seeking feedback can be seen as dependent on multiple factors: (1) learning/workplace culture, (2) relationships, (3) purpose/quality of feedback, and (4) emotional responses to feedback. Both learners and faculty suggest supports and barriers to seeking feedback. Supports include strengthening the workplace learning culture through longitudinal experiences, using feedback forms and explicit expectations for learners to seek feedback, and providing a sense of safety and adequate time for observation and feedback discussions. Barriers include tensions between faculty and learners, learner perceptions of seeking feedback as being related to fear of being found deficient, the emotional costs related to corrective feedback, and perceptions that completing clinical work is more valued than learning.

Additional Steps

Being aware of and understanding the cultural influences discussed in the sections above is a first step to addressing them. It means that while culture surrounds us and is pervasive, we can also enhance our skills at addressing the aspects of a culture we wish to change, to enable the effective provision and use of feedback for learning and development. Seen in this light, culture becomes an actor in the medical education arena and supervisors can take positive steps to counter some of the potentially negative effects and build a more positive culture.[57] For example, if providing constructive feedback does not appear to be valued, supervisors can role-model providing it in an effective way, and can ask colleagues and learners to provide them with feedback to enable learning and improvement. At a systems level, thought is being given to reenvisioning assessment processes.[70] Table 14.3 provides a comprehensive list of strategies for faculty and learners to forward positive change in the culture of feedback and coaching.

Practical Exercises

The first four exercises below are feedback and coaching exercises using demonstration videos of the R2C2 model. The last two are exercises that promote changing the medical education environment to be more supportive of assessment for learning, feedback conversations, and coaching.

Coaching Exercises Using R2C2 Videos

1. Building the relationship and planning with a new learner
   a. Before watching this short video, take a minute and think about what you do to build relationships with new learners when you have little time.
   b. https://youtu.be/13tDGRoHL1g
   As you watch the video, identify the strategies the preceptor used to build the relationship and create a plan with a new clinical clerk, in under 2 minutes.
   c. How might this approach apply to more senior learners, residents, and fellows?
2. Addressing sensitive issues: a learner with a professionalism issue (Part 1)
   a. Before watching Part 1, reflect upon the strategies you use to address a sensitive issue with a learner, one that they probably would prefer not to discuss.
   b. https://youtu.be/GMN9aNhO9_c
   As you watch the video, note the phases of R2C2.
   c. What phrases did the preceptor use to address the sensitive issue that the fellow was uncomfortable with? What strategies/phrases did she use to foster his reflection?
   d. Before viewing Part 2, consider how you would develop a coaching plan for this fellow.
3. Coaching: a learner with a professionalism issue (Part 2): https://youtu.be/p_dND4lo-Y0
   a. What phrases did the preceptor use to pivot the conversation to coaching?
   b. What phrases did she use to engage the learner? To develop the plan and build commitment?
4. Other available annotated videos: as you watch each, consider the R2C2 phase and phrases used by the preceptor. Which do you find helpful?
   a. Coaching the high achiever: https://youtu.be/Cf14-K-jpU
   b. Coaching the "lazy" resident: https://youtu.be/VPxEXx7KRNk

Culture Change Exercise

1. Individual change in your feedback and coaching interactions with learners
   a. Review Table 14.4.
   b. Consider which of these approaches you are currently using and which you would like to adopt.
   c. Decide when you would like to try out the initiative(s) and identify the results you hope to see.

2. Fostering system change
   a. Consider the discussion earlier in this chapter of culture and system factors influencing feedback and coaching and feedback practices (see also Table 14.1).
   b. Reflect upon how you might influence one or two factors in your program/department/workplace that currently limit opportunities for high-quality feedback and coaching interactions with learners. For example, consider committee/working groups/decision-making bodies of which you are a member and strategies you might use to influence their role in positive change.
   c. Develop an action plan for implementing this strategy using the action plan template in Appendix 14.1 and put it into action.

Conclusion

In this chapter, the evolution of the practice of feedback and the incorporation of coaching with feedback have been described. Feedback has evolved from a unidirectional provision of information for improvement to a conversation that engages the learner, promotes their reflection and self-assessment, and, actively and collaboratively with them, coaches the development of a plan for their use of the feedback.

Acknowledgments

We acknowledge the members of the research teams who have contributed to the development and testing of the R2C2 model, the thinking around it, and the various strategies related to using and teaching it:

1. Sargeant J, Lockyer J, Mann K, et al. Performance feedback to inform self-assessment and guide practice improvement: developing and testing a feedback facilitation model. *Acad Med.* 2015;90 (12):1698–1706. (Funded by the Society for Academic CME, Philip Manning Award, 2011–2013)
2. Sargeant J, Mann K, Warren A, et al. Testing an evidence-based model for facilitating performance feedback and improvement in residency education: what works and why? *Acad Med.* 2018 Jul;93(7):1055–1063. (Funded by the NBME Stemmler Award 2014–2016)
3. Armson H, Lockyer J, Zetkulic M, Könings K, Sargeant J. Identifying coaching skills to improve feedback use in postgraduate medical education. *Med Educ.* 2019 May;53(5):477–493.
4. Lockyer J, Zetkulic M, Könings K, et al. In-the-moment feedback and coaching: improving r2c2 for a new context. *J Grad Med Educ.* 2020 Feb;12(1):27–35.

We also extend particular thanks to Marygrace Zetkulic for her creativity in scripting and making the videos and for her generosity in sharing them with the medical education community. Dr. Zetkulic is Program Director of Internal Medicine, Assistant Professor of Medicine, Hackensack Meridian School of Medicine, Department of Medicine, Hackensack University Medical Center, New Jersey.

Annotated Bibliography

1. Gawande A. Personal best: top athletes and singers have coaches—should you? *The New Yorker.* October 2, 2011. Accessed January 16, 2023. www.newyorker.com/reporting/2011/10/03/111003fa_fact_gawande.
   Dr. Gawande is a surgeon who reflects that he has reached a plateau in improving his surgical technique and patient outcomes. In this article he begins by reflecting upon his observation of athletes: "Professional athletes use coaches to make sure they are as good as they can be." He then describes how observation and coaching are used in sports, music, and teaching to enable the players/professionals to see their blind spots and become "as good as they can be." He questions why surgeons and other physicians don't take advantage of having a trusted colleague or teacher observe and coach them, and describes his personal experiences with a coach in the OR. His coach discussed with him a long list of observations, all of which contributed to improving and fine-tuning his critical thinking and decision-making during surgery and his skills. He now invites his coach regularly to observe him, to give feedback on the changes he's made, and to suggest further fine-tuning. He writes and describes his personal experiences in a compelling manner that helps the reader appreciate what coaching is and how it can help practicing physicians as well as learners be "as good as they can be."
2. Heen S, Stone D. Managing yourself—finding the coaching in criticism: the right way to receive feedback. *Harvard Business Review.* January-February 2014:108–111. Accessed DATE URL.
   These authors have spent much of their careers studying difficult conversations, effective communication, and feedback in various workplaces. They write very practically about receiving feedback, removing the emotional investment in feedback, and using it to improve. They provide six strategies with practical examples for receiving feedback that are also readily translated into giving/sharing feedback and leading feedback conversations: (1) Know your tendencies (i.e., how do you generally react to feedback?); (2) Disentangle the "what" from the "who"; (3) Sort toward coaching (i.e., consider feedback as coaching–"Coaching allows you to learn and improve and helps you play at a higher level"); (4) Unpack the feedback (i.e., analyze it and reflect on it); (5) Ask for just one thing; and (6) Engage in small experiments. Their advice is helpful for both faculty and learners.
3. Sargeant J, Lockyer JM, Mann K, et al. The R2C2 model in residency education: how does it foster coaching and promote feedback use? *Acad Med.* 2018 Jul;93(7):1055–1063.
   This paper describes the multisite, multidiscipline research study used to test the R2C2 feedback model in residency education, building on its initial development and testing with physicians published in 2015. The four phases of the model are (1) Build rapport and relationships; (2) Explore reactions to the data and feedback; (3) Explore understanding of the feedback content; and (4) Coach for change. The model, developed from both evidence and theory informing feedback, was well received by the preceptors and residents using it, as was the learning change plan used to guide the coaching phase. The model was reported to be effective in fostering a productive, reflective feedback conversation focused on resident development and in facilitating collaborative development of resident change plans.

References

1. Van de Ridder M, van de Ridder JM, Stokking KM, McGaghie WC, ten Cate OT. What is feedback in clinical education? *Med Educ*. 2008 Feb;42(2):189–197.
2. Archer JC. State of the science in health professional education: effective feedback. *Med Educ*. 2010;44:101–108.
3. Lefroy J, Watling C, Teunissen PW, Brand P. Guidelines on feedback for clinical education: the dos, don'ts, and don't knows of feedback for clinical education. *Perspect Med Educ*. 2015;4(6):284–299.
4. Ajjawi R, Regehr G. When I say … feedback. *Med Educ*. 2019 Jul;53(7):652–654.
5. Tavares W, Eppich W, Cheng A, et al. Learning conversations: an analysis of the theoretical roots and their manifestations of feedback and debriefing in medical education. *Acad Med*. 2020 Jul;95(7):1020–1025.
6. Boud D, Malloy E. What is the problem with feedback? In: Boud D, Molloy E, eds. *Feedback in Higher and Professional Education: Understanding It and Doing It Well*. Routledge; 2013:1–10.
7. Stone D, Heen S. *Thanks for the Feedback*. Penguin Books; 2014.
8. Dweck CS, Yeager DS. Mindsets: a view from two eras. *Perspect Psychol Sci*. 2019 May;14(3):481–496.
9. Richardson D, Kinnear B, Hauer KE, et al. Growth mindset in competency-based medical education. *Med Teach*. 2021 Jul;43(7):751–757.
10. Eva KW, Regehr G. Self-assessment in the health professions: a reformulation and research agenda. *Acad Med*. 2005;80(10 Suppl):S46–S54.
11. Sargeant J, Armson H, Chesluk B, et al. Processes and dimensions of informed self-assessment: a conceptual model. *Acad Med*. 2010;85(7):1212–1220.
12. Robb KA, Rosenbaum ME, Peters L, Lenoch S, Lancianese D, Miller JL. Self-assessment in feedback conversations: a complicated balance. *Acad Med*. 2022 Aug 9 Epub ahead of print.
13. Wolf R, Santen S. Role of informed self-assessment in coaching. In: Deirio N, Hammond M, eds. *Coaching in Medical Education: A faculty Handbook*. American Medical Association; 2017. Accessed January 17, 2023.. https://www.ama-assn.org/system/files/2019-09/coaching-medical-education-faculty-handbook.pdf.
14. Brydges R, Butler D. A reflective analysis of medical education research on self-regulation in learning and practice. *Med Educ*. 2012;46(1):71–79.
15. Brydges R, Law M, Ma IW, Gavarkovs A. On embedding assessments of self-regulated learning into licensure activities in the health professions: a call to action. *Can Med Educ J*. 2022 Aug 26;13(4):100–109.
16. Englander R, Holmboe E, Batalden P, et al. Coproducing health professions education: a prerequisite to coproducing health care services? *Acad Med*. 2020 Jul;95(7):1006–1013.
17. Könings KD, Mordang S, Smeenk F, Stassen L, Ramani S. Learner involvement in the co-creation of teaching and learning: AMEE Guide No. 138. *Med Teach*. 2021 Aug;43(8):924–936.
18. Heen S, Stone D. Managing yourself—finding the coaching in criticism: the right way to receive feedback. *Harvard Business Review*. 2014, January-February:108–111.
19. Gawande A. Personal best. *The New Yorker*. October 3, 2011. Accessed January 17, 2023. www.newyorker.com/magazine/2011/10/03/personal-best.
20. Deiorio NM, Carney PA, Kahl LE, Bonura EM, Miller Juve A. Coaching: a new model for academic and career achievement. *Med Educ Online*. 2016;21(1):5.
21. Van Niewerburgh C. *Coaching in Education: Getting Better Results for Students, Educators and Parents*. Karnac Books; 2012.
22. Ekpenyong A, Zetkulic M, Edgar L, Holmboe ES. Reimagining feedback for the milestones era. *J Grad Med Educ*. 2021 Apr;13(2 Suppl):109–112.
23. Van der Vleuten CP, Schuwirth LW, Driessen EW, et al. A model for programmatic assessment. *Med Teach*. 2012;34(3):205–214.
24. Frank JR, Snell LS, Cate OT, et al. Competency-based medical education: theory to practice. *Med Teach*. 2010;32(8):638–645.
25. The Accreditation Council for Graduate Medical Education in the United States. Accessed January 17, 2023. https://www.acgme.org/acgmeweb/.
26. Royal College of Physicians and Surgeons of Canada. Accessed January 17, 2023. https://www.royalcollege.ca/rcsite/canmeds/canmeds-framework-e.
27. College of Family Physicians of Canada. Accessed January 17, 2023. http://cfpc.ca/Triple_C/.
28. Carraccio C, Englander R, Gilhooly J, et al. Building a framework of Entrustable Professional Activities, supported by competencies and milestones, to bridge the educational continuum. *Acad Med*. 2017 Mar;92(3):324–330.
29. Accreditation Council for Graduate Medical Education. Milestones. Accessed January 17, 2023. https://www.acgme.org/acgmeweb/tabid/430/ProgramandInstitutionalAccreditation/NextAccreditationSystem/Milestones.aspx.
30. Epstein RM, Hundert EM. Defining and assessing professional competence assessing competence. *JAMA*. 2002;287(2):226–235.
31. Holmboe ES, Batalden P. Achieving the desired transformation: thoughts on next steps for outcomes-based medical education. *Acad Med*. 2015 Sep;90(9):1215–1223.
32. Dreyfus S. The five-stage model of adult skill acquisition. *Bull Sci Tech Soc*. 2004;24:177–181.
33. Ericsson KA. Acquisition and maintenance of medical expertise: a perspective from the expert-performance approach with deliberate practice. *Acad Med*. 2015;90(11):1471–1486.
34. Lovell B. What do we know about coaching in medical education? A literature review. *Med Educ*. 2018;52(4):376–390.
35. Sargeant J, Lockyer JM, Mann K, et al. The R2C2 model in residency education: how does it foster coaching and promote feedback use? *Acad Med*. 2018 Jul;93(7):1055–1063.
36. Watling C, Driessen E, van der Vleuten C, Vanstone M, Lingard L. Music lessons: revealing medicine's learning culture through comparison with that of music. *Med Educ*. 2013;47(8):842–850.
37. Watling C, Driessen E, van der Vleuten C, Lingard L. Learning culture and feedback: an international study of medical athletes and musicians. *Med Educ*. 2014;48(7):713–723.
38. Armson H, Lockyer JM, Zetkulic M, Könings KD, Sargeant J. Identifying coaching skills to improve feedback use in postgraduate medical education. *Med Educ*. 2019 May;53(5):477–493.
39. Coaching in Medical Education. In: Deirio N, Hammond M, eds. *A Faculty Handbook*. American Medical Association; 2017. Accessed January 17, 2023. https://www.ama-assn.org/system/files/2019-09/coaching-medical-education-faculty-handbook.pdf.
40. Sargeant J, Lockyer J, Mann K, et al. Facilitated reflective performance feedback: developing an evidence- and theory-based model that builds relationship, explores reactions and content, and coaches for performance change (R2C2). *Acad Med*. 2015;90(12):1698–1706.

41. Kolb DA. *Experiential Learning: Experience as the Source of Learning and Development.* Prentice-Hall; 1984.
42. Boud D, Keogh R, Walker D. Promoting reflection in learning: a model. In: Boud D, Keogh R, Walker D, eds. *Reflection: Turning Experience into Learning.* Routledge Falmer; 1985:19–40.
43. Royal College of Physicians and Surgeons of Canada. Coaching to Competence. Accessed January 17, 2023.https://www.royalcollege.ca/mssites/rxocr/en/story.html.
44. Elwyn G, Nelson E, Hager A, Price A. Coproduction: when users define quality. *BMJ Qual Saf.* 2020;29(9):711–716. https://qualitysafety.bmj.com/content/29/9/711.
45. Ramani S, Könings KD, Mann KV, Pisarski EE, van der Vleuten CPM. About politeness, face, and feedback: exploring resident and faculty perceptions of how institutional feedback culture influences feedback practices. *Acad Med.* 2018 Sep;93(9):1348–1358.
46. Voyer S, Cuncic C, Butler DL, MacNeil K, Watling C, Hatala R. Investigating conditions for meaningful feedback in the context of an evidence-based feedback program. *Med Educ.* 2016;50(9):943–954.
47. Sargeant J, Eva KW, Armson H, et al. Features of assessment learners use for informed self-assessments of clinical performance. *Med Educ.* 2011;45(6):636–647.
48. Holmboe ES, Sherbino J, Long DM, Swing SR, Frank JR. The role of assessment in competency-based medical education. *Med Teach.* 2010;32(8):676–682.
49. Telio S, Regehr G, Ajjawi R. Feedback and the educational alliance: examining credibility judgements and their consequences. *Med Educ.* 2016;50(9):933–942.
50. Holmboe ES, Ward DS, Reznick RK, et al. Faculty development in assessment: the missing link in competency-based medical education. *Acad Med.* 2011;86(4):460–467.
51. Lockyer J, Lee-Krueger R, Armson H, et al. Application of the R2C2 model to in-the-moment coaching and feedback. Acad Med. Submitted and under revision January 2023.
52. Dudek NL, Marks MB, Regehr G. Failure to fail: the perspectives of clinical supervisors. *Acad Med.* 2005;80(10 Suppl):S84–S87.
53. DeNisi AS, Kluger AN. Feedback effectiveness: can 360-degree appraisals be improved? *Acad Manage Perspect.* 2000;14:129–139.
54. Friedson E. *Professionalism Reborn: Theory, Prophecy and Policy.* Cambridge Policy Press; 1994.
55. Teunissen PW, Stapel DA, van der Vleuten C, Scherpbier A, Boor K, Scheele F. Who wants feedback? An investigation of the variables influencing residents' feedback-seeking behavior in relation to night shifts. *Acad Med.* 2009;84(7):910–917.
56. Mann K, van der Vleuten C, Eva K, et al. Tensions in informed self-assessment: how the desire for feedback and reticence to collect/use it create conflict. *Acad Med.* 2011;86(9):1120–1127.
57. Ramani S, Könings KD, Ginsburg S, van der Vleuten CPM. Twelve tips to promote a feedback culture with a growth mindset: swinging the feedback pendulum from recipes to relationships. *Med Teach.* 2019 Jun;41(6):625–631.
58. Watling C, LaDonna K, Lingard L, Voyer S, Hatala R. Sometimes the work just needs to be done': sociocultural influences on direct observation in medical training. *Med Educ.* 2016;50(10):1054–1064.
59. Liakos W, Keel T, Pearlman RE, Fornari A. Frameworks for effective feedback in health professions education. *Acad Med.* 2023 May 1; 98(5):648. doi:10.1097/ACM.0000000000004884.
60. University of Washington Medicine, Graduate Medical Education. Prepare to adapt. Accessed January 17, 2023. https://sites.uw.edu/uwgme/adapt/.
61. Sargeant J, Mann K, van der Vleuten C, Metsemakers J. Reflection: a link between receiving and using assessment feedback. *Adv Health Sci Educ Theory Pract.* 2009;14(3):399–410.
62. Gazelle G, Liebschutz JM, Riess H. Physician burnout: coaching a way out. *J Gen Intern Med.* 2015 Apr;30(4):508–513.
63. Sargeant J. Future research in feedback: how to use feedback and coaching conversations in a way that supports development of the individual as a self-directed learner and resilient professional. *Acad Med.* 2019;94(11S Association of American Medical Colleges Learn Serve Lead: Proceedings of the 58th Annual Research in Medical Education Sessions):S9–S10.
64. Arabsky S, Castro N, Murray M, Bisca I, Eva KW. The influence of relationship-centered coaching on physician perceptions of peer review in the context of mandated regulatory practices. *Acad Med.* 2020 Nov;95(11S Association of American Medical Colleges Learn Serve Lead: Proceedings of the 59th Annual Research in Medical Education Presentations):S14–S19.
65. Roy M, Lockyer J, Touchie C. Family physician quality improvement plans: a realist inquiry into what works, for whom, under what circumstances. *J Cont Educ Health Prof.* 2023.
66. Lockyer J, Armson H, Könings KD, et al. In-the-moment feedback and coaching: improving R2C2 for a new context. *J Grad Med Educ.* 2020 Feb;12(1):27–35.
67. Delva D, Sargeant J, Miller S, et al. Encouraging residents to seek feedback. *Med Teach.* 2013;35(12):e12625–e12631.
68. VandeWalle D, Ganesan S, Challagalla GN, Brown SP. An integrated model of feedback-seeking behavior: disposition, context, and cognition. *J Appl Psychol.* 2000;85(6):996–1003.
69. Crommelinck M, Anseel F. Understanding and encouraging feedback-seeking behaviour: a literature review. *Med Educ.* 2013;47(3):232–241.
70. Holmboe ES, Osman NY, Murphy C, Kogan JR. (in press). The urgency of now: rethinking and improving assessment practices in medical education programs. *Acad Med.*

15 Portfolios

CELIA LAIRD O'BRIEN, PHD, BRIGID M. DOLAN, MD, MED, AND PATRICIA S. O'SULLIVAN, MS, EDD

CHAPTER OUTLINE

Introduction

Portfolios are used in all stages of education,[1-10] ranging from voluntary to mandated and spanning from development and learning purposes to selective purposes.[5] Specific to the health professions, portfolios are used in an array of assessment settings, including preclerkship work, a single student clerkship experience, or the entire range of years of clinical training and across multiple health professions.[10–17] While learners can vary in their engagement with portfolios, literature indicates that over 70% will find value in a portfolio by the end of their time engaging with the process.[18] Therefore portfolios merit consideration as a valuable assessment approach.

However, we acknowledge that *portfolio* is defined in such a variety of ways that there can be confusion as to what it is, how it is to be used, and thus its purpose.[13,19–21] For example, tensions exist between the concept of portfolio as a *process* and portfolio as a *product*.[22] For clarity, we will define a portfolio as a collection of a learner's work, assessments, products, and so forth, accumulated over time, that provides evidence of professional development that is subsequently annotated by the learner's reflection on learning outcomes.[1,2,13,20,23–26] While this definition focuses on the *product*, we note that one cannot examine the portfolio as a product without paying careful attention to the process related to learning that is needed to develop it. We will explore these concepts more in the sections that follow.

One key difference between a portfolio and other types of assessment lies in the learner's engagement with the portfolio as a process of both autonomy and reflection. Learners experience autonomy because they have choice regarding the content they use as exemplars of their learning. Reflection is another critical difference between a portfolio and a logbook or dashboard; through the reflective aspects of the portfolio process, learners convey why they chose a given entry, what they learned from it, and how it can direct their future learning. While some institutions have implemented "reflection" portfolios focusing solely on learners' reflections and not attached to any specific product (often called an *artifact*),[27] a lack of artifacts makes reflection harder to contextualize. While some studies have found value in the reflective portfolio,[24,25,28–30] we agree with the perspectives put forth by Driessen[31] who challenges the value of a reflection-only portfolio because numerous implementations have indicated that learners struggle when reflection is the only purpose; students question the value in the process,[28,29,32] and residents express concern about risks with reflection.[33] Thus, in this chapter we will focus on what is known as a comprehensive portfolio comprising elements identified by the educational program and exemplars selected by learners

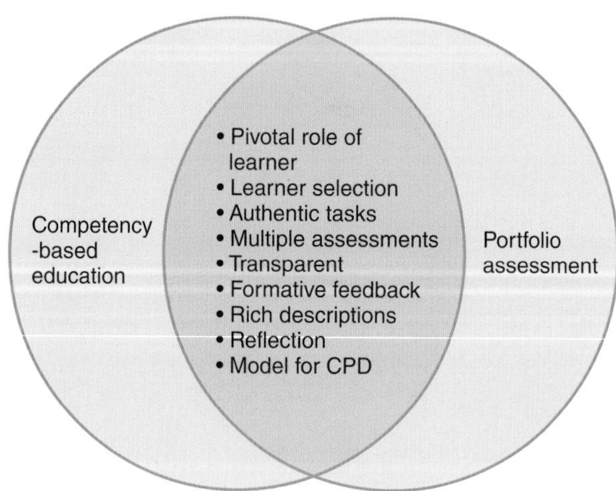

• **Fig. 15.1** Relationship of competency-based education and portfolios. *CPD*, Continuous professional development.

for purposes of assessment, rather than a reflection-only portfolio. In a comprehensive portfolio, reflection remains critical to support learners' need to demonstrate that they are developing their learning and reflective skills.

The use of portfolios in health professions education may now be at a tipping point. The movement toward competency-based education has made portfolios an excellent format for collecting evidence[34,35] (see Fig. 15.1). Portfolio assessment legitimizes the incorporation of judgment that considers the context in which a learner performs, facilitating a fair and defensible process essential in competency-based education.[36] Perhaps more importantly, portfolios align with universal design learning (UDL), a framework derived from models for inclusion of those with disabilities to create inclusivity in pedagogical practices that extend to all learners.[37]

The three key UDL principles are to provide multiple means of access, multiple means of engagement, and multiple means of action expression that can develop learners who are purposeful and motivated; resourceful and knowledgeable; and strategic and goal directed.[38] Fovet[37] argues that the lack of flexibility in assessment formats can be a burden to students, which UDL addresses by offering multiple ways for learners to demonstrate growth, development, and achievements. An implementation of portfolios based on UDL in electrical engineering resulted in creativity not previously seen.[39] Recently, Odukoya and colleagues[40] expanded the concept of UDL to encompass culturally responsive UDL that can be applied to medical education, highlighting the ability to provide learners with diverse ways to demonstrate that one has accomplished learning objectives. As such, portfolios offer an approach to assessment in competency-based assessment while addressing the needs of diverse learners.

The remainder of this chapter will focus on the processes needed for successful implementation and use of comprehensive portfolios that align with rigorous assessment of competencies commonly addressed in medical education as well as a discussion of validity evidence around assessments using portfolios.

Strengths Unique to Portfolios as Assessments

Portfolios contain several potential advantages as part of a robust assessment system. Among these are the alignment of a portfolio system with important assessment goals:

- An approach to encouraging self-regulated learning, featured in many medical education curricula
- The ability to assess difficult-to-measure competencies that frequently are omitted from assessments by using the artifacts in the portfolio
- An emphasis on authentic assessment due to the nature of the artifacts included
- The ability to demonstrate learner development over time

Unlike many assessments, portfolios require the active engagement of trainees in their education, a key component of self-regulated learning. In self-regulated learning, trainees engage in self-assessment by identifying knowledge and skill gaps, set realistic goals, employ adaptive learning strategies, reflect on performance, and adjust as needed.[41,42] These self-directed and lifelong learning skills are foundational for competent physicians, but finding structured ways to teach and assess these skills can be challenging in the health professions despite evidence that doing so fosters these abilities.[43] With structured reflection and supportive coaches (i.e., assigned faculty who provide guidance), portfolios provide a framework for assessment aligned with self-regulated learning and have been shown to increase responsibility for one's learning and reflective capacity.[24] Learners demonstrate engagement via their contribution of artifacts to the portfolio and reflections that often include learning plans supported by coaches' feedback.

This type of assessment incorporating self-regulated learning applies across the continuum of medical education. Given evidence that physicians' performance may decline over time, portfolios can lay the foundation for lifelong professional development and maintenance of competence.[44] The majority of a physician's career will be spent in "independent" (unsupervised) practice and not a structured educational environment, thus engaging in self-assessment and reflection-on-performance are essential lifelong learning skills. In fact, some continuing education programs have embraced this concept using portfolios as a framework for their assessment of competency.[45,46]

Portfolios can also be used to assess skills and competencies that are difficult to measure in other formats. Commonly, portfolios are chosen to assess skills such as critical thinking and problem-solving but they also provide a means to measure self-direction and reflection. Portfolios can also be used to collect evidence demonstrating competence in communication, professional development, and teamwork, frequently seen as challenging to assess.[10]

• BOX 15.1 Summary of 10 Portfolio Advantages

1. Critical learning skills such as self-assessment, reflection, self-directed learning, critical thinking, problem-solving and professionalism can be evaluated.
2. Developmental evidence can be collected longitudinally.
3. Educators can assess trainee progress toward acquiring the desired learning outcomes and goals.
4. Portfolios can provide multiple formative assessment points to build toward a summative assessment.
5. Portfolios provide a method for trainees to receive continuous feedback *and* to document their reactions and subsequent plans in response to that feedback for continuous professional development.
6. Trainees have the important opportunity to contribute evidence of their choosing to the overall assessment process.
7. Portfolios can facilitate better communication between educators and trainees.
8. Portfolios help to remind and encourage trainees that learning and assessment are an interactive two-way process between themselves and educators.
9. Portfolios can potentially stimulate reflective skills, critical to all physicians' lifelong learning and assessment.
10. Portfolios facilitate an integrative approach to both individual assessment and actual medical practice.

Adapted from Friedman Ben-David M, Davis MH, Harden RM, Howie PW, Ker J, Pippard MJ. AMEE Medical Education Guide No. 24: Portfolios as a method of student assessment. *Med Teach*. 2001;23(6):535-551.

The authenticity of portfolio assessment is another key strength. Archbald and Newmann[47] defined authenticity as "the extent to which the outcomes measured represent appropriate, meaningful, significant and worthwhile forms of human accomplishments." Portfolios are seen as "authentic" since the contents of the portfolio reflect a comprehensive collection of evidence of what the trainee *actually does*, not just what they can do. Additionally, when trainees contribute to their portfolio they become invested in interpreting the evidence, reinforcing the authenticity, and making the assessment meaningful. This authenticity enhances the extrapolation of the portfolio—the link between current trainee performance and what they will be capable of doing later in real-world practice.

Finally, unlike other assessment methods, portfolios can be longitudinal collections of evidence over time and therefore capable of demonstrating professional development and progression. Portfolios can include multiple assessments that contribute to a summative judgment of competence, thus providing the structure for a comprehensive assessment system and fulfilling a key component of competency-based education.[31,48]

A 2001 systematic review of portfolios by Freidman Ben-David et al.[1] highlighted strengths still pertinent today that are summarized in Box 15.1.

Use of the Portfolio in Medical Education

Evidence of success for comprehensive portfolios exists in healthcare professions and elsewhere.[10,14–17,23,31] In medical education, the primary purpose of comprehensive portfolios is to demonstrate achievement and progressive professional development along a continuum. Each program must be very clear regarding the purpose(s) the portfolio will have in their educational program, be that formative, summative, or formative leading to summative. Whatever purpose is chosen, learners may have majority control of the contents, with guidance on the types of material or artifacts appropriate for the portfolio. Such content might include a particularly excellent write-up of a patient where they got a difficult diagnosis "right," a video-recorded encounter with a standardized patient, a research presentation, or a journal club write-up, accompanied by a reflection indicating the rationale for selection and what was learned from this evidence to demonstrate a specified skill or competency. One valuable attribute of this "learner-driven portfolio" is that it allows faculty to gain insight into what the trainee believes they did well, which provides a window into their insight and reflective capabilities. Such a portfolio embraces concepts of UDL, allowing learners autonomy in choosing how to represent their progress.

The portfolio approach can be used for formative and/or summative assessment; combining purposes can come at some risk but can be done.[49] Lau[50] provides perspectives on the terms *formative* and *summative*; in medical education formative assessment is often viewed as assessment that provides information to drive future learning (assessment for learning) while building skills toward a summative assessment. However, formative and summative assessments are not purely dichotomous. Rather, the stakes or consequences of an assessment fall along a spectrum. As noted in Chapter 3, no single assessment is sufficient to make a high-stakes decision. When multiple data points are collected through multiple assessment activities, the sum of these can provide a view of competence over time. Thus a portfolio can play an important role across the spectrum of formative and summative assessments. This perspective was highlighted in the 2020 Ottawa conference consensus statements for programmatic assessment that focus on learners' development. Portfolios were included as an opportunity to make decisions on learner progress.[35,51]

Faculty members should address additional considerations if the portfolio is to determine competence (e.g., summative plus formative assessment). The most important consideration will be determination of pass/fail criteria for the learner's portfolio. Traditionally, educators have examined the quality of an assessment method or tool based on psychometric criteria. Holistic methods, like portfolios, present unique challenges to traditional psychometrics. However, research demonstrates that rigorous application of qualitative methodologies can lead to equally high-quality, defensible judgments. Later in the chapter we will explore how both quantitative (psychometric) and qualitative principles can be cast into contemporary assessment frameworks to judge the results of portfolios.

Constructing a Comprehensive Portfolio

The term *comprehensive portfolio* denotes contents that are determined by both the training program and the trainee to maximize outcomes-based assessment in support of societal

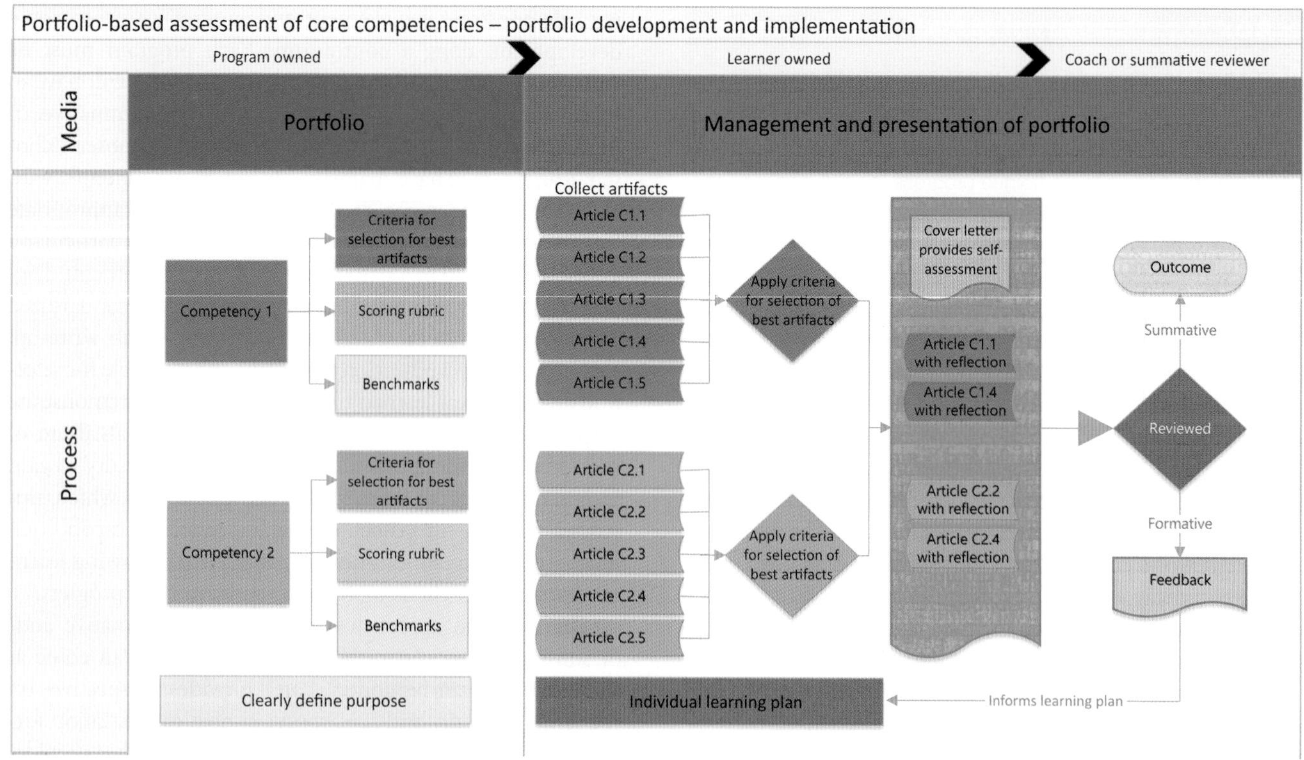

• **Fig. 15.2** Example of portfolio-based assessment of core competencies. Based on Portfolio Process by Patricia O'Sullivan, EdD.

needs. It may also contain what might be considered a "gradebook" component, or dashboard, where learners can reflect on existing data produced by program requirements. The comprehensive portfolio submitted for assessment includes both learner evidence and their critical reflection discussing how the evidence supports their competency achievement. Fig. 15.2 conveys an example of a portfolio process where initial formative processes build toward a summative decision.

When creating a comprehensive portfolio with both learner- and program-selected evidence, important considerations must guide its construction; this both ensures that the portfolio meets its intent and prompts learners to submit materials that align with program expectations. Here we will outline the portfolio design process from the perspective of the program, the learner, and the coach. We will end this section with a discussion of design features that support portfolio use for summative assessment.

Responsibilities of the Program: Defining the Purpose and Articulating the Approach to Evidence

As noted above, the first critical step in designing a portfolio is to articulate a clear purpose, including how it fits into the program of assessment. This purpose commonly serves to measure competencies not easily assessed by other means, such as professionalism, continuous learning and improvement, or teamwork.

Most portfolios currently in use by medical educators possess more structure than the traditional learning portfolio for several reasons. First, portfolios in medical education often are used for summative decision-making, which necessitates a defensible degree of standardization to ensure an acceptable level of validity. Second, medical educators are required to document a trainee's level of competence in specific knowledge, skills, and attitudes. Finally, summative assessment in medical education has implications for public accountability. Given the importance of competency throughout one's career, medical education programs would ideally implement longitudinal portfolios to facilitate competency-based medical practice spanning the continuum from early medical education to clinical practice.[34,52] Thus a portfolio used for summative assessment must not only meet rigorous assessment and research standards but also be credible and defensible to the public.

In the United States, several potential organizing frameworks for portfolios exist, such as the Accreditation Council for Graduate Medical Education (ACGME) competencies and the Association of American Medical Colleges (AAMC) Core Entrustable Professional Activities for Entering Residency.[53] For other educational systems, such as those in Canada and the United Kingdom, the Canadian Medical Education Directives for Specialists (CanMEDS) and Good Medical Practice competencies may guide the organization.[54,55]

Once a clear purpose and framework are articulated, the program will next specify a menu of contents, criteria for how to select evidence, and a rubric demonstrating how the portfolio will be assessed. We present an example based on the ACGME general competencies in Table 15.1 that lists potential assessment tools a program could include in

TABLE 15.1 Examples of Assessment Tools by ACGME Domain of Competence for Residency Training

Domain of Competence	Assessment Tool
Patient Care	• Rotation-specific assessment forms (checklists, global rating scales) • Direct observed history, physical examination, and communication • Critical incidents • Patient and procedure logs • Case log of "best" workups and patient interactions as determined by the trainee
Medical Knowledge	• NBME shelf examinations (medical school) or specialty in-training examinations • Critically appraised topic • Evidence-based medicine journal log • Clinical question log (generated by the trainee) • Chart-stimulated recall
Interpersonal and Communication Skills	• Direct observed history and patient communication • Multisource assessments and surveys • Trainee reflections on peer and patient feedback • Narrative of interview with peer or nursing staff
Professionalism	• Multisource assessments and surveys • Critical incidents and praise cards
Practice-based Learning and Improvement	• Individualized learning plan • Quality improvement project including self-audit of practice • Clinical question logs • Self-assessment and reflection • Web log dialogue and feedback with advisor
Systems-based Practice	• Project on navigating the healthcare system from the perspective of the patient • Project on system error, including critical incident analysis • Microsystem redesign project • Assessment of teamwork skills

a comprehensive portfolio to provide data to both the program and trainee. Benchmark examples help learners select evidence and self-assess.

As demonstrated in the example, portfolios emphasize a multifaceted approach to assessment. An assessment system based solely on global faculty ratings misses opportunities to coach residents to greater competence. Multiple assessment approaches are required to measure the level of competence for trainees,[46,56] and as a general rule each domain of competence should be assessed by more than one method. Assessments can include trainee-produced evidence that can be judged qualitatively and/or with a rubric. We encourage the reader to review the chapters in this book on specific assessment methods and tools to incorporate into a comprehensive assessment system. Within a portfolio, these tools provide competency-based data on which a learner can reflect and develop learning plans. Programs should encourage learners to select multiple types of assessment with perspectives from different assessors; this strengthens the validity evidence supporting portfolio decisions as a summative assessment tool.

In addition to clearly articulating a purpose and providing guidance regarding evidence selection, a program must also ensure that the portfolio process is transparent to the trainee. The learner should "own" the portfolio and its contents, with agreement between the learner and curricular leaders regarding the latter's ability to access parts of the portfolio necessary for assessment. For maximum utility, the program must also ensure that the learner receives sufficient time to thoughtfully prepare and submit a portfolio.

Finally, given the increase in the use of assessment dashboards, we will mention that dashboards can serve as a valuable component of a comprehensive portfolio. Dashboards may improve the ease with which learners and coaches navigate assessment data. However, without learner selection of their exemplar artifacts and critical reflection, dashboards do not constitute a portfolio in and of themselves. As we have highlighted throughout this chapter, portfolios require input, action, reflection, and engagement on the part of the learner.

Role of the Learner: Evidence Selection and Defense

A comprehensive portfolio can be part of a well-designed program of assessment, and a key strength lies in the *learner-centered* components of the process. The first component of this process requires learners to select evidence from authentic artifacts to demonstrate their competency achievement and reflect on how the evidence demonstrates competence and why they have chosen the specific evidence. This process provides a structured framework for the learner to build a self-regulated learning practice.

As noted above, the program will specify content areas and often provide a menu of options that the learner can include when selecting evidence in support of competency achievement. However, for the process to reach full potential, the learner will select a judicious sample of evidence that best supports their own assessment of their level of competency achievement. This evidence is not everything that they have done, but rather is selected to emphasize development of competence. Learners should include only that which supports impact and value on their development. This way, the portfolio requires learner engagement in carefully considering how they are learning and developing.

While graded/existing work may be selected as evidence, ideally this should not be the only data source; as noted by Driessen,[31] portfolios with proscribed data inputs have not demonstrated the same level of positive outcome as portfolios that require a higher level of learner engagement. Pitts and colleagues also cautioned against too much standardization as a threat to the strengths of the portfolio to drive self-directed learning.[57,58] Thus portfolios work best when learners contribute meaningful artifacts demonstrating evidence of professional growth and performance to the structured portfolio beyond assessments completed by others.[5,59,60] Learner autonomy also provides opportunities for coaches to provide feedback on self-assessment skill, a process that will be discussed later in this chapter.

When considering the composition of a portfolio, a variety of artifacts or data sources may support one subcompetency. Snadden and Thomas[59] list a number of items learners could provide including critical incidents of patient events, a reflective journal or diary, written descriptions of typical clinical experiences, video recordings of patient care interaction and experiences, clinical care audits, articles reviewed critically using evidence-based medicine principles, self-selected materials the learner believes demonstrate proficiency, and any materials the learner wishes to keep as a resource for future learning. For example, a resident seeking to demonstrate skill in the subcompetency of interprofessional communication skills may choose to include a sample written note, data from multisource assessments completed by healthcare team members, feedback from a mock-paging exercise, or reflections on the contributions of other team members to the care of mutual patients. Nonclinical activities can also demonstrate key competencies; learners may choose to include research projects or volunteer activities as important contributions to the portfolio as evidence of problem-based learning and improvement or community engagement.

The second critical component of the portfolio is the self-regulated learning process, including self-assessment with reflection. We discuss self-assessment and reflection as activities that occur after learner selection of artifacts, though in reality these processes occur simultaneously and iteratively. Ideally, learners review data, self-assess, reflect on their assessments, and rereview data to support their judgment of their competency achievement in iterative fashion. Driessen[31] and others note that the word *reflection* itself may present challenges for learners, who may associate reflection with emotion or feelings. Instead, one can frame the process as a justification or defense, similar to the process a medical learner engages in when discussing data supporting or refuting a diagnosis in a differential.

Various approaches can facilitate learner reflection and subsequent behavior change. Scholars have used "commitment to change" (CTC) statements, a process that has shown an increased likelihood that individuals will actually change their behavior.[61–63] A second method is simply to use an open-ended written reflection structured by guiding questions. A third approach is to build reflection around an individualized learning plan.[10] This has become a popular approach to organizing the reflection to incorporate action, which aligns with the emphasis on self-regulated learning. We will address additional facilitators and challenges to engaging learners in this process later in the chapter.

Role and Value of the Portfolio Coach: Calibrating Learner Self-Assessment

As noted above, responsibility and management for the portfolio belong to both the individual and program. The program's representative often provides guidance or feedback in helping the learner select and reflect on evidence in support of competency demonstration; we refer to this program representative as a "coach" throughout the chapter, a role strongly advocated for in the portfolio literature.[31] As the comprehensive portfolio can represent a longitudinal process, the learner and coach should interact on a regular basis to ensure sufficient guidance to align the portfolio with its purpose. Student success in learning from assessment data is enhanced when the self-reflection occurs in partnership with a longitudinal coach who serves to enhance the student's ability to create meaningful learner goals that promote continuous improvement.[64] While a full discussion of coaching is beyond the scope of this chapter, we encourage readers to review Chapter 14.

Key among the roles of a coach is to work with the learner to facilitate quality self-assessment and reflection. Portfolios are an ideal format for this process as individuals can review and reflect on data they receive from multiple sources[64,65] to arrive at a conclusion regarding competence. During the self-assessment process, learners may experience "knowledge–performance" discordance: their knowledge about the correct performance is high, the trainee believes they exhibit correct behaviors, but feedback about actual performance demonstrates evidence to the contrary. In these moments, learners appropriately experience emotional discomfort that, with coaching, can provide energy to motivate behavior change to align their actual performance with the desired performance. This experience can also enhance the generation of meaningful reflections.[66] Evidence and the authors' personal experience suggest that when the gap is discovered through self-assessment, it carries more salience and professional reward than one exposed by someone else[63,67] (see Chapter 14). This experience can be improved through review of the performance data with a trusted coach.[64]

When engaging coaches, the authors' experience and the observations of Davis,[75] Eva, and others reinforce the notion that an accurate judgment of performance cannot be made without standard measures based on credible data,[68] as self-assessment in the absence of credible data is unlikely to be of much value. Thus the research around self-assessment lends support for the importance of some level of standardized reflection with a coach instead of in isolation, and clear assessment criteria for portfolios. Tables 15.2 and 15.3 provide a summary of tools to assess reflective ability in undergraduate and post graduate trainees. Faculty may want to consider using these tools with their trainees at the beginning of and during a learning cycle or portfolio process.

TABLE 15.2 **Reflective Ability in Undergraduates**

Assessment Tool	PDRA[a] Professional Development of Reflective Ability	Script Concordance Test[b]	RP[c] Reflective Portfolio	RCV[d] Reflection-evoking Case Vignettes	Structured Worksheet[e]	LEaP[f] Learning Experiences as a Professional
Institution	University of Dundee	Laval University Medical School, Quebec	University of Nottingham	Free University, Amsterdam	University of London	University of California, San Francisco
Course	Professional and Personal Development	Clerkship in Surgery	Communication Skills	Clinical Ethics	Clinical Experience	Multiple Opportunities
Year	Years 4 and 5	Medical students	Year 2	Year 4	Dental therapy students	Years 1–3
Assessment type	Summative	Formative	Summative	Summative	Formative	Formative
Content	The 12 outcome summary sheets	38 clinical vignettes in 4 surgical topics: breast lump; gastrointestinal bleeding; acute abdominal pain; and lump in the thyroid gland	• 800-word reflective commentary • Practical evidence over six practicals ✓ 6 personal reflection forms ✓ 3 peer observation forms ✓ 3 teacher observation forms	Semistructured questionnaire with 4 case vignettes. 1. What are your feelings? 2. What should be the appropriate professional behavior in the case concerned?	• What happened? • Describe your feelings. • Why do you consider this worthy of reflection? • What strengths in your clinical practice did this demonstrate? • What learning did this reveal? • Which one learning need do you address as a priority? • Decide exactly what you would like to achieve. • Complete "target testing."	Written critical reflections on experiences with professionalism and during clinical activities Follows a SOAP format
Structure	Semistructured	Structured	Flexible	Semistructured	Structured	Semistructured
Assessment criteria	Standardized rubric: based on the ability to identify, evaluate, and monitor personal progress		Standardized rubric	Standardized rubric ✓ Overall reflection: 10-point scale. ✓ Perspectives series: 0–2-point scale	Qualitative assessment ✓ Johns' questions ✓ Hatton and Smith's criteria	Standardized rubric 0–6-point scale (when used for research); descriptive feedback when used for formative assessment
Psychometric evaluation	Supports construct validity	Acceptable predictive validity; moderate reliability	Supports construct validity and 0.8 interrater reliability	Supports construct validity and interrater reliability	Good interjudge agreement, especially for Hatton and Smith's criteria	Requires 2 assessors for interrater reliability >.80; has been assessed for construct-irrelevant variance; enhances quality of reflection
Student attitude	Positive		Neutral	Not mentioned	Positive	Neutral with some liking and others feeling restricted by format

[a]From Ker JS, Friedman Ben-David M, Pippard MJ, Davis MH. Determining the construct validity of a tool to assess the reflective ability of final year medical students using portfolio evidence. Members' abstracts, Association for the Study of Medical Education (ASME), Annual Scientific Meeting, 2003, pp. 20-21.

[b]From Brailovsky C, Charlin B, Beausoleil S, Cote S, van der Vleuten CPM. Measurement of clinical reflective capacity early in training as a predictor of clinical reasoning performance at the end of residency: an experimental study on the script concordance test. *Med Educ.* 2001;35(5):430-436.

[c]From Rees C, Sheard C. Undergraduate medical students' views about a reflective portfolio assessment of their communications skills learning. *Med Educ.* 200438(2):125-128.

[d]From Boenink AD, Oderwald AK, De Jonge P, van Tilburg W, Smal JA. Assessing students' reflection in medical practice. The development of an observer-rated instrument: reliability, validity and initial experiences. *Med Educ*. 2004;38(4)368-377.

[e]From Pee B, Woodman T, Fry H, Davenport ES. Appraising and assessing reflection in students' writing on a structured worksheet. *Med Educ*. 2002;36(6):575-585.

[f]From Aronson L, Niehaus B, Hill-Sakuai L, Lai C, O'Sullivan PS. A comparison of two teaching methods to promote reflective ability in third year medical students. *Med Educ.* 2012;46(8):807-814.

Acknowledgment: This table was prepared by Dr. Gominda Ponnamperuma, University of Dundee, Dundee, Scotland. in 2007; updated 2016.

TABLE 15.3 Assessing Reflective Ability in Postgraduates

Assessment Tool	Reflective Personal Development Plans[a]	Pediatric Specialist Registrars Portfolio Assessment[b]	Reflection on Action[c]
Institution	Postgraduate deaneries in the UK	Royal College of Paediatrics & Child Health	University of California, San Francisco
Course	General Practice	Paediatrics	Obstetrics and Gynecology
Year	Continuing professional development	Years 1–5 in postgraduate training	Years 1–4 in postgraduate training
Assessment type	Earlier formative, latterly summative	Summative	Summative for semiannual review
Content	Patient-focused critical incidents, audits, critical reading, patient and peer feedback	Clinical letters and reports, presentation handouts, ethical submissions and parent information leaflets, feedback educational sessions, thank-you letters, course attendance certificates, reports on MSc/MMedSci assignments, group achievements	Reflection on specific experiences related to competencies of Communication and Interpersonal Skills, Professionalism, Practice-based Learning and Improvement, Systems-based Practice
Structure	Semistructured	Unstructured	Unstructured
Assessment criteria	Identification of learning needs, learning plan, assessment plan, understanding, performance	Global and domain-specific ratings on an unsatisfactory–fair–good–excellent rating scale. Domains: clinical, communication, ethics/attitudes, self-learning/teaching, evaluation/creation of evidence, management	Rating on the Reflection on Action scale
Psychometric evaluation	Acceptable content and construct validity; reliability of 0.8 with 7 raters and 0.7 with 3–4 raters	Reliability of 0.8 with 4 raters	Reliability of 0.8 with 2 raters; evidence of relationship to other variables

[a]From Roberts C, Cromarty I, Crossley J, Jolly B. The reliability and validity of a matrix to assess the completed reflective personal development plans of general practitioners. *Med Educ.* 2006;40(4):363-370.

[b]From Melville C, Rees M, Brookfield D, Anderson J. Portfolio for assessment of paediatric specialist registrars. *Med Educ*. 2004;38(10):1117-1125.

[c]From Learman LA, Autry AM, O'Sullivan P. Reliability and validity of reflection exercises for obstetrics and gynecology residents. *Am J Obstet Gynecol.* 2008;198(4):461-468; discussion 461.e8.

Acknowledgment: This table was prepared by Dr. Gominda Ponnamperuma, University of Dundee, Dundee, Scotland, 2007; updated 2016.

Designing a Portfolio to Support Summative Assessment

The endpoint of the process described above will vary by program and need. In a competency-based model, the cycle will repeat until the learner and mentor assess the learner's portfolio as meeting competency standards. In other programs the process remains time based, and the portfolio is submitted for summative review at designated time points in a learner's training, such as between phases of an undergraduate medical education (UME) program[10] or perhaps to a clinical competency committee (CCC) in graduate medical education (GME) (see Chapter 16).

When designing a portfolio to support summative assessment, assessment must follow the principle of "triangulation." We refer to triangulation in two respects. First, if employed effectively and properly, some assessments may be used to assess more than one domain of competence. For example, a mini clinical evaluation exercise (mini-CEX) can capture skill in both patient care and interpersonal communication.[69] Second, building on the work of Davis, Driessen, and others, the assessment of the portfolio itself should involve more than the perspective of a single assessor.[10,13,70] Qualitative methods and the application of computer-based text analysis methods[71] hold promise in evaluating the "descriptive" aspects of the portfolio.[70,72] We will discuss these concepts more in "Reliability and Validity in Portfolio Assessment: Challenges and Opportunities."

To summarize, this section focused on the design of the comprehensive portfolio, and we have addressed the program, the learner, the coach, and summative assessment. The program specifies the purpose and framework for the portfolio. The learner then actively engages in the selection of content to support competency achievement, assembling and reflecting on the content of the portfolio. The learner reviews the comprehensive portfolio with a coach who provides feedback and helps the individual devise and carry out a learning plan. The cycle repeats until the portfolio is submitted for summative review (if a part of the program).

Now that we have reviewed key principles in portfolio design, we will shift to critical components of implementation.

Implementation

We have delineated strengths to a portfolio as an assessment tool. Full realization of these strengths requires thoughtful and continuous attention to implementation with focus on electronic portfolio infrastructure, coach development, learner development, and rater training.

Electronic Portfolio

Implementation of portfolios today relies on electronic platforms. While most of the portfolio literature focuses on the structure for the e-portfolio, Batson[73] argued that e-portfolios were "profoundly disruptive" and expressed concern that few recognized the way technology has changed what we can do and the best way to use this format. When selecting the electronic platform, one must consider how it can influence success.[74,75] In short, the assessment must be clear as to whether or not the technology is a criterion for the assessment or a contributor to irrelevant variance in the assessment.[22] However, a highlight of the disruption Batson refers to is the potential for longitudinal as well as diverse artifacts. Hiradhar and Bhattacharya[75] indicate that e-portfolios have advantages in that they can include multimedia files and have the potential to allow peers to interact with each other's work. The question is what gains the technology gives pedagogically.[22]

In higher education, Walland and Shaw's[22] review showed that e-portfolios were primarily used for self-reflection and for collecting evidence of skills needed for future employment. In Carter's[74] 2021 review of e-portfolios, she notes that assessment e-portfolios in the tertiary education setting provide connections to authentic work where the evidence collected can be unpredictable. Students attest that an e-portfolio helps them critically assess their work and accomplishments and valued peer review to validate competencies.[77]

Guidance exists for implementing e-portfolios in health professions.[78] Faculty need to attend to digital literacy skills and be particularly mindful of the privacy regulations of their country, such as the Health Insurance Portability and Accountability Act (HIPAA) regulations in the United States.[16,79] In addition, technology can lead to ease in plagiarism and schools have turned to programs to ensure originality of portfolio work.[16] Box 15.2 summarizes recommendations related to educational and technical standards that may facilitate successful implementation of any portfolio assessment system.[28,78,80–82] For further considerations, consult the International Journal of ePortfolio (https://www.theijep.com/).

Coach Development

While a full discussion of coaching is beyond the scope of this chapter, its importance in the portfolio process cannot be overstated. As noted by Driessen, "without mentoring [coaching], portfolios have no future and are nothing short of bureaucratic hurdles in our competency-based education programs."[31] Coaches who take a learner-oriented approach can offer new perspectives that help learners realistically assess and value their skills, and enable students to perceive the benefit from portfolio work.[64] A challenge inherent in this approach is that it requires adequate coaching capacity to engage in significant relationship building with learners; in some models, there may be a need to include peer- or near-peer coaching to enhance coaching capacity in a feasible way.

How can coaches motivate students to find benefit in the portfolio process? First, by linking performance examples from the current learning environment placed in their portfolio to future practice. Coaches in the preclinical curriculum can share how current performance may relate to the future clinical environment. In the authors' experience, coaches who are open to normalizing challenges by sharing their own experiences can facilitate learner engagement with the portfolio process. Coaches need to recognize and understand how each student's prior experiences can enhance their learning process, focusing on a strengths-based approach to feedback and reflection. Ideally, coaches will have a strong foundation in facilitating reflection that supports a growth mindset and learning orientation for each learner.[83]

Beyond selecting coaches, for portfolio success significant time and attention is required to train the coaches. In the authors' institution (CLO and BMD), coaches participate in a coaching curriculum. During their first year as coaches, their curriculum includes a 1-day orientation prior to the start of the school year, followed by monthly 1-hour meetings and quarterly 3-hour development sessions to review coaching theory and the philosophy of the portfolio process and to participate in case discussions. Following this, monthly 1-hour sessions continue for the additional 3 years that the coaches are part of the process. The coaches are encouraged to discuss coaching scenarios that arise as a group to continue to develop the coaching skill set.

Learner Orientation

Learners require orientation to and education about the process of critical reflection on progression to competency. As we have discussed above, the purpose of the portfolio and the competencies it will address must be made clear, as clarity of purpose drives the selection of artifacts that will inform summative assessment. Sharing several examples of ways that a learner might select artifacts to demonstrate competency can keep the process learner centered while also providing parameters for what is expected or acceptable. The authors' (CLO and BMD) medical school provides the students a curriculum parallel to what the coaches receive. In four 1-hour sessions over a 6-month period, students learn core concepts in giving feedback, using feedback for growth, devising learning plans, and writing critical reflection of their learning. Their first coaching meeting occurs

• BOX 15.2 Recommendations for Implementation of a Portfolio

Educational Standards

Both the vision and definition of *portfolio* are clearly stated.

There is a match between portfolio goals and their content and structure.

A flexible educational configuration, rather than traditional teacher-directed education, is in place to support a portfolio-driven program of assessment.

Faculty support of the educational innovation/configuration ensures that the portfolio is supported as the appropriate assessment and prevents the portfolio from being the "face" of the innovation.

The learning environment is well suited for challenging students to be self-directed learners acquiring learning in authentic complex task situations, aligning portfolio assessment with learning opportunities.

Learners clearly understand the reasons for developing a portfolio.

Learners maintain intellectual ownership of the portfolio, managing their own learning based on evidence and providing assessment information to meet university expectations.

Learners are empowered to develop a portfolio that allows for creativity while respecting the expectations of the institution for a portfolio demonstrating professional development.

Learners must receive feedback about their portfolio to realize its value or they do not see it meriting the needed time investment.

An advisor, who is generally not an assessor, serves as an advocate and guide who facilitates learning and provides counsel as to which materials best demonstrate developmental progression.

Institutional leadership requires the portfolio as part of the learning and assessment process because it aligns with the learning approach.

Institutional leadership supports portfolio use across the continuum of medical education.

Institutional leadership shows commitment to the portfolio by dedicating curricular time and providing faculty, learner, and staff development as well as educationally appropriate technology and financial resources.

The university or sponsoring institution maintains a portfolio oversight committee including faculty and learners.

Research and scholarship about portfolios is conducted to both improve the functionality and obtain evidence of validity.

Technical

Institutional leadership solicits input from learners on choice or development of electronic portfolio platform.

Adequate resources are available to users, such as hardware, software, personnel for training, and ongoing help during implementation and maintenance phases, respectively.

Selected software, accessible to both faculty and learners, allows for collection, storage, and organization, with an ability to allow or deny sharing of contents by the owner (student).

The electronic portfolio system is available to students when and where needed, and provides a platform that supports the latest web browsers and technologies.

System maintenance and downtimes coincide with low learner use time.

The electronic portfolio system ideally integrates with other key applications used to manage medical education, such as School of Medicine technology platforms that support student learning activities as well as residency management systems, providing a seamless experience for users navigating among the systems.

The electronic portfolio is capable of importing existing student information from other portfolios, institutions, or applications (e.g., undergraduate institutions) and also exporting learner portfolios upon graduation to other portfolio systems (e.g., residency programs, fellowship programs, and Maintenance of Certification [MOC] programs).

The electronic portfolio is robust and scalable, capable of supporting numerous learners.

Learners use the electronic portfolio to assemble and display media-rich evidence of progression.

The electronic portfolio has a user-friendly front end that is easily navigated with minimal training, however it is tagged with metadata that support labeling and organization of evidence on the back end.

The electronic portfolio maintains confidentiality and privacy of the learners; learners are informed about who has access to their portfolios and why.

Generated from the Electronic Portfolio Implementation Committee, University of California San Francisco; Willmarth-Stec M, Beery T. Operationalizing the student electronic portfolio for doctoral nursing education. *Nurse Educ*. 2015;40(5):263-265; Van Tartwijk J, Driessen E, van der Vleuten C, Stokking K. Factors influencing the successful introduction of portfolios. *QHE*. 2007;13(1):69-79; and Siddiqui ZS, Fisher MB, Slade C, et al. Twelve tips for introducing e-portfolios in health professions education. *Med Teach*. 2022:1-6. Epub ahead of print.

during that 6-month period, allowing them to experience the process while learning the basic theories and practices.

While much has been written about the challenges of engaging students in reflective practice, "best practices" are less well defined. Learners can be reminded that this process will continue across their careers as a physician. As health professionals, most individuals will have annual performance reviews or will be tasked with making continuous quality improvement plans based on institutional- or payer-specified metrics. Medical educators may be tasked with maintaining an educator portfolio demonstrating competency and can be used to support academic promotions.[84]

Notably, in their qualitative analysis of student perspectives on a portfolio assessment process, Schrempf et al.[18] found that 73% of students reported benefitting from the process even though only 36.1% fully approved of the process of reflecting on progress in a structured manner. Several participants saw it as an advantage to be able to track their development over time and to be aware of their own progress.[85]

Rater/Evaluator Development

Portfolios require judgment by faculty whether they are used for formative or summative purposes. Thus faculty assessors become a source of error that threatens the "generalizability" of trainee performance. Specific faculty rating issues include the stability of their judgments over time, stability of judgments between different faculty raters, and reproducibility of pass/fail decisions.[1] One of the biggest concerns about using portfolios for summative purposes in medical education is the several studies demonstrating a lack of reasonable reliability, including intra- and interrater agreements that are not as high as with standardized assessments.[57,58,86]

As with any assessment method, reliability can always be improved by using multiple assessors. However, this can be very resource intensive and time consuming. Standardization of criteria is an important first step. Koretz argued that high levels of agreement depend on clear criteria, adequately communicating those criteria to the students, robust student orientation materials, a shared faculty understanding of the assessment purpose, and adequate examiner training.[6] This process is similar to frame-of-reference rater training (discussed in Chapter 5), which emphasizes defining performance standards and allowing for practice and feedback using these standards and has been shown to increase rater reliability.

It is noteworthy that for several of the early studies showing poor reliability in medical education portfolios, little information was provided about faculty training.[57,58,87] One of the few studies of portfolios to demonstrate good reliability and some evidence for validity involved a full day of rater training at the beginning of the project, followed by retraining with the scoring rubrics prior to actual portfolio review.[87,88] O'Sullivan and colleagues, using this faculty training approach for a portfolio in a psychiatry residency, found they could achieve sufficient reliably for relative decisions with just two raters, and achieve a generalizability coefficient of 0.7 with just one additional rater.[88] Gadbury-Amyot and colleagues,[89] using multivariate generalizability theory, found that they needed at least two raters for their portfolio. Additionally, they found that three pieces of evidence within a component of the portfolio was sufficient to obtain a reliable score.

The University of Dundee medical student portfolio contains a broad sampling of the student's work and achievements, including multiple patient and care presentations, log of procedures, special study modules, clinical rotation assessment, learning contracts, and structured reflection reports. Dundee's assessment system provides a substantial amount of structure to the portfolio process with clear criteria and expectation for the students.[13] The University of Dundee has experienced results similar to O'Sullivan; 98% agreement of pass/fail decisions was achieved using two-rater pairs. The Dundee program, like the O'Sullivan program, incorporated substantial rater training.[13]

O'Brien and colleagues[10] also found success using two raters, who were trained using an approach similar to frame-of-reference training. Faculty raters, or reviewers, are first introduced to the competencies assessed in the portfolio, as well as expected performance benchmarks. They then individually review the same two portfolios and return as a group for a consensus-building activity in which results are shared and discrepancies discussed. Reviewers continue to use discussion to reconcile discrepancies throughout the process, as this has been shown to increase reliability during portfolio assessment.[57] If the reviewers are unable to reach agreement using this method, a third rater is brought in to contribute their perspective.

There are limitations to evaluator development. Even trained portfolio raters will still bring different interpretations, heuristics, and biases to their judgments, even if they eventually arrive at the same decisions.[90] Open discussions can make biases and assumptions more explicit and bring transparency to decisions while valuing multiple perspectives, which however idiosyncratic, can also be legitimate and fair.[36,91]

Reliability and Validity in Portfolio Assessment: Challenges and Opportunities

Measurement in medical education has undergone substantive transition in the past 50 years.[48] Historically, we applied the psychometric principles of reliability and validity when judging the quality of an assessment tool. However, recall that the major strengths of the portfolio process include the collection of *descriptive* assessment materials, *written* learner self-assessment and reflection, and the *holistic, composite* nature of a portfolio. Applying psychometric methods to portfolio assessment may be limiting. In contrast, in competency-based education greater emphasis is placed on measuring hard things and with an emphasis on both judgment and validity.[92] Consequently, there have been several

• BOX 15.3 Qualitative Research Strategies to Ensure Credibility and Dependability of Portfolio Assessment

Strategy to Establish Trustworthiness	Criteria	Description	Potential Assessment Strategy
Credibility	Prolonged engagement	Sufficient interaction, over time, from the faculty mentor or others	Training of examiners
	Triangulation	The use of information from different sources about the same construct	Tailored volume of expert judgment based on certainty of information
	Peer examination	Ability of different examiners to arrive at similar decision	Benchmarking examiners through review and feedback
	Member checking	"Test" the data with the member (e.g., trainee) of the group	Incorporate learner view
	Structural coherence	Coherent rationale of judgments	Scrutiny of committee inconsistencies
Transferability	Time sampling	Availability of a broad sample of data across time	Judgment based on broad sample of data points
	Thick description	Depth of narrative details	Justify decisions
Dependability	Stepwise replication	External assessment	Use multiple assessors who have credibility
Confirmability	Audit	Documentation of process	Give learners the possibility to appeal the assessment decision

approaches to clarifying validity evidence for qualitative data. We will share an approach based on guidance from qualitative research[70] and one from an examination of contemporary assessment frameworks.[72] Both examples use a rigorous assessment approach to ensure defensible decisions with qualitative data and are in line with changing trends in assessment in medical education that focus on assessment as judgment and assessment as a system.[48] The second example demonstrates how to apply both the Messick[93] and Kane[94] frameworks for collecting validity evidence, providing guidance on the types of evidence one should accrue when developing and implementing a portfolio.

Example 1: Applying Qualitative Arguments to Portfolio Validity

In the first example, Driessen and colleagues at Maastricht University developed an assessment procedure to judge year-one medical student portfolios using qualitative research criteria[70] of credibility (e.g., internal validity) and dependability (e.g., reliability). Box 15.3 describes their qualitative methodological argument with description and associated assessment strategies to ensure credibility and dependability in judging a portfolio.

The Driessen protocol can be viewed in Fig. 15.3. Using this protocol, 96% of the portfolios were graded without review by the full committee. This early study suggests that complementary, qualitative approaches are possible for assessment of portfolios, and clearly others will need to replicate Driessen's findings with more advanced trainees.

This approach potentially allows educators to "sample through" bias and interrater variation by continuing to sample until a stable judgment can be attained. The importance of sampling cannot be overstated. Much of assessment also depends on the context in which the assessment occurs. The greater the sampling, the more likely the program will gather a more robust picture of trainee competency over multiple domains *and* contexts. This is one of the major potential advantages of portfolio assessment. Similarly, there is a benefit in multiple assessors when possible; assessors often arrive at the same decision but from varying perspectives.[90] This approach also must acknowledge the resource requirements and consider new strategies including natural language processing (NLP) and training individuals from diverse backgrounds as assessors instead of just faculty members.

Example 2: Adapting Messick and Kane's Arguments to Apply to a Portfolio

In the second example, we highlight the approaches advocated by Cook and colleagues using contemporary assessment frameworks. These authors followed Messick's five sources of evidence for validity[93] and Kane's four validity arguments[94] to model how to provide an assessment of validity of qualitative evidence. From Messick, we should develop validity evidence in five categories: content, response process, internal structure, relationship to other variables, and consequences. Kane, on the other hand, emphasizes inferences. He focuses on the argument for validity based on the inferences that can be made concerning scoring, generalization, extrapolation, and implications. These approaches are considering the portfolio as a whole and the goal is an emphasis on competence, so the tasks are likely to be complex and authentic, require a degree of subjectivity or judgment, and thus require a holistic perspective.[95]

The validity evidence of a portfolio is dependent on both the quality of the evidence presented and the process used by assessors (as highlighted in the Driessen strategy). The assessor must be able to determine that the portfolio as a whole demonstrates that the trainee has achieved the

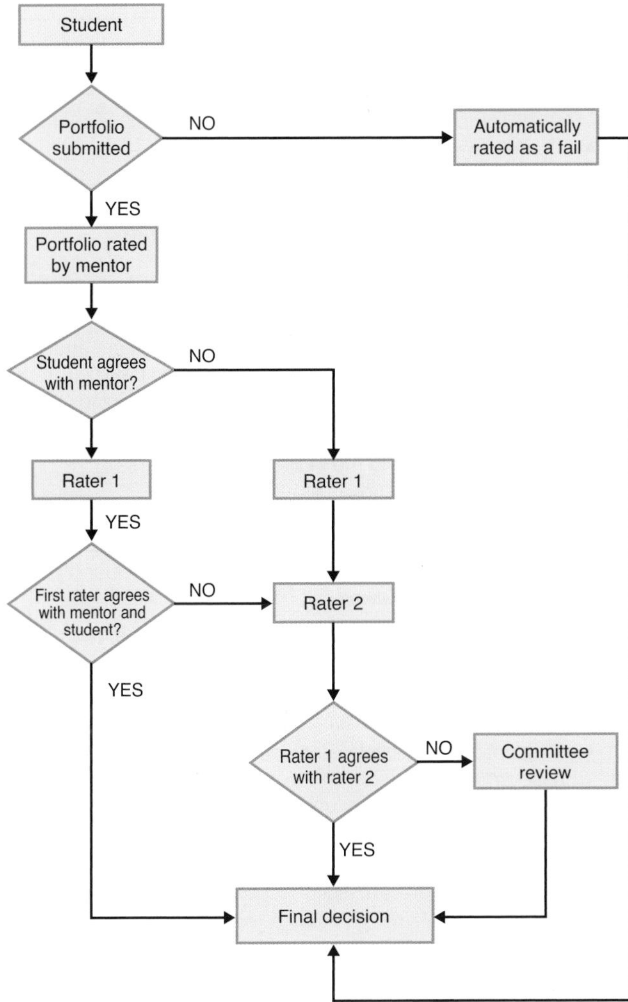

• **Fig. 15.3** Example of a portfolio assessment process that uses qualitative research criteria to reach consensus, including member checking and triangulation. Only a small number of student portfolios causing persistent disagreement are reviewed by the full committee.

specified educational endpoints. We have laid out the psychometric issues using both Messick (see Table 15.4) and Kane (see Table 15.5) to demonstrate validity evidence for portfolio assessments using the two assessment frameworks. Cook and colleagues[72] reviewed portfolios using these two frames. Below we elaborate the kind of evidence expected.

Messick's Framework

Portfolio Content

The evidence of content validity for the descriptive content of the portfolio, such as the trainee-selected evidence, reflections, and narratives, requires specification of basic criteria and structure. This content evidence could include the methods used to word questions regarding how the portfolio content will be assessed and how evidence will be selected for judging the portfolio. For example, a program may ask the trainee to answer a series of questions about a particular experience[63] and the wording of these questions is critical to support appropriate content. In most portfolios there will be learner-selected materials, so the criteria for selecting that evidence will be critically important to contribute to evidence of content validity. Benchmark examples also enhance the content validity. Standardization of portfolio contents can help improve the portfolio assessment process. Standardization comes with the menu that the program specifies as part of elaborating the definition and purpose of the portfolio. This standardization can allow for qualitative and quantitative data. Evidence from review of workplace-based portfolios supports content validity of portfolios.[96]

Response Process

Response process reflects the processes used in the documentation included in a portfolio and the assessor's interpretation. Cook et al.[72] note that having a secure place for documentation relates to response process validity for portfolios. Imagine the challenge should an electronic portfolio tool (e.g., with various types of entry fields) not be sufficient to contain all the narrative evidence a trainee was submitting. Response process validity includes evidence that assessors follow the instructions provided and that the format by which the information was delivered was complete. Earlier in this chapter we detailed training of individuals to be raters as part of the implementation process. The number and qualifications of the assessors also need to be considered. Portfolios are novel in that a learner may also be an assessor (certainly for self, but perhaps for peers) and thus learners must be prepared for this role as part of the validity evidence for response process.

Additionally, it would be important to know the biases and perspective the assessor brings to the responsibility of assessing the portfolio. Assessors are aware of the potential for bias in grading in the clinical environments[97] and the value of unconscious bias training.[98] Programs such as our own require that assessors undergo unconscious bias training that can be applicable for this assessment as well as for others.

A common error in all assessments is failure to adequately train the faculty who provide the ratings and judgment.[99,100] Faculty training in portfolio assessment is essential as we highlighted earlier in this chapter. Much of the response process corresponds to the credibility issues identified when using traditional qualitative approaches.

Internal Structure

Tools (e.g., a self-audit of medical records, objective structured clinical examinations [OSCEs], in-training examinations) can be part of the quantitative self-assessment content for the portfolio.[63] Each tool must also have evidence of validity and one common metric is reliability. For the qualitative data, the assessor might then look for triangulation among the quantitative and qualitative evidence and the narrative analysis and reflection as evidence of validity for internal structure. This should be supported with a description written by the assessor. This is similar to both triangulation and thick description.

TABLE 15.4 Applying Messick's Validity Framework to Portfolios

Type of Evidence	Definition	Examples for Portfolio
Content	How well does the content of the portfolio fit with the constructs it is intended to measure?	• Portfolio menu of contents • Instructions for learners regarding how to select artifacts and guidelines for reflection • Criteria for assessing the portfolio (if summative decisions are included)
Response process	How good is the fit between the construct of the portfolio and the actual processes and procedures applied when implemented?	• Documentation of rater training efforts, including frame of reference training if used • Examples of sample portfolios used to train raters and documentation of discussions raised during training • Unconscious bias training modules or other training materials to identify and address rater bias
Internal structure	How well do the components of the portfolio fit together and support the overarching process?	• Evidence supporting the individual components comprising the portfolio • Number and type of assessments or artifacts supporting each domain of competence assessed • Quantity and quality of narrative description included in the data being reviewed
Relationship to other variables	Do the results of the portfolio assessment correlate (or not correlate) with other measures in the way that might be expected?	• Correlation with clerkship grades, OSCE scores, and NBME shelf exams
Consequences	What is the impact of the assessment? Is there sufficient evidence to justify the consequences if used for summative decision-making?	• Description of possible outcomes of summative assessment • Analysis of positive and unintended consequences of portfolio implementation

NBME, National Board of Medical Examiners; *OSCE*, objective structured clinical examination.

TABLE 15.5 Applying Kane's Validity Framework to Portfolios

Type of Evidence	Definitions[a]	Examples for Portfolio
Scoring	Translating observations and data into one or more scores	• Menu of options for artifact selection ◦ Validity evidence supporting individual tools if included as artifacts • Training processes for learners to create portfolio • Training procedures for raters • Rubric supporting summative judgments
Generalization	Using the scores as a reflection of performance in a test setting	• Consideration of how well artifacts selected provide triangulation supporting a given skill rating • Reflexivity and transparency of the process of review • Consistency of the interpretations and summative assessments of different raters
Extrapolation	Using the scores as a reflection of real-world performance	• Assessment of how well artifacts mirror the authentic work environment • Discussion of how well the portfolio assessment translates to other contexts
Implications	Applying the scores to inform a decision or action	• Evidence of the implications of using portfolio to assess a learner's performance

[a]From Cook DA, Brydges R, Ginsburg S, Hatala R. A contemporary approach to validity arguments: a practical guide to Kane's framework. *Med Educ*. 2015;49(6):560-575.

Relationship to Other Variables

How the assessment from the portfolio relates to other variables is important in all validity frameworks. One should examine how the conclusions from the portfolio assessment associate with other evidence external to the portfolio or to the quantitative elements within the portfolio. Since acquiring validity evidence is an ongoing activity, the relationship to other variables may take time to accumulate.

There is an increasing body of validity evidence of the portfolio process.[72] We highlight several studies that have addressed evidence related to other variables. O'Brien and colleagues[101] studied two groups of students, those whose summative preclerkship portfolios had concerns raised in one or more competencies and those who progressed satisfactorily. Those with concerning preclerkship performance received lower clerkship grades. Gadbury-Amyot and colleagues, in reviewing 15 years of portfolio assessment in dental hygiene, found association between performance and GPA and licensure examination.[102] O'Sullivan and colleagues, in performing a validity analysis of their psychiatry portfolio, found a modest correlation between in-training exam scores and some evidence of increasing portfolio scores with each increasing year of training.[88] One of the main goals of the portfolio process, and one of its greatest strengths, is the promotion of self-directed learning and reflection. O'Sullivan and colleagues performed interviews of the residents about their experience and learned many, but not all, of the residents found the process to be useful personally. Other residents viewed the portfolio as simply a research project. Portfolios are touted as providing the data needed for assessment of Entrustable Professional Activities (EPAs).[49] Research should continue to identify how portfolios can be a robust catalyst for self-directed, lifelong learning.[88]

Consequences

Within the Messick framework the last category of evidence to collect relates to consequences. This includes satisfaction among all stakeholders with the results of the assessment as well as with the efforts to develop and assess the portfolio. Studying five years of the use of a portfolio in a family medicine residency, McEwen and colleagues[26] report the positive impact of portfolios at the individual, programmatic, and institutional levels. A study of portfolios as a form of assessment requires examining both the intended and unintended consequences. Cook et al.[72] point to a number of studies that have assessed consequences both favorable and unfavorable.

Kane's Framework

Above we described how to approach validity from the Messick framework with a strong emphasis on how to collect evidence with qualitative data. Now we would like to highlight points from Kane's framework (see Table 15.5). Kane's framework requires effort in designing the assessment to ensure that purposes, intended use and decision, and necessary evidence to support these decisions are specified. As noted above, the development and successful implementation of a portfolio requires that all of these elements are provided to the learners before assembling a portfolio.

First, applying Kane's framework, we should examine what kinds of evidence assessors provide in support of their scoring.[103] In this case there may be a narrative that accompanies a decision around qualitative data. Additionally, descriptions of preparation and unconscious bias training could be included. Second, the evidence across all elements of either a competency or the entire portfolio (if that is the form for the assessment decision) should allow the assessor to construe an overall impression of the trainee's competence. Also, if more than one assessor is used, the interpretation from the data in the portfolio should be consistent. Third, Kane argues that one should be able to extrapolate from this evidence to a new context. In the case of a portfolio, do the data and the activities of the portfolio reflect real-life activities or future practice? We hope that portfolio developers require authentic work and not evidence contrived for the sole purpose of a portfolio. Will the portfolio assessment apply to other contexts? To what extent does the portfolio assessment associate with other quantitative and qualitative data? As noted by Cook et al.[72] there is little data concerning the relationship between qualitative judgment from portfolios and other judgments. The last of Kane's validity arguments is implications and this argument is similar to consequences. What evidence do we have regarding the implications of using a portfolio to assess performance? Cook et al.[72] show there are positive impacts on study habits, monitoring growth, and setting long-term goals. The negative impacts relate to a sense of burden. O'Brien et al.[10] noted the important implication that the portfolio assessment provided insights not available from other sources.

In reflecting on the use of these two assessment frameworks with portfolio assessment, practices derived from these two frameworks support the use of qualitative data and can be integrated to provide evidence of validity. The frameworks ensure that we provide a rigorous process acknowledging the kind of data required as evidence. The framework from Maastricht requires similar attention to many details to ensure a credible assessment process leading to decisions that will have evidence of validity.

Conclusion

Portfolios can add tremendous value to competency-based assessment systems. They are adaptive to diverse learners and can showcase evidence of achievement beyond traditional measurements. Learners must actively engage with portfolios through the selection of evidence and demonstration of self-regulated learning. There is evidence that portfolios can be beneficial to learners of all levels, from students to practitioners.

Successful implementation of portfolios requires careful planning and sufficient resources. Administrators must commit to clearly defining a portfolio system's purpose, organizing framework, and standards of success. Learners receive the most benefits when guided by a well-trained faculty coach who helps interpret feedback and set plans for growth. If used for summative purposes, raters must be carefully trained to arrive at defendable competency decisions. With these conditions in place, portfolios can be rigorous assessments and valuable additions to more traditional methods.

Annotated Bibliography

1. Driessen E, van der Vleuten CPM, Schuwirth L, van Tartwijk J, Vermunt J. The use of qualitative research criteria for portfolio assessment as an alternative to reliability evaluation: a case study. *Med Educ*. 2005;39(2):214–220.
   Driessen et al. are one of the first groups to demonstrate how systematic, qualitative research methods can be used to evaluate portfolios. The authors focused on the qualitative criteria of credibility and dependability, using the qualitative techniques of triangulation, prolonged engagement, member checking, audit trail, and dependability audit. This approach led to a high degree of agreement between mentors and students, with only a small proportion of portfolio evaluations requiring adjudication by a full committee (9 of 233 portfolios). The key conceptual difference with this approach was the use of additional information during the review process to inform judgment until "information saturation" was achieved (qualitative methodology) instead of looking for consistency across repeated measurements (traditional psychometric/quantitative methodology). This approach to portfolio assessment represents a major shift in the assessment of competence. This study examined portfolios of students early in their training; whether qualitative methods can be used to evaluate competence during later stages of clinical training should be the subject of future studies.
2. O'Brien CL, Sanguino SM, Thomas JX, Green M. Feasibility and outcomes of implementing a portfolio assessment system alongside a traditional grading system. *Acad Med*. 2016 Nov;91(11):1554–1560.
   This study is a current demonstration of portfolios in the United States with a medical school class of 156 students. O'Brien et al. report data from use of portfolios to assess progression toward competency as students entered the clerkship curriculum. Students reflected on their performance in competency domains tagging evidence to support their assessment. Two trained raters reviewed each portfolio (77% initial agreement; 98% after reconciliation); a third rater was brought in if the two raters could not reconcile their agreement (2%). Raters provided narrative feedback to students on areas of strength and areas for continued growth based on portfolio data. The assessment identified 31 students with concerns; four with the expectation of remediation. These students would not have come to the attention of the faculty as early as the portfolios allowed if faculty relied on traditional, non-competency-based, preclerkship assessment methods. Students noted that the portfolio taught them to engage in reflection and demonstrate strengths that otherwise might not be evident. Students did not perceive that learning plans helped them focus improvement efforts or strengthened their abilities to assess their own strengths and weaknesses. The authors shared methods used to ensure the quality of the assessment, drawing from both quantitative and qualitative approaches. Overall, while there are areas for improvement, the portfolio was a beneficial assessment approach.
3. O'Sullivan PS, Reckase MD, McClain T, Savidge MA, Clardy JA. Demonstration of portfolios to assess competency of residents. *Adv Health Sci Educ Theory Pract*. 2004;9(4):309–323.
   Despite weaknesses identified below, this is currently one of the few studies to systematically examine the reliability and validity characteristics of a portfolio and to apply a portfolio to a US-based GME program. The article describes a study involving 18 psychiatry residents over a 4-year period. An important component of the authors' approach was the training of the portfolio raters. Generalizability analysis found that five entries and two raters were sufficient for normative-based decisions. To reach sufficient reliability for absolute decisions, six entries or adding a third rater would be required. Despite the encouraging results on the reliability analysis, the authors noted that they believed the rubric used for scoring the portfolios was somewhat weak, and overall the validity evidence presented was not robust. Regarding validity, the authors did find that portfolio scores improved with increasing years of training but did not correlate with clinical performance. This latter finding is somewhat disappointing given an identified strength of portfolios is their authenticity. However, the authors did find that the portfolios provided valuable information on areas of weakness in the curriculum.
4. Driessen E. Do portfolios have a future? *Adv Health Sci Educ Theory Pract*. 2017 Mar;22(1):221–228.
   Driessen offers a critical review of the use of portfolios in medical education, highlighting the factors that lead to success and the potential pitfalls if these factors are inadequately addressed in implementation. He discusses the resistance portfolios can face from students and faculty; the difficulties with required reflections; and how competency-based education influences learners during workplace-based learning. For comprehensive portfolios to find success, several conditions must be met: adequate mentoring (coaching); an open structure; a supportive learning environment; and the opportunity for direct learning gains for portfolio users. The work of the portfolio must be arranged to foster opportunity to critically review feedback and learning rather than to serve as a "checklist" of competency achievement. The key to achieving benefit from a comprehensive portfolio lies in the dynamic dialogue between a learner and a mentor.
5. Schrempf S, Herrigel L, Pohlmann J, Griewatz J, Lammerding-Köppel M. Everybody is able to reflect, or aren't they? Evaluating the development of medical professionalism via a longitudinal portfolio mentoring program from a student perspective. *GMS J Med Educ*. 2022;39(1):Doc12.
   Schrempf et al. employ qualitative methods to determine how students evaluate the process of longitudinal reflection in their medical education, what aspects influence their perception of reflection, and what opportunities would improve their experience and perception. Notably, the longitudinal process described better matches that of a reflective portfolio than a comprehensive portfolio, which is advocated in this chapter. Nonetheless, the authors share important perspectives on reflection, including that 73% of learners found a benefit to the longitudinal reflection process even though only 36.1% originally approved of the process. Approving students found that reflection provided them an opportunity to track their development over time and to be aware of their own progress. Those who were ambivalent or who rejected the reflection process noted its time-consuming nature in the setting of an already demanding curriculum or a sense that this was a skill that learners had already acquired prior to health professions education. As noted in other studies, authors noted that "the decisive factor for the benefits . . . .was the motivation and trust between the students and the mentors" who facilitated students' process of learning to reflect, provided insights that influenced students motivation to reflect, and helped students realistically assess and value their own performance.
6. Carter S. ePortfolios as a platform for evidencing employability and building professional identity: a literature review. *Int J Work-Integr Learn*. 2022;22(4):463–474.
   Carter notes that the ePortfolio allows students to demonstrate growth mapped over a learning journey and is a tool that provides a "platform for combining the how, the what, and the who in assessment."

Considerations for choosing an ePortfolio are noted, including the need for mobile-friendly access, embedded media, a link to external data, and ease of navigation. The features of two commercially available platforms as of 2020 are compared: PebblePad (paid license) and OneNote (free personal account). Finally, case studies in the fields of nursing and engineering are explored to demonstrate the practical application of the ePortfolio to different settings in higher education.

References

1. Friedman Ben-David M, Davis MH, Harden RM, Howie PW, Ker J, Pippard MJ. AMEE Medical Education Guide No. 24: Portfolios as a method of student assessment. *Med Teach.* 2001;23(6):535–551.
2. Challis M. AMEE Medical Education Guide No. 11 (revised): portfolio-based learning and assessment in medical education. *Med Teach.* 1999;21(4):370.
3. Carraccio C, Englander R. Evaluating competence using a portfolio: a literature review and web-based application to the ACGME competencies. *Teach Learn Med.* 2004;16(4): 381–387.
4. McMullan M, Endacott R, Gray MA, et al. Portfolios and assessment of competence: a review of the literature. *J Adv Nurs.* 2003;41(3):283–294.
5. Smith K, Tillema H. Clarifying different types of portfolio use. *Assess Eval High Educ.* 2003;28(6):625.
6. Koretz D. Large-scale portfolio assessments in the US: evidence pertaining to the quality of measurement. *Assess Educ Princ Policy Pract.* 1998;5(3):309–334.
7. Borgstrom E, Cohn S, Barclay S. Medical professionalism: conflicting values for tomorrow's doctors. *J Gen Intern Med.* 2010;25(12):1330–1336.
8. Gordon JA, Campbell CM. The role of ePortfolios in supporting continuing professional development in practice. *Med Teach.* 2013;35(4):287–294.
9. Chertoff J, Wright A, Novak M, et al. Status of portfolios in undergraduate medical education in the LCME accredited US medical school. *Med Teach.* 2016;38(9):886–896.
10. O'Brien CL, Sanguino SM, Thomas JX, Green MM. Feasibility and outcomes of implementing a portfolio assessment system alongside a traditional grading system. *Acad Med.* 2016;91(11):1554–1560.
11. Duque G. Web-based evaluation of medical clerkships: a new approach to immediacy and efficacy of feedback and assessment. *Med Teach.* 2003;25(5):510–514.
12. Duque G, Finkelstein A, Roberts A, et al. Learning while evaluating: the use of an electronic evaluation portfolio in a geriatric medicine clerkship. *BMC Med Educ.* 2006;6:4.
13. Davis MH, Friedman Ben-David M, Harden RM, et al. Portfolio assessment in medical students' final examinations. *Med Teach.* 2001;23(4):357–366.
14. Bramley AL, Thomas CJ, Mc Kenna L, Itsiopoulos C. E-portfolios and Entrustable Professional Activities to support competency-based education in dietetics. *Nurs Health Sci.* 2021;23(1):148–156.
15. Belousova V, Hassan AK, Lampkin S. Mixed-method study of utilizing portfolios to document and assess co-curricular activities: student and advisor perceptions. *Pharm Basel Switz.* 2019;7(4):E170.
16. Gadbury-Amyot CC, Overman PR. Implementation of portfolios as a programmatic global assessment measure in dental education. *J Dent Educ.* 2018;82(6):557–564.
17. Favier RP, Vernooij JCM, Jonker FH, Bok HGJ. Inter-rater reliability of grading undergraduate portfolios in veterinary medical education. *J Vet Med Educ.* 2019;46(4):415–422.
18. Schrempf S, Herrigel L, Pohlmann J, Griewatz J, Lammerding-Köppel M. Everybody is able to reflect, or aren't they? Evaluating the development of medical professionalism via a longitudinal portfolio mentoring program from a student perspective. *GMS J Med Educ.* 2022;39(1):Doc12.
19. Reckase MD. Portfolio assessment: a theoretical estimate of score reliability. *Educ Meas Issues Pract.* 1995;14(1):12–14.
20. Wilkinson TJ, Challis M, Hobma SO, et al. The use of portfolios for assessment of the competence and performance of doctors in practice. *Med Educ.* 2002;36(10):918–924.
21. Martin-Kniep GO. *Becoming a Better Teacher: Eight Innovations That Work.* Association for Supervision and Curriculum Development; 2000.
22. Walland E, Shaw S. E-portfolios in teaching, learning and assessment: tensions in theory and praxis. *Technol Pedagogy Educ.* 2022;31(3):1–17.
23. Van Tartwijk J, Driessen EW. Portfolios for assessment and learning: AMEE Guide no. 45. *Med Teach.* 2009;31(9): 790–801.
24. Tochel C, Haig A, Hesketh A, et al. The effectiveness of portfolios for post-graduate assessment and education: BEME Guide No 12. *Med Teach.* 2009;31(4):299–318.
25. Buckley S, Coleman J, Khan K. Best evidence on the educational effects of undergraduate portfolios. *Clin Teach.* 2010;7(3):187–191.
26. McEwen LA, Griffiths J, Schultz K. Developing and successfully implementing a competency-based portfolio assessment system in a postgraduate family medicine residency program. *Acad Med.* 2015;90(11):1515–1526.
27. Hughes JA, Cleven AJ, Ross J, et al. A comprehensive reflective journal-writing framework for pharmacy students to increase self-awareness and develop actionable goals. *Am J Pharm Educ.* 2019;83(3):6554.
28. Driessen E, van Tartwijk J, van der Vleuten C, Wass V. Portfolios in medical education: why do they meet with mixed success? A systematic review. *Med Educ.* 2007;41(12):1224–1233.
29. Perlman RL, Ross PT, Christner J, Lypson ML. Faculty reflections on the implementation of socio-cultural eportfolio assessment tool. *Reflective Pract.* 2011;12(3):375–388.
30. Webb TP, Merkley TR, Wade TJ, Simpson D, Yudkowsky R, Harris I. Assessing competency in practice-based learning: a foundation for milestones in learning portfolio entries. *J Surg Educ.* 2014;71(4):472–479.
31. Driessen E. Do portfolios have a future? *Adv Health Sci Educ Theory Pract.* 2017;22(1):221–228.
32. Arntfield S, Parlett B, Meston CN, Apramian T, Lingard L. A model of engagement in reflective writing-based portfolios: interactions between points of vulnerability and acts of adaptability. *Med Teach.* 2016;38(2):196–205.
33. Emery L, Jackson B, Herrick T. Trainee engagement with reflection in online portfolios: a qualitative study highlighting the impact of the Bawa-Garba case on professional development. *Med Teach.* 2021;43(6):656–662.
34. Ten Cate O, Carraccio C. Envisioning a true continuum of competency-based medical education, training, and practice. *Acad Med.* 2019;94(9):1283–1288.
35. Torre D, Rice NE, Ryan A, et al. Ottawa 2020 consensus statements for programmatic assessment–2. implementation and practice. *Med Teach.* 2021;43(10):1149–1160.

36. Valentine N, Durning SJ, Shanahan EM, van der Vleuten C, Schuwirth L. The pursuit of fairness in assessment: looking beyond the objective. *Med Teach*. 2022 Feb 1:1–7. Published online.
37. Fovet F. Using universal design for learning as a lens to rethink graduate education pedagogical practices. In: Jenkins TS, ed. *Advances in Higher Education and Professional Development*. IGI Global; 2021:168–187.
38. Universal Design for Learning Guidelines Version 2.2 (Graphic Organizer). LINCS | Adult Education and Literacy | U.S. Department of Education. Published December 10, 2021. Accessed December 10, 2021. https://udlguidelines.cast.org/more/downloads.
39. Paul RM, Behat L. Assessment as a tool for learning—how portfolios were designed to improve student learning and well being. In: *Incorporating Universal Design for Learning in Disciplinary Contexts in Higher Education*. Taylor Institute for Teaching and Learning; 2021. Accessed December 10, 2021. https://taylorinstitute.ucalgary.ca/resources/incorporating-universal-design-for-learning-in-disciplinary-contexts-in-higher-education-guide.
40. Odukoya EJ, Kelley T, Madden B, Olawuni F, Maduakolam E, Cianciolo AT. Extending "beyond diversity": culturally responsive universal design principles for medical education. *Teach Learn Med*. 2021;33(2):109–115.
41. Clark NM, Zimmerman BJ. A social cognitive view of self-regulated learning about health. *Health Educ Res*. 1990;5(3):371–379.
42. Pintrich PR. Understanding self-regulated learning. *New Dir Teach Learn*. 1995;63:3–12.
43. Sandars J, Cleary TJ. Self-regulation theory: applications to medical education: AMEE Guide No. 58. *Med Teach*. 2011;33(11):875–886.
44. Choudhry NK, Fletcher RH, Soumerai SB. Systematic review: the relationship between clinical experience and quality of health care. *Ann Intern Med*. 2005;142(4):260–273.
45. Campbell CM, Parboosingh JM, Gondocz T, Babitskaya G, Pham BMM. Study of the factors influencing the stimulus to learning recorded by physicians keeping a learning portfolio. *J Contin Educ Health Prof*. 1999;19(1):16–24.
46. Holmboe ES, Hawkins RE. Methods for evaluating the clinical competence of residents in internal medicine: a review. *Ann Intern Med*. 1998;129(1):42–48.
47. Archbald DA, Newmann FM, National Center on Effective Secondary Schools M WI, National Association of Secondary School Principals R VA. Beyond Standardized Testing: Assessing Authentic Academic Achievement in the Secondary School. 1988. Accessed December 8, 2021. https://search.ebscohost.com/login.aspx?direct=true&db=eric&AN=ED301587&site=ehost-live.
48. Schuwirth LWT, van der Vleuten CPM. A history of assessment in medical education. *Adv Health Sci Educ Theory Pract*. 2020;25(5):1045–1056.
49. Heeneman S, Driessen EW. The use of a portfolio in postgraduate medical education—reflect, assess and account, one for each or all in one? *GMS J Med Educ*. 2017;34(5):Doc57.
50. Lau AMS. Formative good, summative bad?" A review of the dichotomy in assessment literature. *J Furth High Educ*. 2016;40(4):509–525.
51. Heeneman S, de Jong LH, Dawson LJ, et al. Ottawa 2020 consensus statement for programmatic assessment–1. agreement on the principles. *Med Teach*. 2021;43(10):1139–1148.
52. Eliasson G, Lundqvist A. [Learning methods in general practice]. *Lakartidningen*. 2019;116:FPT9.
53. Englander R, Flynn T, Call S, et al. Toward defining the foundation of the md degree: core Entrustable Professional Activities for entering residency. *Acad Med*. 2016;91(10):1352–1358.
54. Frank JR, Jabbour M, Tugwell P, Boyd D, Labrosse J, MacFadyen J. Skills for the new millennium: report of the societal needs working group, CanMEDS 2000 Project. *Ann R Coll Physicians Surg Can*. 1996;29(4):206–216.
55. Good Medical Practice. 2001. Published online.
56. Gray JD. Global rating scales in residency education. *Acad Med*. 1996;71(1 Suppl):S55–S63.
57. Pitts J, Coles C, Thomas P, Smith F. Enhancing reliability in portfolio assessment: discussions between assessors. *Med Teach*. 2002;24(2):197–201.
58. Pitts J, Coles C, Thomas P. Enhancing reliability in portfolio assessment: "shaping" the portfolio. *Med Teach*. 2001;23(4):351–356.
59. Snadden D, Thomas M. The use of portfolio learning in medical education. *Med Teach*. 1998;20(3):192–199.
60. Webb C, Endacott R, Gray M, et al. Models of portfolios. *Med Educ*. 2002;36(10):897–898.
61. Mazmanian PE, Mazmanian PM. Commitment to change: theoretical foundations, methods, and outcomes. *J Contin Educ Health Prof*. 1999;19(4):200–207.
62. Jones DL. Viability of the commitment-for-change evaluation strategy in continuing medical education. *Acad Med*. 1990;65(9 Suppl):S37–S38.
63. Holmboe ES, Prince L, Green M. Teaching and improving quality of care in a primary care internal medicine residency clinic. *Acad Med*. 2005;80(6):571–577.
64. Sargeant J, Eva KW, Armson H, et al. Features of assessment learners use to make informed self-assessments of clinical performance. *Med Educ*. 2011;45(6):636–647.
65. Sargeant J, Armson H, Chesluk B, et al. The processes and dimensions of informed self-assessment: a conceptual model. *Acad Med*. 2010;85(7):1212–1220.
66. Maio G, Haddock G. Behavioral influences on attitudes. *The Psychology of Attitudes and Attitude Change*. SAGE Publications Ltd; 2010:131–152.
67. Holmboe ES, Meehan TP, Lynn L, Doyle P, Sherwin T, Duffy FD. Promoting physicians' self-assessment and quality improvement: the ABIM diabetes practice improvement module. *J Contin Educ Health Prof*. 2006;26(2):109–119.
68. Eva KW, Regehr G. Self-assessment in the health professions: a reformulation and research agenda. *Acad Med*. 2005;80(10 Suppl):S46.
69. Norcini JJ, Blank LL, Duffy FD, Fortna GS. The mini-CEX: a method for assessing clinical skills. *Ann Intern Med*. 2003;138(6):476–481.
70. Driessen E, van der Vleuten C, Schuwirth L, van Tartwijk J, Vermunt J. The use of qualitative research criteria for portfolio assessment as an alternative to reliability evaluation: a case study. *Med Educ*. 2005;39(2):214–220.
71. Chan T, Sebok-Syer S, Thoma B, Wise A, Sherbino J, Pusic M. Learning analytics in medical education assessment: the past, the present, and the future. *AEM Educ Train*. 2018;2(2):178–187.
72. Cook DA, Kuper A, Hatala R, Ginsburg S. When assessment data are words: validity evidence for qualitative educational assessments. *Acad Med*. 2016;91(10):1359–1369.
73. Batson T. A Profoundly Disruptive Technology. Campus Technology. Accessed July 5, 2022. https://campustechnology.com/articles/2010/07/28/a-profoundly-disruptive-technology.aspx.
74. Carter S. ePortfolios as a platform for evidencing employability and building professional identity: a literature review. *Int J Work-Integr Learn*. 2022;22(4):463–474.
75. Davis, DA, Mazmanian, PE, Fordis M, Harrison RV, Thorpe KE, Perrier L. Accuracy of Physician Self-Assessment Compared

to Observed Measures of Competence: a systematic review. *JAMA*. 2006; 296(9):1094–1102.

76. Hiradhar P, Bhattacharya A. ICT beyond the classroom: new media and learning. In: Hiradhar P, Bhattacharya A, eds. *ICT in English Language Education: Bridging the Teaching-Learning Divide in South Asia*. SpringerBriefs in Education. Springer; 2022:63–74.
77. Lu H, Smiles R. Course redesign in a capstone course: putting eportfolio into practice. *Int J Res Educ Humanit Commer*. 2022;03(02):216–227.
78. Siddiqui ZS, Fisher MB, Slade C, et al. Twelve tips for introducing e-portfolios in health professions education. *Med Teach*. 2022;0(0):1–6. Epub ahead of print.
79. Nagler A, Andolsek K, Padmore JS. The unintended consequences of portfolios in graduate medical education. *Acad Med*. 2009;84(11):1522–1526.
80. Sowter J, Cortis J, Clarke DJ. The development of evidence based guidelines for clinical practice portfolios. *Nurse Educ Today*. 2011;31(8):872–876.
81. Van Tartwijk J, Driessen E, Van Der Vleuten C, Stokking K. Factors influencing the successful introduction of portfolios. *Qual High Educ*. 2007;13(1):69–79.
82. Willmarth-Stec M, Beery T. Operationalizing the student electronic portfolio for doctoral nursing education. *Nurse Educ*. 2015;40(5):263–265.
83. Bakke BM, Sheu L, Hauer KE. Fostering a feedback mindset: a qualitative exploration of medical students' feedback experiences with longitudinal coaches. *Acad Med*. 2020;95(7):1057–1065.
84. Hong DZ, Lim AJS, Tan R, et al. A systematic scoping review on portfolios of medical educators. *J Med Educ Curric Dev*. 2021;8:23821205211000356.
85. Oudkerk Pool A, Jaarsma ADC, Driessen EW, Govaerts MJB. Student perspectives on competency-based portfolios: does a portfolio reflect their competence development? *Perspect Med Educ*. 2020;9(3):166–172.
86. Pitts J, Coles C, Thomas P. Educational portfolios in the assessment of general practice trainers: reliability of assessors. *Med Educ*. 1999;33(7):515–520.
87. O'Sullivan PS, Cogbill KK, McClain T, Reckase MD, Clardy JA. Portfolios as a novel approach for residency evaluation. *Acad Psychiatry*. 2002;26(3):173–179.
88. O'Sullivan PS, Reckase MD, McClain T, Savidge MA, Clardy JA. Demonstration of portfolios to assess competency of residents. *Adv Health Sci Educ Theory Pract*. 2004;9(4):309–323.
89. Gadbury-Amyot CC, McCracken MS, Woldt JL, Brennan RL. Validity and reliability of portfolio assessment of student competence in two dental school populations: a four-year study. *J Dent Educ*. 2014;78(5):657–667.
90. Oudkerk Pool A, Govaerts MJB, Jaarsma DADC, Driessen EW. From aggregation to interpretation: how assessors judge complex data in a competency-based portfolio. *Adv Health Sci Educ Theory Pract*. 2018;23(2):275–287.
91. Gingerich A, Kogan J, Yeates P, Govaerts M, Holmboe E. Seeing the "black box" differently: assessor cognition from three research perspectives. *Med Educ*. 2014;48(11):1055–1068.
92. Humphrey-Murto S, Wood TJ, Ross S, et al. Assessment pearls for competency-based medical education. *J Grad Med Educ*. 2017;9(6):688–691.
93. Messick S. Validity. In: *Educational Measurement*. 3rd ed. American Council on Education; 1989:13–103.
94. Kane MT. Validation. In: *Educational Measurement*. 4th ed. Praeger; 2006:17–64.
95. Rotthoff T, Kadmon M, Harendza S. It does not have to be either or! Assessing competence in medicine should be a continuum between an analytic and a holistic approach. *Adv Health Sci Educ Theory Pract*. 2021;26(5):1659–1673.
96. Michels NRM, Avonts M, Peeraer G, et al. Content validity of workplace-based portfolios: a multi-centre study. *Med Teach*. 2016;38(9):936–945.
97. Frank AK, O'Sullivan P, Mills LM, Muller-Juge V, Hauer KE. Clerkship grading committees: the impact of group decision-making for clerkship grading. *J Gen Intern Med*. 2019;34(5):669–676.
98. Dillon MP, Puli L, Ridgewell E, Anderson SP, Chiavaroli N, Clarke L. Interassessor agreement of portfolio-based competency assessment for orthotists/prosthetists in Australia: a mixed method study. *Prosthet Orthot Int*. 2021;45(3):276–288.
99. Holmboe ES, Ward DS, Reznick RK, et al. Faculty development in assessment: the missing link in competency-based medical education. *Acad Med*. 2011;86(4):460–467.
100. Dannefer EF, Henson LC. The portfolio approach to competency-based assessment at the Cleveland Clinic Lerner College of Medicine. *Acad Med*. 2007;82(5):493–502.
101. O'Brien CL, Thomas JX, Green MM. What is the relationship between a preclerkship portfolio review and later performance in clerkships? *Acad Med*. 2018;93(1):113–118.
102. Gadbury-Amyot CC, Bray KK, Austin KJ. Fifteen years of portfolio assessment of dental hygiene student competency: lessons learned. *J Dent Hyg*. 2014;88(5):267–274.
103. Cook DA, Brydges R, Ginsburg S, Hatala R. A contemporary approach to validity arguments: a practical guide to Kane's framework. Med Educ. 2015;49(6):560–575.

16

Group Process in Assessment

KAREN E. HAUER, MD, PHD, BENJAMIN KINNEAR, MD, MED, AND ANDEM EKPENYONG, MD, MHPE

CHAPTER OUTLINE

Introduction

Group process for decision-making about learner progress is foundational to high-quality assessment practice in health professions education. Groups such as clinical competency committees, grading committees, and progress committees review, interpret, and synthesize learner performance information to guide future learning and ensure progress toward competence. This chapter provides an overview of the purposes and theoretical underpinnings of group decision-making as part of competency-based medical education (CBME) within programs of assessment. Factors that influence the quality of group decision-making are reviewed, including shared mental models, evidence of validity, and processes for continuous improvement. This chapter presents evidence-based guidance on group composition and the procedures to follow before, during, and after group meetings to maximize the value of the available data. These recommendations are based on literature both within and outside medical education.[1,2] Authors highlight common challenges in group decision-making and strategies to guide educators in conducting effective and efficient meetings. Group process in assessment necessitates an active learner role, along with a coach or advisor, to interpret feedback and plan future learning. Lastly, faculty development for group work is essential. Authors discuss the necessity of faculty training on assessment procedures, the roles and functions of group members, and strategies to reach fair, transparent, and equitable decisions. The chapter concludes with a checklist for group process to optimize this component of assessment.

Purpose of Group Decision-Making

Although group decision-making is ubiquitous, it often occurs implicitly. In healthcare, teams are used to make decisions about patient care to promote higher quality. Similarly, juries are used to make legal decisions that are more defensible or just. In sports, scouts and general managers work together to make decisions when drafting and recruiting players to win. In each example, groups are used because high-functioning groups often make better decisions than individuals.[3–5] "Better" holds different meaning in each context, depending on the purpose and goals of the group. Robust research informs how groups can function optimally to complete tasks and make decisions, drawing from multiple disciplines including sociology, psychology, communication, logic, argumentation, mathematics, and more. In this chapter we draw on select evidence, theories, and frameworks to guide medical education group decision-making.

Group Decision-Making in Medical Education

The benefits of group decision-making extend to medical education and various accrediting bodies have adopted this approach. The Accreditation Council for Graduate Medical

TABLE 16.1 Purposes of Group Decision-making for Learner Assessment in Medical Education

Function of Group Decision-Making	Outcome	Target Individuals Benefiting
Synthesize learner assessment data[55,68,88]	Defensible, valid decisions about learner progress	Learners Public
Generate feedback to learners[53,80,89]	Actionable feedback to guide future learning	Learners
Identify gaps in learning experiences[17,80,90]	Tailor learning experiences to meet learner's needs Identification of areas for curriculum improvement	Learners Program
Determine quality of learner assessment data[14,91,92]	Recognition of need for new assessment tools, improved use of current assessment tools, or faculty development	Teaching faculty Learners Program leaders

Education (ACGME) requires a clinical competency committee (CCC) within each US graduate medical education (GME) training program.[6] Similarly, the Royal College of Physicians and Surgeons of Canada's (RCPSC) Competence by Design initiative requires "competence committees."[7] In undergraduate medical education (UME), grading committees within clinical clerkships or academic progress/promotions committees across courses or clerkships can synthesize learner performance information.[8–10] There are multiple purposes of group decision-making as part of a system of learner assessment, as shown in Table 16.1. Groups can uncover professionalism concerns not previously identified.[11] In GME, clinical deficiencies in the performance of surgical residents not identified by individual faculty members came to light through group discussion.[12] Group discussions prior to the completion of the evaluations of internal medicine residents in continuity clinic resulted in higher reliability.[13] As programs gain experience with group decision-making, they find the process more efficient and effective in gaining insight into learners' progress and providing feedback.[14]

Within a program of assessment, a group of educators is charged with monitoring and making decisions about learner progression.[15] The focus on outcomes that is central to CBME requires commitment to rendering defensible decisions about learners' achievement of competence and supporting learners' ongoing growth.[16–18] Group decision-making affords opportunities for longitudinal review of each learner's assessment information collected from a variety of sources to determine whether the learner is progressing.[19] Groups must weigh evidence, deliberate, and draw conclusions about the learners' achievement of expectations. Groups recognize and support varied learning trajectories, or paths to competence, while also safeguarding the public through adherence to expected outcomes.[20] Assessment of a learner's performance in medical education often involves judgments based on imperfect or incomplete information.[21] Contextual variability in patients, assessors, and the learning environment makes it impossible to standardize all learning and assessment experiences.[22] Accordingly, group members weigh information to render decisions about promotion, remediation, grades, entrustment, and feedback to learners and programs. Group synthesis of learner performance information can generate rich feedback to inform learning plans. The group also serves a quality assurance function by examining the degree to which assessment procedures capture information about learning progress toward desired outcomes. Thus group decision-making contributes to a high-quality assessment program by synthesizing learner assessment data.

Key Concepts in Group Decision-Making

Defining "Group" and "Group Process"

Group decision-making entails individuals working together toward a common goal by sharing and analyzing information to achieve a collective decision. Simply placing multiple individuals together in a physical or social space does not guarantee they will function as a group. Group members may lack a group identity or coherence. In contrast, a group whose communication, interdependence, shared purpose, and structure are aligned experience cohesion in pursuing a common goal.[5,23] A high-functioning group does not imply homogeneity (i.e., all members appearing, thinking, and behaving alike) or exclusivity (i.e., members failing to consider new ideas or perspectives). Rather, as we will see later, diversity of group membership is valuable for group decision-making.[6,24] We draw from social psychology's definition of *group* as "a set of individuals with a shared purpose and who normally share a ... social identity" and *group process* to mean the group's work together on a task.[3] Groups optimize their decisions by using evidence-based approaches, which we review below.

Quality of Group Decision-Making

For group decision-making to achieve its aims of high-quality, fair, and defensible decisions about learners' progress, group members must share mental models of learner outcome expectations, their purpose as a group, their tasks, and the ways they will conduct their work.

Scoring: scores or comments from an observation of the learner	Generalization: data (scores, comments) synthesis represents learner performance	Extrapolation: performance in observation setting represents actual performance in practice	Implications: performance data are used to make justifiable decisions about learners
• Multiple assessment tools • Direct observation by faculty of learners and their work • Training for faculty about assessment tools	• Number of observations or assessments • Sampling of learner work from different settings over time • Blueprinting of assessments to competency framework	• Procedures for data analysis • Standards for performance for individual assessment tools, criterion referenced rather than normative • Interpretation of quantitative and qualitative data	• Standards for overall performance, criterion referenced rather than normative • Agreement among group members • Actions planned based on group's decisions (consequences), such as learner advancing in program or remediation

• **Fig. 16.1** Kane's validity framework applied to group decision-making: key considerations for the group.

They must use strategies and procedures that lead to valid decisions and commit to reflecting upon their work with the goal of continually improving the quality of decisions they render.

Shared Mental Models

Successful group decision-making depends upon the group's understanding of learner outcome expectations, the group's charge, and the procedures they use to generate decisions. These common understandings among group members are termed *shared mental models*,[25,26] *team mental models*, or *team cognition*.[27] Multiple shared mental models support the group's cohesive functioning and successful rendering of decisions about learner progress.[2,28] The group's work depends upon a shared understanding of expected learner performance defined using the program's outcomes language. Commonly these outcome expectations are defined as competencies, milestones, or Entrustable Professional Activities (EPAs).[28] For many faculty, aligning with program outcome expectations requires a departure from personal preferences or expectations from their own training.[29] Group members must share an understanding of how competence is assessed including which strategies are used and what levels of performance signify achievement of competence. Shared understanding of the decisions the group may render and the associated stakes or consequences for the learner is also important. Lower-stakes decisions provide information about progress monitoring for each learner. Higher-stakes decisions certify a learner as ready for advancement or graduation and fulfill the program's accountability to the public. Discussions among group members can facilitate shared understanding of these strategies, the data they generate, and which data to prioritize in assessing outcomes.

Validity

Group members should understand modern approaches to validity and recognize their role in collecting and reviewing relevant evidence about learner performance, drawing inferences, and rendering decisions. We encourage readers to refer to Chapter 2. As shown in Fig. 16.1, Kane's validity framework explicates the key inferences in learner assessment and how they pertain to the work of group decision-making.[30,31] First, at the level of scoring inferences, the group charged with decision-making can examine assessment tools and raters' preparedness to use them and suggest areas for any needed improvement to tools, scoring procedures, or rater training. Second, group decision-making inferences at the generalization level address adequacy of sampling of learner performance—number of observations, variety of contexts, and alignment with program expectations. Group decision-making inferences at the level of extrapolation require consideration of authenticity—types of data that the group is reviewing are known to reflect real-world practice, including workplace-based assessments (WBAs) of tasks that address expected program outcomes. Ultimately, group decision-making generates inferences around implications of assessment results, such as a learner being able to advance to unsupervised practice. Ensuring adequate evidence of validity for decisions rendered fulfills medical education's accountability to train a physician workforce prepared to meet the healthcare needs of patients and populations.[32]

Continuous Improvement

A group charged with assessment decision-making should adopt a mindset of ongoing improvement for learners, the group process, teachers, and the program.[33] A culture of continuous improvement entails involving faculty and learners in reflecting, experimenting, and innovating.[34,35] For example, sharing best practices and enabling teachers, learners, and program leadership to suggest changes constitute the open communication culture necessary for collective improvement.

To achieve this culture of continuous improvement, a group must engage in reflective discussion about its processes and outcomes. Periodic reorientation for returning group members can be structured as an interactive process in which members self-assess regarding their personal contributions and the group's impact.[36] Strategies to optimize group functioning include discussing challenging cases, examining assessment tools and what information they should provide, and reviewing group policies for clarity and any needed updates. For example, a study of CCC implementation cycles in a pediatrics program identified that, though the CCC generated feedback for each resident, the group failed to revisit feedback at subsequent meetings.[37] This group improved their process by asking residents to provide evidence demonstrating how they had addressed prior CCC feedback. Also, a group may identify gaps in curricula that should be remedied to enable learners to demonstrate expected skills. For example, if learners are not seeing certain expected patient types or gaining experience performing particular procedures, the group can recommend changes to learner schedules to ensure access to needed learning experiences. As groups gain experience with assessing learner performance and making judgments about progress, they also become attuned to the quality of the assessment data and where additional or better data may be needed.[14] As end users of assessment data, decision-making groups provide critical feedback to drive assessment improvement efforts.

Establishing the Group

Appointing qualified group members and developing their skills and knowledge is central to the effectiveness of group decision-making. Participation in a group charged with assessment decision-making requires significant commitment of time and expertise development. We, the authors, advocate that faculty be afforded funding to reserve time to participate in these important roles.

Group Chair

The chairperson should have broad expertise in teaching and assessing learners in the program; local assessment tools and strategies; program requirements, policies, and procedures; curriculum content and clinical experiences afforded to trainees; remediation strategies; and expected training outcomes. The chair role also demands expertise in skillful facilitation of group data review and discussion. While a new committee may not have access to a chair with experience in the group decision-making process, over time a committee can prioritize a chair with relevant experience and understanding.

A participative leadership style benefits the group by empowering member participation and using members' input in decision-making.[38] The chair must consider how their leadership style can influence member engagement. Often selected because of their experience and expertise within the program, the chair garners additional power by way of their role within the committee. This status can inhibit member participation.[39] To counteract this risk and engage members, the chair can enact behaviors that lower their own status, often referred to as psychological size.[40] For example, asking questions, allowing and inviting others to speak early and often, demonstrating support for members, and being curious to hear from others rather than sharing one's own opinion reduces one's psychological size and maximize members' input.[41]

Group Membership

Careful selection of group members is foundational to the group's success. As with the chair, members are typically faculty who already have or are willing to develop a nuanced understanding of the desired program outcomes; relevant rules, regulations, and policies pertaining to learner performance and advancement; the system of assessment; and consequences for failing to meet expectations.

Diversity of experiences and characteristics should be sought when constructing a group at any level of medical education. Demographic diversity within the group can broaden the range of perspectives and interpretations while minimizing bias. Members must be willing to share different opinions to enhance the breadth of discussion, a factor known to strengthen group decision-making.[42] Given the known risk of group members to conform to other members' preferences or decisions,[43] members' willingness and motivation to counter this risk by thinking independently and sharing openly is crucial.

Nonfaculty members, such as learners, staff, other health professionals, or public members can strengthen the range of perspectives and skills within the group.[44] Decisions about whether to include learners require consideration of program requirements and confidentiality. Near-peers such as chief residents can provide understanding of the learners' experience while also minimizing confidentiality or conflict of interest concerns that arise with a peer assessing another peer. Key administrative staff bring valuable skills and perspective to the group. For example, an administrative coordinator for the group with skills in data management enables time-efficient information review during the meeting. Administrative staff and interprofessional colleagues bring complementary views of learner performance based on their interactions. Some programs include physician assistants, psychologists, or social workers for their input about performance in competencies such as communication and systems-based practice.[14] Groups may also include public members or patient representatives to ensure that these perspectives are reinforced during discussions about desired patient care outcomes of training. Together, diverse members enhance the range of information considered and opinions shared.

Group Size

The number of group members is influenced by availability of qualified individuals, program size, and policies for the group. Smaller groups have the advantages of reducing the number of qualified members that must be recruited, and individuals may perceive smaller groups as more trustworthy and cohesive than larger groups.[45] However, the smaller the group, the more likely that one individual can dominate and unduly influence decisions.[46] Larger groups can include more diverse opinions and engender more debate and considerations of alternatives.[47] However, members of larger groups may be hesitant to speak, and "social loafing" can

Before	During	After
Group purpose Member roles Group size Ground rules Agenda setting Faculty development	Shared mental models Decision-making Bias Time management strategies Faculty development	Documentation Feedback to stakeholders Learner engagement Continuous quality improvement

• **Fig. 16.2** Approach to addressing group process in assessment before, during, and after a group meeting.

arise, in which members rely on the group rather than their own effort to accomplish work.[48] For maximal function, a group includes approximately 5 to 10 members.[2,49] Larger education programs may be able to engage more faculty through subgroups reporting to the larger group.

Membership Terms

Membership terms ensure a degree of group turnover necessary to minimize the risk of groupthink that can arise through prolonged close engagement of a group lacking fresh perspectives.[50] Term limits may entice individuals to join the group through understanding that service entails a fixed duration commitment. However, term limits may be disadvantageous in smaller programs with an insufficient number of potential new members. Rotating term limits among members provides stability of knowledge of the group's work. Term duration should be defined to enable new members to acclimate to the group and its responsibilities and contribute meaningfully prior to term completion. Defining term durations with opportunities for renewal provides the opportunity to excuse any members who are not engaged and contributing as needed.

Group Procedures

We present this information as a series of factors for groups to consider before, during, and after their meetings (Fig. 16.2). However, these factors can also be considered and reconsidered at any point in the process as groups see fit.

Before the Group Meets

Ground Rules

Ground rules or group agreements articulate expectations and guide the group's work. The goal is to make explicit any assumptions that might otherwise be implicit and thereby variably understood by different members. Ground rules capture the purpose of the group including how data will be used, ways that members will interact to process information and make decisions, and how members will maintain the confidentiality of trainee information. Sample ground rules for a CCC are shown in Table 16.2. The program director or chair should work with members to provide guidance on what types of information can and should be shared within the group during or outside of a meeting. For example, information about learners' protected health information, personal life, or disability status may not be appropriate to share within the group.

Conflicts of Interest

Understanding and identifying potential conflicts of interest are important responsibilities of committee chairs and members. Though experience with trainees will strengthen members' ability to contribute meaningfully to the committee, close interactions with a particular trainee as a mentor, clinician, or family member/friend represents a conflict of interest. Prospective group members may have real or potential conflicts of interest that must be recognized and addressed prior to considering them for the role. For example, a faculty member who has mentoring or coaching relationships with, regularly provides clinical care for, or enjoys close personal relationships with multiple learners has a conflict of interest and may need to recuse themselves from discussion and decision-making for that particular trainee. Members must consider potential conflicts preceding and during periods in which trainees are applying for future training positions or jobs and discuss with the group whether recusal could be appropriate.[51]

Faculty Development

Faculty development is integral to the success of group decision-making. This training begins before the committee meets and continues as part of continuous improvement of the group's procedures. Participating in the group is itself a form of real-time faculty development as members reference learner performance expectations and analyze performance data relative to those expectations. However, despite calls for faculty development, specifically for CCCs,[21,52,53] many groups may not receive adequate training. Faculty development should occur longitudinally as the needs of the committee members and the membership of the group may change over time.[53] Assigning a faculty development leader may facilitate these efforts. However, there are currently no published studies providing evidence of the use of specific approaches for designing faculty development for decision-making groups.

TABLE 16.2 Sample Ground Rules for a Group Charged With Decision-making Regarding Learner Progress in Medical Education[53,55,93]

Responsibility	Expectations for Group Members
Purpose	Review relevant group, committee, or program guidelines/policies/bylaws.
Training	Engage in group member training to understand the group's charge and how it does its work, assessment tools and strategies used in the program, bias, and the training program's curriculum. Training may include reading, online modules, discussions at group meetings, or attendance at separate faculty development sessions.
Preparation	Review materials relevant to any assigned learners in advance of each meeting to be prepared to present or discuss them.
Participation	Attend group meetings; participation is essential and requires clearing one's calendar.
Listening	Listen to and consider other members' opinions with respect.
Data	Use and interpret data to make decisions rather than relying on personal opinion or experience.
Equity and bias	Participate in training on unconscious bias and commit to equitable decision-making practices.
Conflict of interest	Recognize conflicts of interest and adhere to the committee's conflict of interest policy. Conflicts may address one's knowledge of personal or health issues for a particular trainee. Share information appropriately.
Decision-making	Understand and apply the group's approach to or rules for decision-making.
Confidentiality	Maintain confidentiality of group materials and discussions; do not share outside the group except through planned feedback with the resident or faculty.
Improvement	Participate in reflection about the group's work with a commitment to continuously improving the group's function and providing information to improve the training program.

Thus we present suggestions based on the available literature on faculty development and our experience. A scoping review on faculty development in the CBME era suggests that faculty development curricula should:[54]

1) "Be longitudinal, multi-modal, interactive and incorporate feedback" for participants
2) Include "skill development in feedback provision, coaching and facilitated self-direction"
3) Address anticipated barriers such as "lack of time, buy-in and resources."

Table 16.3 presents possible faculty development topics and approaches for assessment decision-making groups. Faculty development before, during, and after group meetings can maximize group members' understanding of their work and effectiveness. Consideration should be given to the experience and training members have had, and what gaps exist in their knowledge and skills related to the group's work.[36] The committee may consist of both new and returning members, those from different practice disciplines, nonphysicians, and junior and more senior faculty. Understanding and sharing their strengths and gaps through group discussion can guide selection of topics and approaches for training. GME programs can look to their specific specialty for appropriate examples, case scenarios, and additional resources.

Conducting a Group Meeting

The information below describes procedures for ensuring a high-quality, productive group meeting. Table 16.4 outlines common challenges that groups experience, possible causes, and mitigation strategies.

Setting the Agenda

Before the meeting, the chair should set goals for the meeting, create an agenda, and distribute it to the members in anticipation of the meeting. The agenda may address follow-up to business from previous meetings and any new contextual information related to curriculum or learner assessment in the program. Approval of prior meeting minutes may be a standing agenda item. The agenda should specify whether all trainees will be discussed or only a subset. Members should be informed in advance about their responsibility to prereview or present information at the meeting. In addition to discussing the trainees, other agenda items may include a short faculty development session (e.g., 10 minutes of a chosen topic—see "Faculty Development" above) and a closing debrief discussion to identify areas to improve the group's processes.

Chair Role

The chair may begin the meeting by reviewing members' roles, desired outcomes of formative feedback to learners, and the consequences of the high-stakes decisions that the group is responsible for making.[55] The chair should guide the group to appoint a timekeeper and clarify who will display learner data during the meeting (typically a staff coordinator).

The chair should conduct meetings using strategies within published guidelines for effective group process[2] (Appendix 16.1). Structured procedures to provide all members the opportunity to share their thoughts maximize the value of the group's wisdom and perspective. To ensure that issues of hierarchy do not stifle participation, the chair should give the most junior members a chance to state their opinions first and ask senior members to follow.[2] The chair

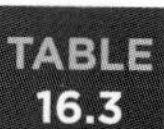

TABLE 16.3 Faculty Development Topics for Groups: Checklist for Chairpersons to Consider

Topic	Consider the Following
Group role(s) and responsibilities	*Has the group discussed its role and responsibilities? Is there a shared understanding about what this is? Is there a written document that captures this?* • The group should take the time to discuss the role and goals of the committee as described by any oversight body (e.g., accrediting body document) and any potential secondary roles that the committee may fulfill (e.g., remediation, faculty development for core faculty, feedback).[55,79,94]
Effective group process	*Has there been a discussion to outline the process that the group plans to use to accomplish its charge? How will decisions be made? Is there a process in place to ensure participation from everyone? What measures will be employed to ensure that junior faculty feel comfortable voicing their opinions? And that all opinions are at least considered?* • Effective group process is the responsibility of the entire group; however, chairs should take the lead in ensuring that issues of hierarchy are addressed and that each member has an opportunity to contribute and to be heard. Individual perspectives need to be elicited and used to reach group judgments and decisions.[2,68] • The group should ensure a standardized process for presenting each trainee, with a concerted effort made to encourage participation from all members. Junior members should be given the opportunity to contribute before more senior members and leaders such as the chair or program director weigh in.[2]
Principles of effective assessment	*What works well in the assessment system, and what could be improved?* • The group should acknowledge that assessment is a "system,"[44] made up of stakeholders, tools, and interconnected processes, not simply a form to complete at the end of a rotation or in a meeting. • Going beyond the assessment of an individual learner, van der Vleuten and colleagues describe six key principles of effective assessment that training programs can use to improve their assessment systems, including the principle that expert judgment, as in group decision-making, is essential for advancement decisions.[15] In addition, they describe the building blocks to implement a program of assessment. Readers should consult chapters of this text re: descriptions (including pros and cons) of different assessment methods. This knowledge can subsequently be used to critique the fit and use of a program's specific assessment tools.[15,95] • For an understanding of the building blocks of a competency-based system, van Melle and colleagues provide a "core competency framework." The framework can be used to evaluate and improve implementation of competency-based medical education.[17]
Developing a shared mental model	*Are all group members on the same page about the expected skills/performance level that trainees are supposed to acquire?* • Developing a shared mental model of competencies and expectations of training, such as milestones,[28] can be accomplished over a series of conversations among the members. • To incorporate faculty development "on the fly" (during the course of a regularly scheduled meeting"), groups can discuss a few milestones at a time (e.g., by core competency). In doing so they can develop a clear description of performance at each level on the scale and determine the frame of reference they are using, such as milestones as a criterion-based framework.[96,97]
Biases	*What biases have been revealed in the group's discussions? What biases is the group at risk for?* • There are multiple biases that can affect CCC decision-making.[76] Although it may not be feasible to avoid biases completely, acknowledging the potential for biases can be an important first step to minimizing them. • Consider performing a "check-in" with the group intermittently (e.g., a couple of times per year) about the issue of bias—as part of a continuous quality improvement process for the group.
Fairness and transparency	*Do key stakeholders know how the group makes decisions? How can the process become more transparent? Are all members empowered to state their opinions? What happens if a trainee does not agree with the group's decision?* • The committee should periodically review its process to ensure that they are fair to both trainees and committee members. Committee members should be made aware of the requirements for due process. This includes notifying learners of their deficiencies, provision of opportunity to cure, and a "reasonable process" to determine if those deficiencies have been cured.[78] Groups should consult their legal departments for laws and requirements specific to their own contexts. • Trainees should be made aware of the group and processes through which decisions are made. Trainees should be referred to the Milestones handbook, or other relevant expectations in the training setting.[98]

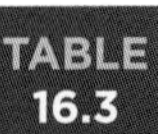

TABLE 16.3 Faculty Development Topics for Groups: Checklist for Chairpersons to Consider—Cont'd

Topic	Consider the Following
Data dilemmas	*Which data do groups process in decision-making? How much data? What is the quality of the data? How do groups synthesize quantitative and qualitative assessment data? What value do groups ascribe to the data generated by different raters? What about the use of "informal" data such as hallway talk, emails?* • Many questions and conundrums arise with respect to which data and the quantity and quality of the assessment data. Program directors and groups contemplate how best to organize assessment data such that it can easily be reviewed. Friedman and colleagues discussed the use of dashboards to facilitate the organization of vast amounts of assessment data that programs continually collect.[60] • Sometimes groups need to figure out how best to use the data they have, even when it is imperfect or incomplete.[21] • "Informal data" can sometimes be introduced into group conversations. Previously undocumented data introduced during the course of CCC meeting discussions can provide context for formal assessments and thus assist CCC members in reaching summative decisions, but must be used judiciously to avoid hearsay, revealing confidential information, or gossip.[71]
Feedback to stakeholders	*What feedback should stakeholders (e.g., trainees, faculty, training programs) receive from these groups? What processes are in place for this to occur?* • Programs should develop a process for engaging trainees in a feedback conversation about their progress; for example, this may take place during semiannual learner progress reviews.[79,80] • Data from the group's decision-making process (e.g., milestones ratings) can be used during annual program review to highlight curricular gaps, trends observed regarding the quality of faculty comments, and other areas for reform. In the United States, CCCs can use milestones data accessed via the ACGME Accreditation Data System to review trends across milestone subcompetencies over time and the variation among trainees.[99] • Groups designed for longitudinal assessment can identify and apply predictors that signal struggles and initiate conversations to uncover reasons for poor performance and develop intervention plans.[19]

ACGME, Accreditation Council for Graduate Medical Education; *CCC*, clinical competency committee.

should also reserve their comments until junior members have voiced theirs. In general, more information sharing leads to better group decisions.[56] Therefore chair efforts to invite members to share information in a structured fashion helps address and analyze all relevant assessment data.[2]

The chair sets the tone for the meeting. Creating a safe and collegial space for members to share their contributions and ask questions is essential.[55] Psychological safety characterizes a high-functioning group within which all members feel able to take the interpersonal risk to share opinions, preferences, and questions without fearing embarrassment or negative personal consequences.[57] For example, the chair can invite members to share differences of opinion or seek clarifications of the rationale for certain interpretations or decisions proposed by other members.

Throughout the meeting, the chair should be mindful of the rules and requirements of their associated oversight body. Ensuring adherence to relevant requirements may entail referring to bylaws and policies during or after the meeting to confirm the appropriateness of committee actions. As needed, the chair may also consult with legal counsel regarding content and wording of letters that communicate about deficiencies to trainees or in response to legal challenges from learners.

Member Role

Group members should maintain familiarity with the group's charge and procedures.[58] During meetings, participating and listening actively and without multitasking on work unrelated to the group maximizes the value of the group process. Members who were assigned trainees to prereview are responsible for arriving with that information available to share a summary with the group. Other members are responsible for listening to identify areas of agreement, conflicting impressions, or additional information relevant to group determinations about each trainee's progress. Sharing relevant information strengthens the group process through enhanced understanding, and conflicting information should be viewed favorably rather than with defensiveness.[56]

Data Management and Organization

To facilitate assessment data collection and organization, many training programs use commercial learner data management systems or create their own. Groups can use dashboards to facilitate the work of displaying assessment data collected from multiple sources over time.[59] Aggregating and reporting assessment data in a convenient, understandable format makes information transparent to the program and each learner. Dashboards should be fit for purpose, aligning with the goals of the group (e.g., formative feedback, summative decisions, etc.) and an overarching assessment framework (e.g., CBME). Accordingly, dashboards may incorporate both quantitative (e.g., examination scores, end-of-rotation ratings) and qualitative (e.g., multisource feedback, end-of-rotation faculty comments, notes of incidents or commendations, patient comments) data.[60]

TABLE 16.4 Common Challenges in Assessment Group Decision-Making

Challenge	Suggestive Signs	Possible Causes	Mitigation Strategies
Unclear agenda or chair role	Discussions jump between learners or topics Little follow-up of prior meeting discussions Persistent confusion about policies and procedures Members unclear which learners will be discussed	Agenda not established or shared with members Lack of clarity about purpose of group	Chair establishes agenda for each meeting Agenda shared in advance of meeting Group debrief about meetings to identify areas for improvement
Lack of data	Difficulty arriving at decisions Reliance on anecdote/personal experience	Underdeveloped program of assessment Poor assessment completion rate	Develop assessment improvement committee Faculty development Incentive program for completion
Poor-quality data	Difficulty arriving at decisions Reliance on anecdote/personal experience	Underdeveloped program of assessment Poor assessor performance	Develop assessment improvement committee Assessor training Feedback on assessment[1,2]
Groupthink	Group reaches quick agreement about all decisions without discussion or debate Sense of group infallibility Individual self-censorship	Lack of group diversity Long-standing membership Hierarchy	Chair invites different opinions Recruit diverse group membership Membership turnover Assign at least one member as a dissenter
Bias/inequitable treatment	May be difficult to detect as often implicit Group discussion dominated by subgroup of members Worse education outcomes for a particular group of learners	Lack of group diversity Lack of implicit bias training	Recruit diverse group membership Implicit bias training Reviewing data (e.g., assessments, scores, etc.) for patterns of inequitable treatment/outcomes
Information cascade	All information is filtered through one group member Lack of discussion	Overreliance on prereview and report-out processes Lack of in-meeting information-sharing processes	Allow in-meeting review of data using dashboards, screen sharing, and handouts Have multiple members complete any prereview and report-outs
Lack of time	Rushed discussions Not addressing all agenda items Meetings running over scheduled time	Scheduled time is too short Agenda is too full Suboptimal time management	Lengthen meetings Increase frequency of meetings Use asynchronous or parallel subgroups to divide tasks Assign a timekeeper

Dashboards facilitate the synthesis of large amounts of data and enable visualization to help groups make sense of each learner's progress. For example, in GME, dashboards are used to generate visualizations summarizing each resident's milestone ratings as trend lines or radar (spider) graphs.[61] More sophisticated dashboard displays can visually represent assessment data in multiple different ways, integrating analytics to help with sense-making.[62] For example, the University of Cincinnati internal medicine residency program uses an Excel-based dashboard to visualize multiple types of data (Fig. 16.3). The dashboard shows longitudinal entrustment data in multiple formats, overlaid with learning analytics that allow committee members to contextualize the data,[63] allowing the committee to "zoom in" to any particular data point in real time. The dashboard also includes self-assessments, 360-feedback from a yearlong ambulatory experience,[64] clinical care measures,[65] and testing data.[66] The work of the group is to use the available quantitative and qualitative data to interpret and summarize each trainee's performance.

Training and continued dashboard development maximize the value of this type of tool. Group members require training on dashboard use and interpretation of displays. Whenever possible, data collection should be designed to autopopulate dashboards, however a group member or administrative support person may be needed to collate, input, or manipulate data to prepare dashboards ahead of meetings. Dashboards may be circulated ahead of time to allow group members to prepare and can be used to augment in-meeting discussions. Groups responsible for decision-making need to monitor the content and visualizations within the dashboard that are driving their decision-making. Members should consider whether the dashboard contains all relevant assessment data, or whether any needed information is missing.[59] As group members use

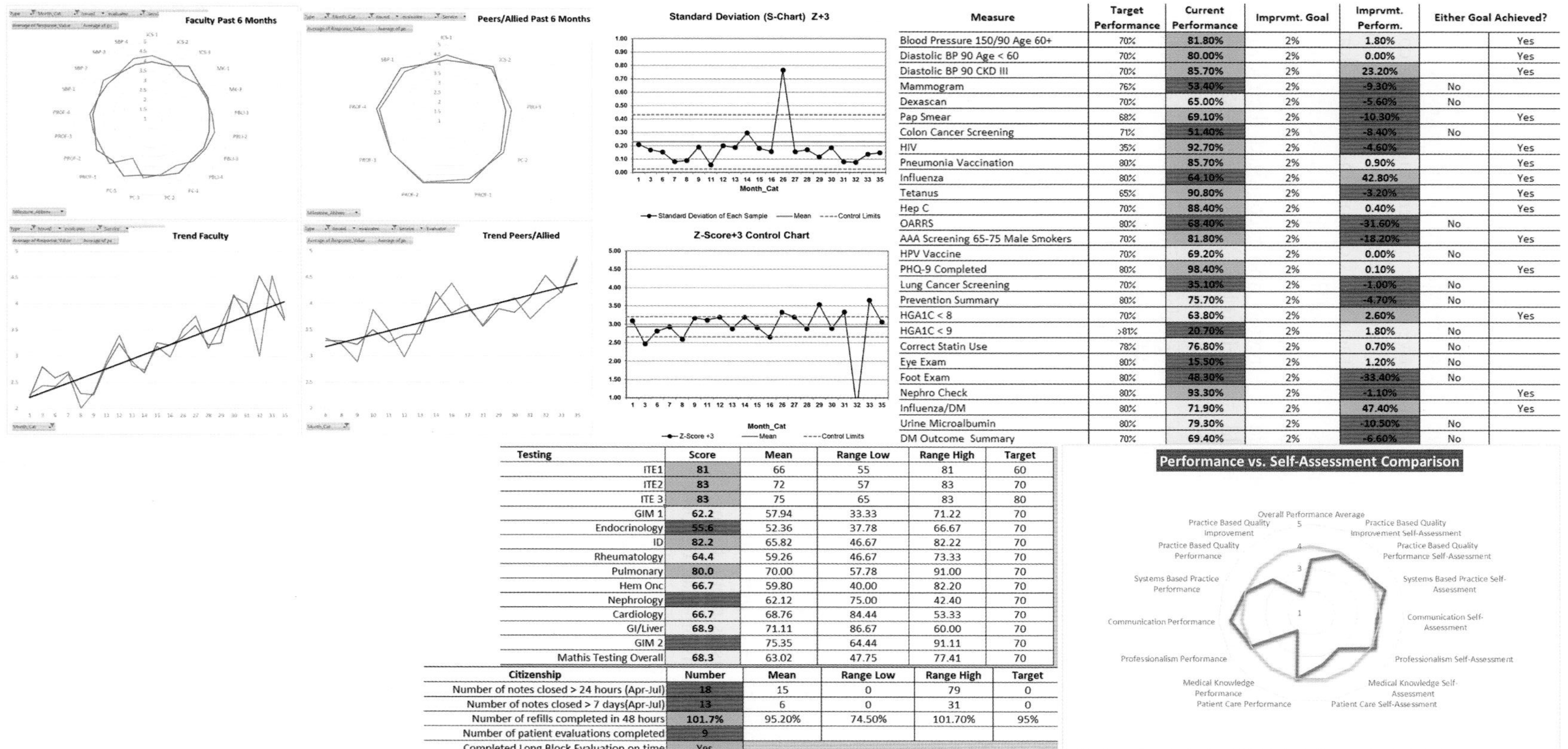

Measure	Target Performance	Current Performance	Imprvmt. Goal	Imprvmt. Perform.	Either Goal Achieved?
Blood Pressure 150/90 Age 60+	70%	81.80%	2%	1.80%	Yes
Diastolic BP 90 Age < 60	70%	80.00%	2%	0.00%	Yes
Diastolic BP 90 CKD III	70%	85.70%	2%	23.20%	Yes
Mammogram	76%	53.40%	2%	-9.30%	No
Dexascan	70%	65.00%	2%	-5.60%	No
Pap Smear	68%	69.10%	2%	-10.30%	Yes
Colon Cancer Screening	71%	51.40%	2%	-8.40%	No
HIV	35%	92.70%	2%	-4.60%	Yes
Pneumonia Vaccination	80%	85.70%	2%	0.90%	Yes
Influenza	80%	64.10%	2%	42.80%	Yes
Tetanus	65%	90.80%	2%	-3.20%	Yes
Hep C	70%	88.40%	2%	0.40%	Yes
OARRS	80%	68.40%	2%	-31.60%	No
AAA Screening 65-75 Male Smokers	70%	81.80%	2%	-18.20%	Yes
HPV Vaccine	70%	69.20%	2%	0.00%	No
PHQ-9 Completed	80%	98.40%	2%	0.10%	Yes
Lung Cancer Screening	70%	35.10%	2%	-1.00%	No
Prevention Summary	80%	75.70%	2%	-4.70%	No
HGA1C < 8	70%	63.80%	2%	2.60%	Yes
HGA1C < 9	>81%	20.70%	2%	1.80%	No
Correct Statin Use	78%	76.80%	2%	0.70%	No
Eye Exam	80%	15.50%	2%	1.20%	No
Foot Exam	80%	48.30%	2%	-33.40%	No
Nephro Check	80%	93.30%	2%	-1.10%	Yes
Influenza/DM	80%	71.90%	2%	47.40%	Yes
Urine Microalbumin	80%	79.30%	2%	-10.50%	No
DM Outcome Summary	70%	69.40%	2%	-6.60%	No

Testing	Score	Mean	Range Low	Range High	Target
ITE1	81	66	55	81	60
ITE2	83	72	57	83	70
ITE 3	83	75	65	83	80
GIM 1	62.2	57.94	33.33	71.22	70
Endocrinology	55.6	52.36	37.78	66.67	70
ID	82.2	65.82	46.67	82.22	70
Rheumatology	64.4	59.26	46.67	73.33	70
Pulmonary	80.0	70.00	57.78	91.00	70
Hem Onc	66.7	59.80	40.00	82.20	70
Nephrology		62.12	75.00	42.40	70
Cardiology	66.7	68.76	84.44	53.33	70
GI/Liver	68.9	71.11	86.67	60.00	70
GIM 2		75.35	64.44	91.11	70
Mathis Testing Overall	68.3	63.02	47.75	77.41	70

Citizenship	Number	Mean	Range Low	Range High	Target
Number of notes closed > 24 hours (Apr-Jul)	18	15	0	79	0
Number of notes closed > 7 days(Apr-Jul)	13	6	0	31	0
Number of refills completed in 48 hours	101.7%	95.20%	74.50%	101.70%	95%
Number of patient evaluations completed	9				
Completed Long Block Evaluation on time	Yes				

• **Fig. 16.3** Sample learner performance dashboard from the University of Cincinnati internal medicine residency program.

dashboards, their needs may change over time. Groups can work with technology experts and statisticians to envision and request enhanced visualization to move from making normative comparisons (comparing learners to one another) to a criterion-based system (comparing learners' performance to predefined standards).[67] Thus dashboards may need to be updated periodically to continue to serve the group's needs.

Decision-Making Process

Members must understand their decision-making process and how performance is judged against expected standards within a system of assessment. Such a system is illustrated in Fig. 16.4. Group procedures for decision-making should indicate the process for rendering decisions. For example, group policy should determine whether different types of decisions are finalized through group consensus or with a vote by the group members. Group procedures may specify requirements for unanimous or majority decisions. Alternatively, the group may be charged with rendering recommendations to the chair or the program director who holds decision-making authority.

Studies to date have shed light on the complexity of the group decision-making process at the GME level. Two studies of CCCs demonstrated varied understandings around either problem identification or supporting and interpreting learner development.[52,69] Others have illuminated the decision-making conundrums that arise for groups. CCC members grapple with how much importance to attach to their personal knowledge of a trainee's performance versus data provided by colleagues via assessment forms.[52] Pack and colleagues described the decision-making process as "effortless" in some cases and "effortful" in others—the latter occurring in situations with inadequate, unclear, or discrepant data.[21] CCCs in the United States vary in how they incorporate assessment data into group decisions, and often find the available data to be insufficient.[69,70] The appropriateness of using previously undocumented data (e.g., summary impressions, contextualizing factors, personal anecdotes, hearsay) for group decision-making remains controversial.[44,71,72] Groups should explicitly discuss which data are acceptable to inform different types of decisions. Taken together, these studies confirm the complexity of group decision-making and underscore the importance of groups discussing and reflecting upon how they do their work, where they see disagreements among members, and how they understand their purpose and procedures.

Risk of Bias and Mitigation Strategies

Just as decision-making by individuals can succumb to bias, so can that of groups. Bias threatens the fairness and validity of a group's decisions. Types of biases include the often unconscious, implicit biases based on individual learners' identities and characteristics, and cognitive biases related to information interpretation and decision-making. Bias often includes an unawareness of automatic patterns in thinking that can be based in harmful stereotypes about individuals or groups. For example, a faculty member may associate higher or lower performance with a learner's gender identity or race/ethnicity.

It is important to recognize and mitigate unconscious bias in a group's decision-making procedures. The risk of unconscious bias affecting impressions of learners should be acknowledged in all group decision-making. In a qualitative study of clerkship grading committees, members identified benefits of the committee process for the quality of their decision-making and felt learners appreciated the fairness of decisions.[8] However, members also identified potential biases within the assessment data available to them for review and recognized their own vulnerability to unconscious bias. Avoiding the use of learner photos or names can decrease biases related to learner appearance or background (gender, skin color, race/ethnicity, or attractiveness).[73,74] Members may review data or hear comments during the meeting that seem to convey bias and should be empowered to call out this information and offer another perspective.

Member training in unconscious (implicit) bias can increase awareness of these automatic, implicit associations. However, the evidence supporting such training is mixed. A systematic review of training interventions about implicit bias in the context of doctor–patient interactions shows variable results: while providers who demonstrate bias against individuals of color have worse doctor–patient relations, the effectiveness of training is shown in some studies but not others.[75] For this reason, unconscious bias training should be seen as a catalyst for reflection and discussion, not as a solution to the issue.

Dickey et al. summarized multiple cognitive biases (heuristics) that may arise within clinical competency committees.[75] These cognitive shortcuts, while efficient to manage a large decision-making workload, can threaten the validity of the decisions rendered.[76] Examples include anchoring (adhering to an initial impression despite newer or differing counter-information) and the framing effect (how information is presented to the group—what is presented first or how it is described—drives group interpretations and decisions). Bias can arise or be averted due to the order in which the committee reviews performance data. For example, showing medical knowledge examination scores can shift committee members' thinking and generate a halo effect that influences their impressions or ratings of other competencies. Strategies to avoid this risk include suppressing older scores that do not reflect current performance (e.g., not showing Medical College Admission Test scores in discussing a student or not showing licensing examination scores from medical school in discussion of a resident).

To capitalize on the benefits of the group process, member training should orient them to strategies for recognizing and counteracting potential cognitive biases. The chair should encourage members to share differing opinions within a psychologically safe space. Groupthink within a cohesive group threatens decision-making because feelings of allegiance to the group supersede sharing or endorsing dissenting information in the effort to achieve unanimity.[50,77] Committee members can engage

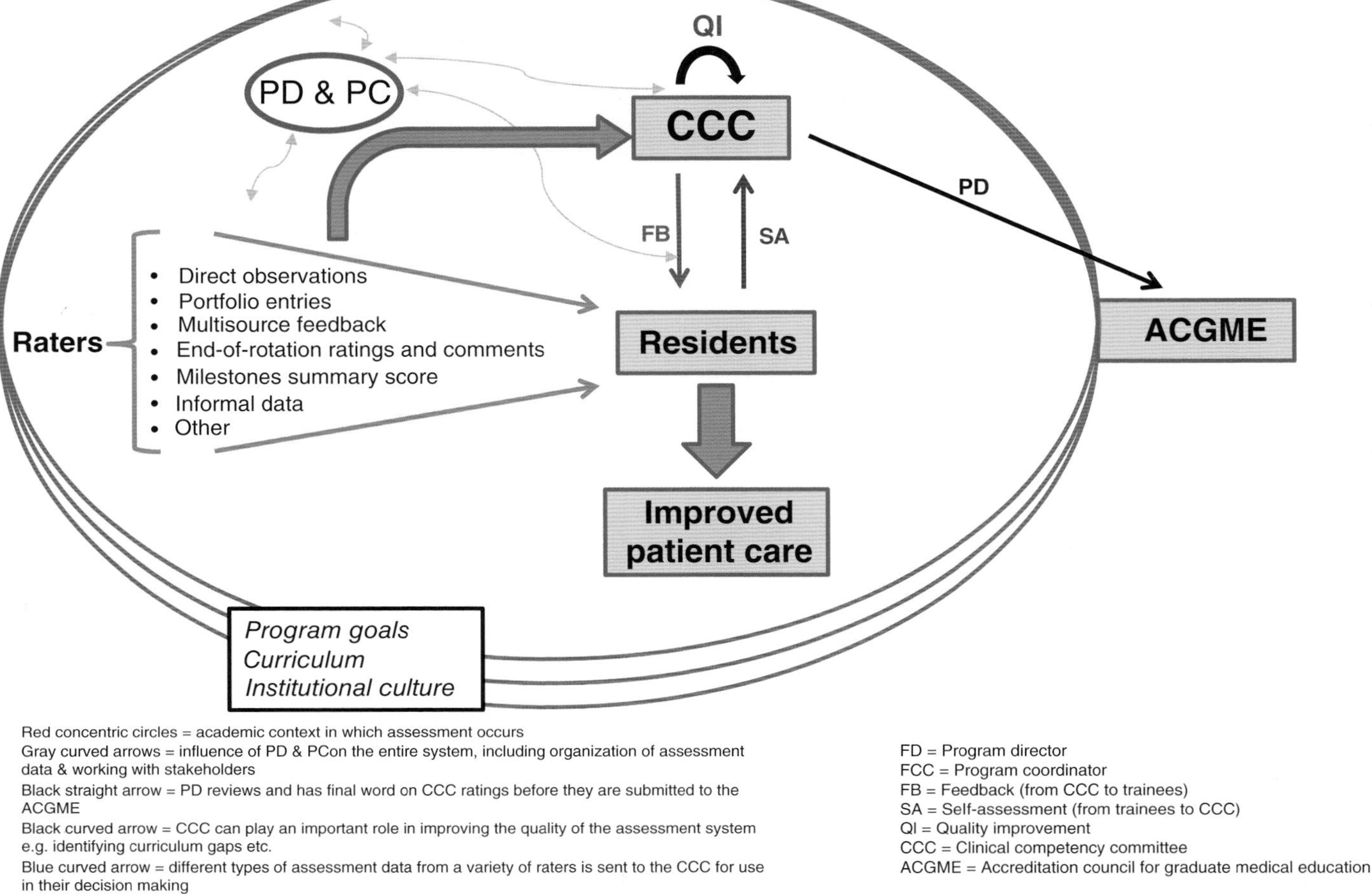

An example of a decision-making group within the context of milestones reporting in graduate medical programs in the United States. Updated from Ekpenyong et al A Textbook of Internal Medicine Programs, 12th ed.[68]

• **Fig. 16.4** Group process as part of a system of assessment.

TABLE 16.5 Time Management Strategies for Group Decision-Making

Time Management Strategy	Benefit(s)	Pitfall(s)
Use of subcommittees	Benefit depends on the focus of the subcommittees; for example: 1) By training level – allows members to become skilled at defining expectations of clinical performance at that specific level 2) By cohort – members can monitor the progress of their cohort longitudinally (over the entire course of training) 3) By core competency – faculty can become content experts	Group may rely too heavily on these subcommittees and not put in place strategies to ensure all trainees are discussed adequately
Increase meeting frequency	Shorter, more focused agenda	May redistribute rather than save time Scheduling more meetings can be challenging
Prereview resident data	Ensures that all learners' performance is reviewed and affords time for in-depth discussion of trainees experiencing various challenges	Prereview process must be robust to avoid situation in which trainees who are performing well are not receiving sufficient attention or feedback for how best to advance further

in reflective discussion after assessing each candidate or at the end of meetings to consider possible biases that may have manifested in their deliberations and generate countermeasures.

Time Management Strategies

Groups should employ approaches to accomplish their agenda within the time allocated for meetings. We elaborate on common time management strategies in Table 16.5. Groups may choose to meet more frequently, although additional meetings may be challenging for members' schedules. Assigning members to do work prior to the meeting by reviewing assessment data for an assigned number of trainees shifts data review tasks outside of meeting time to use group time for discussion and analysis.[55] These faculty perform their review and then present the trainee to the group along with their initial impressions or performance ratings to guide the group's subsequent discussion. Another approach is use of subcommittees.[52,55] Subcommittees may focus on subgroups of trainees based on various factors such as year of training, learning track, or alphabetically. However, these smaller groups need enough members for robust conversation. Their findings and decisions should be presented to the full group for brief endorsement unless there is disagreement necessitating further discussion.

Group chairs should guide group members to maintain focus on the agenda at hand to adhere to the time allotment of the meeting. Time management requires balancing the need to discuss struggling learners in detail with performance review for all learners to assess progress and generate feedback.[69,70]

Virtual Meetings

The COVID-19 pandemic limited in-person meetings and shifted groups to virtual platforms. Some groups may wish to meet virtually for convenience, particularly those with educators spread over multiple campuses. The virtual meeting context necessitates new facilitation skills to manage the chat, administer polling, monitor for questions, and ensure all members' participation. The chair can guide members to establish group agreements for virtual meetings: for example, agreeing that all participants should have their cameras on and use the "raise hand" function to avoid members talking over one another. The chair should anticipate tending to technical requirements of virtual meetings. Appointing someone other than the chair to manage the waiting room and the chat function and monitor for any "raised hands" facilitates members' ability to participate fully. Committee chairs and program coordinators need to ensure that all necessary assessment data are accessible to committee members on a virtual platform and that other data requested during the meeting are easily available for sharing among the members in real time. Committee decisions should be recorded and ideally made visual (e.g., via screen sharing during the meeting). Any audiovisual recording of the meetings should only occur with the consent of all members. The group should decide whether comments or questions in the chat should be included in the meeting minutes.

After Group Meetings

Documentation

Documentation of discussions during group meetings is crucial for providing feedback to different stakeholders (e.g., program leaders, learners, coaches), developing a longitudinal record of past decisions, reviewing and improving group processes, and providing evidence of due process.[78] Each meeting should have a scribe who takes minutes of the meeting's proceedings.[53,55] Scribing should be done by someone other than the group chair to avoid the cognitive load of both facilitating a meeting and documenting meeting events. High-quality minutes succinctly document the group's attendees, process, main discussion points about learners (e.g., strengths, areas for improvement), and decisions reached about promotion and remediation.[79] Minutes should be stored confidentially, accessible to program leadership, and organized in a way that allows for review of learners' longitudinal trajectory through a program. Standardized documentation templates help ensure all necessary information is captured. Minutes should not include known or suspected personal health or medical issues, or verbatim transcripts of comments shared within the committee (especially using colloquial language).[78] Meeting minutes should be used to develop feedback for learners, though they do not necessarily need to be shared verbatim. If previously undocumented data are used in decision-making, they should be summarized and included in the minutes. Transparency in the group decision-making process promotes fairness[44] and may increase acceptability to learners.[80]

Feedback

Learners, program directors, coaches, curriculum designers, assessment leaders, and accrediting bodies are all stakeholders who may receive feedback after group decisions are rendered. A key tenet of CBME is assessment *for* learning,[81–83] and thus learners may be the most important stakeholders to receive feedback. Group decisions should be shared with learners, along with contextual information on which data and processes were used to arrive at those decisions. For example, if narrative observational assessments led to feedback on a particular skill (e.g., more succinct documentation), the learner should be aware of which assessment data informed that feedback. This information allows the learner to reflect on those assessments and incorporate the feedback into real-world tasks. Groups should take a developmental orientation toward decision-making,[69] by providing every learner with feedback on how they can improve, including those who are performing at or above expectations. A fair and transparent process to appeal group decisions should exist for learners to easily access.[44,53,78]

Learner Role Related to Group Decision-Making Within a Program of Assessment

As key constituents in the assessment process, learners should be active participants who are adequately prepared to engage with information and feedback resulting from group decision-making. Successful group decision-making as part of programmatic assessment entails the collection and interpretation of a range of assessment data throughout a period of learning. To maximize the value of assessment for learning, learners must understand the assessment framework and principles behind assessment program design.[80] From the learners' perspective, this approach may be unfamiliar because it may be quite different than the assessment approach and methods used earlier in their education. Key concepts for learners related to group decision-making are shown in Table 16.6. The concept of coproduction is a powerful guide to maximizing the value of group decision-making for learners. Coproduction in learner assessment entails involving learners in the decision, planning, and conduct of the assessment process.[82] Learners are consequently empowered as drivers of their own learning and assessment, rather than just passive recipients of assessment information.[84] Learners may engage in coproduction of assessment data through learning planning or initiating assessments; they may engage in coproduction in the group decision-making process by generating self-assessments or portfolios to showcase their own selection and interpretation of assessment evidence regarding their competence. To achieve coproduction, learners must understand and participate in assessment procedures that contribute to group decision-making.

Orienting Learners to Group Decision-Making

Learner engagement begins with ensuring their clear understanding of the purpose and conduct of group decision-making within the program. Orientation for learners to the assessment program should address the fact that multiple assessment methods are used for the purpose of capturing their progress and performance in the range of skills, knowledge, and attitudes necessary for clinical practice.[80] Understanding this approach provides necessary background for the learner to be prepared to understand the role of the decision-making group and the information generated from their deliberations. Orientation to the program's expectations, typically outlined as competencies and milestones or EPAs, enables learners to target their learning by comparing current to expected performance. Learners will seek to clarify which assessment data are used for what purpose, what decisions may be rendered based on these data, and the "stakes" or consequences attached to those decisions.[85,86] Orienting them to data used as "assessment for learning" illustrates how assessment data can be used by both learners and teachers for the purpose of guiding the supervisors' direct observation of the learner, feedback sharing, and further learner practice. Multiple assessments for learning events, while designed to be low stakes, may be used by a decision-making group as evidence of learning and such use should be clarified for learners. Learners need to understand how assessment of learning entails higher-stakes judgments, and the manner by which groups make decisions.

Continuous Improvement in Group Process

Group process in assessment can drive continuous quality improvement of the assessment system and the overall training program. Detailed analyses of learner assessment data, and gaps in needed data, reveal areas where curriculum and assessment need to be strengthened or expanded.

Groups engaged in review of learner performance should incorporate regular reflection upon their work

TABLE 16.6 Key Concepts for a Learner to Understand Regarding Group Decision-Making

Concept	Definition	Relevance for Group Decision-Making
Competency-based medical education	Outcomes-based approach to the design, implementation, and continuous improvement of medical education curricula including approaches to assessing learner performance[81]	Group decision-making in medical education entails using defined outcomes expectations, commonly including competencies and milestones, to assess learner progress.
Growth mindset	The belief that one can improve through effort and focused practice, ideally guided by a coach[100]	Learners and faculty who embrace a growth mindset encourage and value feedback, reflection, goal setting, and opportunities for practice and reattempting challenging tasks.
Learning goals, learning plan	Learner-generated plans for improvement based on review of performance and program expectations. Goal setting can be supported by introducing learners and their faculty mentors/coaches to the master adaptive learner framework[101] or self-regulated learning theory.[102]	Group can review learner's previously generated goals to determine alignment with group feedback and progress made on achieving the goals, or provide feedback to a learner to use in setting future goals.[103]
Assessment for learning	A process by which learners and their teachers/coaches/mentors seek and interpret information about learner performance to guide decisions about future learning and teaching[85]	Group seeks evidence of learner's response to feedback and demonstration of improvement. Group may generate recommendations about needed future learning opportunities to address gaps in learning.
Assessment of learning	Group decision-making within a program of assessment entails educators reviewing assessment data and applying expert deliberations and judgments to determine learners' achievement of expectations.	Output of group is decision (e.g., regarding readiness to advance, grade earned) or recommendations to program director about achievement of or progress on expectations
Coproduction	Learners and their teachers together create assessment data and use the data to guide future learning.[82,104]	Group may assess learners' participation in generating assessment data and competence in reflection, learning planning
Coaching	A coach in health professions education is an individual paired with a learner for the purpose of guiding that learner to achieve their maximal potential by applying strategies of feedback, learning planning, and reflection.[105]	Before or after group decision-making, a coach can work with a learner to support the learner's interpretation of assessment data, reflection, review of information generated through group decision-making, and generation of learning goals.

through debriefing, discussion with program and institutional leaders as well as other educators and learners, and data review. Review of adherence to institutional and program policies and accreditation requirements contributes to adherence to expectations for the group's assessment work. Defining and monitoring learners' outcomes enables insight into the degree to which the assessment process facilitates achievement of expected learning.[87] The group should identify ongoing faculty development opportunities and needs, as described above. To assist chairpersons and group members in keeping track of these factors that affect the group process and its success, we refer readers to Table 16.7. This table can be used while planning meeting agendas and after meetings to guide continuous quality improvement of the groups process and more.

Conclusion

Group decision-making in medical education serves the purpose of assessing clinical performance as learners embark on their trajectory toward competence and beyond. At the center of group work are the learners and the health and well-being of the public. This chapter describes the various factors that affect group composition and functioning, including key factors for both chairpersons and their group members to consider before, during, and after their meetings. Whether groups are newly formed or well established, their chairs should ensure that these factors are reviewed and discussed by the group periodically to keep the group on target with its goals and maximize its effectiveness.

TABLE 16.7 Group Process Checklist for Use by Group Chairs and Members to Assess and Review the Components and Characteristics of the Group to Achieve Maximum Effectiveness

Decision-making	o Are the assessment data well organized to facilitate decision-making? o How are decisions reached? (e.g., consensus, majority) o Is there a shared mental model among members? o What is the frame of reference used? o Have biases been considered/acknowledged? o Based on valid assessments? o Is there transparency in the decision-making process?
Membership	o Is there an adequate number for robust discussion? o Are diverse perspectives represented? o Do members understand what is expected of them? o Will membership terms be used?
Ground rules	o Has the group established rules by which their meetings will run? (e.g., meeting logistics) o Is certain learner information off limits? (e.g., health information, personal events) o Is there a process for addressing conflicts of interest?
Agenda	o Is a clear agenda set for each meeting? o Is the agenda sent out to members prior to the meeting?
Group process	o Have measures been taken to avoid groupthink and other biases? o Are all members encouraged to voice their opinions? o Are time management strategies employed?
Documentation	o Who is taking minutes during meetings? o Who has access to minutes after meetings? o What template is used to guide minute-taking?
Feedback	o After the meeting, how are group decisions shared with trainees and the training program?
Learner engagement	o Are the learners aware of the group? o Are learners invited to voice their opinions about their assessment? o How do they use and respond to feedback from the group?
Continuous quality improvement	o Does the group periodically review its decisions and processes to make improvements to the efficiency and effectiveness of their work? o Does the group review learner outcomes over time and its own adherence to policies and procedures? o Is faculty development for the members needed? If so, how is this being addressed?

Annotated Bibliography

1. Hauer KE, ten Cate O, Boscardin CK, et al. Ensuring resident competence: a narrative review of the literature on group decision-making to inform the work of clinical competency committees. *J Grad Med Educ*. 2016;8(2):156–164.
This article provides a narrative review of literature on group decision-making, drawing from medical education, psychology, and organizational behavior. The authors cite multiple factors related to group member composition and group processes that can impact the quality of decisions. These factors include member characteristics, group size, group understanding of its work, group leader role, information-sharing procedures, and effects of time pressures. The authors provide multiple practical recommendations for competence committees based on these factors.
2. Hauer KE, Edgar L, Hogan SO, Kinnear B, Warm E. The science of effective group process: lessons for clinical competency committees. *J Grad Med Educ*. 2021;13(2 Suppl):59–64.
This article provides a review of multiple concepts and theories relevant to group decision-making, drawing from fields outside of medical education. The authors review social decision scheme theory, functional theory, groupthink, and the wisdom of crowds. They provide a framework for how these concepts and theories can be employed in competence committee decision-making.
3. Pack R, Lingard L, Watling CJ, Chahine S, Cristancho SM. Some assembly required: tracing the interpretative work of clinical competency committees. *Med Educ*. 2019;53(7):723–734.
This constructivist grounded theory study examined how competence committees at four postgraduate programs in Canada interpret and weigh assessment data when making decisions. The authors found that while some interpretations and decisions were relatively effortless, decisions were much more difficult when "problematic" evidence was present. "Problematic evidence" included assessment data that were ambiguous, data that came from untrusted sources or processes, data that were misaligned with committee expectations of a learner, or data that were absent. These data required more effortful interpretation strategies including unpacking, closer examination, debate, and verification.
4. Frank AK, O'Sullivan P, Mills LM, Muller-Juge V, Hauer KE. Clerkship grading committees: the impact of group decision-making for clerkship grading. *J Gen Intern Med*. 2019;34(5):669–676.
This qualitative study used semistructured interviews with grading committee chairs and members at a single US medical school to explore how members use assessment data to make decisions, as well as the benefits and challenges of a committee approach. Perceived committee benefits included improved grading consistency, fairness, and transparency. Perceived challenges included unconscious bias, tensions when making decisions on learners one knows personally, concerns about data quality, and groupthink.

5. Sapp JE, Torre DM, Larsen KL, Holmboe ES, Durning SJ. Trust in group decisions: a scoping review. *BMC Med Educ.* 2019;19(1):1–13.
In this scoping review, the authors examine what is known about group trust and embark on defining it. They propose a model for group trust, using situated cognition as a theoretical framework, that takes into account individual level factors, group level factors, and the connections between them. Authors define group trust as "group-directed willingness to accept vulnerability to actions of the members based on the expectation that members will perform a particular action important to the group, encompassing social exchange, collective perceptions, and interpersonal trust." Using the factors identified as encompassing group trust, the authors offer practical implications for CCCs. The authors note that this review did not include any papers on group trust in health professions education as none were identified through their search.

References

1. Emmerling T, Rooders D. 7 strategies for better group decision-making. *Harvard Business Review*. September 22, 2020. Accessed June 17, 2022. https://hbr.org/2020/09/7-strategies-for-better-group-decision-making.
2. Hauer KE, Cate OT, Boscardin CK, et al. Ensuring resident competence: a narrative review of the literature on group decision making to inform the work of clinical competency committees. *J Grad Med Educ*. 2016;8(2):156–164.
3. Stangor C. *Principles of Social Psychology – 1st International Edition*. eCampusOntario.
4. Dai P. The conceptual model of influencing factors and influencing mechanism on team decision-making quality mediated by information sharing. *iBusiness*. 2013;05(04):119–125.
5. Johnson DH, Johnson FP. *Joining Together: Group Theory and Group Skills*. 11th ed. Pearson; 2012.
6. Common Program Requirements (Residency). 2020. Published online.
7. Competence committees :: The Royal College of Physicians and Surgeons of Canada. Accessed August 10, 2022. https://www.royalcollege.ca/rcsite/cbd/assessment/competence-committees-e
8. Frank AK, O'Sullivan P, Mills LM, Muller-Juge V, Hauer KE. Clerkship grading committees: the impact of group decision-making for clerkship grading. *J Gen Intern Med*. 2019;34(5):669–676.
9. Green EP, Gruppuso PA. Justice and care: decision making by medical school student promotions committees. *Med Educ*. 2017;51(6):621–632.
10. Hobday PM, Borman-Shoap E, Cullen MJ, Englander R, Murray KE. The Minnesota Method: a learner-driven, Entrustable Professional Activity-based comprehensive program of assessment for medical students. *Acad Med*. 2021;96(7S):S50.
11. Hemmer PA, Hawkins R, Jackson JL, Pangaro LN. Assessing how well three evaluation methods detect deficiencies in medical students' professionalism in two settings of an internal medicine clerkship. *Acad Med*. 2000;75(2):167–173.
12. Schwind CJ, Williams RG, Boehler ML, Dunnington GL. Do individual attendings' post-rotation performance ratings detect residents' clinical performance deficiencies? *Acad Med*. 2004;79(5):453–457.
13. Thomas MR, Beckman TJ, Mauck KF, Cha SS, Thomas KG. Group assessments of resident physicians improve reliability and decrease halo error. *J Gen Intern Med*. 2011;26(7):759–764.
14. Yaghmour NA, Poulin LJ, Bernabeo EC, et al. Stages of milestones implementation: a template analysis of 16 programs across 4 specialties. *J Grad Med Educ*. 2021;13(2 Suppl):14–44.
15. van der Vleuten CPM, Schuwirth LWT, Driessen EW, et al. A model for programmatic assessment fit for purpose. *Med Teach*. 2012;34(3):205–214.
16. Frank JR, Mungroo R, Ahmad Y, Wang M, De Rossi S, Horsley T. Toward a definition of competency-based education in medicine: a systematic review of published definitions. *Med Teach*. 2010;32(8):631–637.
17. Van Melle E, Frank JR, Holmboe ES, et al. A core components framework for evaluating implementation of competency-based medical education programs. *Acad Med*. 2019;94(7):1002–1009.
18. Cooke M. Carnegie Foundation for the Advancement of Teaching. *Educating Physicians: A Call for Reform of Medical School and Residency*. 1st ed. Jossey-Bass; 2010.
19. Holmboe ES, Yamazaki K, Hamstra SJ. The evolution of assessment: thinking longitudinally and developmentally. *Acad Med*. 2020;95(11S Association of American Medical Colleges Learn Serve Lead: Proceedings of the 59th Annual Research in Medical Education Presentations):S7–S9.
20. Pusic MV, Boutis K, Hatala R, Cook DA. Learning curves in health professions education. *Acad Med*. 2015;90(8):1034–1042.
21. Pack R, Lingard L, Watling CJ, Chahine S, Cristancho SM. Some assembly required: tracing the interpretative work of clinical competency committees. *Med Educ*. 2019;53(7):723–734.
22. Gingerich A, Kogan J, Yeates P, Govaerts M, Holmboe E. Seeing the "black box" differently: assessor cognition from three research perspectives. *Med Educ*. 2014;48(11):1055–1068.
23. Lickel B, Hamilton DL, Wieczorkowska G, Lewis A, Sherman SJ, Uhles AN. Varieties of groups and the perception of group entitativity. *J Pers Soc Psychol*. 2000;78(2):223–246.
24. Jönsson ML, Hahn U, Olsson EJ. The kind of group you want to belong to: effects of group structure on group accuracy. *Cognition*. 2015;142:191–204.
25. Cannon-Bowers JA, Salas E, Converse S. Shared mental models in expert team decision making. In: Castellan NJ, ed. *Individual and Group Decision Making*. Lawrence Erlbaum Associates; 1993:221–245.
26. Catholijn M, Jonker MB van R. Shared Mental Models – A Conceptual Analysis. 2010:132–151. Published online.
27. Mohammed S, Dumville BC. Team mental models in a team knowledge framework: expanding theory and measurement across disciplinary boundaries. *J Organ Behav*. 2001;22(2):89–106.
28. Edgar L, Jones MD, Harsy B, Passiment M, Hauer KE. Better decision-making: shared mental models and the clinical competency committee. *J Grad Med Educ*. 2021;13(2 Suppl):51–58.
29. Holmboe ES, Kogan JR. Will any road get you there? Examining warranted and unwarranted variation in medical education. *Acad Med*. March 1, 2022 Published online.
30. Kane MT. Current concerns in validity theory. *JEM*. 2001; 38(4):319–342.
31. Cook DA, Brydges R, Ginsburg S, Hatala R. A contemporary approach to validity arguments: a practical guide to Kane's framework. *Med Educ*. 2015;49(6):560–575.
32. Hodge S. The origins of competency-based training. *Aust J Adult Learn*. 2007;47(2):179–209.
33. Wong BM, Baum KD, Headrick LA, et al. Building the bridge to quality: an urgent call to integrate quality improvement and patient safety education with clinical care. *Acad Med*. 2020;95(1):59–68.

34. Bendermacher GWG, De Grave WS, Wolfhagen IHAP, Dolmans DHJM, Oude Egbrink MGA. Shaping a culture for continuous quality improvement in undergraduate medical education. *Acad Med*. 2020;95(12):1913–1920.
35. Brateanu A, Thomascik J, Koncilja K, Spencer AL, Colbert CY. Using continuous quality-improvement techniques to evaluate and enhance an internal medicine residency program's assessment system. *Am J Med*. 2017;130(6):750–755.
36. Turner J, Wimberly Y, Andolsek KM. Creating a high-quality faculty orientation and ongoing member development curriculum for the clinical competency committee. *J Grad Med Educ*. 2021;13(2s):65–69.
37. Duitsman ME, Fluit CRMG, van Alfen-van der Velden JAEM, et al. Design and evaluation of a clinical competency committee. *Perspect Med Educ*. 2019;8(1):1–8.
38. Burnes B. Kurt Lewin and the Harwood Studies: The foundations of OD. *J Appl Behav Sci*. 2007;43(2):213–231.
39. Magee JC, Galinsky AD. 8 Social Hierarchy: The Self-Reinforcing Nature of Power and Status. *ANNALS*. 2008;2(1):351–398.
40. Salzmann J, Grasha AF. Psychological size and psychological distance in manager-subordinate relationships. *J Soc Psychol*. 1991;131(5):629–646.
41. Rayment M. Your Psychological Size & Leadership Style. Accessed May 20, 2022. https://www.linkedin.com/pulse/your-psychological-size-leadership-style-miche-rayment.
42. Stasser G, Titus W. Effects of information load and percentage of shared information on the dissemination of unshared information during group discussion. *J Pers Soc Psychol*. 1987;53(1):81–93.
43. Beran TN, Kaba A, Caird J, McLaughlin K. The good and bad of group conformity: a call for a new programme of research in medical education. *Med Educ*. 2014;48(9):851–859.
44. Colbert CY, French JC, Herring ME, Dannefer EF. Fairness: the hidden challenge for competency-based postgraduate medical education programs. *Perspect Med Educ*. 2017;6(5):347–355.
45. La Macchia ST, Louis WR, Hornsey MJ, Leonardelli GJ. In small we trust: lay theories about small and large groups. *Pers Soc Psychol Bull*. 2016;42(10):1321–1334.
46. Karotkin D, Paroush J. Optimum committee size: quality-versus-quantity dilemma. *Soc Choice Welfare*. 2003;20(3):429–441.
47. Austen-Smith D, Banks JS. Information aggregation, rationality, and the condorcet jury theorem. *Am Political Sci Rev*. 1996;90(01):34–45.
48. Simms A, Nichols T. Social loafing: a review of the literature. *J Manage*. 2014:15.
49. Laughlin PR, Kerr NL, Davis JH, Halff HM, Marciniak KA. Group size, member ability, and social decision schemes on an intellective task. *J Pers Soc Psychol*. 1975;31(3):522–535.
50. Janis IL. Groupthink. *Psychol Today*. 1971;5:43–46 74-76.
51. Chan T, Oswald A, Hauer KE, et al. Diagnosing conflict: conflicting data, interpersonal conflict, and conflicts of interest in clinical competency committees. *Med Teach*. 2021;43(7):765–773.
52. Ekpenyong A, Baker E, Harris I, et al. How do clinical competency committees use different sources of data to assess residents' performance on the internal medicine milestones? A mixed methods pilot study. *Med Teach*. 2017;39(10):1074–1083.
53. Kinnear B, Warm EJ, Hauer KE. Twelve tips to maximize the value of a clinical competency committee in postgraduate medical education. *Med Teach*. 2018;40(11):1110–1115.
54. Sirianni G, Glover Takahashi S, Myers J. Taking stock of what is known about faculty development in competency-based medical education: a scoping review paper. *Med Teach*. 2020;42(8):909–915.
55. Andolsek K, Padmore J, Hauer KE, Ekpenyong A, Edgar L, Holmboe E. *Clinical Competency Committees: A Guidebook for Programs*. 3rd ed. 2020. Accessed August 9, 2022. https://www.acgme.org/globalassets/acgmeclinicalcompetencycommittee-guidebook.pdf.
56. Dennis AR. Information exchange and use in small group decision making. *Small Group Res*. 1996;27(4):532–550.
57. Nembhard IM, Edmondson AC. Making it safe: the effects of leader inclusiveness and professional status on psychological safety and improvement efforts in health care teams. *J Organiz Behav*. 2006;27(7):941–966.
58. Green EP, Beck Dallaghan GL, O'Hearn DJ, Verduin ML, Zehle CH. Establishing fair and ethical medical student promotions committees. *Med Sci Educ*. 2018;28(3):561–567.
59. Boscardin C, Fergus KB, Hellevig B, Hauer KE. Twelve tips to promote successful development of a learner performance dashboard within a medical education program. *Med Teach*. 2017;0(0):1–7.
60. Friedman KA, Raimo J, Spielmann K, Chaudhry S. Resident dashboards: helping your clinical competency committee visualize trainees' key performance indicators. *Med Educ Online*. 2016;21:29838.
61. Keister DM, Larson D, Dostal J, Baglia J. The radar graph: the development of an educational tool to demonstrate resident competency. *J Grad Med Educ*. 2012;4(2):220–226.
62. Warm EJ, Kinnear B, Kelleher M, Sall D, Holmboe E. Transforming resident assessment: an analysis using Deming's system of profound knowledge. *Acad Med*. 2019;94(2):195–201.
63. Schauer DP, Kinnear B, Kelleher M, Sall D, Schumacher DJ, Warm EJ. Developing the expected entrustment score: accounting for variation in resident assessment. *J Gen Intern Med*. April 4, 2022. Published online.
64. Zafar MA, Diers T, Schauer DP, Warm EJ. Connecting resident education to patient outcomes: the evolution of a quality improvement curriculum in an internal medicine residency. *Acad Med*. 2014;89(10):1341–1347.
65. Warm EJ, Schauer D, Revis B, Boex JR. Multisource feedback in the ambulatory setting. *J Grad Med Educ*. 2010;2(2):269–277.
66. Mathis BR, Warm EJ, Schauer DP, Holmboe E, Rouan GW. A multiple choice testing program coupled with a year-long elective experience is associated with improved performance on the internal medicine in-training examination. *J Gen Intern Med*. 2011;26(11):1253–1257.
67. Thoma B, Bandi V, Carey R, et al. Developing a dashboard to meet competence committee needs: a design-based research project. *Can Med Educ J*. 2020;11(1):e16–e34.
68. Hauer KE, Edgar L, Hogan SO, Kinnear B, Warm E. The science of effective group process: lessons for clinical competency committees. *J Grad Med Educ*. 2021;13(2 Suppl):59–64.
69. Hauer KE, Chesluk B, Iobst W, et al. Reviewing residents' competence: a qualitative study of the role of clinical competency committees in performance assessment. *Acad Med*. 2015;90(8):1084–1092.
70. Ekpenyong A, Edgar L, Wilkerson L, Holmboe ES. A multispecialty ethnographic study of clinical competency committees (CCCs). *Med Teach*. May 30, 2022:1–9. Published online.
71. Tam J, Wadhwa A, Martimianakis MA, Fernando O, Regehr G. The role of previously undocumented data in the assessment of medical trainees in clinical competency committees. *Perspect Med Educ*. 2020;9(5):286–293.

72. Schumacher DJ, Kinnear B. Is the proof in the PUDding? Reflections on previously undocumented data (PUD) in clinical competency committees. *Perspect Med Educ.* 2020;9(5):269–271.
73. Kassam AF, Cortez AR, Winer LK, et al. Swipe right for surgical residency: exploring the unconscious bias in resident selection. *Surgery.* 2020;168(4):724–729.
74. Goldin C, Rouse C. Orchestrating impartiality: the impact of "blind" auditions on female musicians. *Am Econ Rev.* 2000;90(4):715–741.
75. Maina IW, Belton TD, Ginzberg S, Singh A, Johnson TJ. A decade of studying implicit racial/ethnic bias in healthcare providers using the implicit association test. *Soc Sci Med.* 2018;199:219–229.
76. Dickey CC, Thomas C, Feroze U, Nakshabandi F, Cannon B. Cognitive demands and bias: challenges facing clinical competency committees. *J Grad Med Educ.* 2017;9(2):162–164.
77. Mannion R, Thompson C. Systematic biases in group decision-making: implications for patient safety. *Int J Qual Health Care.* 2014;26(6):606–612.
78. Padmore JS, Andolsek KM, Iobst WF, Poulin LJ, Hogan SO, Richard KM. Navigating academic law in competency decisions. *J Grad Med Educ.* 2021;13(2 Suppl):102–108.
79. Ekpenyong A, Padmore JS, Hauer KE. The purpose, structure, and process of clinical competency committees: guidance for members and program directors. *J Grad Med Educ.* 2021;13(2s):45–50.
80. Hall J, Oswald A, Hauer KE, et al. Twelve tips for learners to succeed in a CBME program. *Med Teach.* May 21, 2021:1–6. Published online.
81. Frank JR, Snell LS, Cate OT, et al. Competency-based medical education: theory to practice. *Med Teach.* 2010;32(8):638–645.
82. Holmboe ES. Work-based assessment and co-production in postgraduate medical training. *GMS J Med Educ.* 2017;34(5):Doc58.
83. van der Vleuten CPM, Schuwirth LWT, Driessen EW, Govaerts MJB, Heeneman S. 12 Tips for programmatic assessment. *Med Teach.* November 20, 2014:1–6. Published online.
84. Buttemer S, Hall J, Berger L, Weersink K, Dagnone JD. Ten ways to get a grip on resident co-production within medical education change. *Can Med Educ J.* 2020;11(1):e124–e129.
85. Black P, Wiliam D. Developing the theory of formative assessment. *Educ Asse Eval Acc.* 2009;21(1):5.
86. Schut S, Driessen E, van Tartwijk J, van der Vleuten C, Heeneman S. Stakes in the eye of the beholder: an international study of learners' perceptions within programmatic assessment. *Med Educ.* 2018;52(6):654–663.
87. Schellekens LLH, Slof B, Bok HGJ. Quality assurance of an assessment program. *Understanding Assessment in Medical Education through Quality Assurance.* McGraw Hill; 2022.
88. Griffiths J, Dalgarno N, Schultz K, Han H, van Melle E. Competency-based medical education implementation: are we transforming the culture of assessment? *Med Teach.* 2019;41(7):811–818.
89. Holmboe ES, Sherbino J, Long DM, Swing SR, Frank JR. The role of assessment in competency-based medical education. *Med Teach.* 2010;32(8):676–682.
90. Swing SR. Perspectives on competency-based medical education from the learning sciences. *Med Teach.* 2010;32(8):663–668.
91. Timmerman AA, Dijkstra J. A practical approach to programmatic assessment design. *Adv in Health Sci Educ.* 2017;22(5):1169–1182.
92. Bowe CM, Armstrong E. Assessment for systems learning: a holistic assessment framework to support decision making across the medical education continuum. *Acad Med.* 2017;92(5):585–592.
93. Chahine S, Cristancho S, Padgett J, Lingard L. How do small groups make decisions? A theoretical framework to inform the implementation and study of clinical competency committees. *Perspect Med Educ.* 2017;6(3):192–198.
94. Pack R, Lingard L, Watling C, Cristancho S. Beyond summative decision making: illuminating the broader roles of competence committees. *Med Educ.* 2020;54(6):517–527.
95. van der Vleuten CPM, Schuwirth LWT. Assessing professional competence: from methods to programmes. *Med Educ.* 2005;39(3):309–317.
96. Holmboe ES, Ward DS, Reznick RK, et al. Faculty development in assessment: the missing link in competency-based medical education. *Acad Med.* 2011;86(4):460–467.
97. Hemmer PA, Pangaro L. Using formal evaluation sessions for case-based faculty development during clinical clerkships. *Acad Med.* 2000;75(12):1216–1221.
98. Eno C, Correa R, Stewart NH, et al. *Milestones Guidebook for Residents and Fellows.* Accreditation Council for Graduate Medical Education; 2020:19.
99. Heath JK, Davis JE, Dine CJ, Padmore JS. Faculty development for milestones and clinical competency committees. *J Grad Med Educ.* 2021;13(2s):127–131.
100. Dweck C. What having a "growth mindset" actually means. *Harvard Business Review.* January 13, 2016:1–5. Published online.
101. Cutrer WB, Miller B, Pusic MV, et al. Fostering the development of master adaptive learners: a conceptual model to guide skill acquisition in medical education. *Acad Med.* 2017;92(1):70–75.
102. Sandars J, Cleary TJ. Self-regulation theory: applications to medical education: AMEE Guide No. 58. *Med Teach.* 2011;33(11):875–886.
103. Donato AA, Alweis R, Wenderoth S. Design of a clinical competency committee to maximize formative feedback. *J Community Hosp Intern Med Perspect.* 2016;6(6):33533.
104. Englander R, Holmboe E, Batalden P, et al. Coproducing health professions education: a prerequisite to coproducing health care services? *Acad Med.* 2020;95(7):1006–1013.
105. Lovell B. What do we know about coaching in medical education? A literature review. Med Educ. 2018;52(4):376–390.

17

A Programmatic Approach to Identifying and Supporting the Struggling Learner

WILLIAM IOBST, MD, FACP, AND KAREN M. WARBURTON, MD

CHAPTER OUTLINE

"If you don't know where you are going, any road will get you there."[1]

—LEWIS CARROLL

Introduction

Support for the struggling learner is an expected and essential activity in any competency-based medical education program. As discussed elsewhere in this textbook, effective support, whether in the form of additional specialized evaluation or remediation, requires active participation, or coproduction, of the learner, faculty, and program. Coproduction is essential to achieve desired outcomes and hinges on effective engagement of all key stakeholders when addressing the struggling learner.[2] The responsibilities of learners, faculty, and the program highlighted throughout this chapter reinforce that these interventions are with, and not at or to, the learner and that successful interventions require that all participants must have a shared, mutual understanding of the language, processes, and expected outcomes of any intervention.

Background: Setting the Stage and Definitions

Language Matters

For graduate medical education (GME) programs accredited by the Accreditation Council for Graduate Medical Education (ACGME), program outcomes are defined by the six general competencies with a goal of developing future workforces capable of achieving the Quadruple Aim: improved outcomes; reasonable per-capita cost; improved patient experience; and improved clinician experience (Fig. 17.1). As the medical education community operationalizes a competency- or outcomes-based approach to medical education (CBME/OBME), the approach to the struggling learner must be reconceptualized. Fundamental to CBME is the appreciation that learners are on a developmental journey toward mastery of clearly described outcomes. This journey is made possible by the support provided by programs, faculty, and peers working with those learners to ensure that development follows an expected trajectory. However, for each individual learner the journey is unique, and while program outcomes must ultimately be met, the rate and trajectory of this developmental growth can vary. At times, learners may require additional time or support in the form of further specialized evaluation or remediation. This developmental approach, while not new, is at variance with a more traditional performance-based framing of medical education. Understanding the difference between these approaches to learning is critical. In a developmental mindset to learning, success in achieving an outcome is not automatic or instant, or even guaranteed. Learning is a journey in which success may not be immediate. The learning process is an opportunity for coaching, feedback, and growth. A performance-based approach to learning focuses on demonstrating competence relative to others and seeks immediate success in the task as optimal. To not succeed is to fail. Rather than framing the need for additional support as evidence of failure, as happens in performance-based learning, programs must foster cultures that recognize variable rates of learning as an expected part of developmental, or mastery, learning, even when this requires additional support by the program.

In previous iterations of this chapter, learners identified as needing more support were labeled as "the problem resident" or "the resident with a problem." As we will discuss, language can significantly influence this process, and describing learners as "problems" casts this support in a negative or punitive light that can adversely influence how these interventions are conceptualized by the participants. Furthermore, the term *problem* fails to capture the full picture of the learner's experience at a time of life when many internal and external factors may emerge and impact clinical performance. As such, in this chapter we have dropped use of the term *problem* in favor of *struggling*, a construct that comprises the myriad of circumstances, both at and outside the workplace, in which a learner may fall behind the expected performance trajectory. Support for these learners is presented as an activity that is occasionally, and often predictably, necessary to ensure that all learners achieve desired program outcomes.

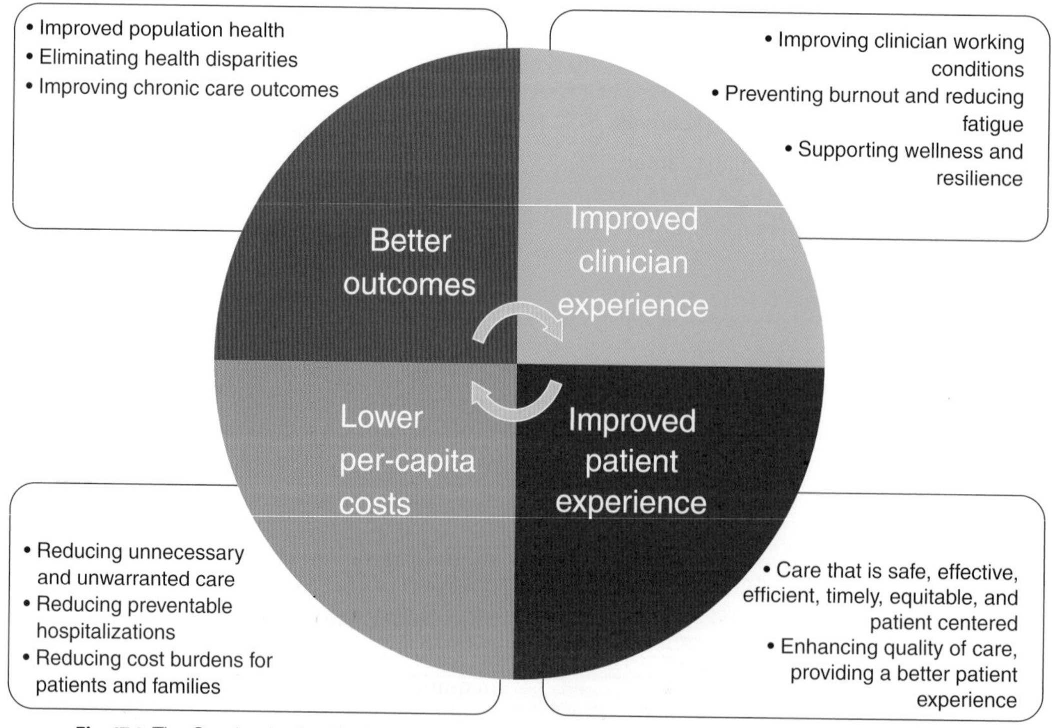

• **Fig. 17.1** The Quadruple Aim. Bodenheimer T, Sinsky C. From triple to quadruple aim: care of the patient requires care of the provider. *Ann Fam Med*. 2014 Nov-Dec;12(6):573-6. doi: 10.1370/afm.1713. PMID: 25384822; PMCID: PMC4226781.

On a basic level, struggling learners can be conceptualized as demonstrating gaps in developmental (academic) growth as defined by expected program outcomes, or they can demonstrate nondevelopmental gaps (misconduct). The interventions targeting these activities are often different and generally fall under the broad categories of remediation or disciplinary action. The first, and most emphasized, concept in this chapter is a developmental framework that characterizes remediation interventions by the term *academic*. The second concept involves issues that are considered nondevelopmental and generates interventions that address misconduct or other behaviors that violate expected societal or professional norms. While this distinction is important, it is notable that performance gaps cannot always be clearly categorized. Programs should recognize that struggles are not always developmental in nature and may reflect the influence of external pressures or internal struggles experienced by the learner. Often, such cases involve lapses in professionalism, which are discussed in more detail later in this chapter. In brief, the learner exhibiting unprofessional behavior may be amenable to interventions to advance developmental growth (remediation) and/or to address such internal or external stressors. However, at times, intervention requires the use of disciplinary action to address misconduct. In addition, this chapter highlights the frequency and importance of mental and physical health issues, often necessitating additional specialized evaluation, that underlie many developmental and nondevelopmental performance concerns.

Documenting why learners are struggling and determining appropriate interventions requires accurate assessment of the learner and well-defined systems for the identification, investigation, classification, intervention, and adjudication of such learners. Struggles can occur in any domain of competence, which, for GME and continuous professional development, is defined by the six ACGME/American Board of Medical Specialties (ABMS) general competencies in the United States and competency frameworks in other countries (see Chapter 1).[3]

In this chapter, off-course learners are described as having a gap between observed and expected performance and requiring programmatic intervention to return them to the expected learning trajectory. Programmatic interventions to assist these learners may include remediation, additional specialized evaluation of potential underlying conditions, disciplinary action, and, for those whose behavior or learning trajectory does not improve, termination. These interventions are defined as follows.

Intervention

> "...*help for a learner who needs more than the standard curriculum to achieve competency in all of the required domains.*"
>
> **JEANNETTE GUERRASIO, MD**[4]

> *The act of facilitating a correction for trainees who started out on the journey toward becoming a physician but have moved off-course.*
>
> **KALET AND CHOU**[5]

Remediation

The meaning and implications of the term *remediation* vary among programs and institutions. Differences center on the threshold for putting a learner on remediation, involvement of the institution's Office of Graduate Medical Education, and type and extent of documentation in the learner's file. Some institutions avoid the term altogether given concerns related to stigma. Remediation is most commonly viewed as a predisciplinary step and is typically not reportable to a licensing board or other regulatory entities. The following definitions[6] provide a reasonable framework for considering the spectrum of remediation. In addition, Kalet and associates have used the term *academic warning* to describe the need for early remediation that, if successful, is not necessarily reportable.[5] However, if the remediation associated with academic warning is unsuccessful, a more significant reportable sanction may be imposed. The importance of this developmental approach is that programs can create learning environments that provide assessment and intervention without long-term punitive consequences.

Informal

Informal remediation—often termed clinical coaching—should be initiated when warning signs exist but are not so significant to warrant immediate formal remediation. This stage serves as a critical opportunity to document the process if the learner fails to improve and there is an ultimate need to escalate the remediation. (Think individualized learning plan!)

Formal

When learners lack buy-in, when efforts to informally coach learners in deficient skills have been unsuccessful, or when struggles are significant enough to impact patient care, formal remediation is a reasonable next step. Institutions differ on policies around remediation, but for most this is a predisciplinary step that requires a written letter of warning in the learner's file, clearly defined objectives, and an outline of the consequences should these objectives not be met within the defined time frame.

Probation

Probation is initiated at some institutions when a learner fails to correct deficiencies during formal remediation or if problems are significant enough to warrant immediate probation (nondevelopmental). Probation is often considered a disciplinary action and may be reportable to the Board.

Termination

Termination occurs when a learner fails to meet the terms of probation or if initial problems are significant enough to warrant immediate dismissal.

In addition to defining these interventions, ensuring that all key stakeholders involved in the support of the struggling learner have a common understanding or shared mental model of the processes is critical and requires that programs work closely with their institutional legal departments to ensure that all appropriate institutional and legal standards are met.

Barriers to Recognition and Remediation of the Struggling Learner

The GME learning climate presents many potential barriers to the timely recognition and acknowledgment of struggling learners. There is often a human element of denial that arises when an educator is faced with a struggling learner. Several articles highlight the notion of "failure to fail,"[7–9] Barriers include logistic constraints that prevent us from directly observing our learners often enough, paucity of time or resources, lack of comfort with remediation, concerns about stigma, and fear of retaliation. While these are all legitimate concerns, they must be weighed against the consequences of ignoring the struggle in specific competencies, which in many cases will not improve without a dedicated remediation effort. More timely recognition of struggling learners often requires a culture change that involves acceptance that a certain proportion of our learners will struggle, that it is our responsibility to help them, and that we put into place the programmatic and institutional resources necessary to do so.

Vignette 1

A third-year resident in a 3-year postgraduate medical education program is referred by her program director in January to her institution's centralized remediation program for help, given significant concerns about her performance in the competencies of Patient Care and Medical Knowledge. The program director notes that "frankly, the concerns have always been there" and admits "we are not sure if this resident is competent and can graduate in June." The resident was encouraged to develop a reading plan several months earlier, but this has not resulted in observable improvement in performance.

Unfortunately, recognition or acknowledgment of deficiency late in training is not uncommon, and unless the faculty members in charge of her remediation plan are able to identify an underlying issue with mental or physical well-being that has led to an abrupt change in trajectory, it is unlikely that remediation of a learner with such significant deficits is going to be successful with only a few months remaining in the training period. This is a common set of circumstances encountered by remediation experts—that is, the delay in recognition or willingness to admit that a learner is struggling.

Vignette 2

A fellow in a 1-year postgraduate specialty training program is identified by his program's clinical competency committee in December to have significant performance concerns in the areas of Professionalism, Medical Knowledge, and Patient Care. The program is worried that he will need to extend his training. The institution has a remediation policy, but the program is reluctant to put the trainee on formal remediation. "We think he will do fine with some informal coaching and don't want to stigmatize him. We will reconvene in three months and assess his progress."

This commonly encountered scenario is risky, because if things do not improve with informal coaching at the three-month mark, it will be challenging to initiate a remediation plan with only three months left in the training program.

Developing clear standards of learner performance, well-defined assessment systems and learning objectives, and a learning culture that embraces assessment as a necessary part of professional development is essential in the anticipation of and preparation for the struggling learner. Developmental frameworks like the ACGME/ABMS Milestones[10] and assessment strategies including the use of Entrustable Professional Activities (EPAs) (see Chapter 1) can provide clarity around program expectations. In addition to defining performance expectations and assessment strategies, program leadership must also promote a culture that encourages ongoing feedback and assessment to advance learner development. Key stakeholders in the educational process charged with the assessment of learners must understand the purpose and outcome of the assessment process. Medical students, residents, fellows, and others, depending on the educational system, must understand undergraduate and graduate medical education is a developmental process leading to progressive levels of competence.

Learners across this continuum must expect and embrace that feedback will be both affirming (reinforcing) and corrective. In fact, they should demand corrective feedback as necessary to enable progress toward the goal of safe and effective unsupervised practice. Faculty completing evaluations must also understand that candid, formative, criterion-referenced feedback should be an expected outcome of assessment (Chapters 1 and 5). Faculty should appreciate that they are typically not making a final or high-stakes assessment of overall or general competence with each evaluation they perform, but rather are contributing an important data point to the comprehensive assessment of the learner by the program. Faculty help determine whether the learner was competent or not competent in that specific context and at that specific time (see Chapter 3).

The determination of general competence is the responsibility of the overall program, and in some countries such as the United States, Canada, Singapore, Qatar, and United Arab Emirates, judgment involves group decision-making processes via a clinical competency committee (CCC).[11] Attesting that a learner can safely progress to the next level of training or enter into unsupervised practice is an essential function of all medical education programs and professional self-regulation. The public rightly expects the medical profession to identify, remediate, and when necessary, discipline struggling learners and practicing physicians. For most educational systems, the overarching assessment framework is grounded in the competencies as described in Chapter 1.

The core attributes of an assessment program that is well equipped to deal with struggling learners include:

1) Clear frameworks defining competency development (e.g., competencies, Milestones, and EPAs, depending on the local educational context and needs).
2) Assessment systems that effectively and accurately generate data defining a learner's developmental stage and trajectory and that inform defensible decisions on learner competence.
3) Robust program structures and processes (e.g., CCCs) that allow for the interpretation and synthesis of assessment data.
4) A safe learning environment that recognizes that learners progress at variable rates and achievement of desired competencies is a developmental process.
5) A strong educational institutional and program culture that supports and empowers feedback and remediation.
6) Clear criteria for determining when an individual's progression deviates significantly enough from expected development that an intervention is required.
7) Clearly defined expectations of the roles and responsibilities of all key stakeholders in the educational and assessment processes. These stakeholders include educators, learners, and patients.
8) Endorsement by the institution's legal department that all policies and procedures are aligned with required legal standards.
9) Courage. Although uncommon, all programs at some point will be faced with the difficult but appropriate decision to dismiss a trainee who does not meet agreed-upon standards of competence (see Chapter 3).

When one of these core attributes is inadequately defined or missing, the ability of the program to effectively address struggling learners is compromised. Further, programs must develop and maintain the structures and processes needed to ensure that desired outcomes are achieved (Table 17.1). This systems approach to designing assessment programs, using structure, process, and outcomes, can help programs effectively develop appropriate pathways for the identification and remediation of struggling learners.

TABLE 17.1 Attributes of Effective Systems Addressing Struggling Learners

Structure	Process	Outcome
Program administration Program faculty Office of Graduate Medical Education Employee Health Services Competency committee Legal counsel Information technology systems	Clearly defined, criterion-referenced processes for: • Defining learning outcomes • Problem identification • Problem verification • Learner assessments • Interventions • Assessments of the intervention • Data synthesis	Successful remediation Unsuccessful remediation Probation Dismissal Continuous quality improvement

Scope of the Problem: Prevalence of Struggling Learners

Struggling learners in medical education are not new, nor are they rare. Prior to the many worldwide initiatives that have defined domains of competence,[12–17] struggle has most commonly been characterized as a problem with medical knowledge or clinical decision-making. Studies examining the prevalence of struggling learners in GME include specialty-specific surveys of program directors[18–22] or retrospective reports from single-center remediation experiences.[23–28] The point prevalence of struggling medical education learners is highly variable, depending on how one defines *struggle* and one's willingness to admit that a learner is struggling, and ranges in these studies between 2% and 22%. This is typically a small proportion of any given program, but these learners typically command a great deal of time and resources, so this should be anticipated.

In 2000, Yao and Wright[18] reported that approximately 94% of US internal medicine residency programs identified at least one resident in difficulty and specifically commented that they feared substantial underreporting of these individuals. In their study, the content areas identified as problematic were insufficient medical knowledge (48%), poor clinical judgment (44%), inefficiency (44%), inappropriate interactions (39%), and the provision of poor skills (36%). Hauer and associates[29] reviewed 13 studies that described single-institution programs designed to remediate problem learners and found that interventions almost exclusively addressed deficits in medical knowledge and clinical skills. In 2012, the American College of Surgeons (ACS) convened a panel of experts who identified four common areas of struggle among surgical residents: the resident who cannot operate; the resident with substance abuse; the inefficient resident; and the resident with poor clinical judgment.[30] In a retrospective review of a single-institution surgery residency program, deficiencies in technical skill was noted in only 8% of the residents who struggled,[24] highlighting the importance of other, nontechnical aspects of a surgical learner's performance.

Other studies evaluating whether current GME graduates can successfully enter into unsupervised practice identify significant competency gaps. To highlight this point, over a full decade after the launch of the ACGME Outcomes Project, Crosson and colleagues[31] identified significant gaps in physicians entering unsupervised practice within the California Kaiser Permanente healthcare system. Similarly, Mattar and colleagues[32] identified substantial gaps in performance in general surgical residents entering fellowship programs.

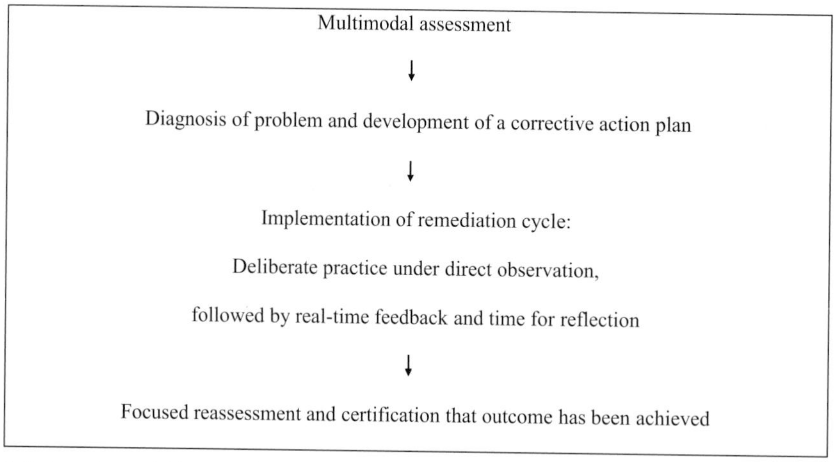

Multimodal assessment

↓

Diagnosis of problem and development of a corrective action plan

↓

Implementation of remediation cycle:

Deliberate practice under direct observation,

followed by real-time feedback and time for reflection

↓

Focused reassessment and certification that outcome has been achieved

• **Fig. 17.2** A basic model for remediation. Modified from Hauer KE, Ciccone A, Henzel TR, et al. Remediation of the deficiencies of physicians across the continuum from medical school to practice: a thematic review of the literature. *Acad Med*. 2009;84(12):1822–1832.

Assessment and Remediation of the Struggling Learner

These studies highlight the importance of completing accurate and meaningful assessments and emphasize the need to, as best as possible, have clearly defined and well-vetted outcomes for all levels of the medical education process. To appropriately meet the healthcare needs of society, such outcomes must not only define expected developmental trajectories for learners at all stages of development but also ensure that terminal graduates can function safely and effectively in the current healthcare delivery system. With this understanding of the scope of the problem and the recognition that a number of learners demonstrate performance gaps in one or more competency domains, the process of remediation must be approached systematically.

In a review highlighting a paucity of evidence to guide best practices, Hauer and associates[29] proposed a stepwise approach, summarized in Fig. 17.2, that provides a useful overarching process. The integrated processes of assessment and remediation of the struggling learner can be characterized by four critical activities: problem identification; problem investigation and classification; determination of an appropriate intervention; and assessment of the success of that intervention.

I. Problem Identification

When a potential struggling learner has been identified, programs should proceed as follows:

1) Confirm that the learner is actually struggling. Traditionally, the identification and confirmation of struggling learners early in training has been difficult. This difficulty has stemmed in part from ill-defined expectations of learners at specific stages of their development. Struggling learners traditionally come to the attention of program leaders in diverse ways. While Yao and Wright[18] identified that struggling learners are most frequently detected through direct observation in the clinical setting, they also reported the struggling resident being recognized via a critical incident or complaint, poor performance in forums such as morning report or on in-training medical knowledge examinations, and as a result of neglected patient care responsibilities. The individuals most likely to bring these concerns to the program's attention included chief residents, attending faculty, or other residents. Written faculty comments identifying struggling learners occurred infrequently. Instead, initial concerns were more likely to be reported verbally or informally. In our experience with hundreds of faculty participating in an assessment course, this paucity of formal reporting by faculty has been frequently attributed to unclear expectations regarding expected performance and consequently a hesitancy to report such concerns to program leadership. Ziring and colleagues investigating professionalism lapses in medical students found student and faculty reluctance to report lapses, lack of faculty training in identifying lapses and in remediation, unclear academic policies, and ineffective remediation strategies impeded reporting.[33] Even when reported, early feedback regarding learner performance is typically poorly defined and is potentially explainable or defensible. An example of such feedback might be, "I realize this was a single incident, but I just have this gut feeling that something may be wrong." As discussed earlier, the propensity for denial when facing a struggling learner is human and is often rooted in discomfort with remediation, lack of resources—most notably time—to carry out effective remediation, concerns about stigma to the learner, and fear of retaliation.

To help better define early concerns once they are identified, programs should consider the learning environment, personal characteristics of the learner, and legal and professional standards. One avenue of early investigation involves review of the learner's application for the program. In a 20-year retrospective review of struggling residents within a single residency program, Brenner and associates[34] found that many problem behaviors were anticipated by the finding of negative comments in the dean's letter or Medical School Performance Evaluation (MSPE) in the United States. Specifically, language such as "nervous, timid, displaying little curiosity or difficulty applying knowledge clinically" did describe those residents who were subsequently identified as struggling residents. While this is a single-institution study, given the difficulties identified with early problem recognition, review of such information should be considered as part of an initial investigation to help guide the diagnosis of the deficiency and remediation plans (see below).

Using a competency framework appropriate to the stage of medical education and locale, programs need to establish when a learner has deviated significantly enough from the normal curve of professional development to merit intervention. If the determination is that the learner is progressing within the normal trajectory and spectrum of learning, remediation may best be framed as individual improvement plans. Systematizing this decision is difficult.

As described by Carraccio and associates over 20 years ago (2002), a successful competency-based education program requires a constant stream of rich formative assessment data and feedback to guide the developmental learning process.[35] Such feedback should include the identification of both strengths and weaknesses and should always include a mutually agreed upon action plan designed to improve some aspect of performance. One opportunity for early detection of a struggling learner could be the failure to act or successfully complete plans of action enacted as part of normal development. In the United States, this is codified as part of the Practice-based Learning and Improvement general competency, with reflective practice now a specific subcompetency in Practice-based Learning and Improvement. Investigators have highlighted that learners must be active participants in the competency-based educational process.[2,35] Learners should be actively engaged in self-directed assessment seeking[36] and reflection that advances their progress toward achieving ongoing competence. Programs should aim to minimize the power differential between educator and learner. Successful engagement of trainees can facilitate learning and remove ambiguity regarding whether expected outcomes are being achieved. However, as Davis et al.[37] and others have written, self-assessment without the guidance of an external reference is suboptimal. Developing formal requirements for learner-driven self-reflection and self-assessment can provide a window into a learner's awareness of their own potential strengths and weaknesses and help avoid the need for more structured programmatic intervention.

2) Determine what role the learner, faculty, and program have played in the genesis of the problem. Assuming that all performance gaps are exclusive to the learner overlooks the potential that some of these problems might actually be related to faculty competence—in the areas of assessment, teaching, and mentorship—program design, or the learning climate. Addressing problems from this broader lens can help avoid falsely labeling a learner as struggling when the issues actually derive from the curriculum or the learning environment. Such review can help focus efforts at faculty development and professional growth or can identify opportunities for program-level improvements when systems issues at the program level are creating undue stress or unrealistic performance expectations for the learner (see Chapter 15). By defining each stakeholder's role in the creation of an identified problem, programs can ensure that the learning environment is continuously assessed and improved. The ACGME's Clinical Learning Environment Review (CLER) program[38] specifically examines the learning and quality environments of the training institution and the effects of the environment on professional development. The CLER pathways can be a useful framework for training programs to examine their institutional culture and learning climate.

3) The role of implicit bias in assessment of learners
Implicit, or unconscious, bias refers to mindsets that develop around certain types of people that influence our understanding and decisions in an unconscious manner.[39] Assessment of a trainee's knowledge, application of knowledge, and professionalism is prone to bias, and this bias has the potential to perpetuate inequities for groups such as underrepresented in medicine (URiM) trainees and women, thus hindering the advancement of these groups.[40,41] Multiple studies have pointed to the importance of more equitable performance assessments that must include acknowledgment of learner identify and learner strengths.[42,43] Equity in assessment according to Lucey et al. "is present when all [learners] have fair and impartial opportunities to learn, be evaluated, coached, graded, advanced, graduated, and selected for subsequent opportunities ... and that neither learning experiences nor assessments are negatively influenced by structural or interpersonal bias related to personal or social characteristics of learners or assessors."[44]

4) Lastly, programs must determine if the event in question actually requires intervention. While programs may have historically demonstrated a tendency to minimize the significance of sentinel events early in the detection and clarification process, effective early intervention has been identified by Evans[45] as the "gold standard for educational supervision." Papadakis and associates[46] have shown that even minor events such as resistance to accepting feedback or immature behavior reported in medical school and residency predict a higher, albeit modest, risk of unprofessional behavior in subsequent unsupervised practice that is significant enough to trigger adverse action by state licensing boards. Likewise, Lipner and colleagues[47] have identified that internal medicine residents who receive lower performance ratings while in residency or fail to attain certification (5%) are also more likely to encounter problems with state licensing boards in practice. While these studies demonstrate higher odds of adverse actions by licensing boards, and the absolute number of learners ultimately disciplined is small, it is still prudent for

• BOX 17.1 Assessment Narrative Content Predicting the Struggling Learner (adapted from Kelleher et al. Perspect Med Educ. 2022)

- Gaps in attention to detail
- Communication deficits with patients
- Difficulty recognizing the "big picture" of patient care
- Feedback as deficiency rather than an opportunity to improve
- Normative comparison that identifies the resident as behind their peers
- Warning of possible risk to patient care

From Kelleher M, Kinnear B, Sall DR, et al. Warnings in early narrative assessment that might predict performance in residency: signal from an internal medicine residency program. *Perspect Med Educ*. 2021 Dec;10(6):334–340. doi:10.1007/s40037-021-00681-w.

programs to take such behaviors and concerns seriously to ensure all future patients receive high-quality care. These studies highlight that attention to what can appear as minor performance or behavioral issues is essential, particularly if there is a pattern of repeated offense.

In the United states and other countries listed above, programs now utilize CCCs to assist in the identification of struggling learners, and effective group process can lead to better judgments (Box 17.1).[11,48] The CCC structure creates a welcome assessment point early enough in a learner's career to ensure that meaningful early intervention can be developed. CCCs additionally provide an opportunity to identify programmatic deficiencies in the design and delivery of curriculum or in the general learning environment (see Chapter 16).

Programs must develop policies that enable the sharing of learner performance information with appropriate faculty. Such information sharing is necessary to maximize the professional development of every learner, to promote a shared understanding of the developmental process by both faculty and learners, and to accurately determine each learner's current and desired level of performance. To achieve such outcomes, the entire medical education community must evolve the culture of medical education to one that welcomes and fosters both formative and summative feedback and recognizes that learners will progress at different rates. Consequently, interventions that take the form of remediation need to be recognized as a normal part of the developmental process. We cannot overstate this: remediation should be seen as a "normal" process within a medical education program.

II. Problem Investigation and Classification

Approaches to investigate and classify struggling learners should respect the developmental nature of competency acquisition and should, with a few caveats, be competency based. A developmental approach recognizes that learners advance in specific competency domains at different rates. Programs need to define when a learner's progress is within expected norms and does not require formal intervention and when intervention is required. When intervention is necessary, programs must next determine whether the learner is safe to continue working in the clinical environment. When impairment is a concern and/or if patient safety is at risk, the learner may need to be removed from the clinical environment while additional investigation is undertaken, and this is discussed later in this chapter.

Programs should characterize gaps in performance using accepted competency frameworks such as the ACGME/ABMS General Competencies and the Canadian Medical Education Directives for Specialists (CanMEDS) roles. (see Chapter 1). Using the CanMEDS frameworks, for example, Zbieranowski[25] identified difficulties in an average of 2.6 roles in struggling residents over a 10-year period. In this study, the competency domains involved, in decreasing order, were Medical Expert, Professional, Communicator, Manager, and Collaborator. Studies investigating struggling learners using the ACGME/ABMS General Competency framework have identified similar results. Figs. 17.3, 17.4, and 17.5 list how often ACGME-accredited internal medicine, general surgery, and pediatric residency programs, respectively, identified the need for remediation in each ACGME general competency.[19,20,49]

a. Importance of the correct "diagnosis"

The general competency domains most frequently identified in struggling learners remain Medical Knowledge and Patient Care.[19,20,29] One reason why Medical Knowledge and Patient Care predominate as the most frequently identified domains is likely a higher degree of skill and comfort among programs in assessing and dealing with these competencies related to others such as Professionalism and Systems-based Practice. Studies have identified that struggling learners typically experience gaps in more than one competency domain[19,25–27].

The correct "diagnosis"—that is, identification of the correct clinical performance deficit(s)—is critical to the success of a remediation plan. Misdiagnosis of the educational deficit leads to implementation of the wrong plan and has the potential to exhaust both the struggling learner and the involved faculty members and may lead to the erroneous conclusion that remediation does not work. Unfortunately, incorrect diagnoses occur frequently,[50,51] and it is especially common for faculty to disproportionately identify medical knowledge as the greatest and most frequent deficit. "Needs to read more" is a phrase commonly found in learner evaluations, especially when evaluators are required to include corrective feedback. Medical educators are conditioned to default to knowledge as the primary problem when confronted with a struggling learner. The phrase "needs to read more" is often a hint that something is wrong, but knowledge is often not the fundamental problem. More commonly, learners struggle with clinical reasoning—that is, the application of medical knowledge. The competency of Patient Care is broad and has been subdivided by remediation experts to include clinical reasoning and organization and efficiency.[26,28]

The Disorganized Learner

Another common phenotype encountered in GME is the "disorganized learner."[52] *Disorganized* and *inefficient* are terms

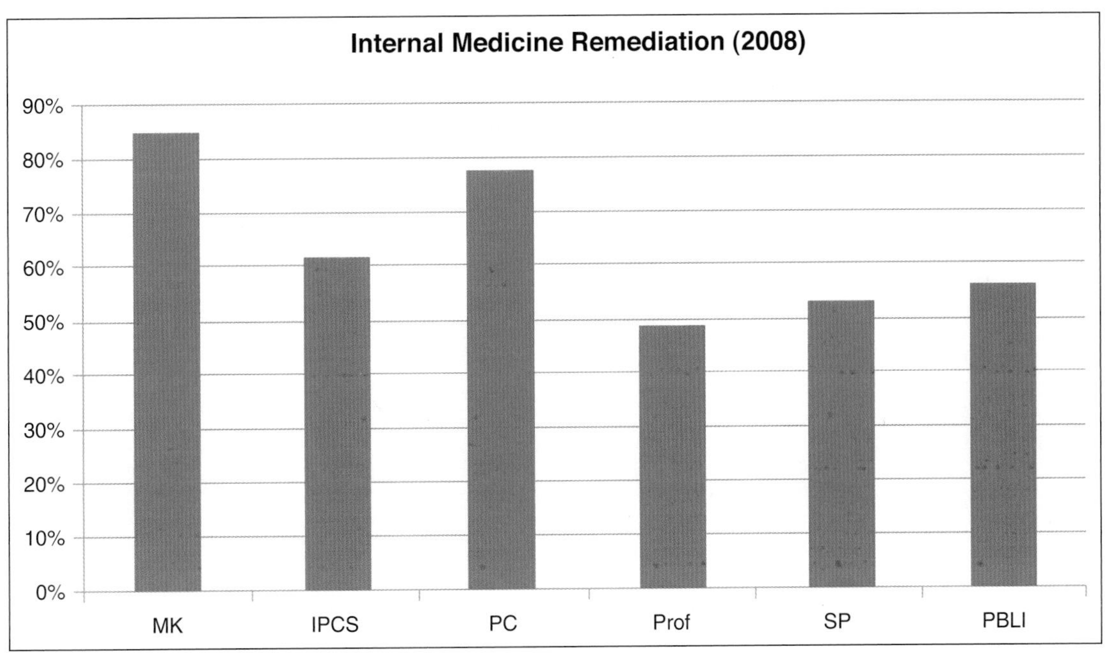

• **Fig. 17.3** Comparison of Reported Competency Deficiency Frequencies Among Internal Medicine Residents with Performance Concerns. Modified from Dupras DM, Edson RS, Halvorsen AJ, Hopkins RH, McDonald FS. "Problem residents": prevalence, problems and remediation in the era of core competencies. *Am J Med*. 2012 Apr;125(4):421–425.

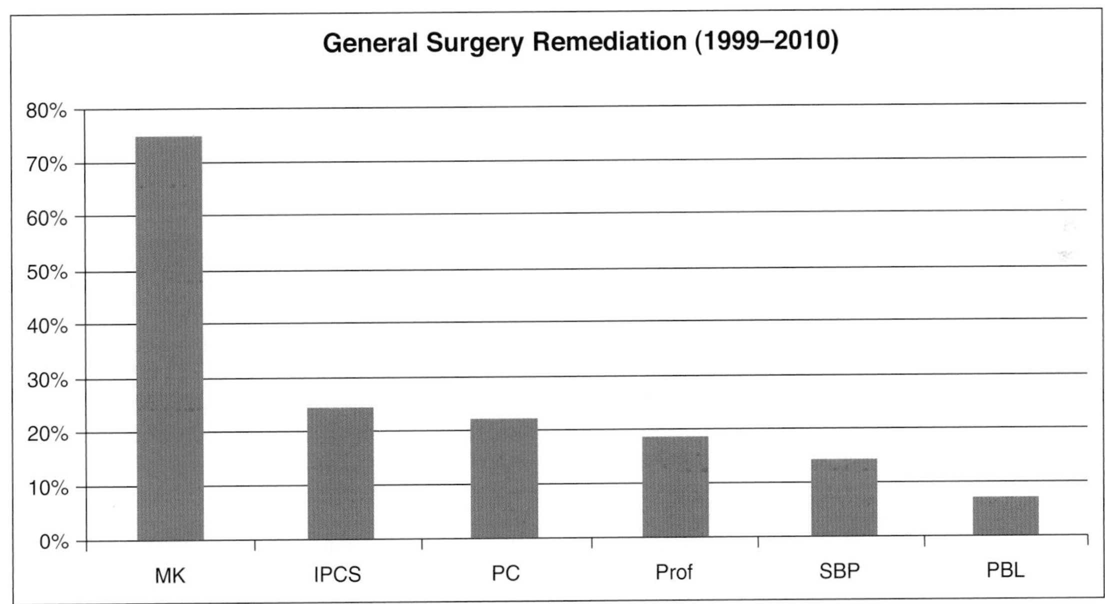

• **Fig. 17.4** 4 Comparison of Reported Competency Deficiency Frequencies Among General Surgery Residents with Performance Concerns. Modified from Yaghoubian A, Galante J, Kaji A, et al. General Surgery resident remediation and attrition: a multi-institutional study. *Arch Surg*. 2012;147(9):829–833.

commonly used to describe struggling learners. These descriptors map to at least four ACGME competencies (Patient Care, Interpersonal and Communication Skills, Professionalism, and Systems-based Practice). Common patterns of behavior include the learner who is consistently late or unprepared for rounds or clinic, the learner who completes their notes late in the day or not at all, and the learner who struggles to keep track of their materials and responsibilities. Disorganized learners typically require considerable supervision, and their struggles often negatively impact the team dynamics and the delivery of safe and timely patient care. A survey of US internal medicine program directors reported that, among residents having difficulty with performance, 41% had trouble with organization and prioritization.[19] Reports from single-center remediation programs suggest that time management and organization are common problems, particularly among resident learners undergoing remediation.[26–28,52] A national survey of US nephrology fellowship program directors cited organization and efficiency as the second most common deficit requiring remediation among nephrology fellows over the

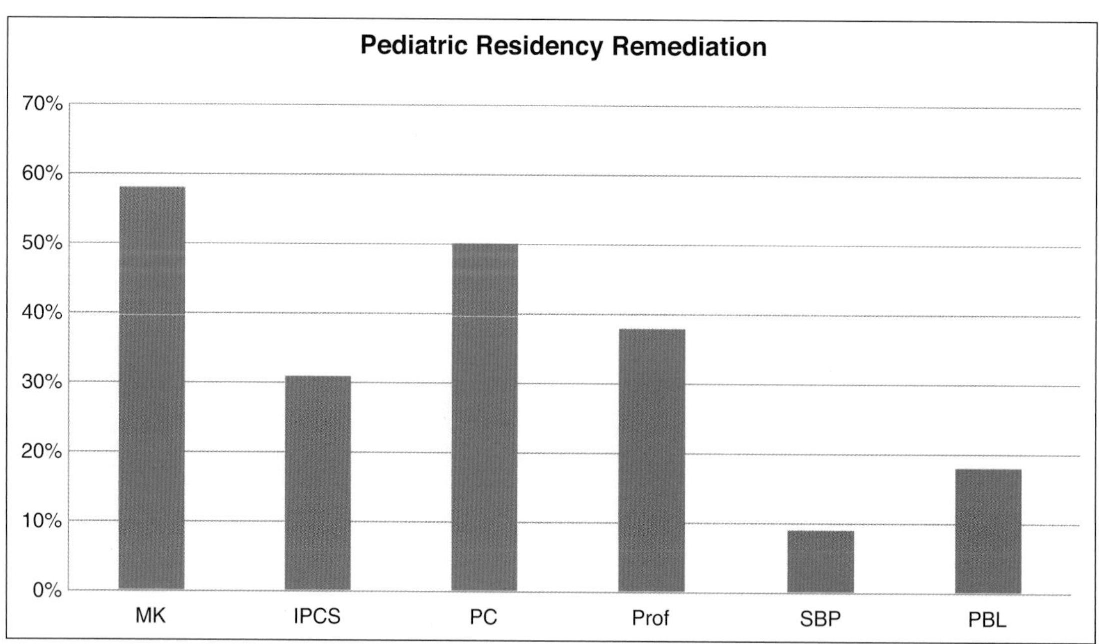

• **Fig. 17.5** Comparison of reported competency deficiencies among pediatrics residents with performance concerns. Modified from Riebschleger MP, Haftel HM. Remediation in the context of the competencies: a survey of pediatrics residency program directors. *J Grad Med Educ*. 2013 Mar;5(1):60–63.

TABLE 17.2 Differential Diagnosis Of The Disorganized Learner

Type of Deficit	Behavioral Clues
I. Organization, efficiency, or time management deficit	• Lacks effective habits, approaches, or systems for completing daily work
A. Global	• Struggles in multiple aspects of life • Difficulty meeting deadlines, bills unpaid, cluttered home or desk • Arrives late to meetings or rounds
B. Specific	• Lack of familiarity with specific information systems (e.g., electronic medical record) • Prior educational/training program did not prepare learner for current program (e.g., size, complexity of patients, different expectations) • Unable to describe systems for evaluating new patients, preparation for rounds
II. Clinical reasoning deficit	• Has not seen all patients prior to clinical rounds, unprepared for rounds in general • Spends an atypically long time evaluating new patients • Struggles to triage tasks in all clinical settings, may lack appreciation of urgency of tasks • Perpetually behind on all work • Scattered history taking or physical exam
III. Mental well-being concern A. Medical impairment (e.g., metabolic disease, neurologic disease, side effect of prescribed medication) B. Significant fatigue C. Substance use D. Depression E. Anxiety F. Cognitive issue (e.g., attention-deficit hyperactivity disorder, learning disorder)	• Other signs of impairment (e.g., unsteady gait; slurred speech; lethargic; agitated; withdrawn; fidgety; inappropriate or uninhibited behavior; memory loss or confusion; disheveled appearance; loud, rapid or nonsensical speech) • Known history of mental health condition(s) • Other issues with performance

last 5 years.[53] Table 17.2 reviews the differential diagnosis of the disorganized learner.[54] It is important to distinguish learners who lack organizational systems from those who appear disorganized because of a primary clinical reasoning deficit. In the former case, remediation centers on providing the learner with effective systems for completing their work. In the latter case, in which learners often lack training and experience in hypothesis-driven data gathering and triaging large amounts of information, remediation involves further assessment to identify the lesions along the diagnostic and management clinical reasoning pathway followed by targeted coaching in these areas.

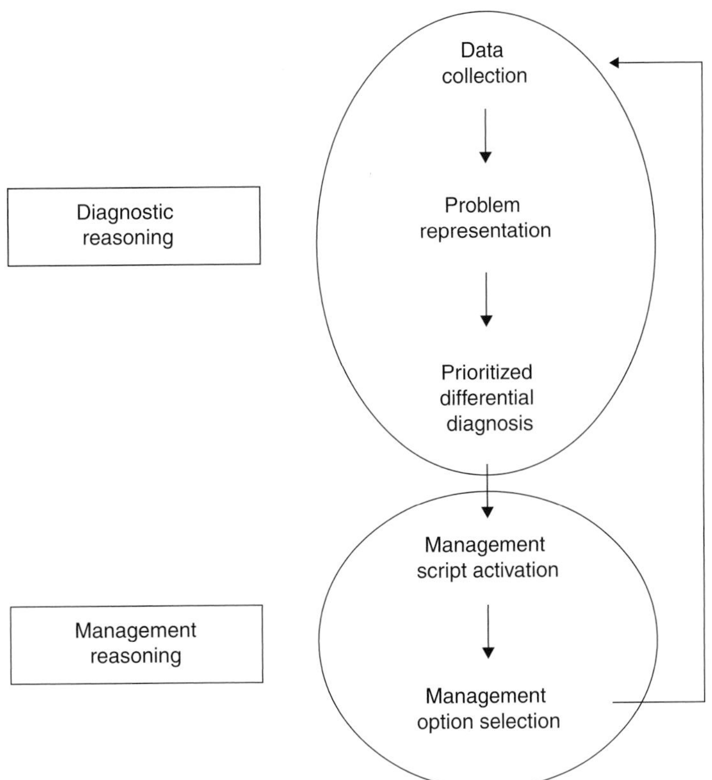

• **Fig. 17.6** The clinical reasoning pathway. Modified from Flaherty JA, Richman JA. Substance use and addiction among medical students, residents, and physicians. *Psychiatr Clin North Am*. 1993 Mar;16(1):189–197.

The Learner With a Clinical Reasoning Deficit

Clinical reasoning involves the integration, organization, and interpretation of information to achieve a working diagnosis and management plan.[55] Medical knowledge is necessary but not sufficient for a learner to reason effectively. The steps of the clinical reasoning pathway are outlined in Fig. 17.6.[56] Commonly used phrases to describe the learner struggling with clinical reasoning are:

- "Difficulty with patient presentations"
- "Cannot see the forest for the trees"
- "Cannot summarize patient in a succinct one-liner"
- "Orders too many tests"
- "Cannot create or prioritize a differential diagnosis or plan"
- "Appears disorganized or overwhelmed"
- "Cannot structure an admission or clinic visit efficiently"
- "Cannot triage a task list, recognize urgency, discern sick versus not sick"

Even seasoned clinician educators may lack the skills and comfort necessary to assess and remediate clinical reasoning,[57,58] leading to a delay in identification or "misdiagnosis" of the learner struggling with clinical reasoning. As noted earlier, the inability to engage in effective and efficient hypothesis-driven data gathering may lead to the appearance that the learner is disorganized and/or inefficient. The observation that a learner is slow to respond in urgent situations may lead an evaluator to be concerned about professionalism, when in fact the primary issue is a deficit in diagnostic or management reasoning. It is critical that educators differentiate a clinical reasoning deficit from those related to medical knowledge, organization and efficiency, and professionalism, as each requires discrete intervention. Clinical reasoning is remediable[26,28,59] and time intensive.[26]

Arrival at the correct "diagnosis" requires a systematic assessment process, once a struggling learner has been identified. A standardized assessment includes an analysis of the learner's complete educational file, direct communication with evaluators, direct observation when logistically possible, an evaluation for underlying medical and/or mental health conditions (discussed later in the chapter), and an interview with the learner.[3] Programs must use high-quality information regarding actual learner performance to clearly define the nature of severity of all performance gaps. Table 17.3 lists assessment methods that can generate performance data in each of the general competencies, and the chapters on specific assessment methods in this book can provide guidance on the right package of assessments needed to make an accurate diagnosis of a learner's performance gaps. The choice of methods to make an accurate diagnosis depends on the nature of the problem. Because it facilitates accurate identification, it is critical to gather data from multiple sources.

b. The overlap between clinical performance and well-being: Assessment of underlying factors

Learners who struggle with clinical performance often have a great deal going on beneath the surface, including stress, physical or mental illness, and burnout. Several

TABLE 17.3 Competency-Based Assessment Methods

General Competency	Potential Assessment Method
Medical Knowledge	Standardized exams Chart-stimulated recall Structured clinical questioning
Patient Care	Direct observation Chart-stimulated recall Standardized patients Multisource feedback Medical records audits Structured portfolio review
Interpersonal and Communication Skills	Direct observation Standardized patients Multisource feedback Structured portfolio review
Professionalism	Direct observation Multisource feedback Structured self-assessment Structured portfolio review
Practice-based Learning and Improvement	Medical records audits Clinical vignettes Structured self-assessment Evidence-based medicine tools Structured portfolio review
Systems-based Practice	Medical records and clinical care Audits Portfolio review Multisource feedback Teamwork assessment

studies have reported the coexistence of mental well-being issues and clinical performance struggles in residents and fellows.[18,19,22,23,26,27] At the University of Colorado, mental well-being concerns were identified in nearly 20% of residents referred to a centralized remediation program,[26] and 38% of medical education learners referred to a centralized remediation program at the University of Virginia had an underlying mental health condition, most commonly anxiety. Among those with an underlying mental health condition, professionalism was the most commonly identified clinical performance deficit,[27] highlighting the relationship between unprofessional behavior and mental well-being. Table 17.4 summarizes factors that may underlie struggles with clinical performance. The assessment of these conditions is a critical part of the assessment of any struggling learner. That said, program faculty must respect that their involvement with learners is as an educator and not a clinician. For ethical and privacy reasons, faculty must not diagnose medical conditions in their learners. Rather, these faculty should focus on identifying specific gaps between expected and observed performance. Programs should put into place a mechanism for reliable, confidential referral for additional evaluation and support of struggling learners who may have underlying mental health conditions.

TABLE 17.4 Factors That May Underlie Clinical Performance Deficits

Fatigue
Psychosocial stress
Anxiety
Depression
Substance use disorder
Medical illness
Cognitive dysfunction, learning disorder
Memory/recall, concentration, executive function, processing, attention-deficit hyperactivity disorder
Unresolved personality adaptations (or disorders)
Burnout
Adverse childhood experiences
Wrong career (or program) choice

Depression

A survey of US internal medicine program directors found that 24% of program directors identify depression as an underlying case in 50% or more of struggling learners.[18] Physicians are at unique risk of depression during training. A meta-analysis of 54 studies involving nearly 18,000 physicians in training revealed that the prevalence of depression or depressive symptoms among residents is 29%, ranging from 21% o 43%.[60] Many studies have highlighted the high rates of depression and suicide among female physicians.[61]

Cognitive Disorders

Cognitive and learning difficulties among struggling medical education learners are not well studied. In a survey of US internal medicine program directors, learning disability was a factor in 6.6% of residents labeled as struggling.[19] A single-center study reported that 17% of learners referred for remediation with a concomitant mental health condition had attention-deficit hyperactivity disorder (ADHD).[27] Among participants surveyed as part of a study assessing the prevalence of self-reported disabilities among residents, 7.5% self-reported a disability, which was most commonly ADHD (67.7%).[62] Many conditions associated with impaired cognition and learning are recognized as disabilities under the Americans with Disabilities Act (ADA) and may warrant accommodation. Educational leaders in other countries also need to understand the laws regarding disabilities in their own jurisdiction. Educational accommodations for a resident with ADHD may include increased supervision, more frequent feedback, coaching in organizational skills specific to the work environment, and adjustment in patient census and rotation schedule.[63] In addition, efforts should be made to ensure that, when warranted, the resident has access to the appropriate pharmacotherapy and cognitive behavioral therapy.

Substance Use Disorders

The prevalence of substance use disorders (SUDs) among physicians is not well defined, but most studies suggest that between 10% and 12% of physicians will develop a problem with substance misuse at some point.[64,65] There is limited information regarding the prevalence and outcomes of SUDs among medical education learners. A retrospective review of a single-center family medicine program over 25 years identified that 7.3% of struggling residents had a SUD.[23] A survey of internal medicine residency program directors identified substance abuse as a factor among <5% of struggling residents.[19] The pattern of substance use varies depending on specialty.[66] Particular attention has been paid to anesthesiologists, and one retrospective study of more than 44,000 residents in anesthesiology training programs found that 0.86% had a SUD during training, and at least 11% of these physicians died of a cause directly related to the SUD.[67]

In some studies, physicians are more likely than the general population to use opiates and other prescribed medications, but alcohol is the most commonly used substance, and women are particularly at risk.[68–70] While the prevalence of SUD among physicians is similar to that of the general population, outcomes are better for physicians. Relapse rates are as high as 60% for nonphysicians versus 22% for physicians, and 71% of physicians with SUD who are enrolled with a physician's health program (PHP) are licensed and practicing medicine at 5 years.[65] This difference in part reflects the existence in most states of physician monitoring programs. Nearly every state has a PHP, and while services vary from state to state, the PHP's role is to both protect the public and assist and/or advocate for physicians in their recovery.

For physicians with SUDs, clues may be subtle, and it is worth remembering that physicians are typically quite good at concealing their symptoms until the problem becomes severe.

Burnout

Burnout is a work-related syndrome characterized by exhaustion, cynicism, and a sense of reduced effectiveness and is tied to depression, substance abuse, medical error, and increased costs to the healthcare system.[71,72] In a national study that assessed burnout using the Maslach Burnout Inventory in 2017, nearly half of practicing physicians met the criteria for burnout.[73] A systematic review and meta-analysis of burnout among more than 4000 medical residents revealed an overall prevalence of 36%.[74] A 2006 study by Rosen[75] identified that 4.3% of interns demonstrated signs of burnout at the beginning of intern year. By the end of that year, the rate had increased to 55.3%. These are pre–COVID-19 pandemic figures, and over the last 2 to 3 years, trainees have endured increased work intensity, redeployment, concerns about personal safety, and isolation. The COVID-19 pandemic has impacted the morale and mental well-being of all physicians, but in particular medical education learners. Table 17.5 outlines the many potential ramifications of burnout among trainees.[76]

TABLE 17.5 Potential Ramifications of Burnout Among Learners[76]

Professional	Personal
• Decreased empathy • Cheating/dishonest behaviors • Dishonesty regarding patient care • Problems identifying and managing conflicts of interest • Decreased altruistic professional values • Inappropriate prescribing behaviors • Decreased personal accountability regarding impaired colleagues • Dropping out of medical school • Influence on specialty choice • Suboptimal patient care • Medical errors • Decreased medical knowledge	• Suicidal ideation • Greater sense of stigma regarding mental health problems • Motor vehicle incidents

A classic model of physician stress offsets the demands placed on us in the workplace with the support provided and the control we have, and, in a more recent modification, with our personal resilience (Fig. 17.7). When the demands outweigh support, control, and resilience, we experience more stress[77] and may be prone to burnout. Key drivers of burnout include excessive workload, inefficiencies in our practice environment, the inability to have a voice or influence change, lack of flexibility and control at work, barriers to healthy work–life integration, and lack of meaning in our work.[78] Each of these drivers is influenced by individual[79] and system factors, and reducing burnout is the shared responsibility of individual physicians and the systems in which they work.[78]

Proposed strategies to improve well-being, at the individual level, include building community, seeking out additional support, and increasing meaning at work. Organizational-level suggestions include wellness curricula, addressing work compression, and access to resources such as mental health support, childcare, financial counseling, and career advising services.

Experts on burnout and physician well-being reinforce the importance of listening to the concerns of trainees before proposing solutions for well-being. Program leadership does not need to have all the answers, nor are they expected to say yes to all requests, but they need to ask what trainees need, and they need to listen and to acknowledge the specific sources of anxiety and fear.[80] It is important to consider the role of burnout among trainees who are struggling with clinical performance. Burnout can be easily assessed using the Maslach Burnout Inventory.[71]

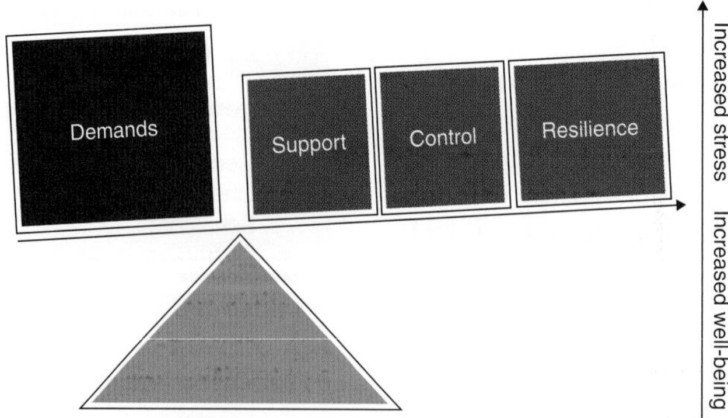

• **Fig. 17.7** The Demands Support Control Model of Physician Stress. Modified from Warde CM, Linzer M, Schorling JB, Moore EM, Poplau S. Balancing unbalanced lives: a practical framework for personal and organizational change. *Mayo Clin Proc Innov Qual Outcomes*. 2019 Feb 26;3(1):97–100.

Adverse Childhood Experiences

Early life trauma, including personally experienced or witnessed physical, sexual, and/or emotional abuse and/or neglect, and/or loss, is linked to medical and mental health issues later in life.[81] A study of trainees and practicing physicians with significant professionalism concerns highlights the relationship between adverse childhood experiences (ACEs) and unprofessional behavior. Among 123 physicians referred for fitness for duty evaluations over a 5-year period, 70% reported at least 1 ACE, while 22% reported ≥4. Types of professionalism concerns associated with ACEs in this cohort included boundary violation, disruptive behavior, and substance misuse.[82] As stressed in Dr. Williams' and colleagues' work, it is important to recognize that learners who are labeled "difficult"—resistant to feedback, emotionally dysregulated, challenging to get along with—may have significant trauma histories and that these difficult behaviors are a response to reexperiencing the pain of early life experiences.[81,82] It is our job as educators to recognize these patterns of behavior, maintain curiosity rather than judgment about these behaviors, and gain comfort in referring our learners for additional evaluation and treatment as part of their remediation plan.

ACGME core program accreditation requirements in the United States state that programs, in partnership with their sponsoring institutions, have the same responsibility to address well-being as they do to evaluate other aspects of resident competence. This responsibility includes attention to scheduling, work intensity, and work compression; assurance of a safe workplace; and policies and programs to support trainee well-being. Residents should have the opportunity to attend medical and mental health appointments, including those scheduled during the working hours.

c. Is the learner safe to practice?

Kogan and associates[83] have provided one approach that can help inform this decision. This method establishes as an outcome that all encounters between learners and patients must result in safe, patient-centered, and effective patient care. This is achieved by balancing the level of learner performance with the level of supervision provided by faculty. If the level of supervision needed for this outcome is not possible, the learner should not continue in the clinical setting until these conditions change. Fig. 17.8 provides an overview of the approach to the struggling learner.

Impairment

In a landmark article in 1973, the American Medical Association (AMA) defined the impaired physician as one who is unable to fulfill professional and personal responsibilities because of psychiatric illness, alcoholism, or drug dependency.[84] This paper was a call to action for our profession to acknowledge that physicians are not immune to impairment and for state medical societies to establish programs to identify and treat impaired physicians. Impairment is often synonymous with substance use disorder, but in reality any mental or medical illness, including severe fatigue, can result in impairment.[61] It is important to know whether you practice in a mandatory reporting state, in which case physicians are obligated to report impaired physicians.

Fitness for Duty Evaluation

If the learner is impaired and/or if there are concerns related to patient safety, the learner must be removed from the clinical environment until a thorough evaluation is completed, and that individual must not return to the clinical environment until a successful intervention has occurred. Programs should have policies in place to evaluate a learner's fitness for duty if concerns arise around the learner's mental or physical ability to effectively perform their required duties. When there is concern about impairment, programs may request a fitness for duty evaluation. To ensure transparency and fairness, the components of the fitness for duty evaluation should be clearly defined, and the evaluation should be performed by an independent practitioner who is not involved in the program leadership. This reduces the risk of alleged discrimination and minimizes the possibility that clinician educators are diagnosing learners. The goal of such an evaluation is to define the type of impairment; thoroughly

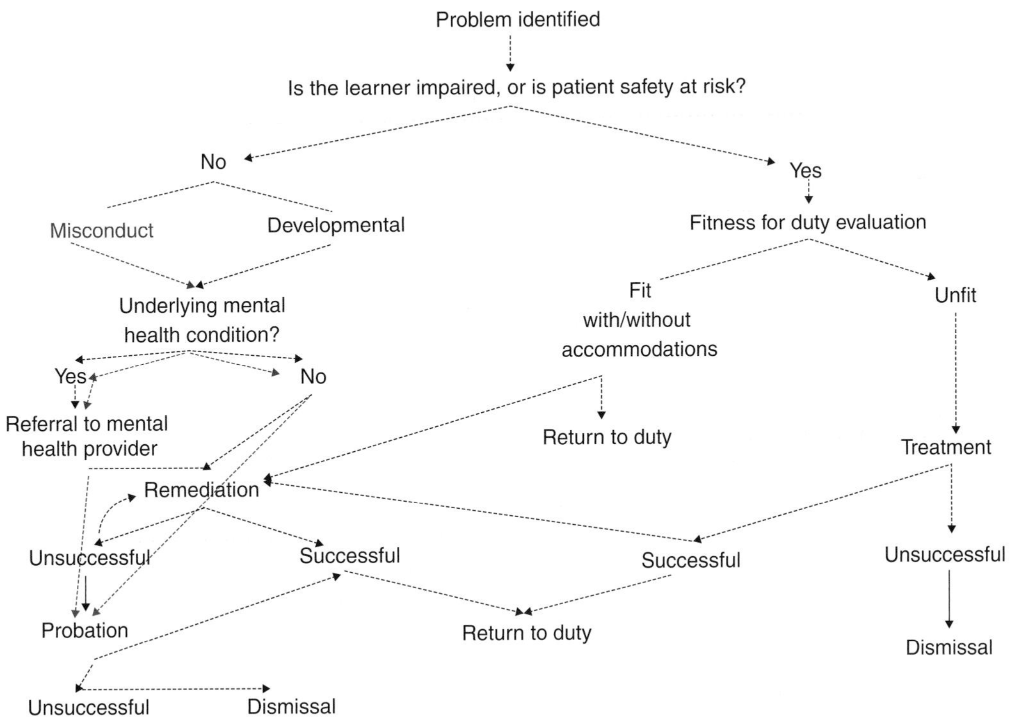

• **Fig. 17.8** Approach to the struggling learner.

evaluate the learner's present physical and mental health; gain an in-depth understanding of the requirements of the job; and propose conditions to ensure safe return to work. Ideally, this is a nondisciplinary process that is not reportable to outside regulatory agencies. The trainee is placed on leave, and a comprehensive evaluation is performed by a qualified independent licensed practitioner with the goal of ensuring that the trainee is able to care for patients in a safe and appropriate manner.

Possible outcomes of this evaluation include a finding that the individual is fit for duty and may return to work without restrictions or modifications. Alternatively, the trainee may require additional evaluation or treatment before they are able to return to work, after which time their fitness may require reassessment. This process may conclude with a request for formal accommodations and/or alterations in the physician's schedule while they are undergoing treatment. Implicit in a determination of fitness is the assurance that the physician is not a danger to self or to patients.

Accommodations

ACGME core program requirements state that the sponsoring institution must have a policy regarding accommodations for disabilities consistent with all applicable laws and regulations. According to the ADA of 1990, a disability is a physical or mental impairment that significantly limits one or more "major life activities."[85] Major life activities are defined to include breathing, walking, talking, hearing, seeing, eating, learning, reading, concentrating, and thinking. Using these definitions, programs should appreciate that all disabilities can be considered impairments, but not all impairments result in disability. For example, while a decrease in visual acuity may be an impairment, it is not necessarily a disability.

Residency programs and medical schools should protect learners by collaborating with institutional officials familiar with the ADA or pertinent laws in other countries, as well as knowledge of state laws that may include additional legislation protecting individuals with disability. A reasonable accommodation is a modification to the job or the work environment that enables the individual with the disability to perform the essential functions of the job. Examples of accommodations for GME include acquisition or modification of equipment or devices, adjustment of work schedules, and adaptation of the work environment. Policy and procedure for request and granting of accommodations vary by institution. Typically, the request for accommodations is made by the learner in conjunction with the learner's treating provider and is backed by medical rationale. Depending on the circumstance, the medical rationale may not be shared with the program director. The program director, in conjunction with the GME office, makes a decision about whether the request is reasonable. This is often an interactive process.

Because the courts in the United States continue to evolve their interpretation of the ADA, programs should actively involve legal counsel in decisions regarding disability and the need to offer accommodations throughout the process. In making this decision, the GME office and program director typically consider requirements of the specialty board, impact of the proposed accommodations on the program, and impact of the proposed accommodations on the learner's ability to achieve competence and succeed in the eventual practice environment. The program must ultimately determine if the proposed accommodation is reasonable and can be implemented without fundamentally changing the educational program, adding undue financial burden to the program, or compromising patient safety. If an employee with a disability needs a reasonable accommodation to gain access to and have an equal opportunity to participate in these benefits and privileges, then the employer must provide the accommodation unless it can show undue hardship. For example, if the proposed accommodation requires that the learner only care for one patient at a time and the program requires that a learner be able to simultaneously care for a minimum of six patients, the accommodation is unreasonable regardless of the underlying problem. The accommodation would fundamentally alter the educational program. Similarly, if the proposed accommodation always requires direct supervision of the learner, such an accommodation is unreasonable for senior residents who are expected to function with progressive levels of independence through reduced levels of supervision.

Any accommodation or modification to the educational program designed to address impairment or disability must ultimately require that the learner in question meet the same program outcomes required of all learners. Programs must also recognize that when a disability or impairment is identified, it does not excuse substandard performance, especially if patient safety is at risk. If appropriate interventions or accommodations do not allow the learner to function at a level required for the delivery of safe and effective patient care, that learner should not continue in the program. In these circumstances programs should recognize that the identified disability has created an impairment. For programs outside the United States, we strongly recommend educational leaders become familiar with local and national laws and policies that affect learners with disabilities and/or impairments.

III. Determination of an Appropriate Intervention

Once a struggling learner has been identified and the cause of the gaps in performance has been determined and categorized, the next decision is whether the corrective action plan requires immediate disciplinary action, such as probation. Early disciplinary action may be appropriate for certain types of misconduct or professionalism lapses, especially if there is a pattern of multiple offenses. This is discussed later in the chapter.

Remediation

For the majority of struggling learners who require intervention, however, remediation is an appropriate next step. The purpose of remediation is to help learners who have fallen behind the expected trajectory in one or more aspects of performance achieve minimum competency in relation to their peers in this/these area(s).

Policies around remediation are unstandardized and vary by institution. In general, remediation refers to additional time and/or supervision and/or resources to allow learners the opportunity to practice the deficient skill(s) under direct observation and be given feedback on their performance in real time. Remediation may occur in many different settings, including but not limited to the clinical learning environment, the office of a peer or faculty member assigned to coach the learner on a specific skill, or a simulation center. The intervention is implemented with the expectation that the learner will show gradual and continuous improvement in those areas targeted for improvement. It is part of the developmental process, but addresses a problem that cannot be addressed through the routine assessment and feedback provided in the normal course of learning. This intervention should not be considered punitive. Depending on the institution, this may be a formal or informal process and may or may not involve a written letter in the file or necessitate involvement by the GME office.

The Remediation Plan

A program director putting a learner on remediation should, in writing:

1. Explain the reason for the remediation
2. Define SMART (specific, measurable, achievable, relevant, time-bound) goals for remediation
3. Outline a plan for remediation, including resources needed to complete the plan
4. Define the timeline for remediation and reassessment
5. Clarify how the learner will be reassessed and by whom
6. Make explicit the consequence if the conditions of remediation are not met

Remediation plans should be documented in writing to optimize outcomes and limit legal liability. Remediation must have a defined timeline and should define clear intermediate as well as ultimate goals that define whether the intervention has been successful. Progress toward achieving these goals is typically gradual and continuous. When the learner is unable to achieve the goals of the remediation plan within the defined timeline, programs will need to consider transitioning the corrective action to a revised remediation plan, probation, or dismissal. It is not recommended that remediation be an open-ended process. It is untenable to ask faculty and programs to continue remediation programs indefinitely, especially if reasonable improvement targets within reasonable time periods have been determined.

Though remediation practices are not standardized across institutions, a remediation plan should adhere to the policies of the institution.

Probation

Initiating probation as the corrective action plan is not part of the typical developmental process and most often reflects that the learner has demonstrated an unacceptable behavior or pattern of behaviors that must cease immediately. Probation can be identified as the initial corrective action or can result from failed remediation. As with remediation, problems that require the initiation of a period of probation should be thoroughly investigated for potential secondary causes. Expected standards of behavior should be reviewed, and counseling should be considered as part of the

TABLE 17.6 Comparison of Corrective Action Plans

	Developmental	Nondevelopmental
Process	Remediation	Disciplinary action (e.g., probation)
Goals	Improvement	Cessation of behavior
Expected progress	Gradual and sufficient	Immediate and sustained
Faculty role	Tutors/coaches/ mentors	Enforcement/clarification of standards/ surveillance
Outcome if unsuccessful	Additional remediation/ extension in training or dismissal	Dismissal

intervention. Table 17.6 provides a comparison of these two types of corrective action plans and contrasts faculty role, goals, and consequences of remediation versus probation.

In all cases, the learner is entitled to due process, meaning that they have a right to receive notice of any action taken by the program and have an opportunity to be heard. Institutions should adhere to due process and apply policies without discrimination.

Reportability

As defined in the US context, remediation is not inherently a reportable program intervention to future employers and licensing or certifying agencies, but programs must take steps to clearly define when such reporting is necessary. What must be reported is generally dictated by the questions that are asked as part of verification requests from boards or future employers. This varies considerably. In general, any intervention that results in an extension of training is reportable. If the trainee's scope of practice had to be modified, this may be reportable. If there is a disciplinary issue such as probation, this is potentially reportable. Institutions should consult with legal counsel when considering any issues related to reporting.

Roles

As much as possible, program directors should resist the temptation to take on the role of remediator. Remediation requires a team approach, with different team members having varying levels of familiarity with the facts of the case and distinct roles. Program leaders should maintain some distance from the detailed knowledge given their role in determining the ultimate outcome for the learner and their duty not only to the resident but also to the program and the patients.[86] Remediation works well when the program director can delegate the remediation oversight to other faculty who can serve in a primarily advocacy role for the learner without these conflicts of interest.

The Importance of Learner Buy-In and Involvement

Adults learn best when they *self-direct* their own learning goals and activities. Successful implementation of a coproduction model for medical education requires that learners take ownership of their performance.[2] Successful remediation hinges on actively engaging the learner when determining the appropriate intervention. Adopting the principles of self-regulated learning can inform strategy for such engagement. Self-regulated learning requires that learners set specific goals, develop strategic plans, and self-monitor and self-evaluate as they participate in the intervention. Self-regulated learning thereby engages learners in the three essential elements of forethought, actual performance, and subsequent self-reflection. Self-regulated learning also requires awareness of the context of the intervention and recognition that how the learner responds to and actually influences that context will affect the impact of the intervention. Self-regulated learning also requires substantial intrinsic motivation. If intrinsic motivation is not a major driver for the struggling learner, the chances of success in remediating the deficiencies become lower. Struggling physicians cannot rely exclusively on extrinsic motivators (i.e., threat of sanctions or discipline) to ensure a successful career strategy. Incorporating the key tenets of self-regulated learning into remediation plans is both logical and supported by educational theory.[87]

Struggling learners often have trouble identifying and actuating feedback, may have blind spots, and often do not learn from the hidden curriculum. In addition to intrinsic motivation, factors that predict success in a remediation intervention include insight, the ability to reflect, honesty, and the capacity to troubleshoot. In our experience, successful engagement of the learner on remediation requires that learners gain comfort in feeding forward, soliciting feedback, and reflecting on this feedback with a coach or mentor. This process allows continued self-reflection and identification of areas for continued work.

To ensure that the educational environment is inclusive, it is important that programs and institutions seek out and address issues of inequity in learning, assessment, and remediation. In particular, it is critical to consider how URiM learners achieve success[42] and design remediation plans to capitalize on the individual strengths and specific learning styles of all learners.

The Unique Challenge of Professionalism

Professionalism as a construct is complex and can be defined by many frameworks. Basic tenets include professional conduct and accountability; humanism and cultural proficiency; emotional, physical, and mental health; and continual personal and professional growth.[88] Unprofessional behaviors include the failure to engage, dishonesty, disrespectful behavior, poor self-awareness,[82] and a variety of other forms of misconduct. Lapses in professionalism impact patient safety,[89] and, when they occur during training, predict later unprofessional behavior and disciplinary consequences.[46,90,91] While most educators "know unprofessional behavior when they see it," determining how to actually define, investigate, and remedy lapses in professionalism can be challenging.

Unprofessional behavior is commonly associated with underlying mental health concerns, including anxiety, depression, addiction disorders, burnout, and unresolved personality factors.[27] It is critical, when devising a remediation plan for the learner struggling with professionalism, to consider that one or more of these issues may underlie the behavior of concern. Additionally, behaviors that appear to be attributable to lapses in professionalism may in fact represent problems with other competencies. The importance of looking beyond the behavior can be illustrated by the following cases.

The Learner Who Is Not Responding Appropriately to Urgent Situations

The resident who is slow to answer, or flat out ignores, pages, or does not seem to appreciate urgency in clinical situations, may appear at first glance to lack accountability or integrity, central character traits associated with professionalism. Probably more commonly, a learner with this behavioral phenotype struggles to appreciate urgency due to a primary deficiency in clinical reasoning or medical knowledge. Lesions at any part of the diagnostic and management reasoning pathway, particularly that of hypothesis generation, may impact the ability to recognize and respond appropriately to clinical urgency (see Chapter 8). Performance anxiety is another common explanation for this type of behavior. Less commonly, learners with neurodevelopmental concerns that lead to the inability to recognize social cues may struggle to appreciate urgency in the clinical learning environment.

The Learner Who Is Habitually Late or Does Not Show Up

Persistent tardiness is generally labeled as a professionalism matter, typically related to accountability and reliability. There are many issues that potentially underlie this behavior, including SUDs, depression, and burnout. Alternatively, learners who have trouble getting to things on time may lack effective organizational systems and could benefit from coaching on time management, or may have a primary issue related to cognitive or executive function that warrants additional evaluation and intervention.

The Learner Who Loses Their Temper Easily or Is Rude to Nurses and Front Desk Staff

Showing compassion and respect for others is integral to professionalism, and there are many reasons why learners may fail to do this in the clinical learning environment, including depression, burnout, and fatigue. Some may have learned this style of communication in their family of origin as a way to get needs met and not recognize that it is counterproductive in their work environment. Others may lack awareness of social norms due to their own cultural or professional background.

In all of these cases, there is a differential diagnosis for the observed behavior, and the remediation plan must be tailored to the root of the behavior, rather than the behavior itself. Oftentimes, additional evaluation is required before a remediation plan can be successfully enacted. There are certainly behaviors that warrant immediate action regardless of the underlying issue, typically severe misconduct issues such as lying, cheating, and stealing. As referenced earlier, Fig. 17.8 illustrates an approach to the struggling learner and takes into account the dichotomy of issues that are academic (developmental) or related to misconduct (nondevelopmental). Finally, in considering unprofessional behavior, program leaders must take into account intent, level of insight, and ability to reflect and self-correct. Fig. 17.8 then presents an approach to intervention based on these and other important features.

As programs grapple with professionalism issues, two additional frameworks that can help conceptualize a learner's professional growth are the professional identity formation trajectory and Rest's Four Component Model of Morality. The American Board of Internal Medicine (ABIM) Foundation Charter on Medical Professionalism can also provide a high-level framework for defining appropriate standards of professionalism. Table 17.7 highlights the principles and commitments. As defined by Kalet and Chou,[5] professional identity formation follows a trajectory that maps to specific

TABLE 17.7 Principles and Commitments of the Physician Charter[16]

<u>Fundamental Principles:</u>
Principle of primacy of patient welfare
Principle of patient autonomy
Principle of social justice
<u>Professional Responsibilities:</u>
Commitment to professional competence
Commitment to honesty with patients
Commitment to patient confidentiality
Commitment to maintaining appropriate relations with patients
Commitment to improving quality of care
Commitment to improving access to care
Commitment to a just distribution of finite resources
Commitment to scientific knowledge
Commitment to maintaining trust by managing conflicts of interest
Commitment to professional responsibilities

goals. Initially, individuals strive to achieve specific goals and gain approval for actions. As professional identity develops, concepts of teamwork, social standards, and balancing work–life issues become a focus and ultimately the individual strives to become a principled individual comfortable with ambiguity and complexity. As a developmental process, this trajectory describes a continuum that is not achieved by all professionals. Rest's Four Component Model of Morality identifies moral sensitivity, judgment, motivation, and implementation as components of behavior that can be ethical or unethical, professional or unprofessional.[92] While beyond the scope of this chapter, each of these components can be measured using standardized testing methods to assess an individual's professionalism to inform potential corrective actions. For a more complete discussion of these frameworks and assessments, the reader is referred to *Remediation in Medical Education: A Mid-Course Correction*.[4]

IV. Assessment of the Intervention

Once a corrective action plan has been implemented, the program must determine if the learner has successfully met the terms of that intervention within a distinct time period. The outcome of all corrective action plans must also be clearly defined. If the learner has met the terms of the intervention, they should return to routine responsibility in the program. While full compliance with the terms of a remediation is the goal, some learners will meet some but not all such goals or may only achieve partial compliance with expectations. When goals have been partially met, programs can choose to extend the period of remediation, extend the required length of training, or place the learner on probation in anticipation of ultimately dismissing the learner from the program. Regardless of the next step, programs must follow defined and established policies and practices (due process) when making the decision, must effectively communicate that decision to the learner, and must document all aspects of the process. If faced with an unsuccessful remediation outcome, it is important to consider that the initial "diagnosis" may have been incorrect and/or that there may be underlying factors that were previously unrecognized.

Legal Principles

While the need for intervention is inevitable for many struggling learners, such intervention will not always have a positive outcome. Some learners are not remediable. Given that these interventions can ultimately lead to a learner being terminated from a program, the potential for legal action initiated by the learner and directed against the program is real. However, legal fears and anxieties are often exaggerated. In the United States, the courts have consistently demonstrated a reluctance to interfere in decisions concerning a learner's competence in specialized fields such as medicine and have established that only professionals in that field are qualified to set competency standards and evaluate whether those standards are met. Courts will not reverse a decision that is based on professional judgment, particularly if that judgment reflects a thorough review of the learner's entire record of performance. As stated by the US Supreme Court, "Courts are particularly ill-equipped to evaluate academic performance." More specifically, courts will defer to a reasonable academic decision if that decision is felt to be fair and equitable and if due process as defined by the program has been afforded the learner.

Minicucci and Lewis[93] reviewed 329 court cases over a 10-year span from 1992 to 2002. In 63% of these cases, the action was initiated by a resident, and 40% of the time a faculty member was identified as a codefendant. In 80% of the claims, the claimant challenged institutional or program actions that resulted in rejection, demotion, or dismissal, and more than half alleged discrimination. In 13% of cases, it was alleged that the institution failed to have or adhere to established policies for reviewing, promoting, disciplining, and terminating. An additional 13% of claims cited a breach of employment contract. In over 90% of these cases, the institutional decision was upheld. This review highlights a consistent message from the legal system that can be characterized by three principles:

1) Judicial deference to professional judgment in reviewing the entire medical record of the student's performance
2) Judicial support of reasoned academic decision-making
3) Judicial nonintervention

While these legal precedents are reassuring, programs must develop and adhere to well-established standards when addressing struggling learners. Padmore and associates have provided a more detailed overview of these standards that is beyond the scope of this chapter but is highly recommended.[94] Examples from Padmore and colleagues are provided in Table 17.8. Educators outside the United States should consult their legal counsel for case law around remediation and probation in their local context.

First and foremost, programs must define and follow due process. This can be defined as academic and nonacademic due process and, in GME, reflects that residents and fellows are both learners and employees. Academic due process applies to those aspects of a learner's performance that reflect the educational process. Nonacademic due process addresses those aspects of behavior that reflect the learner's behavior as an employee. From a legal perspective, GME trainees are protected as students with regard to their educational environment and in clinical settings in which they learn. Typical examples of problems that would be addressed through academic due process include lack of medical knowledge, core competency, specialty training, and even the introspection required for critical self-assessment. When faced with these types of problems, due process has three necessary components: notice of a problem; opportunity to correct that problem; and use of a consistent and deliberative decision-making process. For academic due process, programs should define a standard approach to be used when approaching the problem learner. Academic due process should be the process that is used on a day-to-day basis. If an institution routinely uses a committee such as the graduate medical education committee (GMEC) to review appeals regarding proposed corrective actions or the outcomes of such actions,

TABLE 17.8 **Differences Between Academic Deficiencies and Misconduct**

Performance	Academic Deficiencies	Misconduct in the Academic Setting
Examples	Knowledge-based	Dishonesty/lying
	Deficiency in a core competency[a]	Improper behavior[a] (harassment, retaliation, plagiarism, etc.)
	Technical deficiency	Disruptive behavior
	Lack of insight	Theft
		Violence
What the law requires	Notice (of deficiencies) + Opportunity to cure + Careful and reasonable decision-making process	Notice (of allegation) + Opportunity to be heard + Careful and reasonable decision-making process
	Allows time to remediate and improve after a deficiency is identified	*Does not require time/opportunity to repeat improper behavior*

[a]One of the ACGME core competencies is professionalism; programs must carefully distinguish professionalism, which is "academic," from behaviors, which are really "misconduct."

Modified from Padmore JS, Andolsek KM, Iobst WF, Poulin LJ, Hogan SO, Richard KM. Navigating academic law in competency decisions. *J Grad Med Educ.* 2021 Apr 1;13(2s):102–108.

that practice reflects adequate due process. The key to a defensible process is to adhere to that process for all such cases. It is "the process that you do!"

Nonacademic due process also consists of these three components, but because this process often involves decisions about employee-related rather than education-related standards, adhering to nonacademic due process can be more difficult. Programs should consult with the institution's legal counsel and established policies when addressing cases that fall under this type of due process to ensure that all required standards and regulations have been addressed. Examples of problems falling into this category include misconduct issues such as dishonesty, medical record forgery, harassment, disruptive behavior, theft, and violence. These are all examples of "nondevelopmental" issues highlighted in Fig. 17.8.

Even with an appreciation of this distinction, the appropriate approach to a struggling learner is not always clear. This challenge is further complicated in GME, a professional phase of development in which learners can be considered both students and employees. For the purposes of this discussion, GME learners should first and foremost be considered students. However, from the perspective of tax law, in 2011 the US Supreme Court ruled that teaching hospitals must pay Social Security and Medicare taxes for their medical residents because they are workers and not students. While this may be true regarding tax law, residents and fellows need to be protected as students with respect to the educational environment and the clinical settings in which they learn. This distinction becomes blurry when professionalism issues such as dishonesty surface. In this type of situation, GME learners are routinely held to standards of all employees of the institution and considered in a nonacademic framework. This distinction is important because the required due process afforded the learner as an employee is typically defined by the institution to be compliant with employment law and can be more complex than due process for academic or student issues. All of this highlights the importance of close consultation with the institution's legal counsel, especially when dealing with issues related to misconduct.

Legal Issues: General Guidelines

1. Program directors and offices of GME should have access to legal counsel with expertise in both academic and employee law, and that legal counsel should be consulted early and frequently.
2. Programs must know and adhere to existing guidelines, policies, and procedures. The courts have consistently demonstrated that they will not overturn a reasoned academic decision informed by institutional policies and established due process. However, acting in a manner inconsistent with those policies and due process standards is potentially arbitrary or capricious behavior and will likely not be defensible.
3. Programs must have well-established due process procedures in place, and those procedures must be followed. For academic issues, these procedures need not be complex. Due process can quite literally be "the process that you do." Processes must be fair and applied consistently and without discrimination. The learner must have the opportunity to respond and be heard. There must be an "opportunity to cure," and there must be a reasoned, thoughtful, and standard approach to the adjudication of cases.
4. Programs must provide clear and concise communication of all concerns, problems, expectations, interventions, and consequences of meeting and not meeting the terms of interventions. Everything must be carefully documented, and documentation should include specific comments from individual evaluators. As mentioned

earlier in this chapter, a program's approach to addressing the struggling learner must also be clearly communicated to all stakeholders involved in this process. This includes learner, faculty, program, and institutional administration.

While the specifics of remediation are program specific and will necessarily reflect available resources, programs must ensure that their approach to the struggling learner adheres to all ACGME institutional requirements addressing the promotion, renewal, dismissal, and grievance processes.

Outside the United States

A recent study examined remediation policies and practices in Canada and found that these align well with the existing published best practice guidelines, particularly in their ability to tailor remediation strategies to individual learner needs and promote effective faculty–learner relationships during remediation.[95]

Most of the literature on remediation programs focuses on countries in North America. Outside North America, training programs—and in particular, assessment methods—for medical education learners are often less well defined. In Switzerland, an exploratory study that identified numerous areas for improvement in the recognition and management of residents in difficulty has led to the development of a task force to develop and implement an institutional remediation program at the University of Geneva.[96]

Challenges for the Future

As the approach to the struggling learner continues to evolve, refining standard and criteria-referenced outcomes for specific levels of professional development remains a priority. Medical educators and the profession at large are obligated to define how these criteria reflect development across the continuum of their professional career. Work by Papadakis and colleagues has highlighted the predictive value of what appear to be mild lapses in professionalism in medical students. As a profession, we must enrich our understanding of these types of data. A better understanding of how such behaviors manifest across the entire career of a physician will help catalyze acceptance of why early detection and intervention to correct such behaviors is critical.

Future approaches to the struggling learner must not be reactive processes triggered by happenstance detection of gaps or delays in development. Interventions must be well defined, system based, and grounded in clearly defined standards of expected development and the determination of competence. Throughout this book, we have highlighted the importance of robust *programs* of assessment embedded within functional educational *systems*. Possessing a well-designed assessment program will serve programs well in identifying and working with struggling learners. If CBME is to achieve its full potential, program culture will also need to evolve to a state where requests for remediation would ideally be generated by learners as well as faculty.

In addition, the medical education community will need to work together to develop best practices for remediation so that programs have tools at their fingertips when inevitably faced with a learner who is struggling. These tools should be rooted in a competency-based framework and should also reflect the reality that there are specific phenotypes of learner struggle that require an individualized approach.

Conclusion

In summary, working with struggling learners is a predictable part of undergraduate and graduate medical education. Effectively addressing this group of learners requires successful systems for the identification, investigation, classification, intervention, and adjudication of problems. These systems should:

- Provide interventions that are specific to the identified gaps in performance.
- Define the purpose of the intervention. Remediation should be identified as an improvement opportunity, not a disciplinary or punitive action in the initial phases. In contrast, probation is a disciplinary intervention that typically requires an immediate cessation of a specific problematic behavior or when remediation has failed.
- Outline all responsibilities and steps associated with the corrective action plan.
- Describe a timeline that defines a clear endpoint with specified outcomes and the consequences should that timeline not be achieved. If appropriate, intermediate steps and goals should be identified.
- Provide an advocate or mentor to guide the learner through the remediation process or an individual to monitor compliance if a probationary intervention is deemed necessary.
- Utilize lessons from educational theories such as self-regulated learning to guide corrective action plans.

Finally, all interventions generated by such systems must be effectively communicated to all involved parties in an appropriate manner, be thoroughly documented, protect the confidentiality of all involved parties, and follow appropriate due process.

References

1. http://www.brainyquote.com/quotes/authors/l/lewis_carroll.html#APoie10ogeQtTZyC.99.
2. Englander R, Holmboe E, Batalden P, et al. Coproducing health professions education: a prerequisite to coproducing health care services? *Acad Med*. 2020 Jul;95(7):1006–1013.
3. Accreditation Council for Graduate Medical Education [USA]. 2009 ACGME Outcome Project. Chicago: ACGME. Accessed April 22, 2016. https://www.acgme.org/Outcome.
4. Guerrasio J. *Remediation of the Struggling Learner*. Association for Hospital Medical Education; 2013.
5. Kalet A, Chou CL. *Remediation in Medical Education: A Mid-Course Correction*. Springer; 2014.
6. Smith JL, Lypson M, Silverberg M, et al. Defining uniform processes for remediation, probation and termination in residency training. *West J Emerg Med*. 2017 Jan;18(1):110–113.

7. Santen SA, Christner J, Mejicano G, Hemphill RR. Kicking the can down the road—when medical schools fail to self-regulate. *N Engl J Med.* 2019 Dec 12;381(24):2287–2289.
8. Guerrasio J, Furfari KA, Rosenthal LD, Nogar CL, Wray KW, Aagaard EM. Failure to fail: the institutional perspective. *Med Teach.* 2014 Sep;36(9):799–803.
9. Dudek NL, Marks MB, Regehr G. Failure to fail: the perspectives of clinical supervisors. *Acad Med.* 2005 Oct;80(10 Suppl):S84–S87.
10. Accreditation Council for Graduate Medical Education. Milestones. Accessed April 22, 2016. https://www.acgme.org/acgmeweb/tabid/430/Program_and_Institutional_Accreditation/NextAccreditationSystem/Milestones.aspx.
11. Andolsek K, Padmore J, Hauer K, Holmboe ES. Clinical Competency Committees: A guidebook for programs. 2015. Accessed August 11, 2015. https://www.acgme.org/acgmeweb/Portals/0/ACGMEClinicalCompetencyCommitteeGuidebook.pdf.
12. Accreditation Council for Graduate Medical Education [USA]. 2009a. ACGME Outcome Project. Chicago: ACGME. Accessed May 2, 2016. https://www.acgme.org/Outcome.
13. Frank JR, Snell L, Sherbino J, eds. The draft CanMEDS 2015 physician competency framework. 2015. Accessed December 5, 2015. www.royalcollege.ca/portal/page/portal/rc/common/documents/canmeds/framework/canmeds2015_framework_series_IV_e.pdf.
14. Scottish Deans' Medical Curriculum Group [Scotland]. *The Scottish doctor: Learning outcomes for the medical undergraduate in Scotland: A foundation for competent and reflective practitioners.* 3rd ed. SDMCG; 2009. Accessed May 2, 2016. http://www.scottishdoctor.org.
15. General Medical Council [UK]. Tomorrow's doctors: Outcomes and standards for undergraduate medical education. GMC. 2009. Accessed May 2, 2016. http://www.gmc-uk.org/education/undergraduate/tomorrows_doctors.asp.
16. Graham IS, Gleason AJ, Keogh GW, et al. Australian curriculum framework for junior doctors. *Med J Aust.* 2007;186(7 Suppl):S14–S19.
17. Van Herwaarden CLA, Laan RFJM, Leunissen RRM, eds. *The 2009 framework for undergraduate medical education in the Netherlands.* Utrecht: Dutch Federation of University Medical Centres; 2009.
18. Yao DC, Wright SM. National survey of internal medicine residency program directors regarding problem residents. *JAMA.* 2000;284(9):1099–1104.
19. Dupras DM, Edson RS, Halvorsen AJ, Hopkins RH, McDonald FS. "Problem residents": prevalence, problems and remediation in the era of core competencies. *Am J Med.* 2012 Apr;125(4):421–425.
20. Riebschleger MP, Haftel HM. Remediation in the context of the competencies: a survey of pediatrics residency program directors. *J Grad Med Educ.* 2013 Mar;5(1):60–63.
21. Roback HB, Crowder MK. Psychiatric resident dismissal: a national survey of training programs. *Am J Psychiatry.* 1989 Jan;146(1):96–98.
22. Tabby DS, Majeed MH, Schwartzman RJ. Problem neurology residents: a national survey. *Neurology.* 2011 Jun 14;76(24):2119–2123.
23. Reamy BV, Harman JH. Residents in trouble: an in-depth assessment of the 25-year experience of a single family medicine residency. *Fam Med.* 2006 Apr;38(4):252–257.
24. Williams RG, Roberts NK, Schwind CJ, Dunnington GL. The nature of general surgery resident performance problems. *Surgery.* 2009 Jun;145(6):651–658.
25. Zbieranowski I, Takahashi SG, Verma S, Spadafora SM. Remediation of residents in difficulty: a retrospective 10-year review of the experience of a postgraduate board of examiners. *Acad Med.* 2013 Jan;88(1):111–116.
26. Guerrasio J, Garrity MJ, Aagaard EM. Learner deficits and academic outcomes of medical students, residents, fellows, and attending physicians referred to a remediation program, 2006-2012. *Acad Med.* 2014 Feb;89(2):352–358.
27. Warburton KM, Shahane AA. Mental health conditions among struggling GME learners: results from a single center remediation program. *J Grad Med Educ.* 2020 Dec;12(6):773–777.
28. Warburton KM, Goren E, Dine CJ. Comprehensive assessment of struggling learners referred to a graduate medical education remediation program. *J Grad Med Educ.* 2017 Dec;9(6):763–767.
29. Hauer KE, Ciccone A, Henzel TR, et al. Remediation of the deficiencies of physicians across the continuum from medical school to practice: a thematic review of the literature. *Acad Med.* 2009;84(12):1822–1832.
30. Minter RM, Dunnington GL, Sudan R, Terhune KP, Dent DL, Lentz AK. Can this resident be saved? Identification and early intervention for struggling residents. *J Am Coll Surg.* 2014 Nov;219(5):1088–1095.
31. Crosson FJ, Leu J, Roemer BM, Ross MN. Gaps in residency training should be addressed to better prepare doctors for a twenty-first-century delivery system. *Health Aff.* 2011;30(11):2142–2148.
32. Mattar SG, Alseidi AA, Jones DB, et al. General surgery residency inadequately prepares trainees for fellowship: results of a survey of fellowship program directors. *Ann Surg.* 2013;258(3):440–449.
33. Ziring D, Danoff D, Grosseman S, et al. How do medical schools identify and remediate professionalism lapses in medical students? A study of US and Canadian medical schools. *Acad Med.* 2015 Jul;90(7):913–920.
34. Brenner AM, Mathai S, Jain S, Mohl PC. Can we predict "problem residents"? *Acad Med.* 2010;85:1147–1151.
35. Carraccio C, Wolfsthal SD, Englander R, Ferentz K, Martin C. Shifting paradigms: from Flexner to competencies. *Acad Med.* 2002;77(5):361–367.
36. Eva K, Regehr G. "I'll never play professional football" and other fallacies of self-assessment. *J Cont Educ Health Prof.* 2008;28(1):14–19.
37. Davis DA, Mazmanian PE, Fordis M, Van Harrison R, Thorpe KE, Perrier L. Accuracy of physician self-assessment compared with observed measures of competence. *JAMA.* 2006;296(9):1094–1102.
38. ACGME. The Clinical Learning Environment Review. Accessed February 1, 2023. https://www.acgme.org/What-We-Do/Initiatives/Clinical-Learning-Environment-Review-CLER.
39. Ogunyemi D. Defeating unconscious bias: the role of a structured, reflective, and interactive workshop. *J Grad Med Educ.* 2021 Apr;13(2):189–194.
40. McClintock AH, Fainstad T, Jauregui J, Yarris LM. Countering bias in assessment. *J Grad Med Educ.* 2021 Oct;13(5):725–726.
41. See A, Pallaci M, Aluisio AR, et al. Assessment of implicit gender bias during evaluation of procedural competency among emergency medicine residents. *JAMA Netw Open.* 2022 Feb 1;5(2):e2147351.
42. Teherani A, Hauer KE, Fernandez A, King TE, Lucey C. How small differences in assessed clinical performance amplify to large differences in grades and awards: a cascade with serious consequences for students underrepresented in medicine. *Acad Med.* 2018 Sep;93(9):1286–1292.

43. Klein R, Julian KA, Snyder ED, et al. Gender bias in resident assessment in graduate medical education: review of the literature. *J Gen Intern Med*. 2019 May;34(5):712–719.
44. Lucey CR, Hauer KE, Boatright D, Fernandez A. Medical education's wicked problem: achieving equity in assessment for medical learners. *Acad Med*. 2020 Dec;95(12S):S98–S108.
45. Evans D, Brown J. Supporting students in difficulty. In: Cantillon P, Wood D, eds. *ABC of Learning and Teaching in Medicine*. Wiley-Blackwell; 2010:78–82.
46. Papadakis MA, Hodgson CS, Teherani A, Kohatsu N. Unprofessional behavior in medical school is associated with subsequent disciplinary action by a state medical board. *Acad Med*. 2004;79(3):244–249.
47. Lipner RS, Young A, Chaudhry HJ, Duhigg LM, Papadakis MA. Specialty certification status, performance ratings, and disciplinary actions of internal medicine residents. *Acad Med*. 2016;91(3):376–381.
48. Hauer KE, ten Cate O, Boscardin CK, et al. Ensuring resident competence: a narrative review of the literature on group decision making to inform the work of clinical competency committees. *J Grad Med Educ*. 2016 Mar 9 [Epub ahead of print].
49. Yaghoubian A, Galante J, Kaji A, et al. General Surgery resident remediation and attrition: a multi-institutional study. *Arch Surg*. 2012;147(9):829–833.
50. Winston KA, van der Vleuten CPM, Scherpbier AJJA. Prediction and prevention of failure: an early intervention to assist at-risk medical students. *Med Teach*. 2014 Jan;36(1):25–31.
51. Winston KA, van der Vleuten CPM, Scherpbier AJJA. Remediation of at-risk medical students: theory in action. *BMC Med Educ*. 2013 Sep 27;13:132.
52. DeKosky AS, Sedrak MS, Goren E, Dine CJ, Warburton KM. Simple frameworks for daily work: Innovative strategies to coach residents struggling with time management, organization, and efficiency. *J Grad Med Educ*. 2018 Jun;10(3):325–330.
53. Warburton KM, Mahan JD. Coaching nephrology trainees who struggle with clinical performance. *Clin J Am Soc Nephrol*. 2018 Jan 6;13(1):172–174.
54. Warburton KM, Parsons AS, Yen P, Goren E. Evaluation and Remediation of Organization, Efficiency, and Time Management) Remediation in Medical Education: A Midcourse Correction, 2nd edition. Available at: https://link.springer.com/book/10.1007/978-3-031-32404-8.
55. Waechter D. 2015. LCME Glossary of Terms for LCME Accreditation Standards and Elements 2015-2016. :10. Accessed November 7, 2023. http://changenow.icahn.mssm.edu/wp-content/uploads/sites/13/2017/02/2016-17_Glossary-of-Terms_2016-06-29-1-1.pdf.
56. Parsons AS, Wijesekera TP, Rencic JJ. The management script: a practical tool for teaching management reasoning. *Acad Med*. 2020 Aug;95(8):1179–1185.
57. Barrett JL, Denegar CR, Mazerolle SM. Challenges facing new educators: expanding teaching strategies for clinical reasoning and evidence-based medicine. *Athl Train Educ J*. 2018;13(4):359–366.
58. Daniel M, Rencic J, Durning SJ, et al. Clinical reasoning assessment methods: a scoping review and practical guidance. *Acad Med*. 2019;94(6):902–912.
59. Parsons AS, Clancy CB, Rencic JJ, Warburton KM. Targeted strategies to remediate diagnostic reasoning deficits. *Acad Med*. 2022 Apr 1;97(4):616.
60. Mata DA, Ramos MA, Bansal N, et al. Prevalence of depression and depressive symptoms among resident physicians: a systematic review and meta-analysis. *JAMA*. 2015 Dec 8;314(22):2373–2383.
61. Boisaubin EV, Levine RE. Identifying and assisting the impaired physician. *Am J Med Sci*. 2001 Jul;322(1):31–36.
62. Meeks LM, Pereira-Lima K, Frank E, Stergiopoulos E, Ross KET, Sen S. Program access, depressive symptoms, and medical errors among resident physicians with disability. *JAMA Netw Open*. 2021 Dec 1;4(12):e2141511.
63. Fitzsimons MG, Brookman JC, Arnholz SH, Baker K. Attention-deficit/hyperactivity disorder and successful completion of anesthesia residency: a case report. *Acad Med*. 2016 Feb;91(2):210–214.
64. Goldenberg M, Miotto K, Skipper GE, Sanford J. Outcomes of physicians with substance use disorders in state physician health programs: a narrative review. *J Psychoactive Drugs*. 2020 Jul-Aug;52(3):195-202. doi: 10.1080/02791072.2020.1734696.
65. Dupont RL, McLellan AT, Carr G, Gendel M, Skipper GE. How are addicted physicians treated? A national survey of physician health programs. *J Subst Abuse Treat*. 2009 Jul;37(1):1–7.
66. Hughes PH, Baldwin DC, Sheehan DV, Conrad S, Storr CL. Resident physician substance use, by specialty. *Am J Psychiatry*. 1992 Oct;149(10):1348–1354.
67. Warner DO, Berge K, Sun H, Harman A, Hanson A, Schroeder DR. Substance use disorder among anesthesiology residents, 1975-2009. *JAMA*. 2013 Dec 4;310(21):2289–2296.
68. Hughes PH, Brandenburg N, Baldwin DC, et al. Prevalence of substance use among US physicians. *JAMA*. 1992 May 6; 267(17):2333–2339.
69. Oreskovich MR, Shanafelt T, Dyrbye LN, et al. The prevalence of substance use disorders in American physicians. *Am J Addict*. 2015 Jan;24(1):30–38.
70. Flaherty JA, Richman JA. Substance use and addiction among medical students, residents, and physicians. *Psychiatr Clin North Am*. 1993 Mar;16(1):189–197.
71. Maslach D, Jackson SE, Leiter MP. *Maslach Burnout Inventory Manual*. 3rd ed.. Consulting Psychologists Press; 1996.
72. West CP, Dyrbye LN, Shanafelt TD. Physician burnout: contributors, consequences and solutions. *J Intern Med*. 2018;283:516–529.
73. Shanafelt TD, West CP, Sinsky C, et al. Changes in burnout and satisfaction with work-life integration in physicians and the general US working population between 2011 and 2017. *Mayo Clin Proc*. 2019 Sep;94(9):1681–1694.
74. Rodrigues H, Cobucci R, Oliveira A, et al. Burnout syndrome among medical residents: a systematic review and meta-analysis. *PLoS One*. 2018 Nov 12;13(11):e0206840.
75. Rosen IM, Gimotty PA, Shea JA, Bellini LM. Evolution of sleep quantity, sleep deprivation, mood disturbances, empathy, and burnout among interns. *Acad Med*. 2006 Jan;81(1):82–85.
76. Dyrbye L, Shanafelt T. A narrative review on burnout experienced by medical students and residents. *Med Educ*. 2016;50(1):132–149.
77. Warde CM, Linzer M, Schorling JB, Moore EM, Poplau S. Balancing unbalanced lives: a practical framework for personal and organizational change. *Mayo Clin Proc Innov Qual Outcomes*. 2019 Feb 26;3(1):97–100.
78. Shanafelt TD, Noseworthy JH. Executive leadership and physician well-being: nine organizational strategies to promote engagement and reduce burnout. *Mayo Clin Proc*. 2017 Jan;92(1):129–146.
79. Spickard A, Gabbe SG, Christensen JF. Mid-career burnout in generalist and specialist physicians. *JAMA*. 2002 Sep 25;288(12):1447–1450.
80. Shanafelt T, Ripp J, Trockel M. Understanding and addressing sources of anxiety among health care professionals during the COVID-19 pandemic. *JAMA*. 2020 Jun 2;323(21):2133–2134.

81. Williams BW. Professionalism lapses and adverse childhood experiences: reflections from the island of last resort. *Acad Med.* 2019 Aug;94(8):1081–1083.
82. Williams BW, Welindt D, Hafferty FW, Stumps A, Flanders P, Williams MV. Adverse childhood experiences in trainees and physicians with professionalism lapses: implications for medical education and remediation. *Acad Med.* 2021 May 1;96(5):736–743.
83. Kogan J, Conforti L, Iobst WF, Holmboe ES. Reconceptualizing variable rater assessments as both an educational and clinical care problem. *Acad Med.* 2014;89(5):721–727.
84. The sick physician. Impairment by psychiatric disorders, including alcoholism and drug dependence. *JAMA.* 1973 Feb 5;223(6):684–687.
85. International Classification of Impairments, Disabilities, and Handicaps. Accessed May 2, 2016. http://whqlibdoc.who.int/publications/1980/9241541261_eng.pdf.
86. Smith CS, Stevens NG, Servis M. A general framework for approaching residents in difficulty. *Fam Med.* 2007 May;39(5):331–336.
87. Durning SJ, Cleary TJ, Sandars J, Hemmer P, Kokotailo P, Artino AR. Viewing "strugglers" through a different lens: how a self-regulated learning perspective can help medical educators with assessment and remediation. *Acad Med.* 2011;86(4):488–495.
88. Exploring the ACGME Core Competencies: Professionalism (Part 7 of 7), published January 12, 2017, Accessed January 16, 2023. https://knowledgeplus.nejm.org/blog/acgme-core-competencies-professionalism/.
89. Rostenstein AH. The quality and economic impact of disruptive behaviors on clinical outcomes of patient care. *Am J Med Qual.* 2011 Sep-Oct;26(5):372–379.
90. Papadakis MA, Arnold GK, Blank LL, Holmboe ES, Lipner RS. Performance during internal medicine residency training and subsequent disciplinary action by state licensing boards. *Ann Intern Med.* 2008 Jun 3;148(11):869–876.
91. Papadakis MA, Teherani A, Banach MA, et al. Disciplinary action by medical boards and prior behavior in medical school. *N Engl J Med.* 2005 Dec 22;353(25):2673–2682.
92. Rest JR, Narvarez DF. *Moral Development in the Professions: Psychology and Applied Ethics.* Lawrence Erlbam Associates; 1994.
93. Minicucci R, Lewis B. Trouble in academia: ten years of litigation in medical education. *Acad Med.* 2003;78(10):S13–S15.
94. Padmore JS, Andolsek KM, Iobst WF, Poulin LJ, Hogan SO, Richard KM. Navigating academic law in competency decisions. *J Grad Med Educ.* 2021 Apr 1;13(2s):102–108.
95. Shearer C, Bosma M, Bergin F, Sargeant J, Warren A. Remediation in Canadian medical residency programs: established and emerging best practices. *Med Teach.* 2019 Jan;41(1):28–35.
96. Lanier C, Muller-Juge V, Dao MD, Gaspoz J-M, Perron NJ, Audetat M-C. Management of residents in difficulty in a Swiss general internal medicine outpatient clinic: change is necessary!. *PLoS One.* 2021 Jul 20;16(7):e0254336.

18

Program Evaluation

MICHAEL SOH, PHD, AND STEVEN J. DURNING, MD, PHD

CHAPTER OUTLINE

Introduction

The primary focus of this book is on the assessment of individual learners. However, it is the responsibility of educational leaders to also evaluate the quality of their educational programs with the same degree of rigor that is applied to individual learner assessment. Program evaluation is described by the Accreditation Council for Graduate Medical Education (ACGME) in the United States as the "systematic collection and analysis of information related to the design, implementation, and outcomes of a program, for the purpose of monitoring and improving the quality and effectiveness of the program."[1] In most cases, aggregated data from the assessment of individuals will be useful in contributing to program evaluation. However, assessment data from individual learners is not, in itself, enough to inform rigorous judgments about program performance. Program evaluation involves analyzing the system and all of its interacting parts and making needed changes; an educational system is made up of more than individual learners. Thus many other sources of information may be important in formulating judgments about program quality and informing change and improvement strategies.[2,3]

Program evaluation is an essential activity for any educational enterprise and should be part of core program management activities. Systematically approaching program evaluation will not only help with meeting accreditation standards and meeting one's charge of accountability to the public, learners, and other stakeholders but also should lead to ongoing development and improvement of the program. Indeed, the concepts of "systematic" and "ongoing" are critical to program evaluation success. Further, program evaluation can also provide a venue for scholarship regarding a program's "lessons learned," and when done with rigor and reproducibility can assist *other* programs facing similar challenges. Indeed, program evaluation can be approached using Glassick's criteria (Fig. 18.1),[4] leading to peer-reviewed publications of work.[5]

In this chapter we begin with a discussion of program evaluation purposes, followed by a discussion of a variety of program evaluation models and methods, and then transition to providing practical advice on a variety of general issues concerning program evaluation. We refer the reader to several resources to supplement understanding of this vast and expanding topic in health professions education.

Evaluation Purposes

There are several reasons for evaluating an educational program that are not mutually exclusive.[6,7] Accountability to demonstrate that the program is achieving its stated objectives is one of the primary purposes for evaluation. External bodies, such as the Liaison Committee on Medical Education (LCME), the ACGME, and the Royal College of Physicians and Surgeons of Canada (RCPSC), require evaluation of undergraduate and graduate medical education programs to maintain accreditation. Internal stakeholders, particularly

- Clear goals
  - Purpose clearly stated? Important research question and/or aim?
- Adequate preparation
  - Understand prior scholarship? Resources needed?
- Appropriate methods
  - Appropriate to goals? Effective?
- Significant results
  - Goals achieved? Outcomes significant?
- Effective communication
  - Well written? Appropriate audience? Dissemination?
- Reflective
  - Critically evaluate results? Critical evaluation used to improve quality of future work?

• **Fig. 18.1** Glassick's criteria applied to program evaluation.

those who provide financial support for educational activities, may also expect that educational leaders undertake evaluation to ensure appropriate use of scarce resources. Evaluation of learner achievement and other outcomes, as well as program processes, also serves an important purpose in providing feedback on the program to guide change or ongoing improvement efforts. Information about the quality, outcomes, or impact of the program may be used by a range of "consumers" such as potential applicants to the program or recipients of the program's product (such as residency program directors or hospital administrators).[6] In addition, information gleaned from the evaluation of educational activities or interventions can be used to generate new knowledge about effective practices and innovations, as well as lessons learned, which can be shared with others who are considering or deploying similar activities or interventions in their program(s).[5,7–9]

Overview of Evaluation Models

In developing an evaluation plan, program leaders have multiple models and methods from which to choose. Evaluation models vary to a significant degree with regard to their focus on program outcomes versus processes and the relationship between program elements and, consequently, on their use of quantitative and qualitative methods. At one end of the spectrum are more experimental models such as the goal and measure approach that focuses on program outcomes and deploy quantitative approaches with which most health professions educators are familiar. Health professions educators are generally comfortable with and confident in the results from randomized clinical trials, systematic reviews, statistical analyses of quantitative data, and even semiquantitative survey data as they inform the development of generalizable scientific findings.[10] However, despite the confidence and comfort in the scientific rigor of more quantitative methods, such approaches can be somewhat reductionist in treating the relationship between program elements and outcomes as linear in nature, with expectations that changes in isolated components should lead more or less directly to proportional changes in measured outcomes.[3] Additionally, satisfaction with evaluation models that use quantitative measures focusing almost exclusively on program outcomes has declined because such approaches often yield results showing no or minimal effects of the program, which raises concerns that either our current programming is largely ineffective or we are unable to inadequately capture the effect of our programs.[11,12]

Evolution in thinking about evaluation models has resulted in development of a new paradigm that focuses on the theoretical bases regarding how educational programs lead to change, and identifying how programmatic processes and activities impact its outcomes. Theory-driven evaluation models in general integrate the use of theory in designing, conducting, and interpreting research and look beyond outcomes to better understand and create new knowledge about the causes and contextual determinants of change brought about by programs and interventions.[13] Although such models may use quantitative methods to a variable extent, they rely more on qualitative methods (e.g., focus groups, interviews, ethnographic methods, and narrative) to move beyond a sole outcomes approach to quantifying a program's value and effectiveness and yield information about the internal workings of a program to guide implementation of the program in different contexts and develop generalizable knowledge to inform a range of stakeholders, including other program developers.[10,11]

This examination of the internal workings of a program may rely on a "layered analysis" of philosophies, principles, and techniques that illuminate a program's, and more specifically its interventions', intended function in context.[14] The *philosophy*, defined as the "essence of an intervention," is independent of context but describes its unique conceptual learning conditions that separate it from other interventions. This philosophy is brought to life by its *principles*, or the structural aspects of an intervention that account for context yet embody the philosophy's unique conceptual learning conditions. The realization of these principles leads to *techniques*, or the most context-specific element of an intervention. Chamberland et al.[15] provide an example of layered analysis in action by highlighting the technique of structured reflection in clinical reasoning development within undergraduate medical education. In short, structured reflection requires a number of principles to be in place (i.e., a learner working with a clinical case, a clinically appropriate case based on learner expertise, a systematic progression through clinical reasoning tasks, etc.). These principles, in turn, bring to life two underlying philosophies: the model of reflective practice and the theory of expertise development.

This layered approach to contextualizing a program and its interventions may best be understood by deploying qualitative methods and researchers. Qualitative researchers have developed a number of strategies (triangulation, member checking, pattern matching, negative case sampling, and external audits) that bring rigor to their methods.[16] Evaluation models that are heavily dependent on more qualitative approaches include realist evaluation, the CIPP model, the before, during, after model, and the MRC Complex Intervention Model. These models view the individual programs as complex systems affected by a variety of internal and external factors, with the expectation that outcomes will be highly contextual, based upon the complex interrelationship between program variables[13] and will be covered in this chapter. More participatory, qualitative, or theoretical approaches are necessary to determine the impact of complex, multifaceted initiatives that may have more intricate processes, contextual variables, and uncertain timing with regard to the expected results of a training program.[7,12,13]

Program evaluation models have a rich history that stems primarily from the quality assurance literature. In the next section, we will outline selected models that we believe can be readily implemented to help the director of an academic program anywhere in the continuum of medical education. Indeed, using the same model across the continuum will help facilitate the purposes of program evaluation as well as contribute to a shared mental model for both teachers and learners and a clearer trajectory of goals and expectations for learners.

Evaluators should not feel restricted in their use of models or methods, but should identify aspects from different models that best meet their needs and even how different methods may complement each other by compensating for individual limitations.[10,17] Indeed, many evaluation experts advocate for the use of a "pragmatic approach" that applies mixed methods in the evaluation of social and health services programs.[10,16] An "emergent" approach is very useful, in which the evaluation plan may be adapted or modified based on the evolution or complexity of a particular project or program.[7] It is important to be aware of the limitations of the different models or methods when deciding upon the evaluation approach.[6]

There are some common features in the models described in the next section that are worthy of comment. Program evaluation is a cyclical process that is optimally done in a continual fashion. A variety of measures are incorporated to help inform the evaluator—much like an individual's competency cannot be assessed with a single measure, program evaluation requires multiple measures. Indeed, a recurrent theme of the program evaluation literature is the notion of unexpected findings. The specific model or blend of models chosen is in part driven by program need(s) (e.g., to meet accreditation standards), and given that these needs can vary by phase of training it is not surprising that program evaluation models also vary. As stated earlier in this chapter, program evaluation is more than assessment of learners' performance. A variety of other measures such as program structure and environment are recommended in conducting program evaluation. Finally, there is growing support of moving from psychometric, linear, and outcomes-oriented models to those that are more qualitative, contextual, and relational.

Program Evaluation Models

Goal and Measure

The goal and measure model is a simplification of the before, during, after model that is described below. In this model, one begins with defining a limited number of goals (after measures). Next, the evaluator lists a number of measures (quantitative or qualitative—during measures) that could be used for determining if the goal(s) are met. Determining success is based on having the measures meet acceptable levels of performance as well as the trajectory or improvement over time and overall performance.

For example, one could list proficient procedure performance as a goal. The measures could likely include a procedure log listing procedure type, dates, success, lessons learned, and a faculty member's endorsement of proficiency (signature, level of entrustment on an Entrustable Professional Activity [EPA], or other). Determining success would mean that the procedural log has a sufficient number and quality of entries, expected growth over time, and final endorsement of proficiency. Consistent with this approach, the medical education literature on program evaluation has

TABLE 18.1 Comparison of the Kirkpatrick Model and Moore's Expanded Outcomes Framework

Kirkpatrick	Miller's Pyramid	Moore's Expanded Outcomes Framework	Evaluation Method
		Level 1: Participation	Documentation of attendance
Level1: Reaction		Level 2: Satisfaction	Attendee survey
Level 2: Learning	Knows	Level 3A: Learning: Declarative Knowledge	Self-assessment/self-report Written examination
	Knows how	Level 3B: Learning: Procedural Knowledge	Self-assessment/self-report Written examination (short answer, essay) Case-based discussion
	Shows how	Level 4: Competence	Self-assessment/self-report Direct observation in real or simulated setting
Level 3: Behavior	Does	Level 5: Performance	Self-assessment/self-report Direct observation of clinical practice Multisource feedback Quality-of-care (process) measurement
Level 4: Results		Level 6: Patient Health	Quality-of-care (outcome) measurement (Practice/institution level)
		Level 7: Community Health	Quality-of-care (outcome) measurement (Community/population level)

Modified from Moore DE, Greene JS, Gallis HA. Achieving desired results and improved outcomes: Integrating planning and assessment throughout learning activities. *J Contin Educ Health Prof*. 2009;29;1-15.

several examples of association of two (or more) measures that pertain to a specific goal.

Kirkpatrick Model and Moore's Expanded Outcomes Framework

The Kirkpatrick model describes program evaluation outcomes into one of four levels[18,19]: reaction, learning, behavior, and results. Like the goal and measure model, the Kirkpatrick model was not designed for program evaluation, but rather as a way to capture individual learner or aggregate learner performance. We will illustrate the model using the example of evaluating peer teaching in a residency training program. Level 1 or reaction describes opinions about or reactions to the learning experience. For purposes of program evaluation this could take the form of learners' ratings of peer teachers using a standardized instrument such as an end of month evaluation form. Level 2 or learning (manifest as a change in knowledge, skills, or attitude) could take the form of pre/post self-assessments of teaching competence; for example, with a rating instrument. Level 3 or behavior (change in behaviors or performance in applying learning) might represent videotaping a teaching session with feedback to learners or an OSTE using the peer teacher. Level 4 or results (outcomes) could take the form of improved performance by the recipients of peer teaching.

The literature has demonstrated asymmetry in terms of a preponderance of papers focusing on the lowest Kirkpatrick level (reaction or satisfaction) as opposed to higher-level outcomes. Certainly, collecting learner satisfaction is an important part of program evaluation but should not be limited to this (e.g., necessary but not sufficient). Examples of the use of the Kirkpatrick levels include the evaluation of a clinical scientist program[20] and evidence for Kirkpatrick levels in medical education.[21] Kirkpatrick levels are perhaps most often used in the continuing medical education (CME) world of program evaluation efforts. Shortcomings of the Kirkpatrick model include a focus on outcomes without explicitly including the use of resources, prioritization of measurements, or an integrated framework for assessment. Its strengths include the portability of the levels and transferability to many educational fields. More recently, Moore and colleagues expanded the Kirkpatrick model to specify individual levels of learning that represent the bottom three levels of Miller's pyramid[22] and better capture the impact of CME on physician performance and patient outcomes (Table 18.1).[23] The expanded framework was introduced within a conceptual model for planning and evaluating CME programs, with the intent to drive improvement in CME programming to result in higher-level performance and quality-of-care outcomes. This model, like the original Kirkpatrick model, is commonly considered in CME program evaluation efforts.

Logic Model

The logic model may not be strictly considered an evaluation model or method, per se, but may be viewed more appropriately as an approach to visually representing the interrelationships between program resources, processes, products, and outcomes to support guidance of program planning, implementation, management, and evaluation.[24] Thus a logic model may be useful for program planning and description, as well as evaluation.[3] During development of a logic model, a road map of the program is created that links short- and long-term outcomes to the sequential process and activities that are intended to lead to those outcomes, based on the principles and theoretical assumptions underlying the program.[7,24] Use of a program logic model involves a theory-based approach to evaluation in presupposing that we can learn the most about a program's impact and most influential factors by combining outcomes analysis with methods that help us better understand the processes and context that led to the identified outcomes. Understanding the contextual factors (the how and the why) that impact outcomes allows us to identify the specific targets for change and to fully inform others to seek to implement similar projects or programs.[7]

The logic model approach is designed to be used for evaluation of complex initiatives in which some outcomes may be long term and intangible, such as creating a learning culture in a healthcare system.[7] In the logic model, one of the key structural elements involves impact analysis, which looks at the long-term effects of the program, as opposed to outcomes measurement, which addresses the more immediate or intermediate outcomes.[6]

Although the logic model structure and process may vary depending on the goals and focus of the evaluation, it consists of several key structural elements (Fig. 18.1). The iterative process of filling in the details within each element can be a useful exercise in helping program leaders and evaluators better understand and clarify the logical sequential links and relationships between outcomes; input into the program, activities, processes, and products of the program; and underlying theories and assumptions that link these elements together.[7,25] Furthermore, the process of developing the logic model may help key stakeholders build consensus and a shared understanding about the program and what it intends to accomplish.[7]

The basic logic model structure (Fig. 18.2) begins with *inputs* to the program, which are the human, financial, organizational, and community resources available to be used in the program. Inputs may be either material or intellectual; examples include educational technology, funding sources, and faculty skills and time.[3] Those resources are incorporated into program *activities*, the processes, tools, events, technology, and other actions designed to produce the intended program outcomes. In a sense, the activities comprise the interventions or innovations within the program.[3] Activities may include products (educational materials), services (counseling), and infrastructure that are developed to support attainment of intended change or goals. Together, the inputs and activities constitute the *planned work* of the program (Fig. 18.2). Factors that facilitate or impede change may also be included in the planned work components of the logic model. *Protective factors* include resources such as funding, equipment, facilities, and collaborators. Things that are barriers to change or impede goal attainment, such as restrictive policies and regulations, and lack of resources or support, are considered *risk factors*.[24]

Outputs are the direct results of program activities and may include different types, levels, and targets of services the program seeks to deliver. They represent what actually happened as a result of the program activities and are often described quantitatively in terms of the products and services delivered within the program.[3] Examples would include such items as the number of classes attended, patients encountered, or faculty trained. In the basic logic model described by the W.K. Kellogg Foundation, *outcomes* are divided into short term (1–3 years) and longer term (4–6 years) depending on when achievable outcomes are expected to be attained. Program outcomes are generally defined in terms of changes in individual program participants' knowledge, skills, behavior, and level of functioning or status. In medical education programs, patient outcomes may constitute an important result to measure.[3] *Impact* is generally reserved for broader program outcomes that occur at the level of organizations, systems, and communities, which may not occur until 7 to 10 years after the program is implemented or changed. Together, the outputs, outcomes, and impact comprise the intended results of the program.[24]

In applying the logic model to evaluation, the basic structure can be modified to help focus better on contextual and implementation-related factors that may affect outcomes. For example, contextual factors such as faculty morale may influence interest in participation in various program activities, with a downstream impact on outputs and then outcomes. Implementation factors, such as unexpected lack of access to a critical learning resource or low (or high) patient volume, may lead to problems with learner achievement of key competencies and accreditation problems. These factors can also inform novel approaches for program evaluation, such as Rapid Evaluation, that rely on key aspects of the logic model (context, implementation processes, outcomes, etc.) to in turn provide timely evidence of change.[26] Although the logic model framework is drawn in a linear manner, the relationships between the boxes may be quite complex and recursive over time. It is important to envision feedback as an important process in applying the logic model. In fact, in applying the logic model to program planning, feedback loops back to earlier steps in the model may inform subsequent development and implementation of program activities.

In medicine and medical education, the logic model may be appropriately applied to the evaluation of a number of programs or interventions, including educational interventions, faculty development activities, and public health and research programs.[25,27–29] The logic model may be best applied to evaluation of revision or innovation within a program, particularly if program leaders have an understanding

Using a Logic Model to Assist in the Planning, Implementation, and Evaluation of Educational Programs

Elaine Van Melle, PhD, education scientist, Royal College of Physicians and Surgeons of Canada, and education researcher, Department of Family Medicine, Queen's University

Logic Model Basics

- A logic model is a diagram that shows how a program is thought to work; that is, how resources (inputs) produce key processes (activities), and how the products (outputs) produce desired results (outcomes).
- Logic models can be drawn in numerous ways; they range from fairly simple to more complex.
- A needs assessment sets the scene for educational program design and determination of expected outcomes.

Example of a Logic Model

A Program to Develop Family Medicine Resident Competency in Comprehensive Health Checks for Individuals With a DD

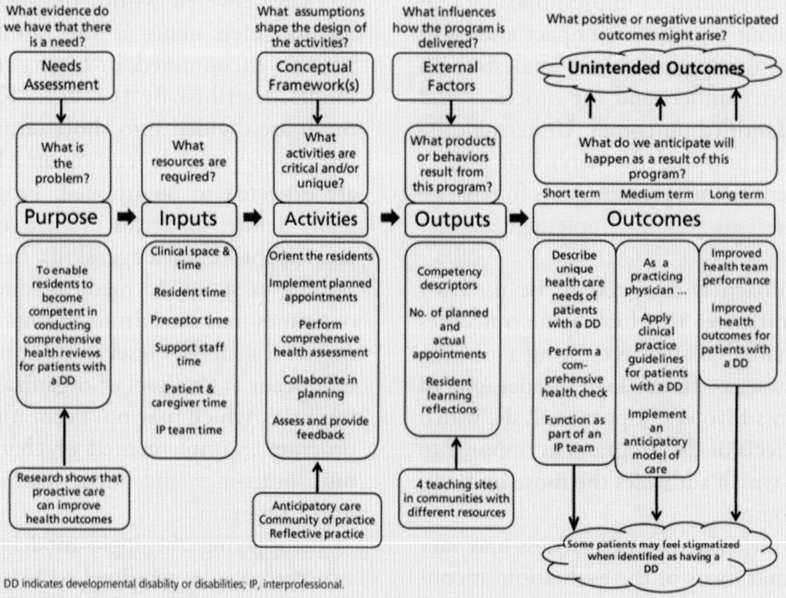

What evidence do we have that there is a need?
Needs Assessment
What is the problem?
Purpose
To enable residents to become competent in conducting comprehensive health reviews for patients with a DD
Research shows that proactive care can improve health outcomes

What resources are required?
Inputs
Clinical space & time
Resident time
Preceptor time
Support staff time
Patient & caregiver time
IP team time

What assumptions shape the design of the activities?
Conceptual Framework(s)
What activities are critical and/or unique?
Activities
Orient the residents
Implement planned appointments
Perform comprehensive health assessment
Collaborate in planning
Assess and provide feedback
Anticipatory care
Community of practice
Reflective practice

What influences how the program is delivered?
External Factors
What products or behaviors result from this program?
Outputs
Competency descriptors
No. of planned and actual appointments
Resident learning reflections
4 teaching sites in communities with different resources

What positive or negative unanticipated outcomes might arise?
Unintended Outcomes
What do we anticipate will happen as a result of this program?
Short term Medium term Long term
Outcomes
Describe unique health care needs of patients with a DD
Perform a comprehensive health check
Function as part of an IP team
As a practicing physician ...
Apply clinical practice guidelines for patients with a DD
Implement an anticipatory model of care
Improved health team performance
Improved health outcomes for patients with a DD
Some patients may feel stigmatized when identified as having a DD

DD indicates developmental disability or disabilities; IP, interprofessional.

Tips for Using and Applying Logic Models

- Involve all key stakeholders (e.g., program leaders, developers, implementers, participants) in creating a draft.
- Develop additional iterations to help create consensus amongst the key stakeholders.
- Use the logic model to identify areas where further program planning may be required.
- Use the final logic model to determine the focus for program evaluation.
- Use the logic model to discover whether an established program is producing the desired outcomes.
- Use the logic model to determine whether a newer program is being implemented as intended.

A good logic model facilitates a common approach to program planning, implementation, and evaluation.

Resources
1. Bordage G. Conceptual frameworks that illuminate and magnify. Med Educ. 2009;43:312–319.
2. Funnell SC, Rogers PJ. Purposeful Program Theory: Effective Use of Theories of Change and Logic Models. San Francisco, Calif: Jossey-Bass; 2011.
3. Kern DE, Thomas PA, Hughes MT. Curriculum Development for Medical Education: A Six-Step Approach. 2nd ed. Baltimore, Md: Johns Hopkins University Press; 2009
4. McLaughlin JA, Jordan GB. Using logic models. In: Wholey JS, Hatry HP, Newcomer KE, eds. Handbook of Practical Program Evaluation. 2nd ed. Hoboken, NJ: Jossey-Bass; 2004.
5. Patton MQ. Essentials of Utilization Focused Evaluation. Thousand Oaks, Calif: Sage; 2012.

Author contact: e-mail: vanmelle@queensu.ca; Twitter: @elainevanmelle

• **Fig. 18.2** Using a logic model to assist in the planning, implementation, and evaluation of educational programs. From Van Melle, E. Using a logic model to assist in the planning, implementation, and evaluation of educational programs. *Acad Med*. 2016;91(10):1464.

regarding how change works within the program. Unlike more quantitative methods, it will not document evidence of any causal effects between program activities and outcomes. But it will support generation of high-quality information and promote a shared understanding of how critical program elements are interrelated that will be useful for both program planning and evaluation and will serve as a reference point for monitoring program process and informing potential modifications.[3,28]

Logic models are typically a representation of program theory, or "an explicit theory of how an intervention is understood to contribute to its intended or observed outcomes," and can be used to capture the two main components of program theory: theory of change and theory of action.[30] Theory of change refers to the "central mechanism by which change [or no change] comes about for individuals, groups, and communities"[30] and can be derived from formal research or unstated understandings. Theory of action explains "how programs or other interventions are constructed to activate their theory of change".[30] However, depending on the type of logic model used, theories of change may not be as explicit. As such, while necessary to focus on inputs, activities, and outputs, a logic model may not be sufficient until processes and causal mechanisms are highlighted to explain how and why outputs are met and outcomes are achieved.

Before, During, After

A commonly used model for purposes of scholarship is the before, during, after approach. This model is derived from the quality assurance literature and divides measures that can be collected for program evaluation purposes into three phases: before starting the program (e.g., baselines), during the program (e.g., process measures), and after the program (e.g., products or outcomes). This model is flexible in terms of giving the evaluator latitude in defining the time frames for the phases, which do not need to be of equal duration. Further, it is acceptable to use the last days, weeks, or months of a program's cycle (e.g., annual) for before or after measures; for example, using the first month of residency as the before phase and the last two months of residency as the after phase. This model proposes that one collects both quantitative and qualitative measures in each phase (before, during, and after) to assist the evaluator with both detecting unexpected results and providing a means for providing some understanding for why associations are observed. It shares features with the logic model derived above; unlike the logic model, the before, during, after model was designed for purposes of program evaluation.

By including baseline measures as controls for the learner at the outset of training, this model can provide more meaningful results than the goal and measure model described above. Further, by using the before, during, after approach, one can define consistency as a success outcome measure be it from year to year or across different geographic sites. This outcome measure (assessing for consistency) can be particularly helpful when instituting a change in the program to determine if there are negative consequences. With using consistency as success, one selects the variable of interest (site, year) as a unit of analysis for outcomes of interest.[31]

A strength of the before, during, after approach is that it reinforces the conception that the eventual product of an educational program depends on both the qualifications of trainees entering the program and the quality of the program itself. In addition to providing important baseline information on trainees, before measures can identify individual learner needs and areas for future curricular emphasis, and can address issues of patient safety as they relate to resident readiness to assume specific clinical responsibilities. Examples of robust, multifaceted assessments, structured in accordance with the ACGME/American Board of Medical Specialties (ABMS) competencies and milestones, have been described in the literature.[32,33]

The before, during, after model is related to the input, process, product model (or Donabedian's structure process, outcome model) from the quality assurance literature. A key difference is that the input, process, product model includes needed resources as the "inputs" but does not explicitly include baseline or before measures. In the context of this model, process measures refer to what we do with learners or what happens during the program (during measures), and products are outcome or after measures. The "process" or "during" measures as defined by this model, however, may include measures that we typically classify as learning and/or patient outcome measures (such as in-training examination performance for a second-year resident, or mean HbA1c levels on patients within a resident panel measured every 6 months during a resident's training). This being said, the before, during, after model does encourage the evaluator to list needed resources as well as consider unexpected outcomes to help inform the before, during, and after measures. An exercise to help educators who wish to use this model is provided in Appendix 18.1.

MRC Model for Complex Interventions

The Medical Research Council's guidance for developing and evaluating complex interventions extends beyond evaluation to offer comprehensive coverage of developing, piloting, implementing, evaluating, and reporting complex interventions to improve health.[12] It is intended to guide researchers in selecting the most appropriate evaluation methods for complex interventions, as well as to help stakeholders understand the methodological and practical limitations of various research approaches and consider their interpretations and decisions based on evaluation results in light of those limitations. Complex interventions, often encountered in healthcare delivery, public health, social policy development, and education, are characterized by the following.[12,34]

- There are several interacting and interdependent components in the intervention.
- It is difficult to standardize the design and delivery of the intervention.
- Flexibility is permitted in tailoring the intervention to different contexts.
- Local context impacts implementation of the intervention.
- Behaviors of those implementing the intervention are variable.
- Potential outcomes of the intervention are numerous and variable.
- Different groups or organizational levels are targeted by the intervention.

Taken together, these characteristics (consistent with the features of many medical education programs) pose significant methodologic and logistical challenges to evaluation of complex interventions, particularly in using standard experimental methods such as randomized controlled trials (RCTs).

TABLE 18.2 Experimental Alternatives to Randomized Controlled Trials for Evaluating Complex Interventions

Method	Rationale for Use	Basic Approach
Cluster randomized trials	Contamination of the control group by the intervention may lead to biased estimates of effect size.	Groups (year groups, classes, schools, residency programs) of individuals are randomly allocated to study or control interventions.
Stepped wedge designs	Practical or ethical objections exist to withholding intervention (e.g., evidence of effectiveness) or intervention is not available to the entire population at the same time.	Intervention is rolled out in phases to different individuals with randomization applied to phasing of the intervention.
Preference trials and randomized consent designs	Recipients of the intervention have strong preferences regarding the intervention.	Recipients are allocated based on preferences, or randomized before consent is obtained.
N-of-1 designs	Recipients are expected to vary in their response to the intervention, or the intervention may work via different mechanisms among recipients.	Recipients receive the intervention in randomized sequence; within and between recipient responses are investigated.

Modified from New framework on complex interventions to improve health, University of Glasgow, UK. For more detailed information, please see https://www.gla.ac.uk/schools/healthwellbeing/research/mrccsosocialandpublichealthsciencesunit/sharingourevidence/news/headline_813090_en.html.

In general, evaluators are encouraged to use the best available method(s) for any evaluation task they are undertaking to minimize bias and optimize generalizability.[35] From this perspective, randomized controlled studies comprise the best method to control for selection or other systematic bias impacting individuals participating in an intervention.[12,34] However, in practice there will exist any number of factors that limit choices regarding evaluation approaches. The MRC model provides a useful perspective on how to use experimental and quasiexperimental approaches when RCTs will not work for a given evaluation plan. Table 18.2 outlines several experimental designs that may be considered depending on the context and appropriateness of using experimental approaches.[12]

The MRC guidance stipulates that there may be times when the randomization requirement for experimental or quasiexperimental methods may be untenable for ethical or political reasons.[12] In this context the "best available" methods may not be the best choice from a theoretical or statistical strength perspective.[34] Factors to consider in deciding on the best method include the timing and size of the expected outcomes. Outcomes that are very large and occur immediately after an intervention (e.g., an educational intervention available to all staff of an accountable care organization coupled with a reminder in the electronic health record results in a 75% increase in colonoscopy requests for all eligible patients within 3 months for staff who completed the intervention) may not be as susceptible to selection bias; therefore randomization may not be necessary and observational approaches with adjustment for confounding variables may be adequate. In addition, alternative approaches to randomization may be appropriate if there is a low likelihood of selection bias, there are ethical or practical reasons for not using experimental methods (such as interventions that are known to be effective or are already in widespread use), the costs for standardized, experimental methods are prohibitive, or selected outcomes are infrequent and not likely to identify used standard experimental approaches.[12,34]

Like other models, the approach outlined by the MRC realizes that determining whether the complex intervention works provides only a partial answer. Understanding whether the intervention will work in other settings and the mechanisms underlying its impact, as well as how different individuals and groups may experience the intervention and have different outcomes, is equally important.[12] The MRC model suggests that "process evaluation" is a valuable complement to outcomes evaluation in detecting variability in implementation of the intervention, identifying contextual factors, and elucidating various causal mechanisms that help explain variation in recipient outcomes.[12,34] The MRC also provides recommendations (Fig. 18.3A and B) for how to plan, design, conduct, and report a process evaluation, highlighting several considerations for building expertise of the evaluation team, clarifying any assumptions of causality, ensuring fidelity of methodology and analysis, and disseminating to appropriate and relevant stakeholders.[36] Interpretation of process evaluation results is linked to intervention outcomes and will help evaluators understand why the intervention led to the identified outcomes and how others may implement it in different contexts.[12,37]

A useful approach espoused by the MRC involves a phased approach to program development and evaluation that utilizes feasibility and pilot studies to focus on key elements, questions, or concerns regarding the complex intervention.[12] Resolution of key questions or uncertainties via pilot studies will allow evaluators to move on to larger-scale exploratory studies and then to more comprehensive evaluation plans in a better informed manner.[34] One or more smaller-scale pilot studies may be particularly useful when there is uncertainty about development, implementation, or

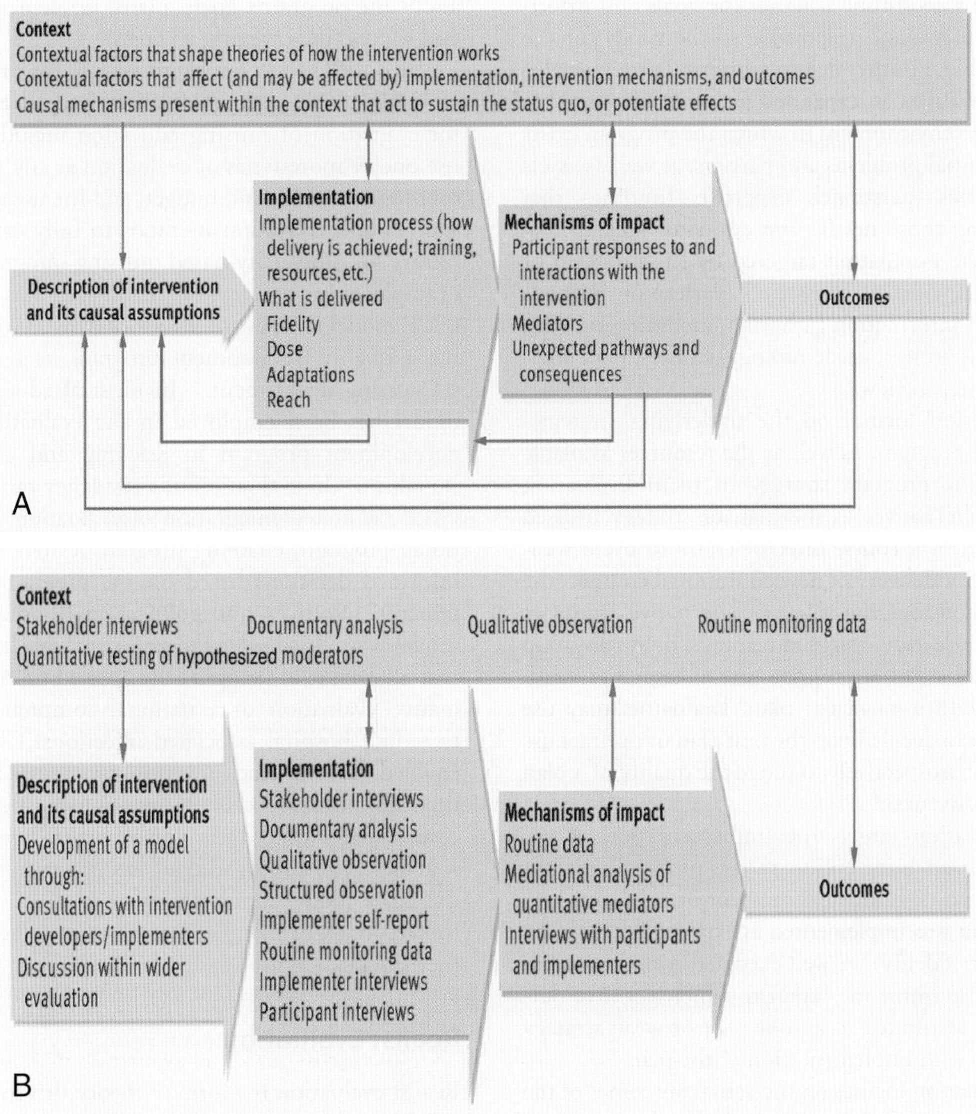

• **Fig. 18.3** (A) Key functions of process evaluation and the relations among them, and commonly used data collection and analysis models for process evaluation. (B) Commonly used data collection and analysis models for process evaluation. (A and B from Moore GF, Audrey S, Barker M, et al. (2015). Process evaluation of complex interventions: Medical Research Council guidance. *BMJ*. 2015;350:h1258.)

acceptance of elements of the intervention or to inform calculations of sample size, response rates, or effect size. Both qualitative and quantitative methods (recipient interviews regarding their understanding of how to engage with the intervention, attendance sheets to gauge recipient participation in intervention activities) may be used to identify barriers to implementation and numerical estimates for subsequent large-scale evaluation studies.[12]

CIPP

The CIPP model was developed related to evolving evaluation and accountability requirements in response to federal programs for reforming education. It was felt that traditional approaches to evaluation using experimental design and objectives-based methods, including the use of standardized achievement tests, were limited in their ability to meet schools' needs. The CIPP model allowed for comprehensive evaluation of educational programs that existed within complex and dynamic real-world conditions. CIPP is an acronym that stands for context, input, process, and product, which are the different types of evaluation used in the model; each could be done independently or combined in various ways depending on evaluator needs and goals. Since its original application the CIPP model has been successfully applied to evaluation of a wide range of disciplines, service areas, programs, and organizations.[8]

In the CIPP model, context evaluation focuses on the needs for the program, or for changes or improvements to the program. Context evaluation can be used to define program goals and priorities to ensure that they address the specific needs or problems of interest, or more retrospectively to determine whether the goals and priorities were appropriate and responsive to the needs for the program or problem it intended to address. Context evaluation can be viewed as an expanded needs assessment that also evaluates the environment in which the program exists to identify potential problems and barriers, as well as assets and opportunities (personnel, expertise, funding) that facilitate meeting those needs. The evaluator seeks information about the population targeted by the program or intervention and which it operates. A variety of methods may be useful in information gathering, including surveys, interviews, focus groups, epidemiologic studies, data analysis, and document review.[8]

Input evaluation focuses on the underlying strategies or plans for the program, as well as the resources available to implement the program strategy or plan. Evaluation may focus on alternatives to the plan or strategy utilized by program (e.g., if a course director chose to use a web-based approach for delivery of new educational content, the evaluator may consider the value of alternative strategies such as a didactic lecture, assigned readings, or small-group activities), as well as the appropriate use of resources (staff, finances, etc.) with a particular plan. Evaluators may use input evaluation to decide upon the best plan or optimal use of resources, or retrospectively to judge the quality of a plan and its cost-effectiveness.[8]

Process evaluation targets the implementation of the program plan or an intervention to the program, including the relevant costs. Evaluators monitor or assess whether the program plan was implemented as expected or required (implementation fidelity). A well-executed process evaluation may help determine the extent to which negative outcomes could be attributed to a poor plan or weak strategy versus problems with implementation of the plan.[8]

Product evaluation focuses on the actual outcomes of the program or changes to the program, including both positive and negative changes, as well as intended and unintended outcomes. Product evaluation addresses the extent to which the goals of the program are being met by targeting a range of short- and longer-term outcomes.[8]

Although the CIPP model focuses on improvement, informing planning and implementation of programs or changes to programs, it may also be applied retrospectively in a summative manner to meet various stakeholder needs.[8] From a formative perspective the CIPP model seeks to answer what needs to be done in terms of planning (context), whether the plan is the right one (input), and whether it is being executed appropriately (process). Questions answered by a summative process focus on whether the goal addresses identified needs (context), whether the plan or strategy was properly designed (input), whether the plan or strategy was effectively implemented (process), and whether the plan or strategy was successful in meeting its goals (product).[8] Essentially, the formative role of CIPP evaluation types is to provide guidance in developing or modifying goals, plans, and implementation activities, whereas the summative role involves making judgments about the program's goals, plans, implementation process, and success in achieving its goals.[8]

The CIPP model has been proposed as a model for application in nursing education. Perceived advantages of CIPP for evaluation of nursing education include the ability to use one or more types of evaluation at any time depending on program needs and budget, and the use of multiple data sources and collection methods to fully capture the complexity of university-based nursing programs.[38] Another example of an application in nursing was the use of the CIPP model to evaluate the process involved in implementing a quality development program in a teaching hospital nursing department.[39] In medical education the CIPP model has been employed in the evaluation of a faculty development program in teaching and assessing professionalism.[40] In evaluation of a residency program the use of CIPP facilitated integration of evaluation into the educational program, enabling program leaders to make better-informed decisions based on the program's unique components, resources, and political environment.[41] The CIPP model was felt to offer the structured yet flexible approach that allowed it to be optimally applied to longitudinal, formative evaluation of a national comprehensive program to reduce hospital associated infections. CIPP users felt it enabled them to track multiple program components over time, monitor the evolving relationship between program components, and continuously gather data from multiple sources.[42] The authors did advise, however, that those using the CIPP model should be aware of the resources required to keep track of many components and the ways in which they interact.

Realist Evaluation

Realist evaluation is a form of theory-driven evaluation that emphasizes the context and processes that impact program outcomes, rather than just the program outcomes, in seeking a deeper explanation regarding how complex programs work.[9] Evaluators using a realist approach are less interested in simply determining whether the program works but are explicitly focused on explaining "what works for whom in what circumstances and in what respects, and how".[43] Implicit in this approach is the assumption that interventions or programs that are implemented in different locations or contexts do not have the same effect at all locations, on all participants, and consistently over time. Programs or interventions are developed and implemented in social systems—which they may, in fact, intend to change—and the program and its impact on participants are affected by those social systems in which they exist. Local culture and relationships, as well as existing infrastructure, policies, and resources, will influence program processes and outcomes. Furthermore, the attitudes and abilities of program participants, as well as those leading and executing program activities, will have an effect on its outputs and outcomes.[43]

From a realist perspective, programs are viewed as complex interventions within an evolving social milieu. Similar to the MRC model described above, Pawson describes characteristics of complex interventions as described by the acronym VICTORE[44]:

- **V**olitions: participants can and often do act on their own volitions. This may affect how programs respond to the intervention.
- **I**mplementation: prone to inconsistency and unintended consequences.
- **C**ontexts: circumstances in which the program is implemented will vary.
- **T**ime: program interventions occur over time.
- **O**utcomes: may vary, including in how they are measured or interpreted.
- **R**ivalry: new interventions may compete or conflict with other programs or policies.
- **E**mergence: effects of the intervention, including adaptations to it, and unexpected consequences will emerge.

Four concepts related to this perspective are put forth to help explain how a program works and allow reflection on any underlying theory on which the program is based: mechanism, context, outcome-pattern, and context-mechanism-outcome pattern configuration.[43]

Mechanism refers to how an intervention or a programmatic component leads to change or a specific outcome, and thus helps explain why a program is successful or fails in meeting its goals. Mechanisms are not the same as program components but may be understood as processes, relationships, or other intangible factors that directly relate to how program resources and activities are received, interpreted, and acted upon by participants to lead to specific program outcomes.[13] They may not be directly visible but can be inferred from observable data showing their impact. Also, the impact of a specific mechanisms is not fixed or constant but is substantially dependent on the context in which it operates.[9,13,45] Generally speaking, a particular intervention may work through multiple possible mechanisms. For example, a web-based intervention designed to help improve population health management may impact learner interest and change because the learner is interested in the technology-based learning format used (mechanism 1), while other participants may be motivated to learn the content because of an emerging interest in public health (mechanism 2), because of an upcoming elective in health services research (mechanism 3), or because it includes an assessment that will impact their grade (mechanism 4).

Context includes the conditions during implementation and conduct of the program that have an effect on how the mechanisms operate.[43] Like individual mechanisms, context can have a positive or negative impact on program activities and outcomes. Contextual factors include the location of the program, as well as its culture, demographics of stakeholders and participants and their relationships, economic conditions, technology, and infrastructure. In medical education programs, contextual factors may have an important impact on the motivation and abilities of both faculty and learners in their respective roles. Elucidating the impact of context on a particular intervention is important in understanding its generalizable, causal pathways and in successfully replicating the intervention in the future and in other settings.[9]

Contributing mechanisms and context vary across programs and over time in individual programs in such a way that the program outcomes are not linear or univariate. Outcome patterns are the end result of the program or intervention as they define the impact of the different mechanisms that are activated within programs and dynamic contextual features on different participant groups.[43] The pattern of outcomes will reflect ultimate differences in participants based on personal, geographic, demographic, temporal, and implementation-related factors. Consequently, multiple evaluation methods will need to be applied to measure those various outputs and outcomes of the program. Such methods will likely include a range of qualitative and quantitative approaches to address both intended and unintended consequences.[43]

Engaging in realist evaluation requires evaluators to develop, test, and refine theories as to why and/or how programs work and achieve specific outcome patterns. Realist evaluators engage in an iterative process that involves observation and investigation of program process and outcomes, constructing theories or explanations regarding how the program works, with such explanations constantly compared against emerging data and explanations revised and enhanced.[11] However, there is no standardized approach, or predefined steps, to conducting realist evaluation and those who have deployed realist methods have utilized different tactics.[13] A commonly used approach to realist evaluation involves developing models to explain program outcomes that facilitate consideration of the potential mechanisms in play, the context in which the intervention is implemented or the program is executed, and how different participant groups may be impacted to cause different outcomes (i.e., patterns of outcomes). These models consist of different context-mechanism-outcome (CMO) pattern configurations that include variations in context and mechanisms and how they may be aligned to explain the range of outcomes.[43] Generation of a CMO configuration provides a useful output of realist evaluation upon which mechanisms, contexts, and outcomes can be closely examined, subsequent theory tested, and other analyses initiated.[46,47] Explanation of the relationships between the three elements within the CMO configurations, through generation of theory propositions, is an important and common goal of realist evaluation.[13,48] Evaluation approaches involve data gathering in support of theories or propositions about the relationship and connections between potential mechanisms, context, and outcome patterns within the CMO configurations. Evaluation results based on the CMO configuration inform revision and refinement of the initial and evolving theories and propositions about how programs achieve specific outcome patterns.[9] Fig. 18.4 demonstrates a potential stepwise process for conducting realist evaluation that is based on separate applications in medical education program evaluation.

The realist evaluation process involves thinking about the program theories that could be tested and then testing

Step 1: Initial Data Gathering

Interview program leaders to understand program goals, resources, activities and outputs, the nature of participant groups (learners, faculty, stakeholders), and contexts and setting in which it will be implemented.

Review relevant documents and literature to supplement information about how the program is expected to work and likely outcomes.

↓

Step 2: Develop a Context-Mechanism-Outcome (CMO) Configuration

Develop an initial CMO configuration to illustrate potential relationships between the different contexts in which the program may be implemented, presumed mechanisms that might explain program outcomes, and expected or actual outcomes of the program (depending upon whether one is conducting a prospective realist evaluation or retrospective or concurrent realist review).

↓

Step 3: Generate tentative explanations (theories, mini-theories, hypothesis, propositions) regarding how program context and mechanism lead to program outcome patterns

Initial explanations should hypothesize how program mechanisms and contexts result in intended or observed outcome patterns (M + C = O)

The primary goal during this step is to generate testable explanations that hypothesize how the program works (*explanations* is chosen here as the operative concept to broadly encompass the range of concepts—theories, mini-theories, middle-range theories, hypothesis, and propositions—that are applied inconsistently and occasionally in a conflicting manner in the emerging literature on realist evaluation in education).

↓

Step 4: Gather data to test the explanations regarding the C + M = O configurations

Qualitative approaches (interviews, focus groups, observational methods, document review, etc.) are used to further understand the potential operative mechanisms and contextual features that impact outcome patterns and also to complement quantitative approaches to outcome measurement (e.g., former participant interviews regarding satisfaction with the program, their learning outcomes, and unintended outcomes of the program).

Quantitative approaches primarily focusing on program outcome to include learner or participant outcomes (self-assessment surveys, licensure or credentialing actions, board scores, program director or employer ratings), patient outcomes, and so forth.

↓

Step 5: Revise and refine CMO configurations and explanations

Data derived from qualitative and quantitative methods inform the accuracy of initial CMO configurations (hypotheses regarding the relationships between context, mechanisms, and outcome patterns) and explanations regarding how they are related in regard to program results.

Steps 2 through 5 are repeated as necessary in achieving program evaluation goals

• **Fig. 18.4** Potential steps of a realist evaluation cycle. (Modified from Salter KL, Kothari A. Using realist evaluation to open the black box of knowledge translation: a state-of-the-art review. *Implement Sci*. 2014;9:115; and Blamey A, Mackenzie M. Theories of change and realistic evaluation. *Evaluation*. 2007;13:439-455.)

various theory-based propositions or hypotheses as to how various mechanisms and contextual variables yield specific program outcomes.[13] As above, a goal of realist evaluation is to refine knowledge and understanding about which mechanisms are activated for which participants and what contextual factors influenced how those mechanisms led to observed changes in participants.[9] What potential mechanisms or contextual variables, or changes to these variables, did or could result in changes in outcome patterns across program participants? The theories could be developed prospectively to understand how planned changes to a program may impact outcomes among its participants and therefore predict the measures that will be necessary to identify outcome patterns. Alternatively, theories could be considered retrospectively to facilitate and drive efforts to understand why interventions or program changes led to different outcomes in selected locations, programs, or within different demographic groups. Hypotheses resulting from theories about program outcomes are framed within the CMO configuration models to fully understand the range of variables impacting outcome patterns.[43] What potential process (mechanism) changes and contextual variables need to be modified to affect a desired change in outcomes or what possible mechanism-related or contextual factor led to the differences in outcome patterns noted?

Realist evaluation has been used in many fields in which complex interventions are deployed, and there is growing experience with its use in healthcare and medical education programming. Examples depicting the application of realist methods in healthcare and medical education include evaluation of a new model of emergency department–based mental health nursing practice[9]; interventions to enhance knowledge translation in clinical practice[13]; factors that engage residents in institutional quality improvement curricula[47]; mechanisms supporting assessment of interpersonal skills[46]; features of internet-based medical education that impact learner satisfaction and outcomes[17]; the effectiveness of faculty development activities[49]; and the effectiveness of a quality improvement program in primary care.[48]

A strength of realist evaluation, like the before, during, after approach, is that it promotes investigation, understanding, and explanation of the important processes, structures, contextual variables, and other (often unanticipated or unintended) factors that impact program outcomes. However, because realist evaluation necessarily involves multiple methods and iterative approaches to developing and refining theories, hypotheses, and knowledge about programs, it may time consuming and resource intensive. In addition, realist evaluation can be intellectually challenging in that no guidance or predefined rules exist to inform its conduct, and it also can be difficult to decide upon and differentiate between mechanisms and contextual variables as well as to formulate initial CMO configurations.[13]

While various program evaluation models are shared here, others exist (RE-AIM, Utilization-Focused Evaluation, Consolidated Framework for Implementation Research, etc.) and may more accurately and appropriately serve a program's intentions, mission, or context. Consultation with an expert in program evaluation may be worthwhile to help determine the best and most relevant program evaluation model to follow.

Constructing an Evaluation Program

It is important to plan carefully in implementing an evaluation plan for an educational program. Thoughtful consideration should focus on what is to be assessed, how it is to be measured, and how results will be used to inform program improvement. Although it will be challenging to design the perfect program evaluation scheme, efforts spent up front to balance the potential competing interests of stakeholder needs, methodological requirements, and resource constraints are likely to decrease the number of surprises and obstacles in moving forward. Evaluators should consider a range of issues in making decision about how to proceed with program evaluation: the distribution of process and structure and/or outcome measures; the use of qualitative and/or quantitative methods; employment of internal and/or external methods and evaluators; measuring short-term (current/intermediate) and/or longer-term outcomes; and allocation of resources.[50]

Constructing a rigorous evaluation program requires a team. In addition to thoughtful consideration of the financial, space, supplies (e.g., computer software), and time needs for conducting evaluation, one should also pay close attention to forming the right team to plan and implement the evaluation. Evaluators should engage individuals with a variety of perspectives and expertise to not only enhance the capabilities of the group but also prevent groupthink that has been described in the group decision-making literature. The team also needs to have a clear vision of what success looks like (outcomes). This may entail combining one or more of the models described above or even creating new models. It is critical that the program evaluation efforts are fit for the program's purposes.

Evaluators should consider the timing of conducting program evaluation. Some aspects of program evaluation are completed on at least an annual basis (such as program director, employer, or graduate surveys) as our learners matriculate and graduate each year and this is an expectation of accreditation bodies. We would recommend, however, that one considers more frequent evaluation with repeating courses, clerkships, or residency rotation (when this is the evaluation unit of analysis) and even more often when starting a new program. During the beginning of a new program the likelihood of important unexpected findings is increased, as such evaluations are the first cycle(s) of evaluation for the program. One means to assist this process is to define flags or early warning signs for individual measures that one collects in their program evaluation efforts. The detection of one or more such flags would lead to an earlier cycle of repeating program evaluation than usual. Accreditation bodies have lists of common program citations to consider including in a program evaluation. Addressing these reasons for citation explicitly in your evaluation plan can help with one's program evaluation efforts.

The following description of the measures and methods used in evaluation programs and the types of information collected emphasize the importance of thoughtful consideration and deliberate planning regarding how various forms of data will be used in supporting evaluation. Attention should be focused on how data will be systematically collected; when and where they will be collected; the sources of the data; how they will be stored, analyzed, and protected; and how they will be used to inform improvement or judgments about the program.[51] Ideally, program leaders should develop a database that includes detailed information about the institution, curriculum, instructional, and assessment methods, faculty, and learners to enable comprehensive evaluation of the program. Experts in medical education research suggest that evaluators should adopt an epidemiologic approach to program evaluation that is facilitated by a comprehensive relational database of program elements.[52,53] Such a database supports conducting high-quality observational (cross-sectional, cohort, case-control, and longitudinal studies) and experimental (RCT and other randomized designs) studies necessary to support systematic and informative evaluation, and contribute to developing an evidence-based body of literature around effective medical education and assessment.[52] There are a number of databases that evaluators can access to close the loop in obtaining important outcomes information on program graduates

TABLE 18.3 Sources of Information Available for Potential Evaluations of Program Process and Outcomes

Organization	Source of Information
Association of American Medical Colleges	American Medical School Application Service data
	Matriculating student questionnaire
	Graduation questionnaire
	Faculty roster
	Medical college admissions test scores
Association of American Medical Colleges/American Medical Association	National Graduate Medical Education census
American Board of Medical Specialties	Board certification status
American Medical Association	Physician master file
Centers for Medicare & Medicaid Services	Medicare claims data
Federation of State Medical Boards	State medical board action database
	Federation credential verification service
National Board of Medical Examiners	United States Medical Licensing Examination pass/fail results and scores
	Subject examination scores

Note: In addition, insurers, healthcare systems and plans, state health departments, and national accreditation agencies may have data on other physician and patient outcomes.

Modified from Cook DA, Andriole DA, Durning SJ, Roberts NK, Triola MM. Longitudinal research databases in medical education: facilitating the study of educational outcomes over time and across institutions. *Acad Med*. 2010;85:1340-1346.

(Table 18.3).[53] Collaboration across programs and institutions to achieve larger sample sizes, include data across the continuum of education and practice, and capture a broader range of contextual factors will contribute to more robust research projects and results and contribute more significantly to the medical education evidence base.[52,53]

Define Evaluation Goals

An important first step in developing the evaluation plan is to identify the goals and objectives of the evaluation. What important questions is the evaluation intended to answer? The following questions might serve as a baseline to begin to elucidate the evaluation plan (adapted from[7]:

1. What do you want your program, project, intervention, etc., to accomplish?
2. How will you know if you have accomplished your goals?
3. What activities and processes will you put in place to accomplish your goals?
4. What factors might help or hinder your ability to accomplish your goals?
5. How will you determine the effect of these factors on your ability to accomplish your goals?
6. What will you want to tell others (such as funders, adopters, and other stakeholders) who are interested in your program, project, or intervention?

Engage Stakeholders

Multiple parties have a stake in undergraduate and graduate medical educational programs and therefore should have the opportunity to shape and participate in processes that measure the quality of such programs.[54] Beyond the immediate evaluation team, anyone who contributes to, influences or is influenced by the program, or is responsible for program performance should be afforded the opportunity to contribute to evaluation planning and administration.[2,28] Those who are recipients of the program graduates have an important perspective to contribute to program planning and change. Ideally, program evaluation should include both internal and external parties. External evaluators, such as educational leaders from another institution, may bring more objectivity and contribute unique or additional insights or perspectives to the evaluation process.[2] It is good to have both complementary and competing views present to ensure a variety of perspectives are heard.[28]

Engaging the learners themselves in the evaluation process is important as well. Students and residents have expectations regarding the quality of their educational experience and are appropriately qualified to provide feedback on specific program performance elements. The faculty who devote time and effort to educational programs deserve to participate in and benefit from program performance assessment. Certainly, it is important to make sure that all stakeholders are provided with feedback from the program evaluation process, particularly those who have participated in providing information as well as those who are the subject of assessment data.[55] This notion informs *coproduction*, or an engagement of all stakeholders, whether they be patients, providers, or the healthcare system, in "both explicit and implicit partnerships" throughout the evaluation process that can improve the overall health and well-being of said stakeholders.[56] Those providing assessment data and opinions regarding program performance need to know that their efforts are appreciated and incorporated into program improvement activities.[57]

There are a number of other benefits from engaging various stakeholders in program evaluation.[28] Involvement in program planning and evaluation promotes ownership and commitment and may encourage buy-in to the program and action based on evaluation results. Involving recipients of an educational intervention in the evaluation process will promote perceptions of fairness and may enhance their support of and participation in the intervention.[12] Furthermore, access to a broad range of perspectives and expertise can only strength the deliberative process of program planning, implementation, and evaluation.[28]

Design and Methods

Borrowing From Various Methods

We described above the most commonly used models for evaluating health professions education programs. In general, a sound, comprehensive evaluation plan will benefit from adoption of elements from more than one model to address the full range of processes and outcomes that are relevant to making judgments about a program's quality. The various models, like conceptual frameworks, are arguably a light and a lens. The structure, measures (described in more detail below), and expected associations can serve as a light. Each model also has assumptions (implicit or explicit) underlying its use, and thus choosing a model at the exclusion of others can be like a magnifying glass where one can "miss" key information for improving the program.

Several of the models described above will include qualitative and quantitative methods to thoroughly test theories about how programs work and measure various program elements. Blending methods from different evaluation models can help compensate for the relative gaps or weakness of each and produce findings that complement or inform each other.[9,12,34] Generally speaking, initial evaluation approaches with these models may be more qualitative in nature; for example, using interviews with program leaders and participants, observational methods, document analysis, and literature reviews to create initial theories regarding how the program functions to achieve is outcomes.[13] Many times, the evaluation process will lead to inconclusive or mixed results, showing partial, variable, or even unanticipated results; the overarching goal of the evaluator may not be to prove whether the program works, but to make sense of evaluation findings in regard to how it works and the contextual factors that explain different outcomes, and to develop theories regarding how they are related.[43,45] Iterative cycles may be required, including rethinking, through reflection and iterative discussion, program theories, adjustments of related hypotheses, changes in research design, and/or modifications or additions to hypotheses and data-gathering approaches.[17] The end result of the evaluation process will not necessarily be a pass/fail decision regarding the program but provisional conclusions with further understanding regarding how and why the program works and guidance regarding the best ways to improve the program and make it more effective.[43]

Use of Quantitative and Qualitative Methods

As briefly discussed above in relation to evaluation models, there is value in using both quantitative and qualitative methods in a complementary manner to best meet program evaluation needs. Quantitative methods such as aggregated data from various written examinations, objective structured clinical examinations (OSCEs), or medical record audits are generally considered superior in providing high-quality feedback to educational leaders; however, qualitative techniques such as focus groups, individual discussion and interviews, and faculty and trainee observation play a useful role in selected aspects of program evaluation.[50] Quantitative methods are typically less labor intensive in data collection and analysis and provide a level of external objectivity that is appreciated by some stakeholders. For example, quantitative outcomes data may be required by accreditation bodies and can provide meaningful benchmarks for program success. Quantitative methods are obviously the first choice when random samples of data or large data sets are readily available for analysis, or when certain confounding variables can be easily controlled to better determine cause-and-effect relationships. However, a heavy focus on outcomes measurement using quantitative methods may overlook key contextual factors that impact outcomes and lead to an impression of neutrality that may not adequately capture the tensions and values that are in play in planning and changing educational programs.[7,13] Research methods that exclude or try to control for contextual and process variables may limit one's ability to understand how programs yield their specific outcomes and why differences in outcomes may be seen among different participant groups over time or within programs that introduced the same intervention.[45] Also, application of quantitative approaches is less desirable if the available outcomes measurements do not align with stakeholders' needs or if the methods or possible outcomes cannot be adapted or made relevant to the needs or contexts to local programs and stakeholder groups.[16]

Qualitative methods are often a better choice for analyzing complex or evolving phenomena, or investigating a program feature (or a limited number of factors) in great depth. Qualitative methods are often needed to explain the how and why of the what: how variability among context, resource, participant, and implementation factors impacts outcome. Qualitative data are valuable when quantitative methods and variables don't meet local program and stakeholder needs and when personal experience is an important outcome. Qualitative techniques are particularly useful when there is some uncertainty about what quantitative measures to select and when it is anticipated that new insights may shape continuing evolution in program development.[50] Qualitative data are also important as programs are "living" entities with a number of stakeholders, microsystems, resources, and so forth that interact in a nonlinear fashion, and thus our standard quantitative measures and analysis may not provide a complete picture of what is happening in the program. Qualitative approaches may allow for more timely collection of data to identify unexpected problems or consequences to inform course correction before serious damage is done, and provide educational leaders a mechanism for continuous communication with learners, faculty, and other stakeholders, thus encouraging stakeholder buy-in and input into evolving program changes. Qualitative approaches may be more time and labor intensive than quantitative methods, may not yield definitive answers regarding specific hypotheses, and may yield results that are perceived as less credible to important stakeholders. Lastly, qualitative methods may fall short of meeting broader stakeholder needs when local program context and/or activities are not generalizable to other programs.[16]

Mixed-method approaches to combining quantitative and qualitative methods are desirable as they give evaluators more flexibility in meeting program evaluation needs, and they help lead to stronger conclusions when narrative information or participant perspectives complement quantitative results and when numerical data add detail or precision to more qualitative, theory-based explanations.[16] Mixed-method approaches allow for a broader range of solutions to determining the effectiveness of a given program and identifying areas where it can be improved. Inclusion of both qualitative and quantitative methods, and addressing the strengths and weakness of individual methods in considering the overall evaluation plan, should help optimize the evaluator's ability to capture the complexities and richness of the project or program. In fact, effective use of mixed methods allows triangulation of results across methods that help confirm, complement, or even support more sophisticated interpretation of program processes and outcomes.[10] Mixed methods approaches also enable evaluators to capture the multidimensional characteristics of most educational programs.[9] Qualitative methods (such as interviews, focus groups, and observation) are particularly helpful in understanding the context of the project or program and help explain the achievement of specific outcomes.[7] On the other hand, engaging in multiple methods may tax the resources and abilities of many evaluators and may be substantially more labor intensive, expensive, and time consuming.[16] As an example, mixed methods were recently used to evaluate a program intended to enhance the physician workforce to improve the healthcare of underserved populations. Quantitative data regarding medical student demographics were enriched by qualitative information (focus groups) regarding pertinent learner experiences and surveys that collected perspectives from key stakeholder groups who were impacted by the program.[58]

Measures

Structure and Process Measures

A current emphasis in program evaluation is on measuring the important or expected outcomes of an educational program or intervention.[51] However, while it is appropriate to emphasize educational and clinical outcome measures in evaluating the quality of the educational experience and informing program improvement, it is also important to understand that program quality can be determined by evaluating program structure and processes, including the elements of the curriculum, comprehensiveness and credibility of the instructional and assessment methods, number and involvement of faculty, and number and kind of patients encountered.[2,55] Evaluation of structure and processes focuses on the effectiveness of the individual activities and materials used within the program, what actually happens within the program, and the extent it reflects the goals of the program.[6] The value of obtaining process and structural information is underscored by the commonly encountered variability in faculty teaching, quality of instructional materials, number and quality of patient encounters during clinical rotations, course and rotation length and intensity, number and ability of colearners, supporting infrastructure, and influence of the informal or hidden curriculum.[59]

Some outcome measures may have uncertain validity as measures of program quality, whereas process measures may add value in predicting specific outcomes.[2] For example, patient volume is an indicator of subsequent learning outcomes such as performance on board certification examinations.[60] Unless some understanding of a program's structure and processes exists, it may be difficult to explain or respond to outcomes data to effect program improvement. Process measures are essential in explaining how or why certain outcomes are obtained[2] and thus are instrumental in identifying where improvement efforts should be targeted in response to specific outcomes.[61] Here, qualitative measures may be more likely than quantitative methods to identify reasons for various outcomes.[2] For example, a negative outcome result may be due to flaws in the design of a particular curricular innovation or may be due to problems in the way it was implemented (e.g., faculty or trainees were not properly oriented prior to introduction); one cannot interpret and properly act upon the outcome without some insights into the relevant processes.[50]

The array of assessment methods and their use within an educational program to provide feedback to learners and inform judgments about their progress comprise structure and process measures. Evaluation should include review of the assessment program itself. Periodic review and critical analysis of assessment approaches is necessary to ensure that assessments are being used properly, in a manner that is congruent with the objectives and curriculum of the educational program and relevant to the total learning experience of the trainee.[62] At the very least, education program leaders should periodically ask themselves a series of questions about individual tools and the entire program (including those questions pertinent to the validity argument described in Chapter 2). To begin, they should question whether the assessment content is appropriate. Are the cases selected for a local OSCE targeting the important cases and tasks? Is the distribution of real patient encounters selected for observation sensible given overall programmatic goals? One must avoid uneven distribution of observations related to the location, preferences, or expertise of core faculty members. Are there an adequate number of faculty observers participating in trainee evaluation? Research suggests that a larger number of raters observing fewer patient encounters each produces a more defensible result than fewer raters observing a larger number of encounters.[63]

Evaluators should compare the results of individual assessments within or across programs to make sure the results make sense. It is reasonable to expect that global ratings, OSCE results, and In-Training Exam (ITE) scores may not correlate as they are measuring different aspects of competence. However, if the results of local multiple-choice examinations are very different from National Board of Medical Examiners (NBME) Subject Examination or ITE results, one should question the purpose and assumptions underlying the local examination as well as its quality. Alternatively, program curricula may not be aligned with national priorities, as reflected by Subject Examination or ITE content.

It is useful to consider the overall performance of a particular examination related to constructs being assessed; that is, whether it is producing results that are consistent with beliefs about the competence being measured and knowledge about the trainees being evaluated. Recognizing that significant variability may exist between trainees at a given level, overall it is reasonable to expect that most assessments will yield better results/higher scores for more advanced or experienced trainees. Beyond the internal assessment discussed here, additional information about the quality of a local assessment program can and should be obtained via periodic review by external parties, either through consultation or occurring as part of formal internal review and external accreditation processes. Lastly, as discussed below, it is important to consider the future performance of graduates as another means of studying the validity of current assessment approaches.[62]

The composition of faculty and faculty development efforts is a core structural measure for educational programs and faculty engagement, and the quality of teaching and assessment is an important process measure. The importance of assaying faculty performance is underscored by research associating the quality of clinical teaching with learner outcomes, including grades/ratings, specialty choice, and examination scores.[59,64] Faculty may be evaluated through various learner or peer surveys or via direct observation of faculty performance by peers or program leaders.[59,65]

Institutional recognition of faculty support of educational programs provides a measure of program success in instilling professional values related to our responsibility to engage in the education and assessment of colleagues and professionals in training, and should be considered a program process measure. As acknowledgment of grant support and research productivity in basic or clinical science results in faculty rewards such as promotion or other forms of recognition, so too should scholarly activity in medical education be rewarded. Do institutions embrace teaching as a valued community (professional) activity? There should be recognition of the diverse nature of scholarship in medical education, ranging from prospective research on teaching and assessment methodology to interpretation and application of existing knowledge into the development of educational programs and teaching approaches.[66]

Outcome Measures

While assessment of structure and processes contributes important information, the ultimate end product of the medical educational process is the learner's achievement of clinical competence and performance in the context of patient care, and in the end the most valuable and informative feedback will be based on measuring educational outcomes.[67] In measuring the efficacy of educational programs, outcomes may be defined from the perspective of the learner and/or from the perspective of the patients or communities they serve.[68] Learner outcomes include measures of competence and performance as reflected by incremental achievement in knowledge, skills, or attitudinal domains; clinical or patient outcomes include measures of the quality of care provided to individual patients or populations of patients.[3,68] Measuring educational or clinical outcomes may present greater methodologic and logistical challenges than evaluation of program structure and processes. It is important to identify which outcomes are reasonable to measure. Although long-term outcomes may be desirable to evaluate, it may not be feasible to do so, and focusing on more immediate or intermediate outcomes may be more helpful in developing a causal link between outcomes and program characteristics and activities.[28] However, in general, evaluator efforts are best applied to focusing on meaningful outcomes that may be hard to measure than focusing on outcomes that are easier to obtain but are less important to key stakeholders.[7]

Increasing adoption of competency-based medical education (CBME) frameworks across the educational continuum furthers the work of program evaluation through their focus on educational outcomes and the requirement for multifaceted assessment programs.[69] Application of a variety of high-quality assessment methods in learner assessment—such as ITEs and NBME Subject Examinations, direct observation tools such as the mini clinical evaluation exercise (mini-CEX), standardized patients (SPs), and other simulation-based methods, chart audits, and multisource feedback—contributes to a robust set of aggregated data that could be used in program evaluation (see Table 18.4). The increasing interest in rigorous workplace-based assessment (WBA) will contribute to more clinically relevant educational outcomes including patient outcomes. National organizations, such as the Association of American Medical Colleges (AAMC) in promoting the development of core EPAs for entering residencies, and the ACGME in requiring resident demonstration of key milestones during residency, are key drivers in moving this field forward.[70,71] Data generated from EPA- or milestones-based assessment

TABLE 18.4 Selected Methods for Assessing the ACGME/ABMS General Competencies Across the Continuum of Education and Practice

Competency	Undergraduate Medical Education	Graduate Medical Education	Continuing Professional Development/Clinical Practice
Medical Knowledge	Locally developed exams NBME subject exams USMLE Step 1 and Step 2 CK	Locally developed exams USMLE Step 3 In-training exams	Board certification exams Maintenance of certification exams Clinical question logs Self-assessment exams
Interpersonal and Communication Skills	Direct observation SP/OSCE Global ratings 360 evaluation Portfolio USMLE Step 2 CS	Direct observation SP/OSCE Global ratings 360 evaluation Portfolio Multisource feedback Unannounced SPs Employer survey	Direct observation SP/OSCE 360 evaluation Portfolio Multisource feedback Unannounced SPs Patient survey Global ratings Employer survey
Professionalism	Direct observation SP/OSCE Multisource feedback Portfolio	Direct observation SP/OSCE Multisource feedback Portfolio Survey Employer survey	Direct observation Multisource feedback Licensing/credentialing actions Unannounced SPs Portfolio Employer survey
Patient Care	Direct observation SP/OSCE Global ratings Medical record audit Chart-stimulated recall Portfolio	Direct observation SP/OSCE Global ratings Medical record audit Chart-stimulated recall Portfolio Employer survey	Direct observation Unannounced SP Global ratings Medical record audit Chart-stimulated recall Multisource feedback Licensing/credentialing actions Maintenance of certification components Portfolio Employer survey
Practice-based Learning and Improvement	Medical record audits Chart-stimulated recall EBM exercises Portfolios SP/OSCE	Medical record audits Chart-stimulated recall EBM exercises Portfolios SP/OSCE QA/PI projects Multisource feedback Employer survey	Medical record audits Chart-stimulated recall EBM exercises Portfolios SP/OSCE QA/PI projects Multisource feedback Unannounced SP Practice improvement modules Employer survey
Systems-based Practice	SP/OSCE Medical record audit Chart-stimulated recall Portfolios	Medical record audits Chart-stimulated recall EBM exercises Portfolios SP/OSCE QA/PI projects Multisource feedback Employer survey	Medical record audits Chart-stimulated recall EBM exercises Portfolios SP/OSCE QA/PI projects Multisource feedback Unannounced SP Practice improvement modules Employer survey

Note: Employer survey = sending a survey to the individual's employer following completion of training (e.g., sending the survey to the program director of the internship following medical school or the fellowship director following graduate medical education or practice supervisor following graduate medical education).

EBM, Evidence-based medicine; *NBME*, National Board of Medical Examiners; *QA/PI*, Quality Assurance/Performance Improvement; *SP*, standardized patient; *OSCE*, objective structured clinical examination; *USMLE*, United States Medical Licensing Examination.

can be used for program evaluation within or at the completion of educational programs. Data from milestones-based assessments have also provided insight into their relationship with performance on qualifying exams and board exams and performance in fellowship on medical knowledge competencies.[72–74]

Learner Outcomes

Program evaluation should include educational outcomes that are measured during the training program and those that reflect the future performance of its graduates. It is also important to obtain baseline data on learner competence to fully understand the impact of the educational experience as much of the explained variance in some educational experiences, such as courses of clerkships, is due to learner characteristics alone.[2,75] Evaluators may involve a wide variety of approaches ranging from analysis of aggregated trainee assessment data (e.g., mean program in-training scores), to surveys (or interviews) of trainees, faculty, and future program directors and employers, milestones, and/or EPAs (see Chapter 1), to studies focusing on healthcare practices and outcomes of current trainees and graduates. The actual program assessment process may comprise inexpensive, broadly applied measures to support continuous monitoring of program performance (employer surveys, monitoring board certification rates or adverse licensure actions) or may involve the deployment of resource-intensive assessment modalities for outcomes assessment of specific program initiatives (e.g., unannounced SPs to measure the success of an intervention to improve screening for domestic violence).

In deciding upon the methods for evaluating educational outcomes it is important to include more than written examinations and course grades or global ratings. In fact, well-designed performance-based assessments such as OSCEs are ideal tools for evaluating important skills and behaviors objectives, and may better predict future performance.[76] Aggregate data from other direct observation-based methods, medical record audits, or conference presentation/participation can also serve as a barometer of program performance in selected competence domains. It is also critically important to include measures of professional attitudes and behaviors beginning early in medical school as performance in this domain may have predictive value for identifying future problems in residency and practice.[77–79] Unfortunately, there is much work that needs to be done to fully understand and develop appropriate instruments to measure several of the important competencies such as teamwork, lifelong learning, patient advocacy, and some aspects of professionalism.

That said, this approach of compiling several different data points to inform and evaluate a learner's performance can yield numerous benefits for assessment practice and more importantly, learner outcomes. In short, a program of, or programmatic, assessment is composed of individual data points that when taken together amount to more than the sum of its parts (see Chapter 3). In programmatic assessment, a learner's program of assessment may include longitudinal data points from course examinations, OSCEs, mini-CEXs, or various other assessment tools. These points are used *for* learning and aid in feedback and mentoring processes. Once the program is complete, however, a summative decision is made—based on these data points—to determine learner competence and readiness. Ultimately, much of the impetus for programmatic assessment is to optimize learning and reflection and drive more informed decision-making of learner performance.[80,81]

Educational leaders should also seek to attain a balance between the use of internal and external measures in assessing educational outcomes. Internal methods, such as the aggregate assessment data described above, or internal evaluators, such as faculty and residents, are likely to be somewhat biased by personal involvement with the program. However, such methods can provide important information and feedback that is enriched by an understanding of program structure, history, goals and objectives, and the constraints under which educational managers operate. External evaluators and methods (such as ITEs) provide for a more objective assessment of program processes and outcomes, often with the additional advantage of providing norm-referenced comparison data, either across several programs or institutions or based on a national cohort of similar trainees and programs.[50]

As in the assessment of individual trainees, comparisons using external measures are more valid if the course or program objectives are matched with the appropriate assessment tool; similarly, comparison between competence and performance at various levels is more appropriately performed through the use of the same or similar assessment tools. Outcome measures that might be applied to assessing the quality of educational programs include both national and local methods. Standardized tests such as the NBME Subject Examinations, the United States Medical Licensing Examination (USMLE), and residency in-training and board certification examinations yield comparisons to national cohorts. Administration of clinical skills examinations through local consortia may provide important information by comparing students and residents to local or regional peer groups. Thoughtful consideration of what one intends to measures versus what various instruments actually measure will inform the selection of appropriate comparison methods. External evaluation processes, such as LCME or ACGME/Residency Review Committee (RRC) reviews, are often conducted by individuals with specific training and tend to have more credibility in influencing institutional change. Of course, despite the quality of the review process, most educational leaders do not wish to rely on such a high-stakes approach for valuable yet critical program assessment information.

Assessment of graduates' performance may target educational or professional outcomes or may focus on the clinical practices and patient health outcomes (covered in the next section) resulting from the care provided by graduates. Outcomes evaluation focusing on the competence and performance of graduates involves logistical and technical challenges. First are the difficulties in collecting information on graduates who may be spread across multiple institutions and geographic locations. Second, there remains uncertainty about the strength of connection between prior educational experiences and achievement and future abilities and practices of graduates.[82] Research has shown that it is difficult to demonstrate a consistent relationship between academic performance in medical school and residency, and the performance of residents and practicing physicians. There are several reasons for this inconsistent relationship; understanding the potential pitfalls in measuring the performance of graduates is critical in informing the development of sound program evaluation processes. While most of the research on educational outcomes has focused on the relationship between learning in medical school and subsequent behaviors and performance in residency and practice, many of the limiting factors also pertain to measuring residency program outcomes in future practice. These limitations have been described by experts in medical education and assessment and include.[83–86]

1. Dissimilarity in constructs between performances at different levels. It is difficult to compare performances at different levels because expectations for the demonstration of competence and performance are different in medical school, residency, and practice. One should not assume that the performance of practicing physicians is an extension of that expected of residents and that the performance of residents represents an extension of that expected of medical students. As one moves along the education–practice continuum the complexity of the practice environment and related situational effects (including clinical specialty) and constraints influence the practice behaviors and performance of physicians. Achievement in medical school reflects more limited and relatively simple domains while performance in practice reflects a complex relationship between knowledge and skills, personal and professional characteristics, and a wide array of patient- and system-related factors. Assessment in undergraduate medical education (UME) largely relates to educational processes and outcomes; assessment of practicing physicians focuses on measure of professional achievement (board certification and Maintenance of Certification [MOC] outcomes) and should ideally focus on compliance with evidence-based processes of care and patient outcomes. The GME environment provides for the transition from educational to clinical outcome measurement.
2. Limitations in assessment methodology. Performance at all levels is measured by instruments that are intrinsically flawed to a variable degree. In addition to the fact that predictor and criterion variables are likely to reflect different constructs, both are measured by imprecise instruments that may be measuring different domains (or different aspects within the same domain), thus raising questions about the validity of interpretations. For example, thorough analysis of scores from an OSCE for fourth-year students may find that they yield valid impressions about trainee communication skills, but history-taking scores (related to local case and checklist development practices) reflect assessment-related interviewing skills rather than their authentic clinical data-gathering practices (see Chapter 5). That predictor variable then may be compared to a sample of intern mini-CEX scores presumed to be measuring the same attributes but actually measuring some combination of cognitive and interpersonal skills. In this situation, one cannot assume that a difference in performance on the OSCE and the mini-CEX reflects improved aptitude; the fact that the two tools are measuring different attributes may explain much of the difference and should be considered. Additionally, assessment methods are to a degree intrinsically biased and can be a reflection of whoever created said assessment or whoever is carrying out said assessment.[87–90] Whether the methods rely on written items or observations, there is inherent subjectivity and bias in item writing or ratings. There can be "power" in subjectivity.[91] Though. and multiple, legitimate viewpoints can inform learner outcomes.
3. Intervening time. The longer one waits between measuring the predictor and criterion variables, the more existing associations will diminish or disappear. This is due to a combination of factors including decay of original knowledge and skills and the introduction of a potentially wide array of educational, professional, and personal events and activities during the intervening time. Such limitations relate to the uncertain correlation between undergraduate education and subsequent practice behaviors and have resulted in a more focused assessment of the intermediate outcomes in GME, such as intern ratings. Concentration on intermediate outcomes in GME is appropriate, though, as the goals and objectives of UME are to prepare graduates for the more limited patient care responsibilities in the supervised environment of GME.[50]
4. Measurement challenges. A variety of measurement challenges affect our ability to detect and accurately quantify relationships that exist across the education and practice continuum:
   a. Range restriction: Relatively speaking, the subjects (students and physicians) being assessed comprise a fairly homogenous group in regard to intrinsic abilities and premedical education. It may be difficult to detect significant differences using traditional correlation and regression-based analyses.
   b. Skewed distributions: The skewed distributions typical of the global rating forms used in assessment obscure our ability to detect correlations.[92]
   c. Nonrepresentative nature of results related to response biases: The voluntary nature of participation in published studies influences their interpretation. The refusal of some students to participate and the failure of subsequent supervisors to return rating forms is related to lower academic achievement in students as well as lower performance in residency.[93,94]
   d. Additional measurement constraints: See Gonnella and colleagues[84] for a more detailed description of additional measurement constraints (nonlinear distribution of ratings, effects of variance of predictor and

criterion variables, relationship between different predictor variables compared to criterion variables).

Despite the above limitations, studies have shown that a relationship exists between performance in medical school and subsequent performance in residency and practice, although the strongest relationships exist for internship performances. For example, students whose academic achievement is extremely low or extremely high are reasonably likely to be classified in similar groups as interns.[95] In various studies, undergraduate measures such as individual and composite clerkship grades, licensure examination scores, faculty clinical ratings, class standing, and history of academic excellence or problems correlate to a variable extent with intern supervisor ratings, licensure and board certification scores, and subsequent academic affiliations.[84] When significant correlations have been observed the magnitude of the relationship has not been particularly large; certainly not enough to endorse strong connections. As expected, stronger relationships exist for conceptually similar measures such as correlations between the separate licensure examination steps and ITE scores, and between clerkship grades and residency supervisor ratings.[95,96]

The data above suggest the potential value and limitations of assessing the performance of graduates as a program outcome measure. This information needs to be thoughtfully incorporated into an overall program evaluation plan. An important objective in designing program evaluation processes is to mitigate the effect of the limitations listed above when deciding upon attributes to be measured and the tools selected to assess them. To the extent possible, the instruments used to measure performance at various levels should be similar with reasonable expectations that they are measuring the same element of clinical competence or performance. One should understand what each tool is actually measuring, as well as its reliability, and apply that knowledge in interpreting results.

Evaluators should consider the ultimate effects and potential endpoints of learning in selecting outcome variables. How will the knowledge and skills acquired at various points in training be manifest in future practice contexts? What assessment methods are reasonably likely to be measuring the same or similar attributes across the continuum of education and practice? Table 18.4 provides some likely combinations of tests that might be associated as long as those performing the comparisons are cognizant of the potential limitations described above and are able to incorporate such understanding into the subsequent interpretation of results. Appropriate methods for comparison are somewhat obvious for the "simpler" domains of Medical Knowledge and Interpersonal and Communication Skills, but are more difficult to imagine for the more complex competencies. For example, how will you be able to distinguish a graduate who is performing well (or poorly) in applying the knowledge and principles of Practice-based Learning and Improvement and Systems-based Practice in their practices?

Educational leaders should address the participation of students and residents in program evaluation, not only as respondents providing input regarding program quality but also as data sources for subsequent analysis. This coproduction of outcomes, and the continuous engagement of trainees, their patients, and those in the healthcare system, is necessary for achieving the "best health and well-being outcomes".[56] This requires that trainees participate in contributing current and future assessment and practice data that inform decisions about program quality and improvement. Informed consent for participation in longitudinal data collection should be obtained early in training so as not to obscure interpretation of future results with nonresponse bias. It is also appropriate to minimize the time after graduation when selected variables are measured, primarily to reduce the effect of confounding variables such as additional educational interventions and evolution in practice context.

Some experts suggest the use of statistical methods that are less affected by the measurement constraints described above. The use of nonparametric (distribution-free) statistics, focusing on outliers, including high and, and in particular, low or marginal performers, is probably more effective in identifying important educational variables.[84] Such an approach would involve categorizing grades or ratings into arbitrary categories. For example, on a 9-point scale ratings of 1 to 3 would comprise the "low" category, 4 to 6 an intermediate category, and 8 and 9 the high category for comparison purposes. One would then compare the frequencies in which graduates fall into the specific categories in areas that constitute important program objectives; alternatively, distribution into various categories using both predictor (current) and criterion (future) assessment measures would provide important validity information regarding the value of selected assessment methods. In general, it makes more sense for program directors to consider those factors that predict subsequent incompetence or poor performance (or vice versa: high academic standing or clinical excellence) as constituting more critical and useful information than factors associated with relatively small correlational differences among graduates. Educational leaders should keep in mind that instruments such as global rating scales, even in the hands of program directors, may not be sensitive in detecting deficiencies and providing accurate feedback to medical school educational leaders.[97] As suggested above, failure of a residency program director or subsequent employer to respond to requests for information on graduates should be followed up as this may indicate cause for concern, and important information may not be communicated.

One of the challenges resulting from limitations in our assessment methods, the intervening time between graduation from the educational program and the influence of other educational activities and experience, is an attribution of the outcome (learner or clinical) to the educational program or specific elements of that program. Evaluators may consider contribution analysis to better define the relationship between the observed results and program activities—to what extent did the program activities or other influencing factors contribute to the measured outcome(s).[98]

TABLE 18.5 The Six Seps of Contribution Analysis

Step 1: Specify the attribution problem to be addressed	Acknowledge the attribution problem. Define the specific cause-effect question being considered. Explore the nature of the program contribution to the expected results and the plausibility of the program contribution to the results. Define other factors potentially influencing the outcome.
Step 2: Develop the theory of change and the risks to it	Build a theory of change to explain how the program produces the desired result(s). Build a logic model/results chain to explicate the contribution of the program to its outputs and outcomes. List the assumptions underlying the theory of change. Consider how other factors may influence the results. Determine how much the theory of change may be contested.
Step 3: Gather existing evidence on the theory of change	Assess the strengths and weaknesses of logic linking the program to observed results and the plausibility of the program's contribution to the results. Gather evidence on: The occurrence of key results (outputs and outcomes) The validity of the assumptions underlying the theory of change The other potential influencing factors
Step 4: Assess the rationale support program contribution	Determine the strength and weakness of evidence linking the program to the observed results. Determine the credibility of the rationale for the program's contribution to the observed results. Obtain stakeholder input regarding credibility of the rationale. Identify the main weakness for further data gathering.
Step 5: Seek out additional evidence	Identify what new data/evidence is necessary. Reconsider and/or adjust the theory of change as appropriate. Gather additional evidence using multiple approaches seeking triangulation to enhance credibility.
Step 6: Revise and strengthen the contribution rationale	Focus on weakness in the rationale; strengthen the evidence to build a more credible rationale linking program activities to results. Process is iterative; return to step 4 as needed.

Modified from Mayne J. Contribution analysis: an approach to exploring cause and effect. ILAC Brief 16, May 2008.

Contribution analysis begins with a clear articulation of the program theory, explaining how the program would lead to the specific outcomes of interest[98] (Table 18.5). A logic model may be developed to create potential causal links between program processes and outputs to immediate, intermediate, and long-term outcomes. Proof of a causal connection may not be definitively achievable, but the contribution analysis seeks to demonstrate a "plausible association" linking outcomes to program activities, and to reduce uncertainty about the connection between the program and results.[99,100] The types of evidence that would support a causal connection between the program and observed results include[100]:

- Results occurring at the expected time relative to program activities
- Temporal variation in results correlating with temporal changes in the level of program activities
- Results correlating with the implementation intensity at different sites
- Alternate explanations regarding other influencing factors being less plausible
- Multiple lines of evidence supporting a causal effect of program activities

Engaging in the contribution analysis may lead to a better understanding of the program elements and how they work and identification of program measures that are better aligned with program goals and more informative regarding program impact.[29,99–101]

Surveys of residents or graduates are a commonly used method for providing feedback on the ability of residency programs to prepare trainees for clinical practice. For the most part, such surveys suggest that programs do a fairly good job preparing graduates to provide care of the clinical conditions pertinent to a particular field, with few exceptions, but may be helpful in detecting areas where graduates are not prepared to deal with some of the content, tasks, or nonclinical requirements of clinical practice. As an example, the responses of senior residents in eight specialties to a survey regarding their preparedness for practice pointed to significant gaps across multiple programs and specialties in preparing them to participate in and contribute to meaningful activities in clinical practice.[102] Residents about to graduate from their programs felt comfortable caring for most of the common conditions seen in their specialty. However, occasional surprises were noted. Residents responded that they were not prepared to care for specific patient conditions or manage patients in certain contexts (e.g., 8% of psychiatry residents were unprepared for diagnosing and treating eating disorders; 29% of obstetrics and gynecology residents were unprepared to care for patients in nursing homes). Across all eight specialty groups surveyed, modest numbers of residents felt unprepared to choose cost-effective treatments, participate in quality assurance, care for populations of patients, collaborate with nonphysician caregivers, and practice in a managed care environment. These findings certainly suggest critical items for inclusion in most program surveys, however the occasional unanticipated results for common specialty-based conditions and patient care contexts indicate that surveys should remain broad and unbiased by unfounded assumptions regarding program quality.

Workforce Outcomes

National conversations regarding GME funding have raised questions regarding the role and contribution of the medical education system to a diverse and competent healthcare workforce. While there is substantial disagreement regarding national workforce projections in general, there is little argument that the current workforce in the United States does not meet national needs in terms of the proportion of trained specialists, allocation of physicians to underserved areas, and extent to which the physician workforce represents the diversity of the US population. In a sense, the recruitment, preparation, and graduation of a diverse set of learners exemplify increasingly important process and outcome measures for our UME and GME programs. In consideration of developing accountability measures for limited federal funding of GME programs, recent research demonstrated that workforce outcome measures are available through national databases for approximately 90% of Medicare sponsoring institutions.[103] Program evaluation efforts, at least at the institution level, should begin including the specialty distribution of graduates, contributions to workforce diversity, and subsequent practice in underserved areas. Additional process measures that should be considered include the demographic composition of matriculants, commitment to underserved populations, and goals for specialty training; structural measures should address the inclusion of educational and faculty development activities that will support attainment of learners' goals such as training in leadership and change management, cultural competence, health equity, social and behavior determinants of health, and population management.[58]

Patient Outcomes

Because the overarching purpose of medical education is to improve the quality of care delivered to patients, and in consideration of the large public investment made in medical education programs, it is important to include educational outcome measures that address the quality of care delivered to the patients and populations cared for by graduates.[104–107] However, the collection of clinical outcomes data to support programmatic evaluation introduces even more significant logistical and measurement challenges than those involved in evaluating learner outcomes. As with the measurement of learner outcomes, the logistical challenges involved in collecting clinical performance data from graduates is especially daunting in that they are likely to be spread across multiple residency programs or practice sites. Beyond the logistical hurdles, evaluators will confront significant measurement challenges, including limitations in the availability and quality of measures focusing on healthcare processes and outcomes; differences in case mix and severity among patient populations; difficulty in achieving adequate sample sizes; attribution challenges due to patient preferences, system factors, and contributions of other clinical team members; and the lag time between the intervention and the outcome measurement.[105,106,108] Skepticism about the relationship between educational processes and clinical outcomes, particularly when there is a period of time separating the two, provides yet another obstacle to the use of clinical data to inform program quality improvement.[106] Practicing physicians perceive little contribution of UME to their later practice performance, but do feel that GME has a more significant effect on their future medical practice.[109]

Nevertheless there are studies demonstrating that there exists a relationship between healthcare outcomes and prior educational experiences, and the impact is measurable.[106] Studies show that the medical school from which a physician graduates impacts their subsequent prescribing practices and related patient outcomes, as well as their ratings by peers, nonphysician colleagues, and patients in selected competency areas.[110–112] Medical school graduates who achieved higher scores on their licensing examination were more likely to engage in more appropriate consultation, prescribing, and preventive care for patients with specific indications.[113] Subsequent research from the United States and Canada also supports the positive relationships between student performance on licensure examinations and the quality of care they provide.[114,115] Similarly, residency program characteristics have been found to correlate with board certifying examination scores, which have then been shown to correlate with subsequent peer ratings of professional competence.[116,117] More recent research shows that the residency program from which an obstetrician graduates predicts their complication rates for vaginal and cesarean section deliveries years into their practice.[104,118] Internists who train in a healthcare system characterized by cost-conscious care delivery are more likely to select appropriate conservative management options on their certifying examination, but retain the ability to choose more aggressive care options when clinically indicated.[119–121] Several studies have evaluated the outcomes of training interventions on resident performance in ambulatory settings, focusing on the cost of care, compliance with preventive healthcare recommendations, counseling skills, and referral practices.[122] A recent large review reported over 90 papers that were published describing a wide range of patient care outcomes for residents during their training including the frequency of medical errors, mortality rates, operating times, and estimated blood loss for surgical procedures, airway management, diabetes control, and interpretation of radiographs. The residency-level clinical outcome studies largely focused on evaluation of progression of competency during training and the impact of educational interventions.[107]

The residency training environment is conducive to evaluating quality-of-care outcomes related to traditional curricular interventions or to experiential learning through involvement in local quality improvement activities.[123,124] Quality-of-care measures (focusing on processes of care, patient experience, or clinical outcomes) are naturally suited to evaluating resident (or student) engagement in institutional quality improvement activities. As an example, Ogrinc and colleagues described improvements in pneumococcal vaccination and venous thromboembolism (VTE) prophylaxis rates, as well as improved hand hygiene and increased smoking cessation rates in one institution as a result of resident participation in an integrated quality improvement curriculum.[47] It is more challenging to use clinical care measures to evaluate student-level achievement in Practice-based Learning and Improvement and Systems-based Practice, given their limited responsibility for patient care outcomes. However, recent focus on exploring value-added roles (such as patient navigator) for medical students provides a context for introducing evaluation of impact on health system performance and patient outcomes.[125]

Although there are a number of studies linking medical education experience to patient clinical outcomes, such studies comprise a significant minority of publications on medical education program evaluation.[105,126] Research on clinical outcomes, as demonstrated by some of the studies described in the previous paragraph, require significant resources, relatively complex designs, and large numbers of participants. Many undergraduate and graduate program leaders will not have access to the resources or expertise to enjoin such large projects. However, authors of the above studies and other measurement experts suggest several approaches that will allow most medical educators to use clinical data to support meaningful program evaluation:

1. One potential way to address the need to obtain data on the performance of program graduates is to combine efforts and resources across multiple programs along the continuum of education and practice, perhaps in the form of research partnerships, networks, or consortia. This may allow for access to additional expertise such as health services researchers, economists, and sociologists who are also interested in patient care outcomes.[105,106]
2. The use of registries, or other databases that allows integration of data across the continuum of education and practice (including electronic health record data), promotes collaboration among stakeholders and facilitates combination and analysis of data linking educational and clinical measures.[127]
3. It makes sense to focus on commonly encountered conditions with a large population impact for which appropriate (or inappropriate) treatment has important and measurable affects.[106] It is also more likely that one can actually obtain such data from healthcare systems or other sources.
4. Alignment with national specialty-based or institutional priorities in selecting quality measures will increase the credibility of the measurement data, allow use of existing performance standards, and increase the likelihood that data will be available for use in measuring educational outcomes.[128]
5. Researchers should focus on identifying sensitive educational outcome measures that are directly related to physician behaviors. Patient activation, for example, is a direct outcome of the patient–physician encounter and provides a validated surrogate measure of patient medical adherence, diabetes outcomes, and health services utilization.[127,129–132]
6. Evaluators should identify other process and learner outcome measures that are associated with and determinants for specific health outcomes. Such measures, which may represent learner knowledge and skills outcomes or patient behaviors or attitudes, may serve as good surrogates for clinical outcomes while not encumbered by some of the above described measurement challenges such as attribution limitations or unnecessarily prolonged lag times.[105,108]
7. Above all, evaluators should have a clear sense of the purpose and objectives in pursuing their research plan and identifying relevant outcomes to target. Clinical outcomes data will be helpful in meeting some but not all measurement needs and goals. In fact, a disproportionate focus on patient outcomes that have a limited range in terms of their coverage of important program goals may result in underemphasis of other educational processes and outcomes that are important to learners.[108]

Learning Environment

It is important to consider the impact of an educational program on the educational and clinical environment in which it resides and, vice versa, the impact of the learning environment and program quality and learner outcomes. In terms of the program's impact on its local environment, evaluation extends beyond accountability for ensuring acquisition of the cognitive and behavioral aspects of competence among trainees and graduates to the larger impact of the educational program on infrastructural and cultural changes in the institutional environment.[66] To what extent does the program influence the teaching and learning experience of faculty and trainees and to what extent do positive (or negative) effects spill over into the local clinical environment? A measure of the efficacy of the educational program can be obtained by measuring the impact on current healthcare outcomes within the home institution.[133,134] For example, patient outcomes such as satisfaction, ratings of health status, or HbA1c levels would be obtained during a resident Practice-based Learning and Improvement project focusing on the quality of routine care provided to diabetics. Of course, in many cases it may be difficult to determine which came first, educational program implementation/innovation or enhancements in institutional culture or educational infrastructure. It is likely that some reciprocal relationship exists between the quality of educational programs and their environment. In fact, the relationship between the quality of medical education and healthcare, in association with a culture supportive of innovation and scholarly pursuit within individual institutions, is an important underlying theme of the Educational Innovation Project sponsored by the Internal Medicine RRC. In return for demonstration of excellence and innovation in education and quality, participating residency programs are offered extended accreditation cycles.[135]

In addition to considering the impact of an educational program on its learning environment, it is also important to understand and measure the influence of the learning environment in which the program is situated on the educational program and its learners' success in achieving key program objectives.[136,137] A number of instruments have been developed to assess medical education learning environments, however there is little consistency within these instruments in terms of the constructs that are measured. Nonetheless. a review of the theoretical frameworks upon which these instruments are derived identified three domains that reflect important components of the learning environment: goal orientation, relationships, and organization/regulation.[136] Thus any instrument chosen to assess a program's learning environment should address one or more of following elements:

1. Goal orientation focuses on how the environment supports learner growth and development through its content and aims; specific elements include the clarity of learning objectives, relevance of the learning content, and use of constructive feedback.
2. Relationship dimensions focus on the openness and supportive nature of the environment; specific elements include open communication, learner cohesion and engagement, and social and emotional support of learners and faculty.
3. Regulation and organizational domains focus on maintenance of and change within the educational program; specific elements include the organization and order within a program; how the program maintains control, articulates expectations, and responds to change; and the roles of faculty and learners.

Schönrock-Adema summarizes how commonly used instruments assessing the medical education learning environment map to these domains.[136]

In GME, the ACGME Clinical Learning Environment Review (CLER) program introduces structured assessment of the learning environment as a requirement for accreditation.[138] The CLER program includes six focus areas: patient safety; quality improvement; transitions in care; supervision; duty oversight, fatigue management, and mitigation; and professionalism. The CLER review focuses on the infrastructure of the program's sponsoring institution learning environment, and the extent to which it supports resident engagement in institutional quality and safety and supports resident learning and development in relation to the six focus areas.[138] This most recent report focused on the impact of the COVID-19 pandemic on the clinical learning environment and highlighted eight overarching themes that will continue to shape GME and healthcare.

Reporting and Feedback

Reports and/or feedback from the evaluation process should be as specific as possible (particularly any recommendations based on the evaluation) and include detailed descriptions of both positive and negative outcomes resulting from the program or particular interventions. The use of multiple formats (presentations, detailed written reports, charts and graphs) may be helpful in describing program results.[12] Reporting of the evaluation outcomes should include as much information about the intervention and the contextual factors impacting its implementation as is needed for stakeholders to ascertain the relevance of its findings to their own program or reproduce the intervention in other settings[12,37] Shortcomings in fully reporting process and outcome analyses and changes or variation in implementation steps or strategies have been a problem with evaluating complex interventions and compromise interpretations or actions based on evaluation results and the adoption of such interventions in other contexts.[34]

Some of these shortcomings, however, can be overcome by utilizing a layered analysis approach, which helps capture the contextual differences in implementation strategies, or by integrating a theory of change in a comprehensive logic model, which aids in explaining how and why outcomes are achieved. Dissemination of program evaluation findings can be of interest and benefit to practitioners and scholars alike, particularly to those attuned to the scholarship of teaching and learning. Guided by Glassick's criteria (Fig. 18.1), documentation of program evaluation results can be rigorous, thoughtful, and translatable and by adhering to these standards, program evaluation reports can be shared with a number of prospective audiences including but not limited to MedEdPORTAL, Academic Medicine (via Innovation Reports), Medical Education (via Really Good Stuff), or Perspectives on Medical Education (via Show and Tell).[139]

Conclusion

Evaluation of educational programs is a core responsibility of the leaders of those programs. Sound evaluation enables educational programs to meet the needs and requirements of various stakeholders, including funders and accreditors, to guide continued improvement efforts and to support development of the evidence base on medical education practices. Various models and methods are available to assist evaluators, who are advised to use the most appropriate elements from among different models in a complementary way to best meet their needs.

Construction of a high-quality evaluation plan begins with a clear definition of the goals of the evaluation and engagement of stakeholders who have an interest in ensuring the success of the educational program. In addition to borrowing from the various models to accomplish their evaluation objectives, evaluators should include a range of structural, process, and outcome measures to develop a comprehensive view the program, including the extent to which it is attaining its goals and how the program can be improved. Lastly, it is important for evaluators to close the loop on the processes by providing accurate, comprehensive, and actionable feedback to the educational program leaders.

Annotated Bibliography

1. W.K. Kellogg Logic Model Development Guide. (W.K. Kellogg Foundation). Updated January 2004. Accessed August 15, 2015. https://www.wkkf.org/resource-directory/resource/2006/02/wk-kellogg-foundation-logic-model-development-guide.
This guide provides a detailed description of the Logic model, with useful examples to illustration key points. It describes the basic Logic model, but also presents different approaches to meet different program needs, whether exploring program theory of change, measuring program outcomes, or focusing on program activities.
2. Craig P, Dieppe P, Macintyre S, Mcihie S, Nazareth I, Petticrew M. Developing and evaluating complex interventions: the new Medical Research Council guidance. *BMJ*. 2008;337:a1655.
This report, prepared on behalf of the Medical Education Council, UK, provides updated guidance on the development, implementation, and evaluation of complex interventions. This report provides useful and detailed information regarding the appropriate application of experimental methods (randomized and nonrandomized designs) in program evaluation. Case studies (14) illustrate the use of various methods in real evaluation contexts.
3. Stufflebeam DL, Coryn CLS, eds. Daniel Stufflebeam's CIPP model for evaluation: an improvement and accountability oriented approach. *Evaluation Theory, Models and Applications*. 2nd ed. Jossey-Bass; 2014:309–339.
This chapter describes the CIPP model of program evaluation including its origins and range of applications in evaluation. It provides detailed information regarding each of the four types of evaluation and illustrates their use in formative and summative roles.
4. Durning SJ, Hemmer P, Pangaro LN. The structure of program evaluation: an approach for evaluating a course, clerkship, or components of residency or fellowship training program. *Teach Learn Med*. 2007;19:308–318.
This paper provides a thorough overview of this three-phrase framework. Examples of methods that may be used during each phase are provided for UME and GME evaluation contexts. Practical guidance is offered for using this model for evaluating different types of educational interventions.
5. Pawson R, Tilley N. Realist evaluation. 2004. http://www.communitymatters.com.au/RE_chapter.pdf.
This paper describes the theory underlying realist evaluation, an introduction to the basic concepts (mechanism, context, outcome patterns, and context mechanism outcome pattern configuration), and a detailed explanation of the strategies and methods used in realist evaluation.
6. Johnson RB, Onwuegbuzie AJ. Mixed methods research: a research paradigm whose time has come. *Educ Res*. 2004;33:14–26.
This paper provides an excellent overview of qualitative, quantitative, and mixed-methods research. It provides a thorough analysis of the strengths and weakness of each, as well as a design matrix and process model for mixed-methods research.
7. Cook DA, Andriole DA, Durning SJ, Roberts NK, Triola MM. Longitudinal research databases in medical education: facilitating the study of educational outcomes over time and across institutions. *Acad Med*. 2010;85:1340–1346.
This article reports on the work of a task force to explore the use of longitudinal databases in medical education research (and program evaluation). It describe the variability in the structure of such databases and different ways in which individual learner information could be used in education research. It also provides a list of sources of learner information that are potentially available for use by researchers.
8. Chen C, Petterson S, Phillips RL, Mullan F, Bazemore A, O'Donnell SD. Toward graduate medical education accountability: measuring the outcomes of GME institutions. *Acad Med*. 2013;88:1–14.
This article provides information on workforce outcomes, including primary care graduates and those electing to practice in underserved areas. It provides a perspective on how workforce accountability measures could be implemented and serve as a means to align GME with national health needs.
9. Findings from the Long-Term Career Outcome Study (LTCOS) and Related Work. *Mil Med*. 2015;180(4):1–172.
This Supplement from Military Medicine contains a variety of program evaluation papers that illustrate examples of models and methods throughout this chapter.

References

1. Accreditation Council for Graduate Medical Education: Glossary of terms. Accessed July 1, 2013. https://www.acgme.org/Portals/0/PDFs/ab_ACGMEglossary.pdf?ver=2015-11-06-115749-460.
2. Durning SJ, Hemmer P, Pangaro LN. The structure of program evaluation: an approach for evaluating a course, clerkship, or components of residency or fellowship training program. *Teach Learn Med*. 2007;19:308–318.
3. Frye AW, Hemmer PA. Program evaluation models and related theories: AMEE Guide No. 67. *Med Teach*. 2012;34:e288–e299.
4. Glassick CE, Huber MT, Maeroff GI. *Scholarship Assessed Evaluation of the Professoriate*. 1st ed. Jossey-Bass; 1997.
5. Durning SJ, Dong T, LaRochelle JL, et al. Findings from the Long-Term Career Outcome Study (LTCOS) and related work. *Mil Med*. 2015;180(Suppl 4):1–172.
6. Goldie J. AMEE Education Guide no. 29: Evaluating educational programs. *Med Teach*. 2006;28:210–224.
7. W.K. Kellogg Foundation Evaluation Handbook. (W.K. Kellogg Foundation). Updated January 2004. Accessed August 15, 2015. https://www.wkkf.org/resource-directory/resource/2010/w-k-kellogg-foundation-evaluation-handbook.
8. Stufflebeam DL, Coryn CLS, eds. Daniel Stufflebeam's CIPP model for evaluation: an improvement and accountability oriented approach. *Evaluation Theory, Models and Applications*. 2nd ed. Jossey-Bass; 2014:309–339.
9. Wand T, White K, Patching J. Applying a realist(ic) framework to the evaluation of a new model of emergency department based mental health nursing practice. *Nurs Inq*. 2010;17:231–239.
10. McEvoy P, Richards D. A critical realist rationale for using a combination of quantitative and qualitative methods. *J Res Nurs*. 2006;11:66–78.
11. Haji F, Morin M-P, Parker K. Rethinking programme evaluation in health professions education: beyond 'did it work? *Med Educ*. 2013;47:342–351.
12. University of Glasgow, 2021. New framework on complex interventions to improve health. Accessed October 6, 2023. https://www.gla.ac.uk/schools/healthwellbeing/research/mrccsosocialandpublichealthsciencesunit/sharingourevidence/news/headline_813090_en.html.
13. Salter KL, Kothari A. Using realist evaluation to open the black box of knowledge translation: a state-of-the-art review. *Implement Sci*. 2014;9:115.

14. Cianciolo AT, Regehr G. Learning theory and educational intervention: producing meaningful evidence of impact through layered analysis. *Acad Med.* 2019;94(6):789–794.
15. Chamberland M, Mamede S, Bergeron L, Varpio L. A layered analysis of self-explanation and structured reflection to support clinical reasoning in medical students. *Perspect Med Educ.* 2021;10(3):171–179.
16. Johnson RB, Onwuegbuzie AJ. Mixed methods research: a research paradigm whose time has come. *Educ Res.* 2004;33:14–26.
17. Wong G, Grenhalgh T, Pawson R. Internet-based medical education: a realist review of what works, for whom and in what circumstances. *BMC Med Educ.* 2010;10:12.
18. Kirkpatrick D. Evaluation of training. In: Craig RL, Bittel LR, eds. *Training and Development Handbook.* McGraw-Hill; 1967:87–112.
19. Kirkpatrick D. *The Four Levels of Evaluation: Measurement and Evaluation.* American Society for Training and Development; 2007.
20. Parker K, Burrows G, Nash H, Rosenblum ND. Going beyond Kirkpatrick in evaluating a clinician scientist programme: it's not "if it works" but "how it works". *Acad Med.* 2011;86(11):1389–1396.
21. Yardley S, Dornan T. Kirkpatrick's levels and education "evidence". *Med Educ.* 2011;46(1):97–106.
22. Miller GE. The assessment of clinical skills/competence/performance. *Acad Med.* 1990(suppl 9):S63–S67.
23. Moore DE, Greene JS, Gallis HA. Achieving desired results and improved outcomes: Integrating planning and assessment throughout learning activities. *J Contin Educ Health Prof.* 2009;29:1–15.
24. W.K. Kellogg Logic Model Development Guide. (W.K. Kellogg Foundation). Updated January 2004. Accessed August 15, 2015. https://www.wkkf.org/resource-directory/resource/2006/02/wk-kellogg-foundation-logic-model-development-guide.
25. Morzinski JA, Montagnini ML. Logic modeling: a tool for improving educational programs. *J Palliat Med.* 2002;5:566–570.
26. Hall AK, Rich J, Dagnone JD, et al. It's a marathon, not a sprint: rapid evaluation of competency-based medical education program implementation. *Acad Med.* 2020;95(5):786–793.
27. Armstrong EG, Barsion SJ. Using an outcomes-logic-model approach to evaluate a faculty development program for medical educators. *Acad Med.* 2006;81:483–488.
28. Sundra DL, Scherer J, Anderson LA. *A guide on logic model development for the CDC's prevention research centers.* Prevention Research Centers Program Office; April 2003. Accessed August 20, 2015. https://www.bja.gov/evaluation/guide/documents/cdc-logic-model-development.pdf.
29. Van Melle E, Hall AK, Schumacher DJ, et al. Capturing outcomes of competency-based medical education: the call and the challenge. *Med Teach.* 2021;43(7):794–800.
30. Funnell SC, Rogers PJ. Purposeful Program Theory: Effective Use of Theories of Change and Logic Models. vol. 31. John Wiley & Sons; 2011.
31. Durning SJ, Pangaro L, Denton GD, et al. Inter-site consistency as a measurement of programmatic evaluation. *Acad Med.* 2003;78(10 Suppl):S36–S38.
32. Hauff SR, Hopson LR, Losman E, et al. Programmatic assessment of level 1 milestones in incoming interns. *Acad Emerg Med.* 2014;21(6):694–698.
33. Lypson ML, Frohna JG, Gruppen LD, Wooliscroft JO. Assessing residents' competencies at baseline: identifying the gaps. *Acad Med.* 2004;79(6):564–570.
34. Craig P, Dieppe P, Macintyre S, Mcihie S, Nazareth I, Petticrew M. Developing and evaluating complex interventions: the new Medical Research Council guidance. *BMJ.* 2008;337:a1655.
35. Eccles M, Grimshaw J, Campbell M, Ramsay C. Research designs for studies evaluating the effectiveness of change and improvement strategies. *Qual Saf Health Care.* 2003;12:47–52.
36. Moore GF, Audrey S, Barker M, et al. Process evaluation of complex interventions: Medical Research Council guidance. *BMJ.* 2015;350:h1258.
37. Campbell NC, Murray E, Darbyshire J, et al. Designing and evaluating complex interventions to improve health care. *BMJ.* 2007;334:455–459.
38. Singh MD. Evaluation framework for nursing education programs: application of the CIPP Model. *Int J Nurs Educ Schol.* 2004;1:1–16.
39. Petro-Nustas W. Evaluation of the process of introducing a quality development program in a nursing department at a teaching hospital: the role of a change agent. *Int J Nurs Stud.* 1996;33:605–618.
40. Steinert Y, Cruess S, Cruess R, Snell L. Faculty development for teaching and evaluating professionalism: from programme design to curriculum change. *Med Educ.* 2005;39:127–136.
41. Hogan MJ. Evaluating an intern/residency program. *JAOA.* 1992;7:912–915.
42. Kahn KL, Mendel P, Weinberg DA, Leuschner KJ, Gall EM, Siegel S. Approach for conducting the longitudinal program evaluation of the US Department of Health and Human Services National Action Plan to Prevent Healthcare-associated Infections: Roadmap to Elimination. *Med Care.* 2014;52(suppl 1):S9–S16.
43. Pawson R, Tilley N. Realist Evaluation. 2004. Accessed July 26, 2016. http://www.communitymatters.com.au/RE_chapter.pdf.
44. Pawson R. *The Science of Evaluation: A Realist Manifesto.* Sage Publications; 2013.
45. Wong G, Greenhalgh T, Westhorp G, Pawson R. Realist methods in medical education research: what are they and what can they contribute? *Med Educ.* 2012;46:89–96.
46. Meier K, Parker P, Freeth D. Mechanisms that support the assessment of interpersonal skills: a realistic evaluation of the interpersonal skills profile in pre-registration nursing students. *J Pract Teach Learn.* 2014;12:6–24.
47. Ogrinc G, Ercolano E, Cohen ES, et al. Educational system factor that engage resident physicians in an integrated quality improvement curriculum at a VA Hospital: a realist evaluation. *Acad Med.* 2014;89:1380–1385.
48. Schierhout G, Hains J, Damin S, et al. Evaluating the effectiveness of a multifaceted, multilevel continuous quality improvement program in primary care: developing a realist theory of change. *Implement Sci.* 2013;8:119.
49. Sorinola OO, Thistlethwaite J, Davies D, Peile E. Faculty development for educators: a realist evaluation. *Adv Health Sci Educ Theory Pract.* 2015;20(2):385–401.
50. Woodward CA. Program evaluation. In: Norman GR, van der Vleuten CPM, Newble DI, eds. *International Handbook of Research in Medical Education.* Dordrecht: Kluwer Academic Publishers; 2002:127–155.
51. Musick DW. A conceptual model for program evaluation in graduate medical education. *Acad Med.* 2006;81:759–765.
52. Carney PA, Nierenberg DW, Pipas CF, Brooks WB, Stukel TA, Keller AM. Educational epidemiology: applying population-

based design and analytic approaches to study medical education. *JAMA*. 2004;292:1044–1050.
53. Cook DA, Andriole DA, Durning SJ, Roberts NK, Triola MM. Longitudinal research databases in medical education: facilitating the study of educational outcomes over time and across institutions. *Acad Med*. 2010;85:1340–1346.
54. Vroeijenstijn AI. Quality assurance in medical education. *Acad Med*. 1995;70(suppl 7):S59–S67.
55. Suwanwela C. A vision of quality in medical education. *Acad Med*. 1995;70(suppl 7):S32–S37.
56. Englander R, Holmboe E, Batalden P, et al. Coproducing health professions education: a prerequisite to coproducing health care services? *Acad Med*. 2020;95(7):1006–1013.
57. Gerrity MS, Mahaffy J. Evaluating change in medical school curricula: how did we know where we were going? *Acad Med*. 1998;73(suppl 9):S55–S59.
58. Sokal-Gutierrez K, Ivey SL, Garcia R, Azzam A. Evaluation of the Program in Medical Education for the Urban Underserved (PRIME-US) at the UC Berkely-UCSF Joint Medical Program: the first 4 years. *Teach Learn Med*. 2015;27:189–196.
59. Kogan JR, Shea JA. Course evaluation in medical education. *Teach Teach Educ*. 2007;23:251–264.
60. Norcini JJ. Current perspectives in assessment: the assessment of performance at work. *Med Educ*. 2005;39:880–889.
61. Christensen L, Karle H, Nystrup J. Process-outcome interrelationship and standard setting in medical education: the need for comprehensive approach. *Med Teach*. 2007;29:672–677.
62. Fowell SL, Southgate LJ, Bligh JG. Evaluating assessment: the missing link? *Med Educ*. 1999;33(4):276–281.
63. Margolis MJ, Clauser BE, Cuddy MM, et al. Use of the mini-clinical evaluation exercise to rate examinee performance on a multiple-station clinical skills examination: a validity study. *Acad Med*. 2006;81(suppl 10):S56–S60.
64. Griffith III CH, Wilson JF, Haist SA, et al. Internal medicine clerkship characteristics associated with enhanced student examination performance. *Acad Med*. 2009 Jul 1;84(7):895–901.
65. Holmboe ES, Hawkins RE, Huot SJ. Effects of training in direct observation of medical residents' clinical competence: a randomized trial. *Ann Intern Med*. 2004;140(11):874–881.
66. Blumberg P. Multidimensional outcome considerations in assessing the efficacy of medical educational programs. *Teach Learn Med*. 2003;15(3):210–214.
67. Stone SL, Qualters DM. Course-based assessment: implementing outcome assessment in medical education. *Acad Med*. 1998;73(4):397–401.
68. Bordage G, Burack JH, Irby DM, Stritter FT. Education in ambulatory settings: developing valid measures of educational outcomes, and other research priorities. *Acad Med*. 1998; 73:743–750.
69. Holmboe ES, Sherbino J, Long DM, et al. The role of assessment in competency-based medical education. *Med Teach*. 2010;32(8):676–682.
70. Association of American Medical Colleges. *Core Entrustable Professional Activities for Entering Residency: Faculty and Learners' Guide*. AAMC; 2014. http://members.aamc.org/eweb/upload/Core%20EPA%20Faculty%20and%20Learner%20Guide.pdf.
71. Holmboe ES, Edgar L, Hamstra S. *The Milestones Guidebook. Version 2016*. Chicago: Accreditation Council for Graduate Medical Education; 2016. https://www.acgme.org/Portals/0/MilestonesGuidebook.pdf.
72. Beinstock JL, Shivraj P, Yamazaki K, et al. Correlations between Accreditation Council for Graduate Medical Education Obstetrics and Gynecology Milestones and American Board of Obstetrics and Gynecology qualifying examination scores: an initial validity study. *Am J Obstet Gynecol*. 2021 Mar;224(3):308.e1–308.e25.
73. Francisco GE, Yamazaki K, Raddatz M, et al. Do milestone ratings predict physical medicine and rehabilitation board certification examination scores? *Am J Phys Med Rehabil*. 2021 Feb 1;100(2S Suppl 1):S34–S39.
74. Heath JK, Wang T, Santhosh L, et al. Longitudinal milestone assessment extending through subspecialty training: the relationship between ACGME internal medicine residency milestones and subsequent pulmonary and critical care fellowship milestones. *Acad Med*. 2021 Nov 1;96(11):1603–1608.
75. Roop SA, Pangaro L. Effect of clinical teaching on student performance during a medicine clerkship. *Am J Med*. 2001;110(3):205–209.
76. Smith SR. Correlations between graduates' performances as first-year residents and their performances as medical students. *Acad Med*. 1993;68(8):633–634.
77. Brown E, Rosinski EF, Altman DF. Comparing medical school graduates who perform poorly in residency with graduates who perform well. *Acad Med*. 1993;68(10):806–808.
78. Papadakis MA, Teherani A, Banach MA, et al. Disciplinary action by medical boards and prior behavior in medical school. *N Engl J Med*. 2005;353(25):2673–2682.
79. Teherani A, Hodgson CS, Banach M, Papadakis MA. Domains of unprofessional behavior during medical school associated with future disciplinary action by a state medical board. *Acad Med*. 2005;80:S17–S20.
80. Hauer KE, O'Sullivan PS, Fitzhenry K, Boscardin C. Translating theory into practice: implementing a program of assessment. *Acad Med*. 2018;93(3):444–450.
81. Van Der Vleuten CP, Schuwirth LWT, Driessen EW, Govaerts MJB, Heeneman S. Twelve tips for programmatic assessment. *Med Teach*. 2015;37(7):641–646.
82. Kassebaum DG. The measurement of outcomes in the assessment of educational program effectiveness. *Acad Med*. 1990;65(5):293–296.
83. Arnold L, Willoughby TL. The empirical association between student and resident physician performances. In: Gonnella JS, Hojat M, Erdmann JB, Veloski JJ, eds. *Assessment Measures in Medical School, Residency, and Practice: The Connections*. Springer; 1993:71–82.
84. Gonnella JS, Hojat M, Erdmann JB, Veloski JJ. A case of mistaken identity: signal and noise in connecting performance assessments before and after graduation from medical school. In: Gonnella JS, Hojat M, Erdmann JB, Veloski JJ, eds. *Assessment Measures in Medical School, Residency, and Practice: The Connections*. Springer; 1993:17–34.
85. Hojat M, Gonnella JS, Veloski JJ, Erdmann JB. Is the glass half full or half empty? A reexamination of the associations between assessment measures during medical school and clinical competence after graduation. In: Gonnella JS, Hojat M, Erdmann JB, Veloski JJ, eds. *Assessment Measures in Medical School, Residency, and Practice: The Connections*. Springer; 1993:137–152.
86. McGuire C. Perspectives in assessment. In: Gonnella JS, Hojat M, Erdmann JB, Veloski JJ, eds. *Assessment Measures in Medical School, Residency, and Practice: The Connections*. Springer; 1993:3–16.
87. Boatright D, Anderson N, Kim JG, et al. Racial and ethnic differences in internal medicine residency assessments. *JAMA Netw Open*. 2022;5(12):e2247649.
88. Hauer KE, Jurich D, Vandergrift J, et al. Gender differences in milestone ratings and medical knowledge examination

scores among internal medicine residents. *Acad Med.* 2021 Jun 1;96(6):876–884.
89. Landau SI, Syvyk S, Wirtalla C, et al. Trainee sex and Accreditation Council for Graduate Medical Education milestone assessments during general surgery residency. *JAMA Surg.* 2021 Oct 1;156(10):925–931.
90. Santen SA, Yamazaki K, Holmboe ES, Yarris LM, Hamstra SJ. Comparison of male and female resident milestone assessments during emergency medicine residency training: a national study. *Acad Med.* 2020 Feb;95(2):263–268.
91. Ten Cate O, Regehr G. The power of subjectivity in the assessment of medical trainees. *Acad Med.* 2019;94(3):333–337.
92. Hawkins RE, Margolis MJ, Durning SJ, Norcini JJ. Constructing a validity argument for the mini-clinical evaluation exercise: a review of the research. *Acad Med.* 2010;85:1453–1461.
93. Verhulst SJ, Distlehorst LH. Examination of nonresponse bias in a major residency follow-up study. In: Gonnella JS, Hojat M, Erdmann JB, Veloski JJ, eds. *Assessment Measures in Medical School, Residency, and Practice: The Connections.* Springer; 1993:121–127.
94. Vu NV, Distlehorst LH, Verhulst SJ, Colliver JA. Clinical performance-based test sensitivity and specificity in predicting first-year residency performance. In: Gonnella JS, Hojat M, Erdmann JB, Veloski JJ, eds. *Assessment Measures in Medical School, Residency, and Practice: The Connections.* Springer; 1993:83–92.
95. Markert RJ. The relationship of academic measures in medical school to performance after graduation. In: Gonnella JS, Hojat M, Erdmann JB, Veloski JJ, eds. *Assessment Measures in Medical School, Residency and Practice: The Connections.* Springer; 1993:63–70.
96. Kenny S, McInnes M, Singh V. Associations between residency selection strategies and doctor performance: a meta-analysis. *Med Educ.* 2013;47:790–800.
97. Lavin B, Pangaro L. Internship ratings as a validity outcome measure for an evaluation system to identify inadequate clerkship performance. *Acad Med.* 1998;73(9):998–1002.
98. Mayne J. Contribution analysis: an approach to exploring cause and effect. *ILAC Brief 16*, May 2008.
99. Kotvojs F. Contribution analysis: a new approach to evaluation in international development. Paper presented at the Australian Evaluation Society 2006 International Conference, Darwin. http://www.aes.asn.au/conference/2006papers/022%20Fiona%20Kotvojs.pdf.
100. Mayne J. *Addressing attribution through contribution analysis: Using performance measures sensibly.* Discussion Paper, Office of the Auditor General of Canada; June 1999.
101. Schumacher DJ, Dornoff E, Carraccio C, et al. The power of contribution and attribution in assessing educational outcomes for individuals, teams, and programs. *Acad Med.* 2020 Jul;95(7):1014–1019.
102. Blumenthal D, Gokhale M, Campbell EG, Weissman JS. Preparedness for clinical practice: reports of graduating residents at academic health centers. *JAMA.* 2001;286(9):1027–1034.
103. Chen C, Petterson S, Phillips RL, Mullan F, Bazemore A, O'Donnell SD. Toward graduate medical education accountability: measuring the outcomes of GME institutions. *Acad Med.* 2013;88:1–14.
104. Asch DA, Nicholson S, Srinivas SK, Herrin J, Epstein AJ. How do you deliver a good obstetrician? Outcome-based evaluation of medical education. *Acad Med.* 2014;89:24–26.
105. Chen FM, Bauchner H, Burstin H. A call for outcomes research in medical education. *Acad Med.* 2004;79:955–960.
106. Tamblyn R. Outcomes in medical education: what is the standard and outcome of care delivered by our graduates? *Adv Health Sci Educ Theory Pract.* 1999;4:9–25.
107. Van der Leeuw RM, Lombarts KMJMH, Arah OA, Heineman MJ. A systematic review of the effects of residency training on patient outcomes. *BMC Med.* 2012;10:65–76.
108. Cook DA, West CP. Perspective: reconsidering the focus on "outcomes research" in medical education: a cautionary note. *Acad Med.* 2013;88:162–167.
109. Renschler HE, Fuchs U. Lifelong learning of physicians: contributions of different phases to practice performance. *Acad Med.* 1993;68:S57–S59.
110. Goldberg M, Tamblyn R, Laprise R, Dauphinee WD, McLeod P. Risk of adverse gastrointestinal events in seniors after prescription of nonsteroidal anti-inflammatory drugs: Does training at specific medical schools affect patient outcome? The Canadian Pharmacoepidemiology Forum. 1995.
111. Lockyer JM, Violato C, Wright BJ, Fidler HM. An analysis of long-term outcomes of the impact of curriculum: a comparison of the three- and four-year medical school curricula. *Acad Med.* 2009;84:1342–1347.
112. Monette J, Tamblyn RM, McLeod PJ, Gayton DC. Characteristics of physicians who frequently prescribe long-acting benzodiazepines for the elderly. *Eval Health Prof.* 1997;20:115–130.
113. Tamblyn R, Abrahamowicz M, Brailovsky C, et al. Association between licensing examination scores and resource use and quality of care in primary care practice. *JAMA.* 1998;280:989–996.
114. Norcini JJ, Boulet JR, Opalek A, Dauphinee WD. The relationship between licensing examination performance and the outcomes of care by international medical school graduates. *Acad Med.* 2014;89:1157–1162.
115. Wenghofer E, Klass D, Abrahamowicz M, et al. Doctor scores on national qualifying examinations predict quality of care in future practice. *Med Educ.* 2009;43:1166–1173.
116. Norcini JJ, Grosso LJ, Shea JA, Webster GD. The relationship between features of residency training and ABIM certifying examination performance. *J Gen Intern Med.* 1987;2:330–336.
117. Ramsey PG, Carline JD, Inui TS, Larson EB, LoGerfo JP, Wenrich MD. Predictive validity of certification by the American Board of Internal Medicine. *Ann Intern Med.* 1989;110:719–726.
118. Asch DA, Nicholson S, Srinivas S, Herrin J, Epstein AJ. Evaluating obstetrical residency programs using patient outcomes. *JAMA.* 2009;302:1277–1283.
119. Chen C, Petterson S, Phillips R, Bazemore A, Mullan F. Spending patterns in region of residency training and subsequent expenditures for care provided by practicing physicians for Medicare beneficiaries. *JAMA.* 2014 Dec 10;312(22):2385–2393.
120. Phillips Jr RL, Petterson SM, Bazemore AW, Wingrove P, Puffer JC. The effects of training institution practice costs, quality, and other characteristics on future practice. *Ann Fam Med.* 2017 Mar;15(2):140–148.
121. Sirovich BE, Lipner RS, Johnston M, Holmboe ES. The association between residency training and internists' ability to practice conservatively. *JAMA Intern Med.* 2014;174:1640–1648.
122. Bowen JL, Irby DM. Assessing quality and costs of education in the ambulatory setting: a review of the literature. *Acad Med.* 2002;77:621–680.
123. Dolan BM, Yialamas MA, McMahon GT. A randomized educational intervention trial to determine the effect of online education on the quality of resident-delivered care. *JGME.* 2015 September:376–381.

124. Hussain SA, Woehrlen TH, Arsene C, Wiese-Rometsch W, Hamstra C, White SR. Successful resident engagement in quality improvement: the Detroit Medical Center story. *JGME.* 2016 May:214–218.
125. Gonzalo JD, Graaf D, Johannes B, et al. Adding value to the health care system: identifying value-added systems roles for medical students. *Am J Med Qual.* 2016;32(3):261–270.
126. Prystowsky JB, Bordage G. An outcomes research perspective on medical education: the predominance of trainee assessment and satisfaction. *Med Educ.* 2001;35:331–336.
127. Kalet AL, Gillespie CC, Schwartz MD, et al. New measures to establish the evidence base for medical education: identifying educationally sensitive patient outcomes. *Acad Med.* 2010;85: 844–851.
128. Haan CK, Edwards FH, Poole B, Godley M, Genuardi FJ, Zenni EA. A model to begin using clinical outcomes in medical education. *Acad Med.* 2008;83:574–580.
129. Kinnear B, Kelleher M, Sall D, et al. Development of resident-sensitive quality measures for inpatient general internal medicine. *J Gen Intern Med.* 2021 May;36(5):1271–1278.
130. Petosa Jr JJ, Martini A, Klein M, Schumacher D. Resident sensitive quality measures for general pediatrics: alignment with existing care recommendations. *Acad Pediatr.* 2021 Aug;21(6):943–947.
131. Schumacher DJ, Holmboe ES, van der Vleuten C, Busari JO, Carraccio C. Developing resident-sensitive quality measures: a model from pediatric emergency medicine. *Acad Med.* 2018 Jul;93(7):1071–1078.
132. Smirnova A, Sebok-Syer SS, Chahine S, et al. Defining and adopting clinical performance measures in graduate medical education: where are we now and where are we going? *Acad Med.* 2019 May;94(5):671–677.
133. Brilli RJ, Jr McClead RE, Crandall WV, et al. A comprehensive patient safety program can significantly reduce preventable harm, associated costs, and hospital mortality. *J Pediatr.* 2013;163(6):1638–1645.
134. Mohr JJ, Randolph GD, Laughon MM, Schaff E. Integrating improvement competencies into residency education: a pilot project from a pediatric continuity clinic. *Ambul Pediatr.* 2003;3:131–136.
135. Accreditation Council for Graduate Medical Education: EIP program requirements. Accessed November 3, 2023. https://www.acgme.org.
136. Schönrock-Adema J, Bouwkamp-Timmer T, van Hell EA, Cohen-Schotanus J. Key elements in assessing the educational environment: where is the theory? *Adv Health Sci Educ.* 2012;17(5):727–742.
137. Thibault GE. The importance of an environment conducive to education. *J Grad Med Educ.* 2016;8(2):134–135.
138. Koh NJ, Wagner R, Newton RC, Kuhn CM, Co JPT, Weiss KB. on behalf of the CLER Evaluation Committee and the CLER Program. *CLER National Report of Findings 2021.* Accreditation Council for Graduate Medical Education; 2021.
139. Colbert-Getz JM, Bierer SB, Berry A, et al. What is an innovation article? A systematic overview of innovation in health professions education journals. *Acad Med.* 2021;96(11S):S39–S47.

Appendix

Chapter 1

Appendix 1.1 Template Based on AMEE Guide 140: Proposed Full Description of an EPA

1. EPA title			
2. Specifications and limitations	*This activity contains or may contain the following elements* *A summative entrustment decision for this EPA does not apply for*		
3. Potential risks in case of failure			
4. Most relevant competency domains[a]	• Medical expert • Scholar • Leader	• Communicator • Professional	• Collaborator • Health advocate
5. Required knowledge, skills, attitudes, and experience	**Knowledge:** **Skills:** **Attitudes:** **Experience:**		
6. Information sources to assess progress and support summative entrustment			
7. When is each entrustment-supervision level expected?			
8. Expiry date			

[a]Choose framework that is applicable in your context.

Appendix 1.2 Carraccio Crosswalk

The "Handover EPA"[a] mapped to competencies and their milestones that are critical to making an entrustment decision, with examples of behaviors associated with the milestone for one of the performance levels[b]

Competencies Critical for Making an Entrustment Decision for This EPA	Milestone Level 1	Milestone Level 2	Milestone Level 3	Milestone Level 4	Milestone Level 5
Patient care. Organize and prioritize responsibilities to provide care that is safe, effective, and efficient.		Organizes the simultaneous care of a few patients with efficiency; occasionally prioritizes patient care responsibilities to proactively anticipate future needs; each additional patient or interruption in work leads to notable decreases in efficiency and ability to effectively prioritize; permanent breaks in task with interruptions are less common, but prolonged breaks in task are still common.			
Patient care. Provide transfer of care that ensures seamless transitions.		Uses a standard template for the information provided during the handoff. Unable to deviate from that template to adapt to more complex situations. May have errors of omission or commission, particularly when clinical information is not synthesized. Neither anticipates nor attends to the needs of the receiver of information.			
Interpersonal and communication skills.		Begins to understand the purpose of the communication and at times adjusts length to context, as appropriate.			
Communicate with physicians and other health professionals.		However, will often still err on the side of inclusion of excess details.			
Interpersonal and communication skills.		Documentation often contains all appropriate data sections, although some information may be missing from some sections or presented in a sequence that confuses the reader (evolution of symptoms is not documented chronologically). Documentation may be overly lengthy and detailed. It may contain erroneous information carried forward from review of the past medical record.			
Maintain comprehensive, timely, and legible medical records.		However, the practitioner at this stage begins to go beyond documentation of specific encounters and may update the patient-specific databases (e.g., problem list and diabetes care flowsheet) where applicable.			
Practice-based learning and improvement.		Documentation is often in the medical record in a timely manner, but may need subsequent amendment to be considered complete. Handwritten documentation is usually legible, timed, dated, and signed.			
Incorporate formative evaluation feedback into daily practice.		Dependent on external sources of feedback for improvement; beginning to acknowledge other points of view, but reinterprets feedback in a way that serves their own need for praise or consequence avoidance rather than informing a personal quest for improvement; little to no behavioral change occurs in response to feedback (e.g., listens to feedback but takes away only those messages they want to hear).			

Competencies Critical for Making an Entrustment Decision for This EPA	Milestone Level 1	Milestone Level 2	Milestone Level 3	Milestone Level 4	Milestone Level 5
Practice-based learning and improvement. Use information technology to optimize learning and care delivery.		Demonstrates a willingness to try new technology for patient care assignments or learning. Able to identify and use several available databases, search engines, or other appropriate tools, resulting in a manageable volume of information, most of which is relevant to the clinical question. Basic use of an EHR is improving, as evidenced by greater efficacy and efficiency in performing needed tasks. Beginning to identify shortcuts to getting to the right information quickly, such as use of filters. Also beginning to avoid shortcuts that lead one astray of the correct information or perpetuate incorrect information in the electronic health record.			

[a]A general pediatrics and common subspecialty EPA: "Facilitate handovers to another healthcare provider either within or across settings."
[b]This chart illustrates the mapping of the pediatrics "handover EPAs" to the competencies (shown in the left-hand column) and their associated milestones for five performance levels (shown in columns 2 through 6). The chart includes descriptions of behaviors for the milestone for level 2 to illustrate how the milestones for the five performance levels are associated with their competencies. Levels 1 to 5 represent progression along a developmental trajectory from novice to advanced beginner, competent learner, proficient learner, and expert learner. The authors caution that labels of the levels (e.g., "advanced beginner") be avoided, to keep the learner and the assessor focused on behaviors rather than labels. The authors propose how assessment in GME, based on EPAs and milestones, can guide both certification and maintenance of certification programs to complete the bridge across the medical education continuum.
EPAs, Entrustable Professional Activities; *GME*, graduate medical education.

Appendix 1.3 Van Melle's Core Components for CBME[a] Worksheet

Component	Description	Assessment of Your Program's Effectiveness
An outcomes-based competency framework	• Desired outcomes of training are identified based on societal needs. • Outcomes are paramount, meaning graduate abilities to function as an effective health professional.	
Progressive sequencing of competencies	• In CBME, competencies and their developmental markers must be explicitly sequenced to support learner progression from novice to master clinician. • Sequencing must take into account that some competencies form building blocks for the development of further competence. • Progression is not always a smooth, predictable curve.	
Learning experiences tailored to competencies In CBME	• Time is a resource, not a driver. • Learning experiences should be sequenced in a way that supports the progression of competence. • There must be flexibility to accommodate variation in individual learner progression. • Learning experiences should resemble the practice environment. • Learning experiences should be carefully selected to enable acquisition of one or many abilities. • Most learning experiences should be tied to an essential graduate ability.	
Teaching tailored to competencies	• Clinical teaching emphasizes learning through experience and application, not just knowledge acquisition. • Teachers use coaching techniques to diagnose a learner in clinical situations and give actionable feedback. • Teaching is responsive to individual learner needs. • Learners are actively engaged in determining their learning needs. • Teachers and learners work together to solve complex clinical problems.	

Continued

Component	Description	Assessment of Your Program's Effectiveness
Programmatic assessment	• There are multiple points and methods for data collection. • Methods for data collection match the quality of the competency being assessed. • Emphasis is on workplace observation. • Emphasis is on providing personalized, timely, meaningful feedback. • Progression is based on entrustment. • There is a robust system for decision-making.	

[a]Adapted from Dr. Elaine Van Melle, Queens University, Canada.
CBME, Competency-based medical education.

Chapter 3

Appendix 3.1 Example of Assessment and Curriculum Matrix for US Competency Milestones

Milestones	Teaching Methods	Major Rotation/ Learning Experiences (Goals)	Assessment Methods and Tools (e.g.)							Questions, Reflections and Issues in Assessment for this Competency
			Direct Obs. Tools	Faculty Evals (Global Assmt)	Clinical Reasoning Assess (CSR)	Medical Record Audit and/or Review	Multisource Feedback (i.e., 360)	Simulation	Other	
Patient Care										
PC___										
PC___										
PC___										

Milestones	Teaching Methods	Major Rotation/ Learning Experiences (Goals)	Assessment Methods and Tools (e.g.)							Questions & Realizations
			Direct Obs. Tools	Faculty Evals (Global Assmt)	Clinical Reasoning Assess (CSR)	Medical Record Audit and/or Review	Multisource Feedback (i.e., 360)	Simulation	Other	
Medical Knowledge										
MK___										
MK___										
MK___										

Milestones	Teaching Methods	Major Rotation/ Learning Experiences (Goals)	Assessment Methods and Tools (e.g.)							Questions & Realizations
			Direct Obs. Tools	Faculty Evals (Global Assmt)	Clinical Reasoning Assess (CSR)	Medical Record Audit and/or Review	Multisource Feedback (i.e., 360)	Simulation	Other	
Professionalism										
Prof___										
Prof___										
Prof___										

Milestones	Teaching Methods	Major Rotation/ Learning Experiences (Goals)	Assessment Methods and Tools (e.g.)							Questions & Realizations
			Direct Obs. Tools	Faculty Evals (Global Assmt)	Clinical Reasoning Assess (CSR)	Medical Record Audit and/or Review	Multisource Feedback (i.e., 360)	Simulation	Other	
Interpersonal Skills and Communication										
ISC___										
ISC___										
ISC___										

Milestones	Teaching Methods	Major Rotation/ Learning Experiences (Goals)	Assessment Methods and Tools (e.g.)							Questions & Realizations
			Direct Obs. Tools	Faculty Evals (Global Assmt)	Clinical Reasoning Assess (CSR)	Medical Record Audit and/or Review	Multisource Feedback (i.e., 360)	Simulation	Other	
Practice-based Learning and Improvement										
PBLI___										
PBLI___										
PBLI___										

Continued

Milestones	Teaching Methods	Major Rotation/ Learning Experiences (Goals)	Assessment Methods and Tools (e.g.)							Questions & Realizations
			Direct Obs. Tools	Faculty Evals (Global Assmt)	Clinical Reasoning Assess (CSR)	Medical Record Audit and/or Review	Multisource Feedback (i.e., 360)	Simulation	Other	
Systems-based Practice										
SBP___										
SBP___										
SBP___										

Appendix 3.2 Consolidated Framework for Implementation of Competency Milestones Version 2.0 in the United States

Element/Topic	Description	Implications for Milestones 2.0
I. Intervention characteristics		
Intervention source	Perception of key stakeholders about whether the educational intervention is externally or internally developed	Milestones 2.0 was developed through a collaborative, community-based process, but Milestones 2.0 will likely be seen as an "external" process by GME programs and PDs.
Evidence strength and quality	Stakeholders' perception of the validity of evidence supporting the belief that the educational intervention will produce desired outcomes	While there is a growing body of validity evidence for the Milestones approach, continued work is needed to continually build validity evidence in Milestones 2.0.
Relative advantage	Stakeholders' perception of the advantage of implementing the intervention versus an alternative solution	At the moment, the only alternative is a historical one—competencies without Milestones. Prior work noted that implementation of the competencies without Milestones was difficult. Even EPAs, seen by some as an "alternative" to Milestones, are actually dependent on competencies for their proper construction and use.
Adaptability	The degree to which an intervention can be adapted, tailored, and/or refined to meet local needs	Local contextual factors have and will continue to affect the use of Milestones 2.0 in all specialties. The Supplemental Guides are designed to allow programs to add local examples to facilitate adaptation to local context and circumstances.
Trialability	The ability to test the educational intervention on a small scale and reverse course if warranted	While trialability was initially used in the early days of Milestones 1.0, there is limited trailability with Milestones 2.0. To allow for continued improvement, Milestones are part of the CQI, formative part of accreditation in the United States designed to enable ongoing refinement. A CQI mindset can enable an iterative approach to implementation.
Complexity	Perceived complexity, reflected by duration, scope, radicalness, disruptiveness, centrality, and intricacy and number of steps required to implement	As noted earlier, there is no question Milestones is a complex educational intervention with a long journey and broad scope, and requires multiple steps and components.
Design quality	Perceived excellence in how the educational intervention is bundled, presented, and assembled	Milestones Version 2.0 has undergone a number of changes across the specialties and now comes with a supplemental guide. It will be important to continually interact and learn from the GME community to see if the changes are helpful and impactful.

Element/Topic	Description	Implications for Milestones 2.0
Cost	Cost of the educational intervention	The biggest cost of the Milestones are time, requiring better assessment, the use of CCCs, and more engagement on the part of the fellow. There are also costs associated with learning management systems and potentially costs with assessment tools.
II. Outer Setting		
Cosmopolitanism	Degree to which an organization is networked with other external organizations	Robust learning networks are essential to moving innovation and change forward. Unfortunately, this is an area where GME continues to struggle, rarely reaching across specialty lines and learning from each other. Milestones 2.0 is an opportunity to enhance networks, both within a specialty but also across other specialties and health professionals.
Peer pressure	Mimetic or competitive pressure to implement an educational intervention	Interestingly, this has not been a major driver for innovation or change in GME.
External Policy and Incentives	A broad construct that includes external strategies to spread interventions including policy and regulations, external mandates, and recommendations.	Milestones are an external mandate from ACGME. The key policy position is that Milestones are a formative, developmental, descriptive rubric to guide curriculum and better assessment. Remember, Level 4 (proficiency) is a goal, not a requirement.
III. Inner Setting		
Learner needs and resources	The extent to which learner needs, as well as barriers and facilitators to meet those needs, are accurately known and prioritized by the organization	Research in Milestones 1.0 helped reveal key facilitators and barriers around learner needs. For example, we know learners need to be active agents in their learning and assessment. Creation of individualized learning plans is essential. A philosophy of coproduction can also help to advance the use of Milestones 2.0.
Structural characteristics	The social architecture, age, maturity, and size of the organization	As noted above, the use of Milestones is embedded in multiple, complex social settings. The size of a program and institution can have profound impact on implementation of the Milestones.
Networks and communications	The nature and quality of webs of social networks and the nature and quality of formal and informal communications within an organization	There are multiple actors and agents involved with Milestones 2.0. The strengths and quality of the interactions and interdependencies are crucial to the ability of Milestones 2.0 to enhance GME programs.
Culture	Norms, values, and basic assumptions of a given organization	Culture eats strategy. For Milestones 2.0, programs need to believe and buy into the importance of fellowship as an intensely developmental process, thereby necessitating the need for developmental assessments to support Milestones 2.0.
Implementation climate	The absorptive capacity for change, shared receptivity of involved individuals, and extent the use of the educational intervention will be rewarded, supported, and expected within the organization	A major issue for Milestones 2.0 as there is unquestionably a risk for change fatigue. Milestones 2.0 was approached from the perspective of improving the content and process of the Milestones, but ongoing surveillance and refinement will be needed.
• Tension for change	The degree to which stakeholders perceive the current situation as intolerable or needing change	Research from Milestones 1.0 has clearly shown this perception ranges across and within specialties. There was clearly some unhappiness with the design of Milestones 1.0, and initial reactions to Milestones 2.0 has been more favorable but will require ongoing, longitudinal research.
• Compatibility	The degree of tangible fit between meaning and values attached to the educational intervention, how those align with the individuals' (e.g., PDs) own norms, values, and perceived risks and needs, and how the intervention fits with existing workflows and systems	This characteristic highlights the centrality and critical importance of PD leadership and buy-in around the use of Milestones 2.0. Given Milestones are embedded in complex clinical and educational systems, a systems-thinking approach to implementing Milestones 2.0 is needed.
• Relative priority	Individuals' shared perception of the importance of the implementation within the organization	For Milestones 2.0, share mental models and shared perceptions of the importance of Milestones is essential. If programs detect a mismatch here, closing the gap will be an important step for the program.

Continued

Element/Topic	Description	Implications for Milestones 2.0
• Goals and feedback	The degrees to which goals are clearly communicated, acted upon, and fed back to staff and alignment of that feedback with goals	It is essential that learners and faculty understand the goals of Milestones, and that feedback loops for both the learner and program are robust and continuous. The Milestone Guidebooks can be very helpful.
Learning climate	A climate in which (a) leaders express their own fallibility and need for team members' assistance and input; (b) team members feel that they are essential, valued, and knowledgeable partners in the change process; (c) individuals feel psychologically safe to try new methods; and (d) there is sufficient time and space for reflective thinking and evaluation	The clinical learning environment has clear effects on both educational and clinical outcomes. Psychological safety for learners is essential to empowering them to seek assessment and feedback, and to engage in coproduction with faculty. Faculty and program leaders must also create safe spaces and time for reflection and evaluation of how the program is performing, including the use of Milestones.
Readiness for implementation	Tangible and immediate indicators of organizational commitment to its decision to implement an intervention	Given Milestones are required for accreditation, the key issue here is to ensure that the institution and department are committed to advancing educational improvement and using the competencies and Milestones as one part of the educational system.
• Leadership engagement	Commitment, involvement, and accountability of leaders and managers with the implementation	Leadership is critical in implementing change. Research is clear that implementation tends to be more successful with the presence of a thoughtful, committed opinion leader.
• Available resources	The level of resources dedicated for implementation and on-going operations, including money, training, education, physical space, and time	Always a major challenge for GME programs writ large. Time is always at a premium. In addition, faculty development around the Milestones and, especially, assessment is essential for outcomes-based education. Resources for faculty development can be limited, but the regional hub faculty development program in assessment may be helpful to GME faculty.
• Access to knowledge and information	Ease of access to digestible information, and knowledge about the intervention and how to incorporate it into work tasks	All GME communities continue to learn and struggle with using Milestones as they are a fundamental shift in how we teach and assess. The CCC and Milestones Guidebooks, the National Milestones Data Report with predictive analytics and other metrics, and the Milestones bibliography can all help.
IV. Characteristics of Individuals		
Knowledge and belief about the educational intervention	Individuals' attitudes toward and value placed on the intervention as well as familiarity with facts, truths, and principles related to the educational intervention	Faculty and learner understanding of the Milestones continues to evolve. For PDs, it is really important to engage fellows and faculty early in learning about the new specific Milestones and the pedagogical principles and science that underlie both CBME and the Milestones.
Self-efficacy	Individual belief in their own capabilities to execute courses of action to achieve implementation goals,	Faculty and learners do not like to feel incompetent or incapable about their work. Teaching, assessment, feedback and coaching are no different. As noted above, coproducing change with the fellows can enhance their self-efficacy, along with encouraging guided self-assessment, reflection with advisors, and the creation of individualized learning plans. Faculty development is also essential to build self-efficacy and skills.
Individual stage of change	Characterization of the phase an individual is in, as they progress toward skilled, enthusiastic, and sustained use of the intervention	The stages of change model can be very helpful in guiding implementation of educational changes. The stage of the individual, from precontemplative to action, will help guide the approach to helping each individual use Milestones.
Individual identification with organization	A broad construct related to how individuals perceive the organization, and their relationship and degree of commitment with that organization	PDs may want to assess how their learners and faculty perceive the department and institution in regard to supporting educational change and innovation. Are they supportive and enthusiastic, or will the GME program need to "build the case?"

Element/Topic	Description	Implications for Milestones 2.0
Other personal attributes	A broad construct to include other personal traits such as tolerance of ambiguity, intellectual ability, motivation, values, competence, capacity, and learning style	Systems depend on interactions between multiple individuals who bring varying degrees of motivation, tolerance for uncertainty, competence in various educational skills, capacity for change, and learning style preferences that can impact the implementation of Milestones.
V. Process		
Planning	The degree to which a scheme or method of behavior and tasks for implementing an intervention are developed in advance, and the quality of those schemes or methods	GME programs should build on lessons learned in Milestones 1.0, such as effective CCC group process, individualized learning plans, and programmatic assessment, while preparing to implement the new specialty-specific patient care and medical knowledge competencies, and the four new harmonized Milestones.
Engaging	Attracting and involving appropriate individuals in the implementation and use of the intervention through a combined strategy of social marketing, education, role modeling, training, and other similar activities	All of these recommendations apply to the implementation of Milestones 2.0, including using the principles of coproduction with fellows.
• Opinion leaders	Individuals in an organization who have formal or informal influence on the attitudes and beliefs of their colleagues with respect to implementing the intervention	Opinion leaders, most often through role modeling and active engagement, can substantially enhance implementation efforts.
• Formally appointed internal implementation leaders	Individuals from within the organization who have been formally appointed with responsibility for implementing an intervention as coordinator, project manager, team leader, or other similar role	Implementation, like all of medicine, requires interprofessional team effort, even for educational interventions. Be sure to identify a group of individuals, including fellows, to manage and improve curriculum and assessment during the Milestones 2.0 process.
• Champions	"Individuals who dedicate themselves to supporting, marketing, and 'driving through' an [implementation]," overcoming indifference or resistance that the intervention may provoke in an organization	Champions are by definition highly active agents in helping others adopt a change and implement that change effectively.
• External change agents	Individuals who are affiliated with an outside entity who formally influence or facilitate intervention decisions in a desirable direction	Specialty societies can be facilitators in the implementation of Milestones 2.0. It is also strongly encouraged that all programs take advantage of the multiple educational resources at ACGME, including the Milestones guidebook for residents and fellows.
Executing	Carrying out or accomplishing the implementation according to plan	This is obviously a complex, longitudinal task that will require ongoing evaluation and refinement.
Reflecting and evaluating	Quantitative and qualitative feedback about the progress and quality of implementation accompanied with regular personal and team debriefing about progress and experience	Ongoing evaluation of the GME program, using all available data sources such as the Milestones data, the national Milestones data, the resident and faculty surveys, and local evaluation efforts to continuously improve the program. This is one of the major goals of the annual program evaluation.

ACGME, Accreditation Council for Graduate Medical Education; *CBME*, competency-based medical education; *CCC*, clinical competency committees; *CQI*, continuous quality improvement; *EPAs*, Entrustable Professional Activities; *GME*, graduate medical education; *PDs*, program directors.
Modified from Damschroder LJ, Aron DC, Keith RE, Kirsh SR, Alexander JA, Lowery JC. Fostering implementation of health services research findings into practice: a consolidated framework for advancing implementation science. *Implement Sci*. 2009;4:50. doi:10.1186/1748-5908-4-50.

Chapter 4

Appendix 4.1 The RIME Evaluation Framework: A Vocabulary of Professional Progress

We describe performance goals for trainees using the following progression: Reporter, Interpreter, Manager, Educator (RIME). The framework emphasizes a developmental approach and distinguishes between basic and advanced expectations. Each step represents a synthesis of skills, knowledge, and attitude—a final, common pathway of professional competencies—and is useful for setting *minimal* expectations for a learner. A learner's progress toward higher steps is usually apparent in the basic stages. Trainees might function at a reporter level for a complex problem and at a higher level for problems that are more common. RIME can be applied to single patient encounters or to overall level of consistency.

Reporter: The learner can and does accurately gather and clearly communicate the clinical facts on their own patients and can answer the "what" questions. Proficiency in this step requires the basic skill to do a history and physical examination and the basic knowledge to know what to look for. The step emphasizes day-to-day reliability; for instance, being on time or following up on a patient's test results. Implicit in the step is the ability to recognize normal from abnormal and the confidence to identify and label a new problem. This step requires a sense of responsibility and "ownership," achieving consistency in bedside skills in dealing directly with patients. These skills are often introduced to students in their preclinical years, but by the third year they must be mastered as a "passing" criterion. This level is a nonnegotiable expectation for interns for all patients.

Interpreter: Some transition from reporter to interpreter is an essential step in the growth of a clerkship student, and is often the most difficult. At a basic level, a student must prioritize among problems they have identified. The signs of diagnostic reasoning, such as active use of pertinent positives and negatives, and key findings that imply differential diagnosis become apparent and penetrate the process of reporting. Problem lists give syndromes and not merely repetition of findings. The next step is to offer an explicit differential diagnosis, explicitly supported. Because a public forum can be intimidating to beginners and third-year students cannot be expected to have the "right answer" all the time, we define student success as offering at least three reasonable diagnostic possibilities for new problems, but they must take public ownership of the process of clinical reasoning. Follow-up of tests provides another opportunity to interpret the data (especially in the clinic setting). This step requires a higher level of knowledge, more skill in stating the clinical findings that support possible diagnoses, and applying test results to specific patients. A learner must emotionally make the transition from bystander to seeing themselves as an active participant in patient care and taking ownership of answering what Hemmer calls the "why?" questions. Interns should be able to interpret, though for unusual problems, their knowledge may limit them.

Manager: Managing patient care takes even more knowledge, more confidence, and more judgment in deciding when action needs to be taken, and to propose and select among options; to answer the "how?" questions for getting things done. We cannot require novices to be right with each suggestion, so we ask students to include at least three *reasonable* options in their diagnostic and therapeutic plan, but they must take ownership of the process of clinical decision-making. Finishing interns should be able to manage common problems they will see; advanced residents should be proficient at managing atypical and complex cases and using the full resources of the specific practice setting. An essential element is working with each particular patient's circumstances and preferences; that is, to be patient centered, which depends upon interpersonal skills and the ability to educate patients.

Educator: This is part of being a manager, and the action is focused on a learning plan for the physician and the patient. Success in each prior step depends on self-directed learning and on a mastery of basics; but to be an educator in the RIME scheme means to go beyond the required basics, to read deep, and to share new learning with others; in other words, to take ownership of the process of self-evaluation and improvement. Having the drive and time management skills to look for hard evidence on which clinical practice can be based and knowing whether current evidence will stand up to scrutiny are qualities of an advanced trainee; to share leadership in educating the team (and even the faculty) takes maturity and confidence. Systematically learning from one's own practice experience and being an educator are generally expected of residents.

Modified from Pangaro, LN. Evaluating professional growth: a new vocabulary and other innovations for improving the descriptive evaluation of students. *Acad Med.* 1999 Nov;74: 1203-1207. doi:10.1097/00001888-199911000-00012.

Appendix 4.2

INTERNAL MEDICINE RESIDENT EVALUATION FORM

Resident's Name | Rotation Name

Attending's Name | Rotation Period | Evaluation Date

In evaluating the resident's performance, use as your standard the level of knowledge, skills, and attitudes expected from the clearly satisfactory resident at this stage of training. **For any component that needs attention or is rated a 4 or less, please provide specific comments and recommendations on the back of the form.** Be as specific as possible, including reports of critical incidents and/or outstanding performance. Global adjectives or remarks, such as "good resident," do not provide meaningful feedback to the resident.

	Unsatisfactory	Satisfactory	Superior	
1. Patient Care Incomplete, inaccurate medical interviews, physical examinations, and review of other data; incompetent performance of essential procedures; fails to analyze clinical data and consider patient preferences when making medical decisions ❑ Insufficient contact to judge	**1 2 3**	**4 5 6** ❑ Performance needs attention	**7 8 9**	Superb, accurate, comprehensive medical interviews, physical examinations, review of other data, and procedural skills; always makes diagnostic and therapeutic decisions based on available evidence, sound judgment, and patient preferences
2. Medical Knowledge Limited knowledge of basic and clinical sciences; minimal interest in learning; does not understand complex relations, mechanisms of disease ❑ Insufficient contact to judge	**1 2 3**	**4 5 6** ❑ Performance needs attention	**7 8 9**	Exceptional knowledge of basic and clinical sciences; highly resourceful development of knowledge; comprehensive understanding of complex relationships, mechanisms of disease
3. Practice-Based Learning Improvement Fails to perform self-evaluation; lacks insight, initiative; resists or ignores feedback; fails to use information technology to enhance patient care or pursue self-improvement ❑ Insufficient contact to judge	**1 2 3**	**4 5 6** ❑ Performance needs attention	**7 8 9**	Constantly evaluates own performance, incorporates feedback into improvement activities; effectively uses technology to manage information for patient care and self-improvement
4. Interpersonal and Communication Skills Does not establish even minimally effective therapeutic relationships with patients and families; does not demonstrate ability to build relationships through listening, narrative, or nonverbal skills; does not provide education or counseling to patients, families, or colleagues ❑ Insufficient contact to judge	**1 2 3**	**4 5 6** ❑ Performance needs attention	**7 8 9**	Establishes a highly effective therapeutic relationship with patients and families; demonstrates excellent relationship building through listening, narrative, and nonverbal skills; excellent education and counseling of patients, families, and colleagues; always "interpersonally" engaged

Continued

Appendix 4.2—cont'd

	Unsatisfactory	Satisfactory	Superior	
5. Professionalism Lacks respect, compassion, integrity, honesty; disregards need for self-assessment; fails to acknowledge errors; does not consider needs of patients, families, colleagues; does not display responsible behavior ❑ Insufficient contact to judge	1 2 3	4 5 6 ❑ Performance needs attention	7 8 9	Always demonstrates respect, compassion, integrity, honesty; teaches/role models responsible behavior; total commitment to self-assessment; willingly acknowledges errors; always considers needs of patients, families, colleagues
6. System-Based Learning Unable to access/mobilize outside resources; actively resists efforts to improve systems of care; does not use systematic approaches to reduce error and improve patient care ❑ Insufficient contact to judge	1 2 3	4 5 6 ❑ Performance needs attention	7 8 9	Effectively accesses/utilizes outside resources; effectively uses systematic approaches to reduce errors and improve patient care; enthusiastically assists in developing systems' improvement
Resident's Overall Clinical Competence in Internal Medicine on Rotation	1 2 3	4 5 6 ❑ Performance needs attention	7 8 9	

Attending's Comments

____

____

____

____

____

____

Signatures: Resident's __________________________ **Attending's** __________________________

Appendix 4.3

MEDICINE CLERKSHIP EVALUATION FORM

Student Name: ______________________ Dates: From ______________ To: ______________

Circle one: MIDPOINT or FINAL Site: ______________ Evaluator: ______________

For each area of evaluation, please check the appropriate level of ability. Qualities should be cumulative as rating increases, e.g., an outstanding rating for physical exam skills assumes that major findings are identified in an organized, focused manner AND that subtle findings are elicited. Indicate the level at which the student consistently performs.

OUTSTANDING	*ABOVE AVERAGE*	*ACCEPTABLE*	*NEEDS IMPROVEMENT*	*UNACCEPTABLE*
		DATA GATHERING		
Initial History/Interviewing Skill			If Not Observed, Check Here o	
o Resourceful, efficient, appreciates subtleties, prepares for management.	o Precise, detailed, appropriate to setting (ward or clinic), focused/selective.	o Obtains basic history. Identifies new problems. Accurate data gathering.	o Inconsistent reporter. Incomplete or unfocused. Inconsistent data gathering.	o Unreliable reporter. Inaccurate, major omissions, inappropriate.
Physical Examination Skill			If Not Observed, Check Here o	
o Elicits subtle findings	o Organized, focused, relevant	o Major findings identified	o Incomplete, or insensitive to patient comfort	o Unreliable exam; misses major findings
		DATA RECORDING		
Written Histories & Physicals			If Not Observed, Check Here o	
o Concise, reflects thorough understanding of disease process & patient situation	o Documents key information, focused, comprehensive, reporting implies interpretation	o Accurate, complete, timely reporting. Takes ownership of reporter role.	o Often late; poor flow in HPI, lacks supporting detail, labs, or incomplete problem lists. Gaps in reporting.	o Inaccurate data about patient or disease. Major omissions. Unreliable reporting, recording.
Progress Notes/Clinic Notes			If Not Observed, Check Here o	
o Analytical in assessment and plan	o Precise, concise, organized	o Identifies ongoing problems & documents plan	o Needs organization, omits relevant data	o Reports incorrect or inaccurate data
Oral Presentations			If Not Observed, Check Here o	
o Tailored to situation (type of rounds); emphasis and selection of facts teaches others key points	o Fluent reporting; focused; good eye contact; selection of facts implies interpretation; uses minimal notes	o Maintains format, includes all basic information	o Major omissions, often includes irrelevant facts, rambling	o Consistently ill-prepared, does not know facts about patient, reports inaccurate information
		KNOWLEDGE		
In General			If Not Observed, Check Here o	
o Understands therapeutic interventions, broad-based	o Demonstrates thorough understanding of diagnostic approach; consistently able to interpret data	o Demonstrates understanding of basic pathophysiology	o Struggles to interpret data; demonstrates marginal understanding of basics.	o Major deficiencies in knowledge base
Relating To Own Patients			If Not Observed, Check Here o	
(check as consistently applicable) o Broad textbook mastery o Directed EBM search o Educator of others	o Provides expanded differential diagnoses, able to discuss minor problems; sufficient to suggest management	o Knows basic differential diagnoses of active problems in own patients; actively seeks knowledge	o Inconsistent and/or insufficient understanding, to be able to interpret consistently on own patients	o Lacks knowledge to understand own patients' problems; rarely sufficient to interpret
		DATA INTERPRETATION		
Analysis				
o Understands complex issues, interrelates patient problems	o Consistently offers reasonable interpretation of data	o Constructs problem list, applies basic, reasonable differential diagnosis	o Frequently reports data without analysis; problem lists need improvement	o Cannot interpret basic data; problem lists inaccurate/not updated
Judgment/Management				
o Insightful approach to management plans	o Diagnostic decisions are consistently reasonable	o Appropriate patient care, aware of own limitations	o Inconsistent prioritization of clinical issues	o Poor judgment, actions affect patient adversely
		MANAGEMENT SKILLS		
Patient Care Activities			If Not Observed, Check Here o	
o Negotiates with patients, coordinates health care team	o Efficient & effective, often takes initiative in follow-up (clinic or ward)	o Monitors active problems, maintains patient records, fulfills duty toward patient	o Needs prompting to complete tasks; follow-up is inconsistent	o Unwilling to do expected patient care activities; unreliable
Procedures			If Not Observed, Check Here o	
o Proficient and skillful; engages patient in informed consent process	o Careful, confident, compassionate, participates in informed consent process	o Reasonable skill in preparing for and doing procedures; reports indications	o Awkward, reluctant to try even basic procedures. Cannot relate indications	o No improvement even with coaching, insensitive toward patients

April 2008

Continued

Appendix 4.3—cont'd

PROFESSIONAL ATTITUDES

Reliability/Commitment

o Accepts full personal ownership in education & patient care	o Seeks responsibility as manager; views self as active participant in patient care	o Fulfills responsibility, accepts ownership of essential roles in care	o Often unprepared, not consistently present, not reporting accurately	o Unexplained absences, unreliable. Makes no promise of duty.

Response to Instruction/Feedback

o Continued self-assessment leads to further growth; insightful reflection	o Seeks and consistently improves with feedback; self-reflective.	o Takes ownership for improvement; generally improves with feedback	o Inconsistent, does not sustain improvement	o Lack of improvement; defensive/argumentative; avoids responsibility

Self-Directed Learning (knowledge and skills)

o Outstanding initiative, consistently educates others	o Sets own goals; reads, prepares in advance when possible	o Reads appropriately, and accepts ownership for self-education	o Needs prompting, not consistently improving expertise	o Unwilling, lack of introspection. Makes no effort to improve expertise

PROFESSIONAL DEMEANOR

Patient Interactions

o Preferred provider; seen as care manager by patients/teachers	o Gains confidence & trust, duty is evident to patient/health care team	o Sympathetic, respectful, develops rapport, gains trust	o Occasionally insensitive, inattentive; not trusted as advocate, reporter	o Avoids personal contact, tactless, rude, disrespectful

Response to Stress

o Outstanding poise, constructive solutions	o Flexible, supportive	o Appropriate adjustment	o Inflexible or loses composure easily	o Inappropriate coping

Working Relationships

o Establishes tone of mutual respect & dignity	o Good rapport with other hospital staff	o Cooperative, productive member of own team	o Lack of consideration for others	o Antagonistic or disruptive

DESCRIPTIVE COMMENTS: (Written descriptive comments are also required. **What is the "next step" for this student?**)
Please check each step the student has consistently reached: o Reporter o Interpreter o Manager o Educator

Recommended Grade: _____ Midpoint or Final (circle one) Have you discussed this report with the student? _____

Printed Name ____________ Signature ____________ Date ____________ Intern ____ Resident ____ Attending ____ Preceptor ____

Our System is Based on Performance Criteria Rather Than Percentages. Please Use These to Describe Current Level of Student Work

PASS: (Reporter) Satisfactory performance. Obtains and reports basic information completely, accurately, reliably; is beginning to interpret. Works professionally with patients, staff, colleagues. Distinctive personal qualities should be recognized in descriptive comments.

HIGH PASS: (Interpreter) Clearly more than typical work in most areas of evaluation. Consistently offers reasonable interpretations without prompting; good working fund of knowledge; an active participant in care. Consistent preparation for clinics. Promises of duty/expertise evident.

HONORS: (Manager/ Educator) Outstanding ratings in most major areas of evaluation. Fourth-year level of patient care, actively suggests reasonable management options; excellent general fund of knowledge, outstanding (broad/deep) knowledge on own patients. Strong qualities of leadership and excellence in interpersonal relationships. Able to take the lead with patients/families/professionals on solutions. Promises of duty and growing expertise clearly evident and exceptional.

LOW PASS: Overall marginal performance - performs acceptably in some areas but clearly needs improvement in others. Has shown evidence of progress and may be able to perform acceptably as an intern following additional experience in medicine during fourth year without having to repeat the entire third-year clerkship.

FAIL: Overall inadequate performance or unacceptable performance in any major area of evaluation. Little improvement with guidance. A recommendation of Fail means additional medicine rotation(s), usually at the third-year level, is/are needed to address deficiencies.

April 2008

Chapter 5

Appendix 5.1 Examples of Rater Training Workshops

1.5-Hour Workshop

Rater Training Content	Explanation	Time
Introductory lecture	• Rationale for direct observation • Sources of poor reliability of assessments	20 minutes
Demonstrate poor interrater reliability	• Participants watch and rate trigger video (5 minutes) • Discuss observations and ratings (10 minutes)	15 minutes
Barriers to direct observation	• Participants describe barriers to frequent, high-quality direct observation	5 minutes
Performance dimension training exercise	• Participants develop framework for skill (10 minutes) • Participants review evidence-based framework for skill (10 minutes) • Participants apply framework to video (10 minutes)	30 minutes
Frame of reference training	• Participants encouraged to shift to criterion-referenced assessment • Participants identify the behaviors needed for competence	10 minutes
Brainstorm direct observation snapshots	• Participants identify brief observations that would be valuable for learners and patients	10 minutes
Wrap-up	• Questions	5 minutes

3-Hour Workshop

Rater Training Content	Explanation	Time
Ice-breaker activity	• Discuss experiences being observed and doing observation	10 minutes
Introductory lecture	• Rationale for direct observation	20 minutes
Barriers to direct observation	• Group identifies barriers to direct observation	10 minutes
Demonstrate poor interrater reliability	• Participants watch and rate trigger video (5 minutes) • Discuss observations and ratings (10 minutes) • Discuss sources of poor reliability of assessments (15 minutes)	30 minutes
Break		10 minutes
Performance dimension training exercise	• Participants develop framework for skill (10 minutes) • Participants compared to evidence-based framework (10 min) • Participants apply framework to video (10 minutes)	30 minutes
Frame of reference training	• Participants describe standard used to select rating • Participants taught to shift to criterion-referenced assessment and enstrustment • Participants identify what is required for satisfactory performance • Participants apply framework to two additional videos of the same skill	40 minutes
Preparation for direct observation	• Discuss preparing learner, preparing patient for direct observation • Teach concept of triangulation	10 minutes
Brainstorm how to do snapshots of observation	• Participants identify brief observations that would be valuable for learners and patients while not necessarily taking extra time for faculty	10 minutes
Wrap-up	• Questions	10 minutes

Continued

Full Day Workshop. The workshop additions can be added to the 3-hour workshop to create a full day training experience in direct observation.

Workshop Additions

Rater Training Content	Explanation	Time
Feedback	Review how to give feedback	60 minutes
Direct Observation Simulation Workshop (see Appendix 5.5 for details)		
Overview	Review goals of simulation	10 minutes
Station 1	Clinical Skill 1 Observation and Feedback	40 minutes
Station 2	Clinical Skill 2 Observation and Feedback	40 minutes
Break		10 minutes
Station 3	Clinical Skill 3 Observation and Feedback	40 minutes
Station 4	Clinical Skill 4 Observation and Feedback	40 minutes
Debrief	Discuss perceptions of day	15 minutes

Spaced Longitudinal Practice

Timing	Content	Time[a]
6 weeks after initial workshop	• Skill 1: watch 2–3 videos, rate independently then discuss as group or compare to expert • Skill 2: watch 2–3 videos, rate independently then discuss as group or compare to expert	30–45 minutes 30–45 minutes
6–8 weeks later	• Skill 1: watch 2–3 videos, rate independently then discuss as group or compare to expert • Skill 2: watch 2–3 videos, rate independently then discuss as group or compare to expert	30–45 minutes 30–45 minutes
6–8 weeks later	• Skill 1: watch 2–3 videos, rate independently then discuss as group or compare to expert • Skill 2: watch 2–3 videos, rate independently then discuss as group or compare to expert	30–45 minutes 30–45 minutes
Annual	• Skill 1: watch 2–3 videos, rate independently then discuss as group or compare to expert • Skill 2: watch 2–3 videos, rate independently then discuss as group or compare to expert	30–45 minutes 30–45 minutes

[a]Spaced learning can be done asynchronously using a learning management platform.

Appendix 5.2 Faculty Guide to Training Videos

As part of this textbook, you have access to a set of nine training videos of recorded learner–patient encounters that can help facilitate faculty development programs focusing on improving direct observation and feedback skills in medical interviewing, physical examination, and counseling. These videos can be used in conjunction with the training methods discussed in this chapter. The medical interviewing and counseling videos come from an effort by the Accreditation Council for Graduate Medical Education (ACGME) in the United States to improve faculty skills in direct observation. The ACGME provides an open-access (i.e., free) faculty toolkit for direct observation under the assessment tab at Learn@ACGME (Assessment [acgme.org]). Readers are encouraged to check out this resource that provides over 30 videos with answer keys for your own faculty development.

This appendix provides descriptions of the training scenarios. The scenarios are scripted to depict three levels of performance. Learner and clinical care deficiencies are demonstrated in each level—none of the videos are designed to demonstrate mastery-level performance. There are three scenarios for each clinical skill of medical interviewing, physical examination, and counseling; each successive scenario displays progressively better aspects of performance. Finally, a video is provided of what *not* to do when performing an observation (described later; Video Scenario 5.10). This can be a very useful video to include in workshops.

However, as discussed in this chapter, the ultimate question the rater, or judge, must ask themselves is whether the patient received safe, effective, patient-centered care.

Answering this question first logically informs decisions around entrustment and supervision of the learner moving forward. Key deficiencies, or "errors," for each clinical encounter scenario are outlined in the materials provided. It is important to note that the deficiencies range from minor to more severe; the judgment of the faculty is an important component of the training exercises. You can use this guide to help you discuss and calibrate your own faculty in workshops. We recommend you review the scenarios carefully on your own with the guidelines to become comfortable with the clinical encounters before using them in workshops with your own faculty. Finally, frameworks for data gathering and informed decision-making are provided at the end of this appendix as potentially useful tools for you to use in faculty development. We encourage you to use these frameworks as guides or evidence-based frames of reference, and not as checklists, when viewing and judging these videos as part of your own and your program's faculty development.

Facilitator Key to the Clinical Scenarios

As noted previously, the videos are scripted to illustrate varying levels of learner development and competence; all scenarios contain at least some deficiencies. The scenarios were developed iteratively for use in research studies on direct observation. Separate appendices are provided that describe and highlight the deficiencies deliberately scripted for each encounter. You may not agree with all of them; this could be a rich source for dialogue with your workshop group. Some deficiencies are more blatant than others; the key simply denotes the presence or absence of the deficiency, not the degree or magnitude of the deficiency. There may be other deficiencies you detect that could also serve as a rich source of dialogue and exploration during a workshop. As we noted throughout this chapter, faculty judgment is important. However, research has also clearly demonstrated that *informed, evidence-based judgment* is paramount. Many of your faculty will likely also possess some deficiencies in their own clinical skills. Faculty development in direct observation, using many of the tools provided in this chapter, can become a "twofer" experience: help faculty improve their own clinical skills while learning to enhance their observation, rating, and feedback skills. All of these videos can be used for direct observation of competence training described in this chapter. The facilitator key is provided in the format of an abstraction instrument. The key can be used to assess faculty performance in direct observation, and to provide feedback to the faculty. The criteria are based on an absolute (criteria, not a relative [normative-based]) scale for optimal patient care. Again, to reiterate, the primary frame of reference for an observation is whether (or not) the patient received safe, effective, patient-centered care. Your faculty may have different points of view depending on the level of learner you choose for your direct observation exercises.

How Faculty Should Conduct an Effective Observation (Scenario 5.10)

A separate video (Video 5.10) is provided to illustrate important concepts in direct observation. The focus of this scenario is on the faculty physician performing the observation of a resident or student. This scenario provides multiple examples of what not to do when performing an observation. A few points should be noted about this direct observation by the faculty attending:

1. The faculty member is late, disrupting the flow of the trainee–patient encounter.
2. He does a poor job of explaining to the patient what his role will be during the observation and was not explicit with the trainee about what he will do during the physical examination.
3. His positioning to observe the physical examination is poor; he is seated behind the patient and in front of the trainee. This makes it very difficult for him to see if the physical examination maneuvers were done correctly, and having the observer right in front of the patient may be distracting to the trainee.
4. He disrupts the blood pressure measurement by trying to wash his hands during the measurement.
5. He disrupts the eye examination by moving around and inserting himself into the examination process. One reason this may have distracted the trainee was the lack of explanation by the faculty physician on what he would do during the examination (see item 2).
6. He further disrupts the examination by asking the patient questions during the trainee's examination of the lungs. This could have been avoided had the faculty physician reviewed the patient's history and presenting concern with the trainee before observing the physical examination. The medical history presentation could have been done at the bedside. This would have cued the faculty physician on what he should be looking for during the physical examination.
7. The faculty physician is distracted by a knock at the door. This distraction causes him to miss a critical component of the examination: the cardiac examination in a patient presenting with syncope.

These are the major take-home points from this direct observation encounter. Some basic principles for effective direct observation are:

- Prepare for the observation.
- Faculty: Know what you are looking for.
- Resident: Let them know what to expect.
- Patient: Let them know why you are there.
- Minimize intrusiveness—correct positioning using "triangulation," when possible.
- Minimize interference with the trainee–patient interaction.
- Avoid distractions.

Appendix 5.3 Steps for Performance Dimension Training

- Participants watch a stimulus video of a learner taking a history from or counseling a patient and complete a rater assessment form. The learner is scripted as requiring indirect supervision.
- Participants share their ratings, the rationale for their ratings, and the standard they used to select their rating.
- Participants work in small groups of four to eight to develop a list of behaviors that constitute aspirational history taking or counseling (e.g., what should be asked, done, conveyed, and how). The list of items should be behavioral and observable.
- Groups review an evidence-based framework of behaviors associated with effective history taking or counseling and compare the framework to the list of behaviors they identified.
- Groups apply their framework back to the video.

Appendix 5.4 Overview of Frame of Reference Training

- Participants develop/are given descriptions for each dimension of competence. They then discuss what the qualifications are for each dimension.
- Participants define what constitutes superior skill (the most effective criteria and behaviors) from the perspective of optimal patient outcomes.
- Participants define and reach consensus on the minimal criteria for satisfactory performance, defined as safe, effective, patient-centered care (competent). Once the satisfactory criteria are set, marginal criteria are defined. Everything else by default is unsatisfactory performance.
- Participants are asked to make a prospective entrustment decision using their framework.
- Participants are shown videos demonstrating performance from unsatisfactory to average to outstanding and asked to differentiate levels of performance.
- Participants write narrative assessments and provide an entrustment rating.
- Session trainer/facilitator shares the expert narrative assessment and expert consensus rating with rationale.
- Training session concludes with a discussion about the discrepancies between the participants' ratings and the expert ratings.

Appendix 5.5 Materials for Direct Observation and Feedback Practice With Standardized Residents and Patients

Facilitator Guide: Direct Observation of Clinical Skills Simulation Workshop

Prior to Arriving to the Workshop

1. Review the scenario you have assigned.
2. Review the framework for the skill associated with your station.
3. Review the resident instructions for satisfactory/unsatisfactory performance. Think of specific behaviors the resident can portray to further demonstrate satisfactory/unsatisfactory performance.
4. Review the resident instructions for receiving feedback. Think about specific behaviors the resident can portray to demonstrate insight/lack of insight/receptivity to/lack of receptivity to feedback.
5. Remind yourself of the concepts of performance dimension training, frame of reference training, inference, and principles of effective feedback.

Workshop Overview

Faculty will be divided into groups of four to six. There are (INSERT #) of stations. The stations are (INSERT CONTENT OF STATIONS). Each station lasts 40 to 60 minutes. The goals for each station are to discuss the skill (performance dimension training), let faculty observe an encounter, have faculty discuss their observations and ratings, let a faculty participant give the resident feedback, and discuss the feedback. The structure of each station is described in more detail in the following sections.

Meeting Your Resident and Practicing With Them

1. You will have 30 minutes to meet with your resident and standardized patient (SP) on the morning of the workshop prior to the start of the session.
2. Ask the resident if they have any questions about the case, training materials, or skills they are being asked to portray.
3. Watch the resident practice the case with the SP. Let them run through the case at least twice (satisfactory/unsatisfactory). Provide suggestions for skills to include/exclude. SPs often have helpful suggestions as well.
4. Remind the resident/SP to keep the encounter to less than 10 minutes.

Facilitator Role

1. As your group enters the room, ask the resident/SP to leave the room.

2. Tell your group what the station skill is (e.g., history, counseling, breaking bad news, etc.).
3. Do brief performance dimension training. Ask the group what behaviors are important for the skill. Make sure everything is behaviorally described (how could you tell someone is being empathic or listening?).
4. Distribute the framework for the skill. Let participants review it. (STEPS 3/4=5 minutes)
5. Identify which participant will be the "preceptor." Walk the preceptor out of the room to meet the resident. Have the SP return to the room. Tell the resident/preceptor to come back into the room when ready.
6. Have the group watch the encounter. Call a timeout if the encounter is running long. The encounter should be less than 10 minutes. When the encounter ends, send the resident and SP out of the room.
7. Given the group a minute to rate the resident using the rater assessment form. Ask participants to write their observations and a summary statement and to select an entrustment rating.
8) Ask the preceptor to discuss their observations and rating. Encourage the group to share observations. Highlight when the group is making inferences. Highlight the frame of reference being used (i.e., normative, self). Ask whether they would entrust the resident with their skill. (STEPS 6/7=5–8 minutes)
9. Have the resident/SP come back into the room. (Note to the group that the patient would obviously not be present for feedback.)
10. Ask the preceptor if they are ready to give feedback. Ask the preceptor if there is anything they will want feedback about. Let the preceptor give feedback to the resident. (APPROX 5–8 minutes)
11. Debrief the preceptor feedback. *Remind the group to use best practices when giving feedback and be respectful.* Ask the preceptor to self-assess their feedback or ask what they want feedback about. Moderate the group giving feedback to the preceptor (10 minutes). *Your job as facilitator is to protect the faculty preceptor if they are receiving critical feedback or if it looks like they are becoming upset. Be attentive and monitor the group dynamic.*
12. Ask the resident to provide additional feedback to the faculty member. You can prompt the resident with specific questions. For example, in scenarios where the resident is resistant to feedback, you can ask the resident what might have worked to make them less resistant. For the resident who performed unsatisfactorily and cannot be entrusted to perform the skill unsupervised the next time, ask the resident if that was clear from the feedback.
13. For stations 3 and 4, the resident will portray the scenario once but the feedback will be role-played twice (the resident will take on a different personality for the second feedback). This way every participant has the chance to give feedback.

Example Schedule/Station Overview

7:15–8:00: Arrival of residents, facilitators, and SPs; facilitators train resident with SP
7:45–8:05: Faculty arrival/review goals of session
8:05–8:10: Move to first station
8:10–8:50: Station 1:
Resident performance: Satisfactory
Resident feedback personality: Insightful/receptive
8:50–8:55: Move stations
8:55–9:35: Station 2:
Resident performance: Unsatisfactory
Resident feedback personality: Insightful/receptive
9:35–9:55: Break
9:55–10:55: Station 3 (2 feedback role-plays)
Resident performance: Satisfactory
Resident feedback personality 1: Insightful/overly receptive (the perfectionist)
Resident feedback personality 2: Lacks insight/not receptive (checked out resident)
10:55–11:00: Move stations
11:00–12:00: Station 4 (2 feedback role-plays)
Resident performance: Unsatisfactory
Resident feedback personality 1: Lacks insight/receptive
Resident feedback personality 2: Lacks insight/not receptive

Resident Instructions: Direct Observation of Clinical Skills Simulation Workshop

Thank you very much for volunteering to assist in our workshop on direct observation of clinical skills. We wanted to provide you with information on the goals of the workshop, a workshop overview, your role, and the schedule for the day.

Goals of the Workshop

The workshop you will be participating in is designed to teach faculty how to improve the assessments they make and the feedback they give when they observe trainees with patients.

Workshop Overview

Faculty participants will be in groups of (INSERT # of faculty per group). There are (INSERT # of stations), each with a different standardized patient clinical case focusing on a different clinical skill (e.g., history taking, reviewing the plan, breaking bad news, motivational interviewing). Each station lasts 40 to 60 minutes and there is a facilitator for each station.

In each station, faculty will observe an interaction between the resident (you) and the standardized patient. Given the short duration of each station, the resident standardized patient interaction will only be a part of a clinical encounter (i.e., just the history, just the counseling). The clinical interaction should take about 10 minutes. The facilitator may end the interaction in the interest of time. After the encounter, you will be asked to step out of the room. Faculty will then discuss how the resident performed (strengths, areas for improvement). You will be asked to return to the room and one of the faculty participants will give you feedback. Again, the facilitator may end the interaction in the interest in time. The group will then discuss how the feedback went. You may be asked to contribute to that conversation. If there is time, the process may repeat itself. There will be a proctor who will provide 10-minute and 5-minute warnings for each station.

Your Role

You will play the resident in the case. Your station facilitator will ask you to portray (to the best of your ability) different levels of skill (i.e., satisfactory (S) or unsatisfactory (U)). Be reassured that you are playing a role and it doesn't matter how exact you are since the goal is for faculty to practice observation and feedback. The faculty will know you are acting! Additionally, your station facilitator will also ask you to portray a "resident personality" when receiving feedback. You will be asked to alter your level of insight (I) into your performance (accurate self-assessment, mixed self-assessment, inaccurate self-assessment) and your receptivity (R) to feedback (receptive vs. defensive).

Example of Resident Script

Fatigue Case
RESIDENT TASK: History taking only
PATIENT'S NAME: XXX

PRESENTING SITUATION: Patient is a 32-year-old female with fatigue. She describes feeling tired all over for 6 to 12 months and it has gotten progressively worse. She is particularly tired at the end of the day. She describes irritability, difficulty sleeping (interrupted sleep and early morning awakening).. She does snore. No problem with concentration. The patient describes no energy, never feels refreshed, and unable to exercise secondary to fatigue.

GYNECOLOGIC HX:

- Pregnancies: 2 (4-year-old and 2-year-old twins)
- Last exam and pap smear: about 1 year ago
- LMP 1 month ago. Irregular (every 40 days), dysmenorrhea, heavy, lasts 7–8 days with 7 pads on a heavy day

PAST MEDICAL HISTORY

- Reflux 9 months ago–resolved. On omeprazole.
- Iron deficiency 3 years ago. Stopped iron secondary to side effects.
- Depression after birth of twins. Treated with fluoxetine–self-d/cd because felt better and too busy to see physician.
- Never hospitalized for psychiatric illness.

PAST SURGICAL HISTORY: Appy 10 years ago
MEDICATIONS:
Prilosec (20 mg once a day)
ALLERGIES: none
SOCIAL HISTORY: No tobacco, no ETOH, no drugs, married, bookkeeper, + stress at home
FAMILY MEDICAL HISTORY:

- Mother: age 60, thyroid disorder
- Father: age 64, HTN, CAD, MI age 60
- Sister: age 36, thyroid disorder
- Brother: age 30, healthy

Resident Scripting

Encounter Performance

Satisfactory: You should take a relatively accurate history, though you should jump around regarding the questions you are asking (it shouldn't be completely hypothesis driven but you should ask all the right questions). You are the blind squirrel that finds the nut. Look at the list of interpersonal skills below; do most of them. Do not agenda set at the beginning of the visit. Make sure you start with an open-ended question, but after one or two open-ended questions become more focused in your questioning. Don't leave too much silence and do not ask the patient what she thinks symptoms are from. Essentially, we developed this case as an early resident who completed a relatively accurate history but did so by simply modeling what he had seen other faculty do while they were a medical student. The resident really had no understanding of why the questions asked were appropriate.

Feedback

Insight/Receptivity: You have insight and are receptive: Identify one or two things you did wrong but don't identify everything. You are receptive to the feedback, take ownership, and want to improve.

Insight/Overly Receptive: You have insight. When asked what you did well, immediately jump to what you know you did wrong. When they ask what you did well, perseverate on what went wrong. You are the perfectionist. You worry that you were ineffective. You can say you worry you are never going to be as good as some of the amazing physicians you have worked with. When you get constructive feedback, interpret it as if you did a terrible job.

No Insight/Not Receptive: You lack insight and you aren't receptive. You've taken histories since you have been a third-year medical student. It has seemed to go well. Essentially, you are a checked-out intern. When asked what you did well, you can identify a superficial skill you did well, but you can seem disinterested during feedback. In general, you have rarely found faculty feedback particularly helpful. It seems like a "checkbox" activity to you and you haven't really bought in to direct observation.

Encounter Performance

Unsatisfactory: When you take the history, you should demonstrate premature closure (have a narrow differential and miss many pertinent positive/negatives). You should also dismiss the patient's concerns and lack empathy and supportive listening.

Insight/Receptive: You didn't do much outpatient medicine as a medical student. You find it difficult to think on your feet in the office and you don't have the ability to read and go back to ask the patient additional questions. You cannot collect a history well in the outpatient setting and you are terrified you will cause harm. When asked what you didn't do well, you can admit you weren't sure what else to ask. You are sure there are more things on the differential but you found it hard to think of everything. Of note, your lack of empathy, supportive listening is related to the fact that you are just trying to think about what questions to ask (you are so focused on the content you forget to think about process/interpersonal skills). You are very receptive to feedback and suggestions.

No insight/Receptive: When getting feedback, you think you did a good job. If pressed for something you didn't do well, say something that has nothing to do with the significant errors made. You are convinced you got the right diagnosis, so you don't believe there was premature closure. You don't realize you were dismissive and lacked empathy. When the faculty provides you with feedback, you are open to their suggestions.

No insight/No receptivity: If pressed for something you didn't do well, say something that has nothing to do with the significant errors made. You are convinced you got the right diagnosis, so you don't believe there was premature closure. You don't realize you were dismissive and lacked empathy. When you get feedback, be resistant and defensive. Come up with reasons why you think what you did was fine, find ways to externalize blame (you have seen others do it this way, clinic is busy there are several other patients waiting, you can just get labs anyway to figure out what is wrong with the patient, etc.).

Example of Schedule for Simulation Session

Station	Fatigue	Hypertension	Handoff	Breaking Bad News
1	Group A: S/+I/+R	Group B: S/+I/+R	Group C: S/+I/+R	Group D: S/+I/+R
2	Group D: U/+I/+R	Group A: U /+I/+R	Group B: U/+I/+R	Group C: U/+I/+R
3	Group C: S/+I/+R (overly) then S/-I/-R	Group D: S/+I/+R (overly) then S/-I/-R	Group A: S/+I/+R (overly) then S/-I/-R	Group B: S/+I/+R (overly) then S/-I/-R
4	Group B: U/-I/+R then U/-I/-R	Group C:U/-I/+R then U/-I/-R	Group D: U/-I/+R then U/-I/-R	Group A: U/-I/+R then U/-I/-R
5	Group A: S/+I/+R	Group B: S/+I/+R	Group C: S/+I/+R	Group D: S/+I/+R
6	Group D: U/+I/+R	Group A: U /+I/+R	Group B: U/+I/+R	Group C: U/+I/+R
7	Group C: S/+I/+R (overly) then S/-I/-R	Group D: S/+I/+R (overly) then S/-I/-R	Group A: S/+I/+R (overly) then S/-I/-R	Group B: S/+I/+R (overly) then S/-I/-R
8	Group B: U/-I/+R then U/-I/-R	Group C:U/-I/+R then U/-I/-R	Group D: U/-I/+R then U/-I/-R	Group A: U/-I/+R then U/-I/-R
	1. PDT for skill			
	2. Faculty observe performance/rate resident			
	3. Discuss observations using framework/facilitator highlight inferences			
	4. Discuss rating and frame of reference (self, normative, criterion referenced)			
	5. What is needed to entrust?			
	6. Feedback			
	7. Debrief (a) faculty self-assess their feedback; ask faculty if areas they want feedback about; (b) group input			

S = Satisfactory resident performance.
U = Unsatisfactory resident performance.
+I =Resident insightful during feedback.
-I = Resident not insightful during feedback.
+R = Resident receptive to feedback.
-R =Resident not receptive to feedback.

Appendix 5.6 Tips for Increasing Direct Observation

- **SAMPLING**
  - It's OK to watch part of an encounter (i.e., history OR exam OR counseling).
    - It's even OK to watch part of a part (part of the history [i.e., agenda setting]; part of the exam [i.e., cardiovascular or shoulder exam]).
  - Sampling should align with learner goals and program milestones.
- **OUTPATIENT SETTING**
  - **HISTORY TAKING**
    - Watch first 5 minutes of an encounter to observe agenda setting.
    - Each clinic, observe the first learner–patient encounter of the session (usually no learner is ready to present in the first 10 minutes of clinic).

- Ask the learner who is the most challenging patient on their schedule (e.g., tangential patients, patients requesting pain medications, patients whose history is difficult to elicit; patients who have low adherence). Observe those encounters. Learners can find feedback on "challenging clinical encounters" helpful.
- Consider focusing observation on specific topics or skills: assessment of the geriatric patient, medication reconciliation, assessment of health literacy, use of a translator, telehealth.

- **PHYSICAL EXAM**
  - Tell the learner to take a history but request observation for the physical exam. This strategy is helpful to encourage observation of pelvic and musculoskeletal exams.
- **COUNSELING**
  - Tell the learner to wait to discuss the plan of care with the patient until the assessor can observe counseling (i.e., discussion of tests to be ordered, starting a medication, etc.).
  - Consider watching a learner counsel a patient on behavioral change (weight loss counseling, smoking cessation counseling).

- **INPATIENT SETTING**
  - **HISTORY TAKING**
    - Watch part of an admission history. Since attendings need to see the patient at some point, this is a "two for one."
    - Come in early to observe a learner preround, which facilitates observation of history, exam, and counseling. Observation early in the day can substitute for seeing the patient later in the day.
    - Ask the learner to take the history in a night float or handover patient.
  - **PHYSICAL EXAM**
    - Watch the physical exam during prerounding (see above).
    - Take the team to the bedside and ask a team member unfamiliar with the patient to lead the exam on the patient (i.e., cardiovascular exam and assessment of volume status in patient admitted with heart failure; neurologic exam in patient admitted with stroke or change in mental status).
    - Have a team member lead the physical exam on a night float or handover patient.
  - **COUNSELING**
    - Watch counseling during prerounding.
    - When a patient needs to be updated on the care plan (i.e., it changed on rounds), watch the learner review the plan with the patient.
    - Observe important counseling skills such as informed consent for a procedure, breaking bad news, goals of care discussions, code status discussions, and discharge plans.
- **MAXIMIZING OBSERVATION**
  - Identify situations when observation can help the learner and the patient.
    - Observe history taking works for a learner who frequently runs late in clinic. Observation can help clarify how the learner uses their time.
    - Ask learners what skills they need feedback on (i.e., a geriatric assessment, the musculoskeletal exam, starting insulin in a poorly controlled diabetic, advanced directives, family meeting, etc.).
- **CREATE A SYSTEM FOR TRACKING**
  - Consider using electronic systems to track workplace-based assessment using online assessment platforms or QR codes.
  - Make a word document with three columns (see example below). Column one lists all the learners in clinic or on service. Column two lists the target number of observations. Column three is a place to tally when an observation is done. Staple the document to a folder that contains the mini-CEX (or other direct observation tool). Hang the folder in the clinic precepting room or conference room. Tally observations as you go. Start each clinic/day by looking to see who needs to be observed.

Residents in Clinic/Service	Target # of Observations	Observation is Complete

- **OTHER TIPS FOR DIRECT OBSERVATION**
  - Encourage observations that inform the competencies and goals of the educational program.
  - Try to embed the observation in the work being done.
  - Observe trainees multiple times to improve the generalizability of the assessments.
  - Follow direct observation with meaningful feedback that includes an action plan: what steps can the learner take to improve in a particular area?
  - Help learners take ownership of the need to have direct observation.
  - Divide and conquer: use different rotations to observe different skills.

Chapter 6

Appendix 6.1 Modified SEGUE[1] Communication Skills Checklist with a behaviorally anchored rating scale (BARS) from Northwestern University Feinberg School of Medicine.

This checklist includes Communication Skills that fall under the following Northwestern University Feinberg School of Medicine Competency Standards (https://www.feinberg.northwestern.edu/md-education/curriculum/assessments-evaluations/index.html)

- **Listening** (ECIS-1): Listen empathically and effectively to patients, colleagues, and teachers.
- **Sharing Information** (ECIS-3): Communicate information clearly to patients, colleagues, and teams. Demonstrate closed-loop communication skills.
- **Shared Decision-Making** (ECIS-5): Utilize shared decision-making to promote patient-centered communication by eliciting and incorporating patient preferences.
- **Respect/Compassion** (PBMR-3): Display honesty, integrity, respect, and compassion toward others (patients, families, faculty, staff, etc.), regardless of gender, race, religion, ideology, socioeconomic status, disability, age, national origin, sexual orientation, or ability to pay.

Communication Skills Checklist

	1	2	3	4	5
EYE CONTACT (ECIS-1)	*Student uses minimal eye contact/is more focused on notes than on patient/uses uncomfortable amount of eye contact.*		*Student makes eye contact that fosters patient connection most of the time.*		*Student makes consistent eye contact, which fosters patient connection throughout interview.*
BODY LANGUAGE (ECIS-1)	*Student has distracting body language throughout much of the interview (e.g., twiddles pen, strokes hair, slouches, etc.).*		*Student's body language fosters connection. Very few distractions.*		*Body language greatly facilitates connection, (e.g., angles toward patient, leans forward, no distractions).*
VERBALIZES UNDERSTANDING OF HISTORY (ECIS-1) (ECIS-3)	*Student does not verbalize their understanding of patient's story.*		*Student reflects, clarifies, or summarizes the history at times during the interview.*		*Student reflects, clarifies, or summarizes the history frequently during the interview.*
ENCOURAGES PATIENT TO TELL STORY (ECIS-1)	*Student almost exclusively uses closed-ended questions/ does not use facilitating remarks.*		*Student uses facilitating remarks or open-ended questions at points in the interview.*		*Student uses many facilitating remarks and open-ended questions throughout the interview.*
LANGUAGE AND VOCABULARY (ECIS-1) (ECIS-3) (ECIS-5)	*Student uses medical jargon frequently without explanation OR uses slang that is jarring.*		*Student usually explains medical terms when using them; student can always explain terms if prompted.*		*Student avoids medical terminology or explains without prompting; student adjusts information to suit patient's level of understanding.*

Continued

Communication Skills Checklist

	1	2	3	4	5
WRAP-UP (ECIS-1) (ECIS-3) (ECIS-5)	*Student ends encounter abruptly without soliciting questions or explaining immediate next steps.*		*Student solicits some questions and/or partially explains immediate next steps.*		*Student solicits all questions, acknowledges patient's emotions, and thoroughly explains immediate next steps.*
CLARITY OF EXPLANATION (ECIS-3) (ECIS-5)	*Student does not share information about the diagnosis or plan.*		*Student provides fairly clear information about the diagnosis or plan.*		*Student provides exceptionally clear information about the diagnosis and plan.*
ASSESSED PATIENT RESPONSE TO DIAGNOSIS AND PLAN (ECIS-3) (ECIS-5)	*Student does not assess patient's emotional response to or agreement with the diagnosis or plan OR student does not share a diagnosis or plan.*		*Student briefly assesses patient's emotional response to or agreement with the diagnosis and plan.*		*Student thoroughly assesses patient's emotional response to or agreement with the diagnosis and plan, creating a patient-centered environment.*
CHECKED FOR UNDERSTANDING (ECIS-3) (ECIS-5)	*Student does not ask patient to state their understanding of the diagnosis or plan.*		*Student briefly asks patient to state their understanding of the diagnosis or plan.*		*Student asks patient to thoroughly state their understanding of the assessment and plan.*
ELICIT AND INCOPORATE PATIENT PREFERENCES (ECIS-3) (ECIS-5)	*Student offers no invitation for patient to speak about their ideas, solutions, or preferences.*		*Student elicits some of patient's ideas and solutions and/or includes some of patient's preferences when developing a plan.*		*Student consistently elicits patient's ideas and solutions and fully incorporates patient's preferences into the plan.*
RESPECT (PBMR-3)	*Student lacks professional demeanor during history and physical (e.g., minimally acknowledges patient beyond the chief concern or often touches before talking).*		*Student usually acknowledges patient beyond chief concern and uses talk before touch.*		*Student consistently interacts with patient using utmost respect (e.g., shows a lot of interest in patient beyond chief concern; consistently talks before touch).*

Communication Skills Checklist

	1	2	3	4	5
INTEREST AND ENGAGEMENT (ECIS-1) (PBMR-3)	*Student's facial expressions (or lack of expression) create a disconnect.*		*Student's facial expressions convey interest/ engagement at times (e.g., nods, changes expression appropriately in response to information).*		*Student's facial expressions convey consistent, genuine, appropriate interest and engagement throughout the encounter.*
COMPASSION (PBMR-3)	*Student does not offer either verbal or nonverbal empathic responses.*		*Student shows empathy and compassion at times during encounter through words and nonverbal behaviors.*		*Student consistently displays empathy and compassion throughout (verbal and nonverbal behaviors).*

	YES	NO
ELICITS PATIENT PERSPECTIVE **(ECIS-1)** **(ECIS-5)** *Note to standardized patient: This must be an open-ended question, not yes or no. Examples include: "What do you think might be causing this?" "What are you worried this could be?" "How is this problem affecting your life?" "How do you feel about this problem?" This must happen during the information gathering phase, not after the diagnosis or plan is shared by the student.*		

[1]Makoul G. The SEGUE Framework for teaching and assessing communication skills. *Patient Educ Couns*. 2001 Oct;45(1):23-34. doi:10.1016/S0738-3991(01)00136-7.

ECIS, Effective communication and interpersonal skills; *PBMR*, professional behavior and moral reasoning.

Chapter 8

Appendix 8.1 Strength of Assessment Methods for Measuring the Different Components of Clinical Reasoning

Strength is indicated by shading: ■ = poor; □ = average; ■ = good; ■ = very good

Assessment methods	Information Gathering	Hypothesis Generation	Problem Representatio	Differential Diagnosis	Leading Diagnosis	Diagnostic Justification	Management
Non-workplace-based assessments							
Clinical or comprehensive integrative puzzles: An extended matching crossword puzzle designed to assess a learner's ability to relate clinical vignettes to specific diagnoses and diagnostic or therapeutic interventions.	poor	poor	average	good	very good	poor	good
Concept maps: A schematic method for learners to organize and represent their knowledge and knowledge structures through a graphical illustration of the complex processes and relationships between concepts within a subject domain.	poor	poor	good	average	poor	average	average
Extended matching questions: A written exam format consisting of a lead-in question (vignette) followed by multiple answer options in a list where more answer options are given than in multiple choice questions (i.e., > 5).	poor	poor	poor	average	very good	poor	good
Key feature examinations: Problems typically consist of a clinical vignette followed by 2–3 questions that assess the critical elements ("key features") or challenging decisions that clinicians must make.	average	poor	poor	good	good	average	good
Multiple-choice questions: A clinical vignette is followed by up to 5 alternatives. Questions may take the following formats: single best alternative, matching, true or false, and combinations of alternatives.	average	poor	poor	average	very good	poor	very good
Modified essay questions: A method wherein serial information about a case is presented chronologically. After each item, the learner documents decisions and they cannot preview subsequent items until decisions are made.	good	good	average	very good	very good	good	very good
Oral examinations: A verbal examination conducted by one or more faculty members through unscripted or semi-scripted questions that assess clinical reasoning and decision-making abilities, as well as professional values.	good	good	good	very good	very good	very good	very good
Patient management problems: A clinical scenario is presented in real-life settings with specific resources available for diagnosis or management. The learner chooses among multiple alternatives. The results of actions (e.g., labs, images) are provided.	very good	average	poor	good	very good	average	very good
Script concordance tests: Clinical scenarios with uncertainty are followed by a series of questions (e.g., if you are thinking X and you find Y, the answer becomes more likely, less likely, or neutral). Responses are compared to those of experts.	poor	average	average	average	good	average	good
Short or long answer (essay) questions: A clinical vignette is followed by one or more questions. Learners provide free text responses that range in length from a few words to several sentences.	average	good	good	very good	very good	very good	very good
Assessments in simulated clinical environments							
Objective structured clinical examinations: Performance-based evaluations comprised of multiple stations where examinees execute different clinical tasks, incorporating standardized patients, observer ratings, written notes, etc.	very good	good	good	very good	very good	good	very good
Technology-enhanced simulation: An educational tool or device with which the leaner physically interacts to mimic an aspect of clinical care. Tools range from high-fidelity mannequins to dynamic virtual reality patients.	very good	average	poor	good	very good	average	very good
Workplace-based assessments							
Chart stimulated recall: A hybrid assessment format that combines review of a written note from an actual patient encounter and an oral examination to probe the learner's underlying thought processes, with feedback to improve decision-making.	good	good	good	very good	very good	very good	very good
Direct observation: A method that involves an instructor watching a learner in the workplace environment. Assessment tools for this include the mini-clinical evaluation exercise (mini-CEX).	very good	good	good	very good	very good	good	very good
Global assessment: Individual judgment or preceptor gestalt of learner clinical reasoning performance, often expressed on clinical rating forms (e.g., end-of-shift, end-of-clerkship).	good	average	good	very good	very good	good	very good
Oral case presentation: A structured verbal report of a clinical case. The learner makes deliberate choices about what to include, what not to include, the order in which data are presented, and the structure and content of the assessment and plan.	good	good	very good	very good	very good	very good	very good
Self-regulated learning microanalysis: A structured interview protocol designed to gather in-the-moment, task-level information on a learner's thoughts, actions, and feelings as they approach, perform, and reflect on a clinical activity.	good	very good	very good	very good	very good	very good	very good
Think aloud: A method in which participants are given a task and asked to voice their thoughts in an unfiltered form while completing or immediately after completing the task.	good	very good	very good	very good	very good	very good	very good
Written notes: A structured written report about a patient case. Post-encounter notes are one specific format with expectations for expressing clinical reasoning in the form of a summary statement, problem list, prioritized differential diagnosis, etc.	good	average	good	very good	very good	very good	very good

From Daniel M, Rencic J, Durning SJ, et al. Clinical reasoning assessment methods: a scoping review and practical guidance. *Acad Med*. 2019 Jun;94(6):902-912. doi:10.1097/ACM.0000000000002618.

Appendix 8.2 and 8.3 ART and ART-R Tools

ASSESSMENT OF REASONING TOOL™

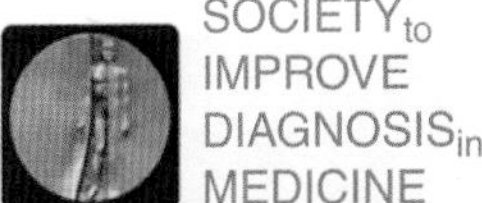

SOCIETY to IMPROVE DIAGNOSIS in MEDICINE

Learner: ______________ Evaluator: ______________

Did the Learner...	Assessment		
	Minimal	Partial	Complete
Collect/report history and examination data in a **hypothesis-directed manner?**	• Non-directed in questioning and exam • Asked questions without clear focus on potential dia noses	• Questioning and exam generally reflective of potential diagnoses, but less relevant or tangential questions ☑	• Followed clear line of inquiry, directing questioning and exam to specific findings likely to increase or decrease likelihood of specific diagnoses
Articulate a complete **problem representation** using descriptive medical terminology?	• Included extraneous information • Missed key findings • Did not translate findings into medical terminology	• Generally included key clinical findings (both positive and negative) but either missed some key findings or missed important descriptive medical terminology ☑	• Gave clear synopsis of clinical problem • Emphasized important positive and negative findings using descriptive medical terminology
Articulate a **prioritized differential diagnosis** of most likely, less likely, unlikely, and "can't miss" diagnoses based on the problem representation?	• Missed key elements of differential diagnosis, including likely diagnoses or "can't miss" diagnoses	• Gave differential diagnosis that included likely and "can't miss" diagnoses but either missed key diagnoses or ranked them inappropriately	• Gave accurately ranked differential diagnosis including likely and "can't miss" diagnoses ☑
Direct evaluation/treatment towards **high priority diagnoses?**	• Directed testing and treatments toward unlikely/unimportant diagnoses • Did not order tests or treatments for most likely/ "can't miss" diagnoses	• Major focus of evaluation and treatment was likely and "can't miss" diagnoses but included non-essential testing ☑	• Efficiently directed evaluation and treatment towards most likely and "can't miss" diagnoses • Deferred tests directed towards less likely or less important diagnoses
Demonstrate the ability to **think about one's own thinking** (metacognition)? *Consider asking: is there anything about the way you are thinking or feeling about this case that may lead to error?*	• Not able to describe the influence of cognitive tendencies or emotional/ situational factors that may have influenced decision-making ☑	• Can name one cognitive tendency or emotional/situational factor that may have influenced decision-making	
OVERALL ASSESSMENT	**NEED IMPROVEMENT** ☐	**MEETS COMPETENCY** ☐	**EXCELLENCE** ☐

Comments:

"Complete" descriptors adjusted to form the "Minimal" and "Partial" anchors in the original ART

Original ART 5-Domain Rubric 15 Descriptors for "Complete"

ART-D 5-Domain 15-Item 5- Point Likert Scale

Did the Leaner	Assessment			ART-D
	Minimal	Partial	Complete	
Collect/report history and examination data in **hypothesis-driven manner?**	Non-directed in questioning and exam Asked questions without clear focus on potential diagnoses	Questioning and exam generally reflective of potential diagnoses, but some irrelevant or tangential questions	Followed clear line of inquiry, directing questioning and exam to specific findings likely to increase or decrease likelihood of specific diagnoses	→ Item 1 → Item 2 → Item 3
Articulate a complete **problem representation** using descriptive medical terminology?	Included extraneous information Missed key findings Did not translate findings into medical terminology	Generally included key clinical findings (both positive and negative) Either missed some key findings or missed important descriptive medical terminology	Gave clear synopsis of clinical problem Emphasized important positive and negative findings using descriptive medical terminology	→ Item 4 → Item 5 → Item 6
Articulate a **prioritized differential diagnosis** of most likely, less likely, unlikely, and 'can't miss diagnoses' based on the problem representation?	Missed key elements of differential diagnosis including likely diagnoses or "can't miss" diagnoses	Gave differential diagnosis that included some likely and "can't miss" diagnoses but either omitted key diagnoses or ranked them inappropriately	Gave accurately ranked differential diagnosis including likely and "can't miss" diagnoses	→ Item 7 → Item 8 → Item 9
Direct evaluation/treatment towards **high priority diagnoses?**	Directed testing and treatments toward unlikely/unimportant diagnoses Did not evaluate or treatments for likely/can't miss diagnoses	Major focus of evaluation and treatment was likely and "can't miss" diagnoses but included non-essential testing	Efficiently directed evaluation and treatment towards most likely and "can't miss" diagnoses deferred tests directed towards less likely or less important diagnoses	→ Item 10 → Item 11 → Item 12
Demonstrate ability to **think about one's own thinking** (metacognition)?	Not able to describe the effect of cognitive tendencies or emotional/situational factors that may have influenced decision-making	Can name one cognitive tendencies or emotional/situational factors that may have influenced decision-making		→ Item 13 → Item 14 → Item 15

Appendix 8.4 Diagrams Illustrating Situated and Distributed Cognition

Situated Cognition: Clinical Reasoning and Error are Context Dependent

Michelle Daniel, Steven J Durning, Eric Wilson, Emily Abdoler, Dario Torre

Situated cognition posits that clinical reasoning and error are the result of a multitude of a dynamic, context-specific, bidirectional interactions between individual(s) and the environment.[1] Cognition is thought to unfold through a complex and evolving interplay of participants (i.e., patients and providers) within a specific physical, sociocultural and conceptual environment. Patient factors, practice factors and provider factors thus all influence clinical reasoning outcomes (e.g., diagnosis or management).

Consider the following: A 28-year-old woman presents to her family physician in California (CA) complaining of headache (HA), fever and a rash. She recently went camping in Connecticut (CT) and reports a tick bite. She knows Lyme disease is prevalent on the East Coast and felt this was important to mention. The medical student performs an initial evaluation and sees a bullseye rash on the patient's back. She consults *Up to Date* for images of Lyme rashes and notes the similarities. She discusses the case with the attending who wonders if the patient's fever and HA need further evaluation for Lyme meningitis, since she read the treatment for meningitis is intravenous (IV) instead of oral. The attending has only seen one prior case of Lyme disease as it isn't prevalent in CA.

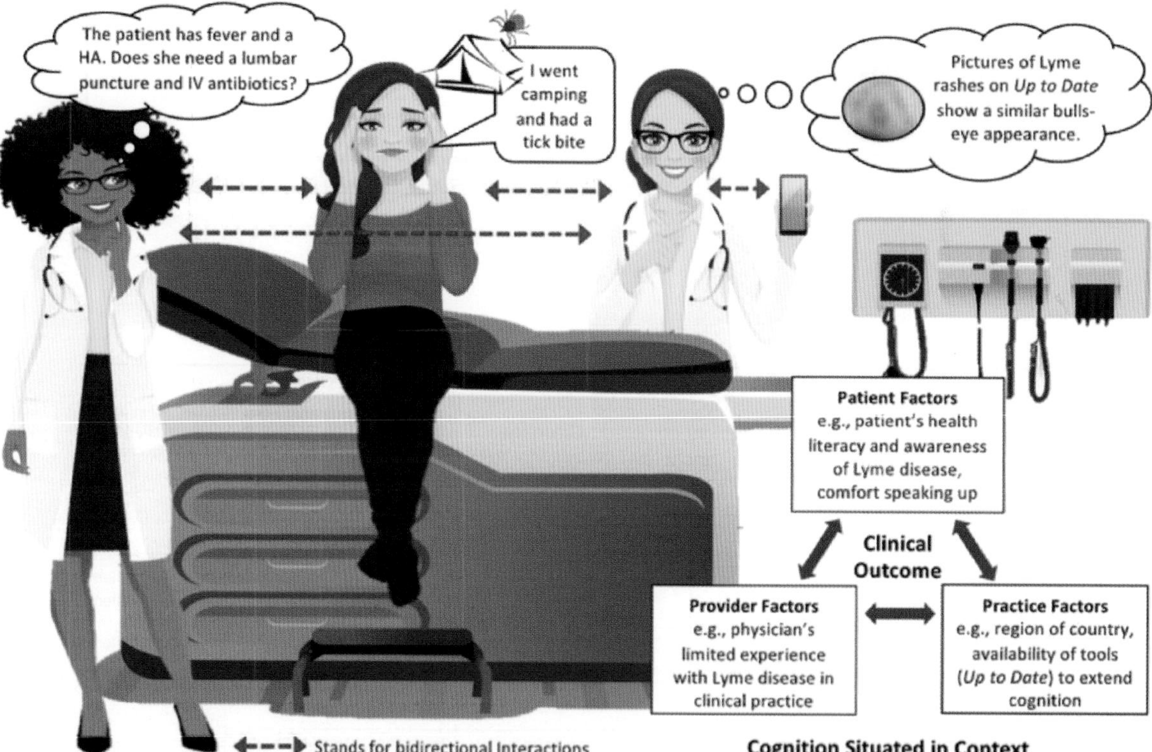

In this example, the physician interacts with the patient who mentions a tick bite and the student who finds a typical image of a Lyme rash on her smart phone. This interplay among agents is fully embedded in the environment, and the cognitive processes of patient, student and physician cannot be understood in isolation (i.e., cognition is situated). The patient's health literacy influences the history she communicates, prompting the clinicians to investigate Lyme disease, which may not have been considered based on low prevalence in CA. The student's use of an on-line resource exemplifies how tools can extend clinical reasoning, aiding in identification of the patient's rash. The attending physician's limited experience with Lyme disease is a direct result of her training and practice in a region where Lyme disease is less common, accounts of situated cognition related to Lyme disease are lacking. This impacts her diagnostic and therapeutic reasoning, leading her to consider a lumbar puncture (LP) and a course of IV antibiotics. If she had more experience with patients with early localized (Stage 1) Lyme disease, she might realize that HA and fever are common, and an LP is unnecessary. This illustrates how situated reasoning results from a complex interplay between individuals and a specific situation or context, influencing cognition and leading to diagnostic accuracy or error.

References: 1) Durning SJ, Artino AR. Situativity theory: a perspective on how participants and the environment can interact: AMEE Guide no. 52. Med Teach. 2011;33(3):188-99.
Disclaimer: The views expressed herein are those of the authors and not necessity those of the Department of Defense or other federal agencies.

Appendix 8.4—cont'd

Distributed Cognition: Interactions Between Individuals and Artifacts

Eric Wilson, Colleen Seifert, Steven J Durning, Dario Torre, Michelle Daniel

In *distributed cognition,* bidirectional interactions between *individuals* and *artifacts* (i.e., medical charts, computers, imaging technology) facilitate medical decision making. Because cognition is dispersed among team members and their work tools, the system has greater capacity for developing complex diagnostic and treatment plans. Additionally, the distributed nature of cognitive processes allows information to be accessed and modified by multiple individuals, teams, and information systems across space and time. However, access to certain elements of the distributed cognitive system can also be limited by an individual's *horizon of observation*; that is, their ability to directly interact with specific providers and patients, access to clinical notes and records, and testing data such as imaging.

Example: A 25-year-old male is brought to a local hospital after a motor vehicle collision (MVC) in which he was the unrestrained driver. The paramedics report significant vehicle damage and a prolonged extraction. He is complaining of severe chest and abdominal pain and has parasternal, abdominal and thoracic spine tenderness on initial exam. The emergency physician (EP) obtains a pan-CT. The radiologist notes multiple rib fractures and an aortic dissection. The EP arranges air-medical transfer to a trauma center. The chart, but not the original images, are sent with the patient. On arrival at the trauma center, the patient is tachycardic and hypotensive. The receiving EP discusses the case with the trauma surgeon, and the patient is rushed to an operating room (OR). Post-operatively, the patient is paraplegic and a T7 burst fracture is found.

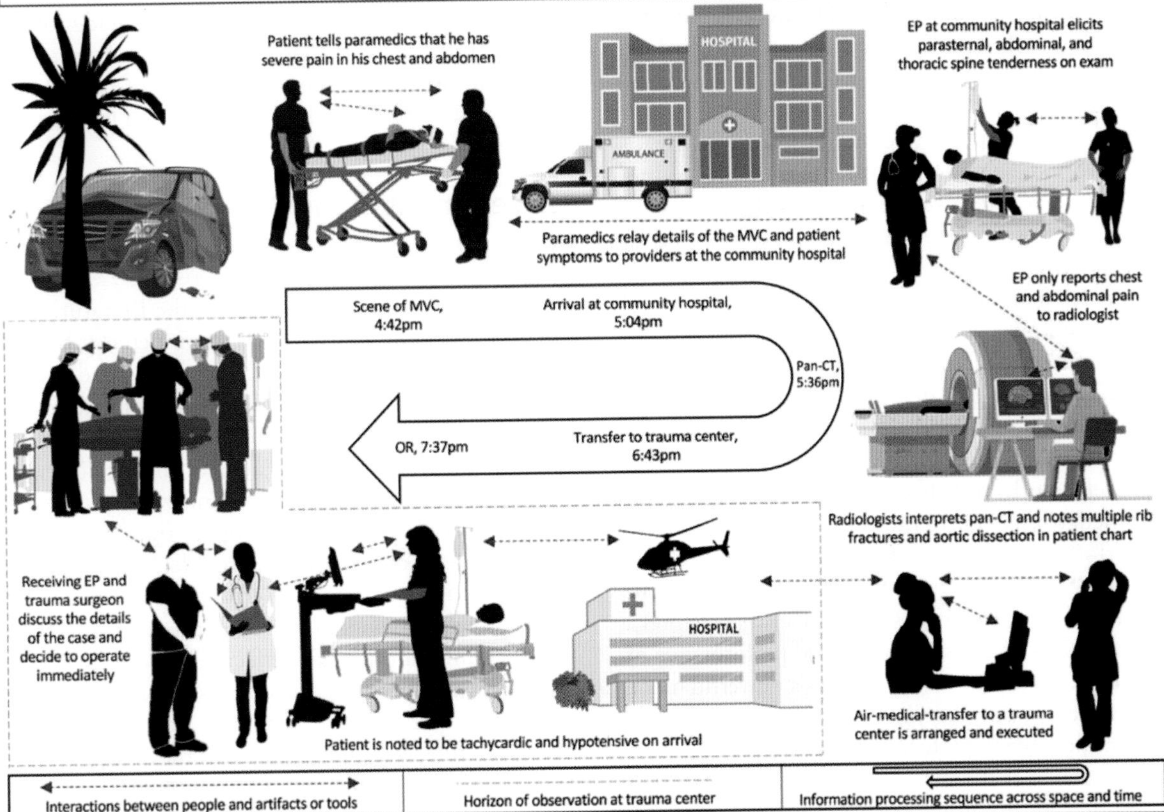

In this example, a distributed cognitive network (DCN) is created as individual healthcare workers (i.e., paramedics, EPs, radiologist, trauma surgeon) gather historical (i.e., chest and abdominal pain), physical (i.e., parasternal, abdominal, and thoracic spine tenderness), and imaging (i.e., pan-CT) data that is exchanged via team interactions and/or externally represented through artifacts (i.e. patient chart, CT images). Individual providers can expand the DCN by documenting their impressions (i.e., radiologist dictates multiple rib fractures and traumatic aortic dissection in patient's chart) or verbalizing their thoughts with others (i.e., EP reports chest and abdominal pain, but fails to mention thoracic spine tenderness to the radiologist). Ultimately, details from the scene of the MVC provided by the paramedics, signs and symptoms noted by the EP at the community hospital, and the radiologist's interpretation of the pan-CT are communicated to the receiving EP and surgeon at the trauma center. The boundaries of the DCN span space and time, enhancing the ability of providers at the trauma center to act. However, because the CT images were not delivered to the trauma center, the providers develop a treatment plan based on the radiologist's note in the chart. Their limited *horizon of observation* (i.e., inability to view CT images) causes them to miss the T7 burst fracture until they note his paraplegia post-operatively.

References: 1) Hutchins, E. (1995). *Cognition in the wild.* Cambridge, MA: The MIT Press.
Disclaimer: The views expressed herein are those of the authors and not necessarily those of the Department of Defense or other federal agencies.

Chapter 9

Appendix 9.1 Issues Concerning the Broader Context of Assessment

Assessment is a very important part of medical education. It is also a complex topic. In the world of education, the terms *assessment* and *evaluation* mean different things. Assessment refers to judging an individual learner's progress, whereas evaluation refers to judging the effectiveness of a program or curriculum. Almost all assessment instruments are made up of a series of individual items. The quality of the assessment instrument depends on the quality of the individual items that comprise it, and the process of developing (or editing) items should not be taken lightly. Two common forms of items include (1) broad statements of performance, such as "The candidate maintained an efficient flow during the procedure in the context of competing demands on their attention" (anchored by a 5-point Likert scale), or (2) simple checklist items, such as "Keeps edges of the wound everted while closing the skin—done/not done." There is extensive literature on the process of writing items to test for knowledge or for application of knowledge to a clinical problem. One of the best guides to writing items is a manual published by the National Board of Medical Examiners,[93] and it should be consulted when assessing the quality of items in a prospective assessment tool or when attempting to develop your own assessment tool. Item writing, and critical appraisal of items on existing assessment tools, is a learned skill, and with practice it can be done efficiently and effectively.

For knowledge tests, one of the key concerns is to ensure that test performance is not a function of highly developed test-taking strategies (this would be a good example of construct-irrelevant variance; see earlier in this chapter). Although this is less of an issue for tests of performance or skill, it is helpful to realize that any test has a powerful motivational influence on the student, and it is human nature to use any means possible to perform well in a high-stakes test. Given this tendency, it is your responsibility to ensure that the test measures what you intend it to measure, not irrelevant test-taking skills. *This concept forms the core of validity.*

The Importance of Variance

When you are assessing performance in any domain, you need to see variation in scores. This is a simple but critical assertion. If there were no variance in the scores produced by an assessment exercise, all individuals would be deemed to be identical in the domain of interest and there would therefore be no need to have used an assessment instrument. Stated another way, one of the reasons why an assessment instrument is used is to discriminate (in a good way) between individuals with differing levels of skills or performance. Note that many measures of competence used in resident assessment, such as end-of-rotation evaluations, produce results with relatively little variance.[94-96] Fortunately, many of the tests described in this book show good variation across a wide spectrum of performance and have demonstrated evidence of validity. Another problem in the field of assessment is the tendency for "grade inflation;" it can be difficult to get faculty to rate learners on the bottom end of a scale. The development of construct-aligned scales described earlier in the chapter can help mitigate this tendency.

Assessment in the Broader Context of Competency-Based Medical Education

Another major factor influencing the literature on assessment is the rapid move toward a competency-based framework for medical education, including the detailed specification of essential subcompetencies and milestones for achievement during residency training. This framework, now being widely adopted around the world, emphasizes the detailed regular tracking of individual residents' competence as they proceed through training. Despite the commitment of healthcare providers to practice at the highest standards, medical errors do occur. The ultimate goal of valid assessment-based decisions is increased public accountability in how effectively we train our learners and prepare them for unsupervised practice. This places enormous pressure on individual core faculty as well as program directors and residents as they attempt to provide valid evidence for decisions around progression and graduation from training programs. This book is intended to provide guidance for program directors and core faculty in meeting this challenge.

Chapter 10

Appendix 10.1 Internet EBP Education Resources

Centre for EBM (Oxford)	www.cebm.net/
Centre for EBM (Toronto)	https://ebm-tools.knowledgetranslation.net/
Educational prescription (Toronto Centre for EBM)	https://www.cebm.net/
The Fresno EBP Test[a]	http://bmj.bmjjournals.com/cgi/content/full/326/7384/319/DC1
The Berlin Test[b]	http://bmj.bmjjournals.com/cgi/content/full/325/7376/1338/DC1
General Practitioners' Perceptions of the Route to Evidence Based Medicine survey[c]	http://bmj.bmjjournals.com/cgi/content/full/316/7128/361/DC1
An instrument to characterize the environment for residents' evidence-based medicine learning and practice[d]	https://fammedarchives.blob.core.windows.net/imagesandpdfs/fmhub/fm2012/February/Misa98.pdf

[a]For more information, see Ramos KD, Schafer S, Tracz SM. Validation of the Fresno Test of competence in evidence based medicine. *BMJ*. 2003 Feb 8;326(7384):319-321. doi:10.1136/bmj.326.7384.319.

[b]For more information, see Fritsche L, Greenhalgh T, Falck-Ytter Y, Neumayer HH, Kunz R. Do short courses in evidence based medicine improve knowledge and skills? Validation of Berlin questionnaire and before and after study of courses in evidence based medicine. *BMJ*. 2002 Dec 7;325(7376):1338-1341. doi:10.1136/bmj.325.7376.1338.

[c]For more information, see Downing SM, Haladyna TM. Validity threats: overcoming interference with proposed interpretations of assessment data. *Med Educ*. 2004 Mar;38(3):327-333. doi:10.1046/j.1365-2923.2004.01777.x.

[d]For more information, see Mi M, Moseley, JL, Green ML. An instrument to characterize the environment for residents' evidence-based medicine learning and practice. *Fam Med*. 2012; 44(2):98–104.

Appendix 10.2 Examples of Educational Prescriptions

1. Educational prescription example.

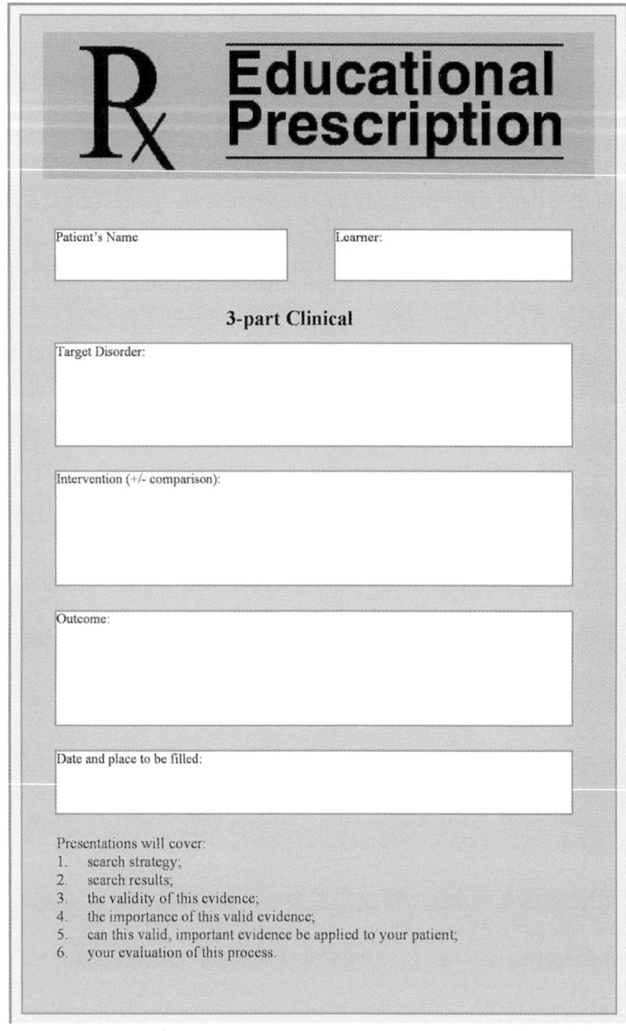

Rx Educational Prescription

Patient's Name

Learner:

3-part Clinical

Target Disorder:

Intervention (+/- comparison):

Outcome:

Date and place to be filled:

Presentations will cover:
1. search strategy;
2. search results;
3. the validity of this evidence;
4. the importance of this valid evidence;
5. can this valid, important evidence be applied to your patient;
6. your evaluation of this process.

From Knowledge Translation Program: University of Toronto Educational Prescription. Accessed February 23, 2022. https://ebm-tools.knowledgetranslation.net/educational-prescription

2. Educational prescription example.
   From Green ML. Evaluating evidence-based practice performance [editorial]. *ACP J Club*. 2006;145(2):A8-A10. Reprinted with permission.

Centre for Evidence-Based Medicine, University of Toronto. Educational Prescription. Accessed April 2015. https://www.cebm.net/.

Resident(s): ______________	**Faculty:** ______________	**"Rx" date** ____________ **"Fill" date** ____________

1. Rotation:	Wards	Elective	Geriatrics	Continuity clinic	Ambulatory office	Other:
	ICU	Emergency	Night float		Ambulatory specialty	

2. Context	Question conference	EBM curriculum	Resident report	General patient care	Other:

3. Clinical scenario:

4. Question			
Patient	Intervention	Comparison	Outcome

5. Clinical task:	Clinical findings	Differential diagnosis	Prognosis	Prevention
	Etiology/harm	Diagnostic testing	Therapy	Manifestations of disease

6. Information source that provided answer:	Clinical evidence	EBM on call	MEDLINE original study
	Cochrane Library/DARE	UpToDate	MEDLINE meta-analysis
	ACPJC online	PIER	MEDLINE narrative review
	Rational clinical exam	Textbook	Consultant/colleague
	Info retriever (POEM or other source: _______)		Other:

7. The evidence (reference)

8. Your answer/results:

9. What did you learn from this experience? How will it change your clinical practice, if at all?

Faculty

Date returned: ________________

Describe the main teaching point (EBM slice) you made for this exercise:

▯ None	
▯ Ask	
▯ Acquire	
▯ Appraise	
▯ Apply	

From Green ML. Evaluating evidence-based practice performance (editorial). *ACP J Club.* 2006 Sep-Oct;145(2):A8–A10. Reprinted with permission.

Chapter 11

Appendix 11.1 List of Useful Resources for Quality Improvement and Patient Safety

- Institute for Healthcare Improvement Open School
  - Online courses in quality and patient safety (www.ihi.org/IHI/Programs/IHIOpenSchool/)
- Choosing Wisely (ABIM Foundation)
  - Provides five diagnostic and/or therapeutic interventions that have little to no benefit to most patients across multiple specialties (www.choosingwisely.org/)
  - Useful videos: http://modules.choosingwisely.org/modules/m_03/default_FrameSet.htm
- Choosing Wisely Canada
  - Choosing Wisely Canada is source of information and guidance for reducing unnecessary tests and treatments in Canada (https://choosingwiselycanada.org)
- High Value Care
  - Initiative of ACP: https://www.acponline.org/clinical-information/high-value-care
  - Helpful toolkit and resources for programs
- Discovering Value-Based Health Care (modular training with useful videos)
  - Free from UT Austin Dell School of Medicine; four modules in all (https://vbhc.dellmed.utexas.edu/)
- World Health Organization (WHO) Patient Safety Curriculum Guide
  - Provides a number of free resources, including guide and slides
    - For medical schools: WHO patient safety curriculum guide for medical schools (https://www.who.int/publications/i/item/9789241598316)
    - Multiprofessional: Patient safety curriculum guide: multi-professional edition (https://www.who.int/publications/i/item/9789241501958)

Appendix 11.2 Sample Medical Record Abstraction Form for Diabetes

Date of Abstraction	
Abstractor Initials	
Abstraction Time (in minutes)	

Physician Name		
First visit with this MD?	YES	NO
First visit to this clinic?	YES	NO

Demographics		
1.	Patient Name (First, MI, Last)	
2.	Patient Identification (MRN) #	
3.	Gender	a. Male b. Female
4.	Race/Ethnicity *(circle all that apply)*	a. White b. Black c. Hispanic d. Asian e. Other f. Not Documented
5.	Date of Birth (MM/DD/YYYY)	__ __/__ __/__ __ __ __

Chart Information			
6.	Does the chart contain a problem list?	Yes	No
7.	Does the chart contain a preventive services checklist?	Yes	No
8.	Does the preventive services checklist have ***any*** entries?	Yes	No

Conditions Present			
9.	Hypertension	Yes	Not Documented
10.	Coronary Artery Disease	Yes	Not Documented
11.	Heart Failure	Yes	Not Documented
12.	Conduction Disorder/Bradyarrhythmia	Yes	Not Documented
13.	Aortic Stenosis	Yes	Not Documented
14.	Chronic Obstructive Pulmonary Disease/Asthma	Yes	Not Documented
15.	Cerebrovascular Disease	Yes	Not Documented
16.	Peripheral Vascular Disease	Yes	Not Documented
17.	Chronic Renal Disease	Yes	Not Documented
18.	Chronic Liver Disease	Yes	Not Documented
19.	Diabetes Mellitus	Yes	Not Documented
20.	Dyslipidemia	Yes	Not Documented
21.	Breast Cancer	Yes	Not Documented
22.	Colon Cancer	Yes	Not Documented
23.	Dementia	Yes	Not Documented
24.	Bleeding Disorder/Risk	Yes	Not Documented
25.	Peptic Ulcer Disease	Yes	Not Documented
26.	Anemia	Yes	Not Documented

Continued

Appendix 11.2—cont'd

Physical Examination		
27.	Height	________ Inches Not Documented
28.	Date of most recent height	__ __/__ __/__ __ __ __ N/A
29.	Weight	________ Lbs. Not Documented
30.	Date of most recent weight	__ __/__ __/__ __ __ __ N/A

Physical Examination			
31.	Record all blood pressures from the last three visits during the observation period (Insert period).		
Date	Blood Pressure	Date	Blood Pressure
1. __/__/____	______/______	7. __/__/____	______/______
2. __/__/____	______/______	8. __/__/____	______/______
3. __/__/____	______/______	9. __/__/____	______/______
4. __/__/____	______/______	10. __/__/____	______/______
5. __/__/____	______/______	11. __/__/____	______/______
6. __/__/____	______/______	12. __/__/____	______/______

Counseling/Prevention		
32.	Was an assessment of tobacco use performed?	Yes Not Documented
33.	Is patient a current smoker?	Yes No Not Documented
33a.	Was smoking cessation counseling offered?	Yes Not Documented N/A
34.	Was a foot exam performed? (*insert observation period*)	Yes Not Documented
34a.	Was a monofilament test for neuropathy performed?	Yes Not Documented
35.	Has the patient ever received Pneumovax?	Yes Not Documented

Labs/Diagnostic Studies:

For all questions pertaining to labs/diagnostic studies, review the record from 6/30/2001 back to 7/1/1999 (if necessary). Record the most recent date that the test was performed prior to 6/30/2001 and the value.

Lab Test/Diagnostic Study	Test Performed	a. Date Performed	b. Value
36. Blood Urea Nitrogen	36. Yes Not Documented *If yes, record the date and value.*	36a. __/__/____	36b. ____________ (Normal range 6–19 mg/dL)
37. Creatinine	37. Yes Not Documented *If yes, record the date and value.*	37a. __/__/____	37b. ____________ (Normal range 0.6–1.4 mg/dL)
38. Blood Sugar	38. Yes Not Documented *If yes, record the date and value.*	38a. __/__/____	87b. ____________ (Normal range 70–105 mg/dL)

Appendix 11.2—cont'd

Lab Test/Diagnostic study	Test Performed	a. Date performed	b. Value
39. Was blood sugar recorded as fasting?	39. Yes Not Documented		
40. Albuminuria Test	40. Yes Not Documented	40a. __/__/____	40b. Albumin present? Yes Not Documented
41. Hemoglobin A1C	41. Yes Not Documented *If yes, record the date and value*	41a. __/__/____	41b. ___________ (Normal range 3.0%–6.5%)
42. Total Cholesterol	42 Yes Not Documented *If yes, record the date and value.*	42a. __/__/____	42b. ___________ (Normal range 120–220 mg/dL)
43. HDL Cholesterol	43. Yes Not Documented *If yes, record the date and value.*	43a. __/__/____	43b. ___________ (Normal range 44–55 mg/dL)
44. LDL Cholesterol	44. Yes Not Documented *If yes, record the date and value.*	44a. __/__/____	44b. ___________ (Normal range 40–170 mg/dL)
45. Triglycerides	45. Yes Not Documented *If yes, record the date and value.*	45a. __/__/____	45b ___________ (Normal range 40–150 mg/dL)
46. Potassium	46. Yes Not Documented *If yes, record the date and value.*	46a. __/__/____	46b. ___________ (Normal range 3.3–5.1 mEq/L)
47. ECG performed	47. Yes Not Documented *If yes, record the date and findings.*	47a. __/__/____	47b. ECG findings: *Select all recorded findings:* a. Myocardial infarction (any age) b. Atrial fibrillation c. LVH d. LBBB e. None of the above f. No interpretation

Continued

Appendix 11.2—cont'd

Treatment

48.	Does the chart contain a current list of medications?	Yes Not Documented
48a.	Are the patient's medications documented at the last visit to this physician?	Yes Not Documented

49.	Record all medications that the patient was taking or that were prescribed at the end of the observation period (*insert observation period).* Use hospital discharge summaries, consultation notes, phone conversations, etc., if necessary.

Medication	Dosage
1.	
2.	
3.	
4.	
5.	
6.	
7.	
8.	
9.	
10.	

50.	Does the chart contain a medication allergy section?	Yes Not Documented

Office Visits (Measurement Year):

51. Record all dates on which the patient was seen at this office during the observation period.		
1. __/__/____	11. __/__/____	21. __/__/____
2. __/__/____	12. __/__/____	22. __/__/____
3. __/__/____	13. __/__/____	23. __/__/____
4. __/__/____	14. __/__/____	24. __/__/____
5. __/__/____	15. __/__/____	25. __/__/____
6. __/__/____	16. __/__/____	26. __/__/____
7. __/__/____	17. __/__/____	27. __/__/____
8. __/__/____	18. __/__/____	28. __/__/____
9. __/__/____	19. __/__/____	29. __/__/____
10. __/__/____	20. __/__/____	30. __/__/____

Created by Qualidigm and the Yale Primary Care Program.

Chapter 12

Appendix 12.1 Exemplary Examples

The examples selected provide good descriptions of how the instruments were developed and assessed. They provide either full copies of the instrument or sufficient detail that the constructs and items can be determined.

A Tool for Assessing Undergraduate Medical Student Performance

These articles describe the development and testing of an MSF initiative for undergraduate medical student performance in the clinical context. The articles describe how the instruments were developed and assessed using Messick's six aspects of validation: (1) content validity, (2) substantive/cognitive validity, (3) structural validity, (4) generalizability, (5) external validity, and (6) consequential validity.

- Prediger S, Fürstenberg S, Berberat PO, Kadmon M, Harendza S. Interprofessional assessment of medical students' competences with an instrument suitable for physicians and nurses. *BMC Med Educ*. 2019 Feb 6;19(1):46. doi:10.1186/s12909-019-1473-6.
- Prediger S, Schick K, Fincke F, et al. Validation of a competence-based assessment of medical students' performance in the physician's role. *BMC Med Educ*. 2020 Jan 7;20(1):6. doi:10.1186/s12909-019-1919-x.

A Tool for Assessing ACGME Milestones for Pediatric Trainees

These articles profile the development and assessment of an MSF initiative designed to assess milestones for pediatrics residents. Impacts of the MSF assessments were provided by learners and site leads.

- Schwartz A, Margolis MJ, Multerer S, Haftel HM, Schumacher DJ; APPD LEARN–NBME Pediatrics Milestones Assessment Group. A multi-source feedback tool for measuring a subset of Pediatrics Milestones. *Med Teach*. 2016 Oct;38(10):995-1002. doi:10.3109/0142159X.2016.1147646.
- Hicks PJ, Margolis MJ, Carraccio CL, et al. A novel workplace-based assessment for competency-based decisions and learner feedback. *Med Teach*. 2018 Nov;40(11):1143-1150. doi:10.1080/0142159X.2018.1461204.
- Hicks PJ, Margolis M, Poynter SE, et al. The Pediatrics Milestones Assessment Pilot: development of workplace-based assessment content, instruments, and processes. *Acad Med*. 2016 May;91(5):701-709. doi:10.1097/ACM.0000000000001057.

A Tool for Assessing PGME Program Directors

This article describes the development and testing of a set of MSF tools to assess program director effectiveness by trainees, the GME director, and the chair/chief of the specialty department (e.g. surgery). The online version of the article provides copies of the instruments and the evaluation forms used to assess the effectiveness of the program.

- Goldhamer ME, Baker K, Cohen AP, Weinstein DF. Evaluating the evaluators: implementation of a multi-source evaluation program for graduate medical education program directors. *J Grad Med Educ*. 2016 Oct;8(4):592-596. doi:10.4300/JGME-D-15-00543.1.

A Tool for Assessing Interprofessional Professionalism

This article describes the development and testing of a 26-item questionnaire to measure observable behaviors of healthcare professionals in training who demonstrate professionalism and collaboration when working with other healthcare providers in the context of person-centered care. The complete questionnaire is provided within the publication.

- Frost JS, Hammer DP, Nunez LM, et al. The intersection of professionalism and interprofessional care: development and initial testing of the interprofessional professionalism assessment (IPA). *J Interprof Care*. 2019 Jan-Feb;33(1):102-115. doi:10.1080/13561820.2018.1515733.

Literature Review

Many reviews of MSF have been undertaken. Stevens provides a synthesis of eight reviews evaluating the validity of MSF published between 2006 and 2016. In terms of validity evidence, each review demonstrated evidence across at least one domain of the American Psychological Association's validity framework. Evidence of assessment validity within the domains of "internal structure" and "relationship to other variables" has been well established. However, the domains of content validity (i.e., ensuring that MSF tools measure what they are intended to measure), consequential validity (i.e., evidence of the intended or unintended consequences MSF assessments may have on participants or the wider society), and response process validity (i.e., the process of standardization and quality control in the delivery and completion of assessments) remain limited.

- Stevens S, Read J, Baines R, Chatterjee A, Archer J. Validation of multisource feedback in assessing medical performance: a systematic review. *J Cont Educ Heal Prof*. 2018 Fall;38(4):262-268. doi:10.1097/CEH.0000000000000219.

Chapter 13

Appendix 13.1 List of Simulators and Their Characteristics

	Simulator[a]	Features	Specialty	Cost[b]	Comments
Part-Task Trainers	Venipuncture Arms[116] www.limbsandthings.com	Adult-sized arm that provides functional anatomy of upper extremity veins filled with mock blood for intravenous access skills	Surgery Emergency Medicine Critical Care Internal/Family Medicine OB/GYN	$	Inexpensive task trainer that provides hundreds of assessment opportunities.
	CVC Insertion Simulator II[117] www.kyotokagaku.com	Partial adult-sized task trainer that provides functional (and ultrasound-compatible) anatomy of neck and upper chest with landmarks for subclavian and internal jugular vein catheterization	Surgery Internal Medicine Critical Care	$$	Newer task trainer that allows assessment of central venous catheter insertion technique (and complications—pneumothorax, arterial puncture) with or without ultrasound guidance.
	Eye Examination Simulator[118] www.kyotokagaku.com	Partial adult-sized task trainer that provides functional anatomy of external and internal eye with normal and abnormal retinal findings	Internal/Family Medicine Ophthalmology	$$	Inexpensive task trainer that provides opportunities to assess funduscopic exam technique and identification of normal and common abnormal retinal findings.
	Ear Examination Simulator II[119] www.kyotokagaku.com	Partial adult-sized task trainer that provides functional anatomy of external and middle ear with normal and abnormal findings	Internal/Family Medicine Otolaryngology	$$	Inexpensive task trainer that provides opportunities to assess otoscopic exam technique and identification of normal and abnormal middle ear findings.
	Breast Examination Trainers[120] www.limbsandthings.com	Partial adult-sized task trainers that provide functional anatomy of female upper chest and breasts with normal and abnormal findings	OB/GYN Internal/Family Medicine	$$	Simple strap-on task trainers that provide opportunities to assess breast exam technique and identification of pathologic findings.
	Airway Management Trainer[121] www.laerdal.com	Various sized head-neck-torso trainers that simulate a variety of upper airway anatomic variations and conditions	Anesthesiology Critical Care Emergency Medicine Internal Medicine Pediatrics	$$	Relatively low-cost airway mannequins that serve as tools for assessment of various airway management skills, including difficult airway scenarios.

Simulator[a]	Features	Specialty	Cost[b]	Comments
Resusci Anne[122] www.laerdal.com	Adult-sized, medium-fidelity, portable task trainer that provides functional anatomy for critical life-saving skills; optional built-in assessment system that evaluates adequacy of chest compressions and ventilations	Critical Care Emergency Medicine Internal/Family Medicine	$$	Inexpensive mannequin for assessing critical life-saving skills. Numerous studies provide evidence of reliability, validity, and feasibility of using the simulator as an assessment tool.
Advanced Epidural and Lumbar Puncture Model[124] www.limbsandthings.com	Partial adult-sized, ultrasound-compatible task trainer that provides functional anatomy and landmarks for lumbar puncture and various spinal injections	Neurology Internal Medicine Anesthesiology	$$	Relatively inexpensive task trainer that provides opportunities to assess technique of lumbar puncture and epidural injection with or without ultrasound guidance. Water can be added to simulate CSF, allow measurement of CSF pressure, and provide feedback regarding correct needle placement.
Pediatric Lumbar Puncture Simulator II[125] www.kyotokagaku.com	Infant-sized task trainer that provides functional anatomy and landmarks for lumbar puncture technique	Pediatrics Neurology	$$	Inexpensive task trainer that provides opportunities to assess identification of anatomic landmarks and technique of lumbar puncture. Water can be added to simulate CSF, allow measurement of CSF pressure, and provide feedback regarding correct needle placement.
MamaNatalie Birthing Simulator[126] www.laerdal.com	"Wearable" pregnant abdomen/perineum containing neonate-sized task trainer with simplified but representative maternal and fetal/neonatal anatomy, permitting manual control of labor progression and delivery	OB/GYN Pediatrics	$$	Simple strap-on task trainer used for hybrid simulations that can assess vaginal delivery technique and management of birthing complications, such as maternal postpartum hemorrhage or neonatal resuscitation.

Continued

	Simulator[a]	Features	Specialty	Cost[b]	Comments
	PROMPT Flex Birthing Simulator[128] www.limbsandthings.com	Partial adult-sized task trainer that provides functional anatomy of female lower abdomen/pelvis and vagina with articulating thighs, plus neonatal model with cord/placenta	OB/GYN	$$$	Medium fidelity simulator that can be used to assess individual and team skills during management of a wide range of obstetric scenarios, ranging from normal manual to device-assisted deliveries, and including various neonatal presentations and complications, such as shoulder dystocia. Several studies provide validity evidence for simulator, including translation of skills to real-world improvement in patient outcomes.
	Male Rectal Examination Trainer – Advanced[129] www.limbsandthings.com	Partial adult-sized task trainer that provides functional anatomy of male buttocks, anus, rectum, and prostate	Urology Surgery Internal/Family Medicine	$$	Relatively inexpensive task trainer that provides opportunities to assess exam technique and identification of normal and pathologic findings of the rectum and prostate.
	Clinical Female Pelvic Trainer Mk 3 – Advanced[130] www.limbsandthings.com	Partial adult-sized task trainer that provides functional anatomy of female lower abdomen, perineum, vagina, and rectum	OB/GYN Internal/Family Medicine	$$$	Partial task trainer for assessing recognition of appropriate landmarks, vaginal and bimanual exam, cervical smear, and digital rectal exam. Evaluates ability to identify normal and abnormal uterine and ovarian findings.
Computerized Task Trainers	METI Pelvic ExamSIM[139]**	Partial adult-sized, high-fidelity female pelvic simulator that functionally simulates a variety of gynecologic findings and automatically and objectively tracks user examination technique	GYN Internal/Family Medicine	N/A**	Several studies have provided validity evidence to support use as an assessment tool. **Retired by CAE (which had acquired METI); no longer commercially available as stand-alone simulator.
	Harvey, the Cardiopulmonary Patient Simulator[146] www.gordoncenter.miami.edu	Adult-sized high-fidelity mannequin that provides comprehensive cardiac and pulmonary physical findings	Internal/Family Medicine Pediatrics Critical Care Emergency Medicine Surgery	$$$$	Longest continuous high-fidelity simulator with numerous studies providing validity evidence for use as an assessment tool; has been used in high-stakes national board certification exams.

	Simulator[a]	Features	Specialty	Cost[b]	Comments
Computer-Enhanced Mannequin (CEM) Simulators	CAE HPS: Human Patient Simulator[159] www.caehealthcare.com	Adult-sized, high-fidelity mannequin that functionally simulates all organ systems and responds physiologically to procedures and medication administration	Anesthesiology Critical Care Emergency Medicine Internal/Family Medicine	$$$$$$	Numerous studies provide validity evidence to support use of simulator as an assessment tool. Well suited for assessing multiple competencies including team skills, often used in a "theater" setting.
	PediaSIM HPS[159] www.caehealthcare.com	Small child-sized, high-fidelity mannequin that functionally simulates the anatomy and physiology of a 6-year-old (17-kg) child and responds appropriately to interventions	Pediatrics Emergency Medicine Anesthesiology Family Medicine	$$$$$	Newer simulator that uses much of the same technology as the HPS, but is designed to function and react differently than an "adult."
	CAE Ares[161] www.caehealthcare.com	Adult-sized, high-fidelity mannequin that is more portable than the HPS and is programmed for more emergency (especially trauma) scenarios; less sophisticated physiologic responses to interventions	Critical Care Emergency Medicine Trauma Surgery	$$$	Newer simulator that uses much of the same technology as the HPS, but is designed to be more rugged and portable so that it can be used in numerous environments.
	CAE Luna[164] www.caehealthcare.com	Neonate-sized, high-fidelity mannequin that functionally simulates the anatomy and physiology of a newborn infant and responds appropriately to interventions	Pediatrics Anesthesiology Critical Care Emergency Medicine	$$$	Newer simulator that is wireless/tetherless and designed to function with physiologic responses appropriate for an infant up to 4 weeks old.
	SimMan 3G[166] www.laerdal.com	Full-sized adult male, high-fidelity mannequin that is wireless and portable and provides functionally realistic anatomy for performing multiple life-saving techniques and other clinical procedures	Emergency Medicine Critical Care Anesthesiology Internal/Family Medicine Surgery	$$$$-$$$$$	Multiple studies provide evidence of validity and feasibility of simulator use as an assessment tool. One of the most widely used high-fidelity simulators for evaluating individuals and teams across a broad range of clinical skills and scenarios.
	SimMom[173] www.laerdal.com	Full-sized adult female, high-fidelity mannequin that simulates a range of normal and complex delivery scenarios; neonate model is a simple, but realistic-appearing task trainer without computerized elements	OB/GYN Pediatrics	$$$$-$$$$$	Newer simulator that facilitates assessment of ability to perform many critical interventions and life-saving procedures relevant to pregnancy and childbirth.

Continued

	Simulator[a]	Features	Specialty	Cost[b]	Comments
	SimNewB[176] www.laerdal.com	Neonate-sized, computerized mannequin that provides functional anatomy and physiologic responses for a range of critical interventions required to care for newborn babies	Pediatrics Anesthesiology Critical Care Emergency Medicine	$$$	Newer simulator that allows evaluation of ability to perform general life-saving procedures (such as airway management), as well as techniques specific to the care of neonates (such as vascular access via umbilical vein/artery).
	HAL[183] www.gaumard.com	Full-sized adult, high-fidelity mannequins that are tetherless, portable, and programmed for emergency scenarios; have operational and monitoring components that come in the form of a wireless tablet computer. Newest models simulate emotions and neurologic findings through dynamic facial expressions and can follow simple commands.	Emergency Medicine Critical Care Internal Medicine Neurology	$$$$-$$$$$$	Portable and durable high-fidelity simulators suited for a wide range of emergency scenarios from prehospital environments to the emergency department to the intensive care unit. The newest models begin to fill the gap in mannequin-based simulation of neurologic conditions like stroke.
	VICTORIA[187] www.gaumard.com	Adult- and neonate-sized high-fidelity simulators that provide functional anatomy and physiologic responses for myriad scenarios, including complete delivery and postnatal care	OB/GYN Pediatrics	$$$$-$$$$$	Newer simulators with computer-enhanced components in both mother and fetus/newborn mannequins that offer interactive and automated features for more complicated pregnancy and delivery scenarios; built-in sensors can track user actions during delivery maneuvers.
Virtual Reality (VR) Simulators	ARTHRO Mentor[253] www.simbionix.com	VR simulator with haptic components combined with anatomic models of various joints (shoulder, knee, hip) that simulates many arthroscopic procedures	Orthopedic Surgery	$$$$$	Users can train to overcome orientation and instrument handling problems as well as hand–eye coordination difficulties. This system tracks data for performance assessment including time to locate structures, efficiency of scope movement, and errors.

Simulator[a]	Features	Specialty	Cost[b]	Comments
Eyesi Surgical[277] www.vrmagic.com	Mannequin head with artificial eyes, realistic foot pedals for equipment control, position-tracking instruments, and a surgical microscope that receives virtual stereo images of the operation	Ophthalmology	\$\$\$\$\$-\$\$\$\$\$\$	There are several different procedure modules that permit simulation with objective assessment of a range of intraocular surgical skills.
Minimally Invasive Surgical Trainer-Virtual Reality (MIST-VR)***	VR-based simulator that consists of a structural frame supporting two mechanical arms that hold standard laparoscopic instruments linked to a computer monitor; provides training and assessment of fundamental laparoscopic skills	General Surgery Trauma Surgery GYN Urology	N/A***	One of the most extensively studied VR simulators. The system records multiple parameters for performance evaluation. Several studies have demonstrated transfer of skills from simulator to real patients. ***Retired by Mentice. The MIST is no longer manufactured, but limited parts and support might be available for existing users.
URO Mentor[309] www.simbionix.com	VR task trainer that supports the use of flexible and rigid endoscopes with working channels for tool insertion; the user can control instruments with actual handles that function realistically while viewing virtual images of the procedure on a simulated display	Urology	\$\$\$\$\$	A versatile simulator that provides a range of diagnostic and therapeutic endourologic procedures. The system tracks multiple parameters to aid in performance assessment, including time to complete task, X-ray exposure time, and number of errors; it is probably the most evaluated/validated VR system for assessment of endourologic skills.
PERC Mentor Suite[321] www.simbionix.com	VR simulation platform that supports different task trainers with corresponding software modules to simulate performance of various image-guided percutaneous procedures, including thoracentesis, central line placement, pericardiocentesis, and upper extremity nerve blocks	Interventional Radiology Critical Care Emergency Medicine Cardiology Anesthesiology	\$\$\$\$\$	The simulator has built-in capability to record data for use in assessment exercises, including number of puncture attempts and complications.

Continued

Simulator[a]	Features	Specialty	Cost[b]	Comments
ANGIO Mentor[322] www.simbionix.com	VR trainer that uses haptic components to mimic the use of guidewires, balloons, stents, and other devices during myriad endovascular procedures; includes dynamic indicators of patient status that change with drug administration and procedural maneuvers	Cardiology Interventional Radiology Vascular Surgery Neurology Neurosurgery Nephrology	$$$$-$$$$$$	Embedded tracking system allows assessment of user's medical decision-making and management skills. The simulator tracks a set of parameters and generates statistical reports on individual or group performance.
Vascular Intervention Simulation Trainer (VIST)[324] www.mentice.com	VR simulator that enables the user to manipulate real tools and devices passed through an introducer while performing multiple endovascular techniques; haptic mechanisms reproduce tactile feedback with simulated fluoroscopic images displayed on a monitor	Cardiology Interventional Radiology Vascular Surgery Neurology Neurosurgery Nephrology	$$$$-$$$$$	In addition to renal, iliac, aortic, and carotid artery endovascular techniques, the system also simulates a range of interventional cardiology procedures—angiography, angioplasty/stenting, pacemaker placement, electrophysiologic studies, and transcatheter aortic valve implantation. It became the primary simulator to train and assess clinicians before using the first FDA-approved carotid stent. It contains a sophisticated tracking system that measures time to complete tasks, efficiency of movement, and errors.
BRONCH Mentor[339] www.simbionix.com	VR haptic system that allows users to manipulate modified endoscopes with ports for passing real instruments to simulate a range of bronchoscopic diagnostic and therapeutic procedures, with realistic tactile experience and virtual graphic displays	Pulmonology Critical Care ENT	$$$$-$$$$$ (higher end of price range for combo unit with GI Mentor)	System allows assessment of basic skills such as airway navigation and inspection, as well as numerous techniques for specimen collection; built-in system can provide performance metrics for self-assessment or evaluation of competence prior to real patient practice; can be used as stand-alone system or combined on same platform with GI Mentor.

	Simulator[a]	Features	Specialty	Cost[b]	Comments
	GI Mentor[340] www.simbionix.com	VR haptic system that allows users to employ modified endoscopes with ports for passing real instruments to simulate a range of upper and lower GI endoscopic techniques for diagnosis and treatment, with realistic tactile experience and virtual graphic displays	Gastroenterology Surgery ENT	$$$$-$$$$$ (higher end of price range for combo unit with BRONCH Mentor)	System allows assessment of basic skills such as navigation, inspection, and instrument handling, as well as numerous procedures including biopsy and polypectomy; built-in system can provide performance metrics for self-assessment or evaluation of competence prior to real patient practice; can be used as stand-alone system or combined on same platform with BRONCH Mentor.
Augmented Reality Trainer	SonoSim LiveScan[189] www.sonosim.com	Augmented VR system that utilizes a special simulated ultrasound probe and proprietary sensor tags placed on live humans or mannequins to create realistic hybrid simulations, whereby a linked computer screen displays realistic virtual sonographic images of normal and pathologic internal human anatomy	Almost any specialty that would perform examinations or procedures using ultrasound, especially: Radiology Emergency Medicine Trauma Surgery Critical Care OB/GYN Internal/Family Medicine Cardiology	$$$-$$$$ (depends on number of probes and licenses for modules, which are offered on an annual subscription basis)	Simulation system can reproduce myriad clinical scenarios for evaluation of technical (ultrasound exams or guided procedures) and nontechnical (communication) skills when combined with standardized patients; optional system tracks performance metrics.

[a]Superscript numbers next to product names correspond to references within main chapter text and link to websites where specific product information can be found. Homepage for general manufacturer websites also provided here.

[b]Estimates (as of April 2023): $, <$1,000; $$, $1,000–$5,000; $$$, $5,000–$35,000; $$$$, $35,000–$75,000; $$$$$, $75,000–$150,000; $$$$$$, >$150.000.

CSF, Cerebrospinal fluid; *FDA*, US Food and Drug Administration.

Chapter 14

Appendix 14.1 Learning/Change Plan or Action Plan

First priority

Change and Specific Goals	Specific Actions	Timeline (1)	Timeline (2)	Resources Required	Challenges	Identifiable Results and Follow-up
Describe specific, observable changes that you intend to make as a result of this feedback. **For each, what is your goal?**	What do you need to do to achieve your goal?	When will you begin?	When do you think you will see results?	Identify the resources you will use. Who will help you? What resources will you need? What learning will you need?	What will get in the way of you accomplishing change?	How will you know the results have been attained? With whom will you follow up?

Adapted from Wakefield J, Herbert CP, Maclure M, et al. Commitment to change statements can predict actual change in practice. *Contin Educ Health Prof.* 2003;23(2):81–93.

Appendix 14.2 ADAPT Model

Second priority

Learner Initiates Feedback		Coach Initiates Feedback
• Reflect on learning goals. • Communicate your goals.	**PREPARE** **for the observation**	• Reflect on program and learner goals. • Orient learner to expectations.
• Try to be natural.	**PERFORM** **the observation**	• Try to be neutral.
	DEBRIEF **With the ADAPT Conversation**	
• Reflect on the observation. • Ask for feedback.	**ASK**	• Reflect on learner readiness. • Ask for their thoughts about the observation.
• Have a conversation about the activity.	**DISCUSS**	• Coach observed, modifiable, specific behaviors related to the task(s).
• Ask for clarification.	**ASK**	• Ask learner to clarify points, as necessary.
• Plan next steps with your coach.	**PLAN TOGETHER**	• Plan next steps with your learner.
Follow through with the plan.		***Follow up with learner, if possible.***
	LEARNER ***Improved Future Work Performance*** ***and Better Patient Care***	

Appendix 14.3 R2C2 "In the Moment" Trifold

Third priority

Setting the stage

To prepare for a session, ensure you have reviewed previous learning goals.

Present the R2C2 ITM approach as an ongoing conversation about observations and co-creation of learning goals.

Coaching micro-skills* are applicable in all phases.

Phases may not always be linear but often are iterative. You might find you need to return to an earlier phase.

Phase 1. Build relationship

Goal: To engage the learner and build mutual respect and trust.

Relationship building is central. It may have been established previously (if longitudinal experience) but must be maintained throughout the session.

Phrases and strategies:

How has this rotation/clinic been for you? What do you enjoy? What challenges you?

What are a couple of areas you have been working on and what would you like me to focus on today?

Confirm what you are hearing, show respect, build trust.

*open-ended questions, active listening, promoting self-reflection, clarifying questions, paraphrasing, summarizing,

Phase 2. Explore reactions and reflections

Goal: To foster learner self-reflection, address emotions and begin to develop shared understanding of the experience.

Phrases and strategies:

Encourage self-assessment: *How was that experience for you? What went well? What were challenges for you? Did anything surprise you?*

Understand learners' perspective & integrate preceptor observations:

Can you tell me about your thoughts on this?

I'm curious, when you decided to do [Y], what was your intent?

When I watched you, I observed [X].

I thought you did [X] well, but you seemed [upset, frustrated, flustered] by [Y]. Can you tell me more about that?

When there are significant gaps in performance:

What things do you wish you had done differently?

Phase 3: Confirm content

Goal: To enable learner and preceptor to summarize and reach agreement on the focus for coaching.

Phrases and strategies:

So, let's summarize what we have discussed so far.

Is there anything we discussed that isn't clear?

Would you like to add anything at this point?

Given our conversation, what areas would you like to focus on moving forward?

For learner who does not identify a priority: *We talked about x, y & z, what would you like to focus on?*

Example: I think we agree that you need to focus on communication skills.

Appendix 14.3—cont'd

Phase 4: Coach for change and co-create an action plan

Goal: To ensure learner and preceptor agree on a specific learning goal and co-create an achievable action plan.

Phrases and strategies:

Set a goal: *Now that we have established a focus for learning, what specific goal should we work on now?*

Example: Now that we have decided to work on communication skills, I hear you say that you want to specifically focus on delivering bad news.

For learner who is having difficulty coming up with a specific goal: *It seems you may be unsure about what you want to work on; can I suggest that you work on [X]. Will that work for you?*

Action Plan

Describe a specific, observable change you intend to make.

What will you do to achieve this goal?

When will you begin?

What will you need for support? Knowledge, experiences, resources, people?

What might get in the way of making the changes?

Determine the follow-up plan

Who are you working with next? Could they help you?

When do you think you will see results?

How will you ensure you are on track?

Adapted from: Sargeant et al., Academic Medicine, 2015, 2018; Armson et al., Medical Education, 2019; Lockyer et al., JGME,2020.

Further information about the R2C2 model, watch the 'in-the-moment' videos and print the tri-fold:
https://medicine.dal.ca/departments/core-units/cpd/faculty-development/R2C2.html

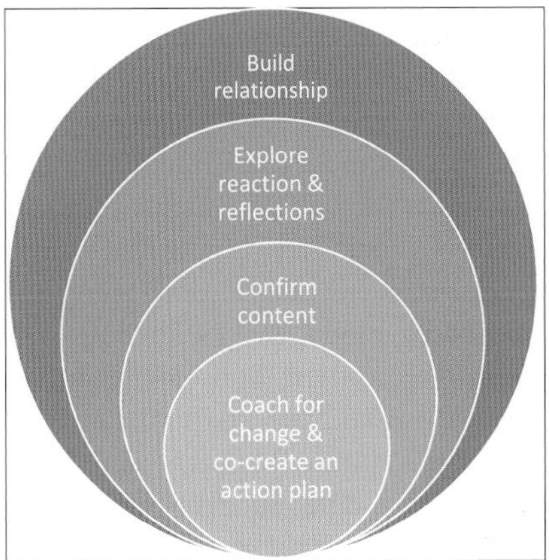

R2C2

Evidence-Informed Facilitated Feedback and Coaching

"In the Moment" Version

Appendix 14.4 R2C2 Research Publications

Developing and Testing by R2C2 Group

Armson H, Lockyer JM, Zetkulic M, Könings KD, Sargeant J. Identifying coaching skills to improve feedback use in postgraduate medical education. *Med Educ.* 2019;53(5):477–493.

Lockyer J, Armson H, Könings KD, et al. In-the-moment feedback and coaching: improving R2C2 for a new context. *J Grad Med Educ.* 2020 Feb;12(1):27–35.

Lockyer J, Lee-Krueger R, Armson H, et al. Application of the R2C2 model to in-the-moment feedback and coaching. *Acad Med.* 2023 Apr 14. Epub ahead of print.

Sargeant J, Lockyer J, Mann K, et al. Facilitated reflective performance feedback: developing an evidence- and theory-based model that builds relationship, explores reactions and content, and coaches for performance change (R2C2). *Acad Med.* 2015;90(12):1698–1706.

Sargeant J, Mann K, Manos S, et al. R2C2 in action: testing an evidence-based model to facilitate feedback and coaching in residency. *J Grad Med Educ.* 2017;9(2):165-170.

Sargeant J, Lockyer JM, Mann K, et al. The R2C2 model in residency education: how does it foster coaching and promote feedback use? *Acad Med.* 2018;93(7):1055–1063.

Empirical Research on Using R2C2 Conducted by Other Groups

Arabsky S, Castro N, Murray M, Bisca I, Eva KW. The influence of relationship-centered coaching on physician perceptions of peer review in the context of mandated regulatory practices. *Acad Med.* 2020 Nov;95(11S Association of American Medical Colleges Learn Serve Lead: Proceedings of the 59th Annual Research in Medical Education Presentations):S14–S19.

Farrell L, Cuncic C, Hartford W, Hatala R, Ajjawi R. Goal co-construction and dialogue in an internal medicine longitudinal coaching program. *Med Educ.* 2022 Oct 1. Epub ahead of print.

Graham R, Beuthin R. Exploring the effectiveness of multisource feedback and coaching with nurse practitioners. *Nurs Leadersh (Tor Ont).* 2018;31(1):50-59. https://www.longwoods.com/content/25472/nursing-leadership/exploring-the-effectiveness-of-multisource-feedback-and-coaching-with-nurse-practitioners

Murthy V, Sethuraman KR, Choudhury S, Shakila R. Application of Practice Oriented-Peer Review for Prosthodontics (PRO-PReP)—a qualitative study. *Int J Psychiatry Med.* 2022;57(2):117–133.

Roy M, Lockyer J, Touchie C. (in press). Family physician quality improvement plans? A realist inquiry into what works, for whom, under what circumstances. *J Cont Educ Health Prof.* 2022;4.

Safavi AH, Papadakos J, Papadakos T, Quartey NK, Lawrie K, Klein E, Storer S, Croke J, Millar BA, Jang R, Bezjak A, Giuliani ME. Feedback Delivery in an Academic Cancer Centre: Reflections From an R2C2-based Microlearning Course. *J Cancer Educ.* 2022 Dec;37(6):1790–1797. doi: 10.1007/s13187-021-02028-9. Epub 2021 Jun 24. PMID: 34169464.

Pooley M, Pizzuti C, Daly M. Optimizing multisource feedback implementation for Australasian physicians. *J Contin Educ Health Prof.* 2019;39(4):228–235.

Roy M, Kain N, Touchie C. Exploring content relationships among components of a multisource feedback program. *J Contin Educ Health Prof.* 2021 Oct 1. Epub ahead of print.

Sebok-Syer SS, Shaw JM, Sedran R, et al. Facilitating residents' understanding of electronic health record report card data using faculty feedback and coaching. *Acad Med.* 2022 Aug 9. Epub ahead of print.

Chapter 18

Appendix 18.1 Exercise in Program Evaluation

Exercise in Program Evaluation

Consider one specific challenge that you're facing with your existing educational program or program innovation/new program—either something is not going as well as you'd like, or you don't really know how things are going.

Step 1: Goal statement related to <u>this</u> challenge. Finish this sentence: "I would feel good about my program if I knew that…" or "I need to know whether…" or "I would be embarrassed if I discovered that…"

Step 2: What "outcome" or "**AFTER**" measures will help you determine "success" in answering your question? Please list as many as you think might help. List both immediate and long term. (*** = those you feel are essential)**

<u>Immediate Outcome Measures</u> <u>Longer-term Outcome Measures</u>

Step 3: What measurements (assessments) will you make/gather **DURING** the program? These measures should be in line with the outcome you're interested in.

- Some things to consider about these measures: feasibility (can you do it), reliability, and validity of assessment methods.
- Think of whether the measures are process or product measures; quantitative or qualitative; essential or sesirable?
- We will come back to the resources you need to do this.

MEASURES DURING THE PROGRAM	Process or Product?	Quant or Qual?	Essential or Desirable?	RESOURCES (Time, Money, Human Resources)

Step 4: What baseline or "**BEFORE**" measures are needed? [Helps you compare intervention and control groups, correct for baseline differences in performance, understand what is a result of the program.]

- Think of whether the measures are quantitative or qualitative; essential or desirable?
- We will come back to the resources you need to do this.

MEASURES "BEFORE" THE PROGRAM	Quant or Qual?	Essential or Desirable?	RESOURCES (Time, Money, Human Resources)

Step 5: Identify "Yellow and Red flags" for this evaluation—What will make you lose sleep if you find it is occurring (i.e., specific accreditation issues)? Try to list measures that are quantifiable (numeric), qualitative (words), process (content), and product measures.

Yellow Flags (Concerning, warrants more frequent "sampling" of data if you find it)	Red Flags (You Must Do Something immediately if you find it)

Step 6: Go back to **steps 3–5**. Is there any additional information that you will need to gather ("what to evaluate"—"before," "during," and/or "after" measurements) based upon your red and yellow flags?

Step 7: Go back to **steps 3–6**, and in the right-hand margin, write down "**needed resources**" (consider time, human resources, funding) and potential barriers for each step.

Step 8: What are possible unexpected outcomes with this intervention and how might you detect these outcomes?

Index

Note: Page numbers followed by '*b*' indicate boxes, '*f* indicate figures and '*t*' indicate tables.

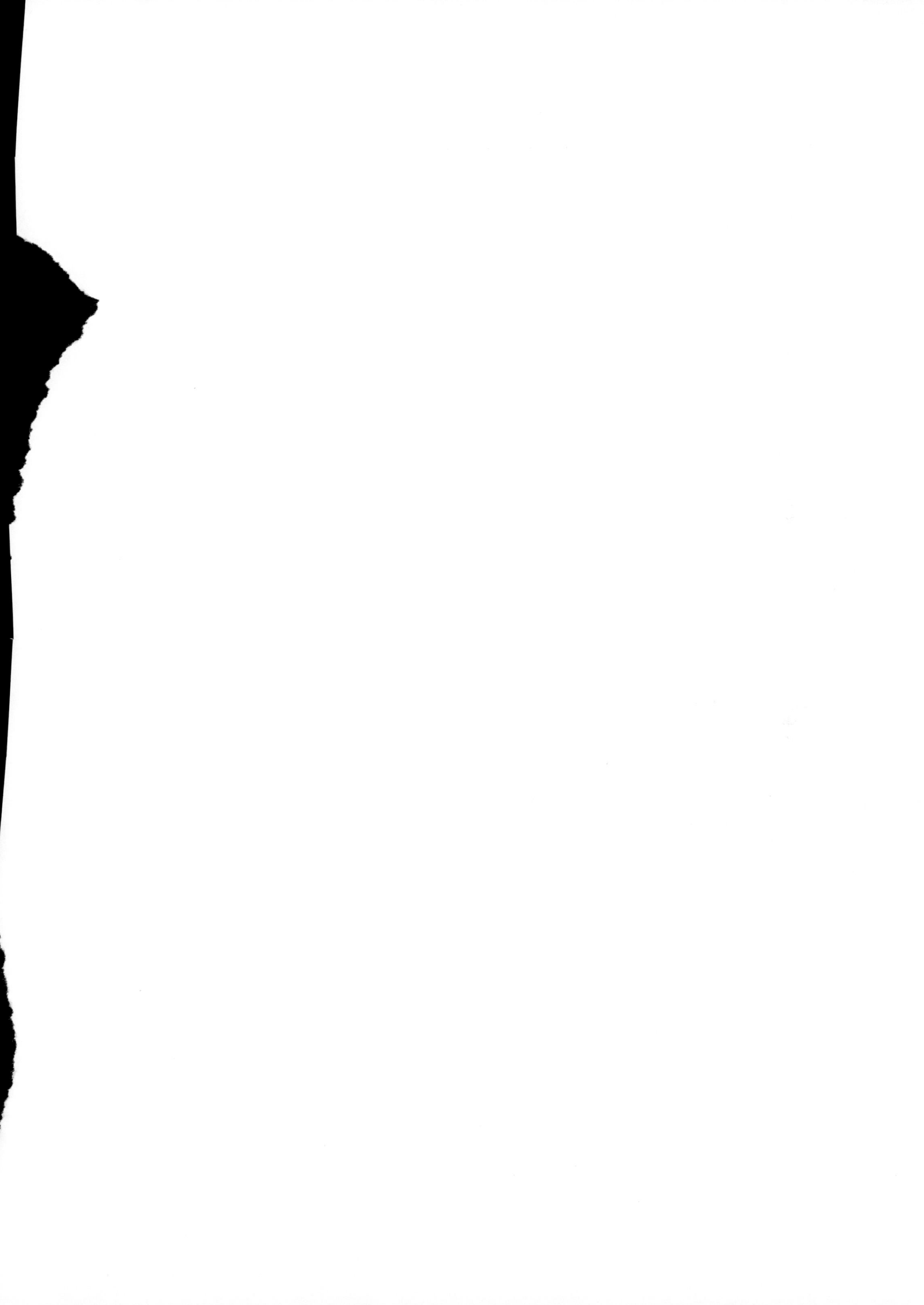